Current Opinion in DERMATOLOGY

1995

Editors

Mark V Dahl
Department of Dermatology
University of Minnesota Medical School
Minneapolis, MN

Peter J Lynch
Department of Dermatology
University of Minnesota Medical School
Minneapolis, MN

Editorial board

CONTENTS

Inflammatory diseases
Bruce H Thiers

Surgery
Duane C Whitaker

Neoplasms
Pearon G Lang, Jr

Photobiology, photodermatoses, and photoaging
John Hawk

Pigmented and adnexal disorders
Jean L Bolognia

Therapy
Ralph Coskey

Systemic diseases
Warren W Piette

Clinical research
Mark Pittelkow

Pediatrics and genodermatoses
Moise Levy

Infections and infestations
Neil A Sadick

Philadelphia office

Editor: Joseph Barron   Typesetting: Colleen Ward
Acquisitions Editor: Steven Rusche   Subscriptions: Sean McGlinchey
Advertising: Steve Miller

400 Market Street, Suite 700, Philadelphia, PA 19106-2199
Tel 215 574 2266   Fax 215 574 3533

London office

Electronic Database: Martin Buckmaster   Subscriptions: James Wendel
Bibliography: Neelam Shah   Advertising: Helen Dixon

34–42 Cleveland Street, London W1P 5FB
Tel (0)71 323 0323   Fax (0)71 580 1938

Current Opinion in Dermatology subscription information

Current Opinion in Dermatology is published annually by Current Science (Philadelphia, PA). Each volume consists of approximately 325 pages.

1995 Subscription rates	USA and Canada* $US (+ postage)	Rest of World $US (+ postage)	United Kingdom £UK (+ postage)	Europe† £UK (+ postage)	Rest of World £UK (+ postage)	Japan Yen (+ postage)
Personal	99.95 (3.50)	99.95 (16.00)	68.50 (9.00)	68.50 (15.00)	68.50 (24.00)	§
Institutional	215.00 (3.50)	215.00 (16.00)	140.00 (9.00)	140.00 (15.00)	140.00 (24.00)	§
Students/residents‡	55.95 (3.50)	55.95 (16.00)	42.00 (9.00)	42.00 (15.00)	42.00 (24.00)	§

*Canadian residents must add GST.
†Subscribers within the EC may be liable to a European tax.
‡Students/residents must give the name of their institution or school, plus the name of the residency director or department chairman, to qualify for the discounted rate. Students/residents rate is available for a maximum of 2 years.
§Yen prices are not available.
All prices are subject to change without notice.

Orders should be placed with a bookseller or subscription agent, or sent to Current Science: *In the USA and Canada:* Current Science, 400 Market Street, Suite 700, Philadelphia, PA 19106, USA, or call TOLL FREE 1-800-552-5866 (in PA 215-574-2266; fax: 215-574-3533). *In Japan:* Nankodo Co Ltd, Tokyo International, PO Box 5272, Japan. *Rest of the world:* Current Science, 34-42 Cleveland Street, London W1P 5FB, UK. Second class postage paid at Philadelphia, PA and at additional mailing offices. Postmaster send address corrections to Current Science, 400 Market Street, Suite 700, Philadelphia, PA 19106, USA. Cancellations on renewed subscriptions will not be accepted after the first issue has been shipped.

ISBN 1-85922-686-8 ISSN 1068–381X

Film originated in Italy by Sele & Color.
Printed in Korea by Sung in Printing Co., Ltd.

Contents

Continued

Pediatrics and genodermatoses
edited by Moise Levy

Surgery
edited by Duane C. Whitaker

Photobiology, photodermatoses, and photoaging
edited by John Hawk

Therapy
edited by Ralph Coskey

Continued

Clinical research
edited by Mark Pittelkow

Infections and infestations
edited by Neil A. Sadick

Cover illustration: Corticosteroid-induced acne rosacea and perioral dermatitis in a 38-year-old woman who had been using desoximetasone for 1 year. Flaring erythema and papules and fine scaling are seen 4 days after withdrawal of desoximetasone. (*From* Wells and Brodell, *Postgrad Med* 1993, 93:225–230; with permission.)

Editorial

Never has the explosion of new information seemed so real to us. Both of us are writing second editions of textbooks, and so both of us have had to search out new knowledge about a variety of subjects. We almost pray for good review articles to simplify our task.

Current Opinion in Dermatology provides such review articles. Our section editors worked with us to identify important topics. They enlisted experts to bring us up to date. We sent each expert a list of new, relevant articles. The expert simply placed a check mark next to important articles, and we made sure he or she received a copy of each. This system worked extremely well, as you will see. It encouraged our authors to focus on new findings and to highlight evolving concepts of diseases and treatments. A short turnaround time for processing manuscripts at the publisher ensured that *Current Opinion in Dermatology* is indeed current.

In the bibliography at the end of each review, articles of particular interest are highlighted and annotated, to help you decide if you want to read them for yourself.

Enjoy and learn!

Mark V. Dahl, MD
Professor of Dermatology

Peter J. Lynch, MD
Professor and Chairman, Department of Dermatology

University of Minnesota Medical School
Minneapolis, Minnesota, USA

Inflammatory diseases

Edited by

Bruce H. Thiers

Medical University of South Carolina
Charleston, South Carolina, USA

CURRENT SCIENCE

Recent developments in the pathogenesis and treatment of atopic dermatitis

Israel Eckman, MD, and Matthew J. Stiller, MD

Massachusetts General Hospital, Boston, Massachusetts, USA

Recent advances in the pathogenesis and treatment of atopic dermatitis (AD) are reviewed. Although the exact pathogenesis of AD remains unknown, several immunologic abnormalities including enhanced production of IgE and increased selective T-cell activation are recognized in patients with AD. The role of Langerhans cells as a link between IgE hypersensitivity and increased T-cell activation in the pathogenesis of AD has received much attention. Recruitment of eosinophils by various lymphokines and mediators may contribute to the late inflammatory skin reaction characteristic of AD. Treatment of AD remains a challenge, because no single safe, effective therapy exists. Both topical and systemic corticosteroids and oral cyclosporine are effective in the treatment of AD. However, serious side effects of long-term treatment have resulted in the introduction of alternative therapies. Phototherapy with high-dose ultraviolet A1 is effective in the treatment of patients with severe AD. Interferon gamma therapy is also effective in producing clinical improvement during treatment, although relapse is common after discontinuing treatment. Other immunomodulatory agents including subcutaneous thymopentin and interferon alfa have limited efficacy and may be used as adjunctive therapies in the management of severe AD.

Current Opinion in Dermatology 1995:3–9

Atopic dermatitis (AD), a chronic inflammatory skin disorder, usually has its onset during childhood. The exact pathogenesis of AD remains unknown, but it is associated with several immunologic abnormalities including enhanced production of IgE and impaired delayed-type hypersensitivity responses [1]. Corticosteroids, both topical and systemic, remain the cornerstone of treatment, but no specific therapy exists at this time. Phototherapy continues to be valuable in severe, recalcitrant AD. In addition, interferon (IFN) gamma and thymopentin have recently been used successfully in severe AD.

Pathogenesis

IgE dysregulation

Atopic dermatitis is characterized by overproduction of IgE, which may result from an imbalance of interleukin (IL)–4 and IFN-γ production observed in AD patients. These patients demonstrate increased IL-4 production and decreased IFN-γ levels [2•]. IL-4 is a potent enhancer of IgE production, inducing class switching to the IgE isotype in B lymphocytes, while IFN-γ inhibits this effect. In addition, IL-4 inhibits the production of IFN-γ at the level of transcription [3,4]. Renz et al. [5•] observed enhanced IL-4 production and IL-4 receptor

expression in patients with AD. Byron et al. [6] demonstrated that in vitro production of IFN-γ by peripheral blood mononuclear cells was reduced. This reduction closely correlated with the disease severity in AD patients.

T helper cell subsets 1 and 2

The aforementioned immunologic imbalance may be related to differences in the type of T helper (T$_H$) cell subsets present in the lesional skin of AD patients. Two types of T$_H$ cell subsets have been described in a murine model and are defined by the lymphokine profiles they release upon activation. The T$_H$1 subset secretes IL-2, IFN-γ, and tumor necrosis factor and mediates macrophage activation and delayed-type hypersensitivity response [7]. The T$_H$2 subset releases IL-4, IL-5, IL-6, and IL-10, which stimulate B-cell activation. The T$_H$1 and T$_H$2 subsets are mutually inhibiting, so that IL-4 inhibits T$_H$1-type responses, and IFN-γ inhibits T$_H$2-type responses, (Fig. 1) [8••,9,10]. Similar T$_H$1 and T$_H$2 subsets have been found in humans, with release of the identical lymphokine profiles observed in the murine model [1]. The majority of T-cell clones from atopic human lymphocytes resemble the murine T$_H$2 cell that produces IL-4, whereas very few clones produce IFN-γ [6,11]. Therefore, the selective expression of the T$_H$2 subset with subsequent production of IL-

---

Abbreviations

AD—atopic dermatitis; ECP—eosinophilic cationic protein; IFN—interferon; IL—interleukin; T$_H$—T helper; UVA—ultraviolet A; UVB—ultraviolet B.

4 and decreased levels of IFN-γ–producing cells could lead to preferential enhancement of IgE production.

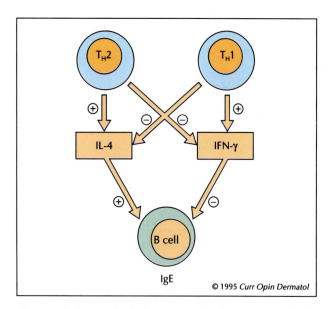

Fig. 1. Imbalance of T helper (T$_H$) cell subsets 1 and 2 leads to enhanced IgE production in atopic dermatitis (AD). Two types of T$_H$ cell subsets have been described in humans, similar to those described in a mouse model. The T$_H$2 subset releases interleukin (IL)–4, a potent stimulator of IgE production and B-cell activation, whereas the T$_H$1 subset secretes interferon gamma (IFN-γ), which inhibits IL-4–induced IgE expression. These two subsets are mutually inhibitory, so that an imbalance leads to preferential enhancement of one subset response over the other. In fact, atopic lesional T-cell clones reveal predominantly the IL-4–producing T$_H$2 subset, with a reduction of the T$_H$1 subset and IFN-γ production. This increased proportion of T$_H$2 cells may lead to the uninhibited IL-4 release with enhanced IgE production that is characteristic of AD.

Cell-mediated dysfunction

Atopic dermatitis reflects a state of increased T-cell activation and proliferation that contributes to the inflammatory process. Specifically, CD4+ T cells are the major infiltrating cell found in lesions of AD [12•]. Furthermore, a proportional increase in circulating activated and unactivated CD4+ lymphocytes is observed in AD, with an associated reduction in the percentage of CD8+ suppressor cells. The increase in proportion of activated and unactivated CD4+ cells and decrease in proportion of CD8+ cells have been shown to correlate with disease severity. These findings support the notion that selective activation and proliferation of circulating CD4+ lymphocytes occur in severe AD [13].

Increased T-cell activation

The association between T-cell activation and disease activity is further supported by the increased serum levels of soluble IL-2 receptors in AD patients during flares of dermatitis. This receptor can be used as a marker for clinical improvement. Increased *in vitro* production of IL-6 by peripheral blood T cells in patients with AD has been observed and reflects increased activation of T cells. Elevated T-cell IL-6 production *in vitro* may reflect selective predominance of the T$_H$2 subset *in vivo* with subsequent dysregulation of IgE production as IL-6 potentiates IL-4 stimulation of IgE production.

Langerhans cells

Recent studies investigating the histopathology of AD have revealed increased numbers of dermal Langerhans cells with hyperstimulatory antigen-presenting activity in lesional skin of AD [8••]. Epidermal Langerhans cells express a low-affinity Fc receptor (CD23) for IgE and upon binding of allergen to cell membrane–bound IgE, dermal T-cell activation and proliferation occur with subsequent lymphokine production. As a result, eosinophils are recruited to the dermal lesional site and release their granular contents, including major basic protein and eosinophilic cationic protein (ECP), culminating in a severe local inflammatory reaction [14•].

Eosinophils

Increased peripheral blood eosinophilia is common in patients with AD, suggesting a role for eosinophils in the pathogenesis of AD. Although biopsies of dermatitic skin typically do not demonstrate increased eosinophil levels, they do reveal large amounts of eosinophilic major basic protein [14•]. Furthermore, increased ECP serum levels are observed in patients with AD and correlate with disease activity, reflecting the presence of activated eosinophils in AD [15]. Increased serum ECP levels may represent the activation state of the whole eosinophilic pool [16••]. Clinical improvement correlates with a decrease in serum ECP levels, which may serve as a marker for monitoring disease activity in AD [16••].

Eosinophils from patients with AD are thought to be in a preactivated state in the circulation as a result of exposure to the activated T cell–mediated cytokines IL-3, IL-5, and granulocyte macrophage-colony stimulating factor [17]. IL-5 in particular is a selective and potent eosinophilic chemotactic factor. Mast cells may also release IL-3, IL-5, and granulocyte macrophage-colony stimulating factor, and there is evidence that Langerhans cells generate, directly or indirectly, an eosinophilic chemotactic factor [15]. These factors result in recruitment of eosinophils to the lesional site and continuation of the inflammatory cascade. Activated eosinophils may therefore play a major role in the allergic inflammatory process of AD (Fig. 2) [16••].

Treatment

Topical or systemic corticosteroids continue to be the cornerstone of AD therapy, acting as immunosuppressive and anti-inflammatory agents. As a result of the well-known serious side effects long-term corticosteroid treatment can produce, alternative therapies for AD have been developed with variable success. Most of these newer treatments are immunosuppressive or immunomodulatory agents that affect some component of the immune mechanism thought to be responsible for the lesions in AD. Oral cyclosporine has been

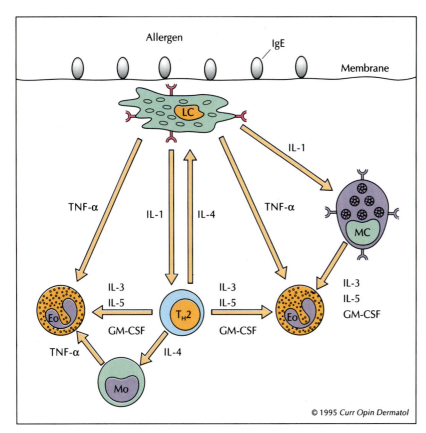

Fig. 2. Proposed pathway of lymphokine interaction resulting in eosinophil (Eo) recruitment in atopic dermatitis (AD). Upon the binding of an allergen to cell membrane–bound IgE, Langerhans cells (LCs) release interleukin (IL)–1, leading to T helper subset 2 (T$_H$2) cell activation and proliferation with expression of several lymphokines, among which IL-3, IL-5, and granulocyte macrophage-colony stimulating factor (GM-CSF) are potent chemotactic factors for Eos. Mast cells (MCs) likewise may release IL-3, IL-5, and GM-CSF, thus enhancing Eo recruitment. Finally, LCs and monocytes (Mos) may directly release an eosinophilic chemotactic factor, which together with IL-3, IL-5, and GM-CSF contributes to the migration and influx of Eos and the inflammatory response characteristic of AD. Tumor necrosis factor-α (TNF-α) activates Eos.

shown, at a dosage of 5 mg/kg daily, to be highly effective in the treatment of recalcitrant AD, with reduction of disease extent and severity scores [8••,18]. Some of the more recent therapies reviewed include phototherapy, IFN-γ and IFN-α therapy, thymopentin, allergen-antibody complexes, traditional Chinese herbal therapy, and nonsedating H$_1$ antihistamines (Table 1).

Phototherapy

Both psoralen and ultraviolet A (UVA) and ultraviolet B (UVB) therapy have limited therapeutic efficacy in the treatment of AD [19]. Combined UVA-UVB irradiation has proven to be more effective than UVB alone [20•]. A recent clinical trial has demonstrated the superiority of high-dose UVA1 therapy (340 to 400 nm) in the treatment of AD. Krutmann *et al.* [20•] observed significant clinical improvement in the management of patients with acute exacerbation of AD compared with those receiving conventional UVB or UVA-UVB therapy. Significant clinical improvement occurred after only 1 week of therapy without any serious side effects, and elevated serum ECP levels decreased markedly. However, whether this latter finding is the result of the effect of UVA1 on eosinophil function directly or a marker for clinical improvement needs to be further elucidated [19]. A single exposure to high-dose UVA1 light has been reported to alter human Langerhans cell number and function [20•,21,22]. Krutmann and Schopf [19] observed that the number of IgE-bearing Langerhans cells was significantly reduced following high-dose UVA1 therapy. Thus, high-dose UVA1 therapy is capable of modulating both eosinophil function and Langerhans cell surface marker expression. Langerhans cells may serve as its treatment target.

Interferon gamma

As a result of the imbalance of decreased IFN-γ but high IL-4 production observed in AD patients, recent study has focused on the effect of IFN-γ in the treatment of severe AD. Reinhold *et al.* [23•] found significant clinical improvement in patients treated with recombinant IFN-γ for 6 weeks. Subcutaneous injections of 100 mg of IFN-γ were given daily for 5 days during the 1st week of treatment, followed by three injections per week for the next 3 weeks and, finally, two injections per week for the last 2 weeks. However, no reduction in serum IgE levels was observed following IFN-γ treatment. In a double-blind, placebo-controlled trial, Hanifin *et al.* [24•] reported the effectiveness of recombinant IFN-γ in reducing symptoms and lesion severity in severe AD. The patients in this study received daily subcutaneous injections of 50 μg/m^2 recombinant IFN-γ for 12 weeks. The mean eosinophil count was significantly reduced, although serum IgE levels remained elevated during therapy. Although the exact mechanism of action of IFN-γ is not understood, it may function by inhibiting the proliferation of IL-4– and IL-5–producing T$_H$2 cells. IFN-γ has been shown to selectively inhibit the proliferation of T$_H$2 cells but not T$_H$1 cells in the murine model described earlier [24•]. Recombinant IFN-γ is effective in the treatment of AD, although the long-term benefit needs to be further investigated.

Table 1. Treatment modalities for atopic dermatitis

Treatment	Approval status*	Mechanism of action	Advantages	Disadvantages and side effects	Route of administration	Efficacy
Corticosteroids	Approved	Immunosuppressive	Effective in severe AD	Adverse effects with long-term treatment	Systemic Topical	Excellent
Cyclosporine	Experimental	Immunosuppressive	Effective in severe AD	Does not reduce allergic response to inhalant allergen Adverse effects with long-term treatment Disease recurs upon discontinuation	Oral	Excellent
Phototherapy UVA-UVB	Approved	Reduction and in-activation of Langerhans cells	More effective than UVB treatment	Slight erythema	Irradiation	Good to excellent
High-dose UVA1	Approved	Reduction and in-activation of Langerhans cells	Immediate clinical improvement	Photoaging of skin Risk of skin tumors	Irradiation	Excellent
Interferon Gamma	Experimental	Inhibition of IL-4–induced IgE expression, IL-4 receptor expression, and IL-4–induced proliferation of T cells	Clinical improvement within 1st week of treatment	No major adverse effects	Subcutaneous injections	Good
Alfa-2b	Experimental	Inhibition of IL-4–induced IgE expression and IL-4 receptor expression	Favorable safety profile	No significant adverse reactions Flulike syndrome	Subcutaneous injections	Poor
Alfa-2a	Experimental	Inhibition of IL-4–induced proliferation of T cells	Favorable safety profile	No significant adverse reactions Flulike syndrome	Subcutaneous injections	Limited
Thymopentin	Experimental	Suppression of IL-4 production and enhancement of *in vitro* inter-feron gamma production	Decreased histamine-releasing factor and plasma histamine concentration	No serious side effects	Subcutaneous injections	Limited
Allergen-antibody complexes	Experimental	Suppression of immune response toward allergens contained in complexes	Includes allergens with ubiquitous distribution and persistence throughout the year	Autologous antibody required No serious side effects	Intradermal injections	Fair to good
Traditional Chinese herbal therapy	Experimental	Immunosuppressive Anti-inflammatory Antimicrobial Sedative	Ease of oral administration	Unpalatability of decoction Potential toxic effects including hepatotoxicity	Oral decoction	Good
Nonsedating H$_1$ antihistamines	Approved	Blocking of H$_1$ receptors	Limited efficacy in reducing pruritus with favorable safety profile	Interaction with frequently prescribed drugs	Oral Topical	Questionable

*For drug therapies, status refers to approval of US Food and Drug Administration; for nondrug therapies, status refers to approval of the scientific community.
AD—atopic dermatitis; IL—interleukin; UVA—ultraviolet A; UVB—ultraviolet B.

Interferon alfa

Interferon alfa, like IFN-γ, inhibits IL-4–induced IgE production by normal human lymphocytes as well as the spontaneous *in vitro* IgE production of mononuclear cells from atopic patients [25,26]. Jullien *et al.* [25] reported no effect of IFN-α2b in the short-term treatment of AD. IFN-α2b was administered by subcutaneous injections in doses of 90 to 150 U/wk for a period of 4 to 8 weeks. Paukkonen *et al.* [27] observed no clinical improvement following IFN-α2b treatment administered by subcutaneous injection of 3 to 9 MU IFN-α2b three times a week for 6 to 14 weeks. However, significant reduction in blood eosinophils was observed. Torrelo *et al.* [28] observed a moderately beneficial therapeutic effect with recombinant IFN-α2a, although serum IgE levels remained the same. The patients received 3×10^6 IU of intramuscular recombinant IFN-α2a, three times a week for 4 weeks. If no response was observed at that time, the dosage could be doubled or remain the same [28]. Recombinant IFN-α therapy provides limited if any benefits in the treatment of AD.

Combined interferon alfa and interferon gamma

Pung *et al.* [29••] reported on two patients with severe AD who received sequential treatment of IFN-γ and IFN-α with subsequent dramatic improvement of AD lesions and significant reduction of the severity score. Both patients were treated initially with IFN-γ (0.05 mg/m² thrice weekly). After 12 weeks, IFN-γ was replaced by IFN-α (3 MU/m² thrice weekly) for an additional 20 weeks in patient 1, because IFN-γ therapy failed to lead to complete resolution of the disease. Following a flare-up in disease activity at the 4th week, the IFN-γ dosage was increased to 0.1 mg/m² in patient 2. After 6 weeks, IFN-γ was discontinued, and patient 2 received 20 weeks of therapy with IFN-α (0.5 MU/m² thrice weekly) [29••]. Both patients demonstrated marked clinical improvement following the conclusion of the trial. Further study of sequential or combined usage of IFN-α and IFN-γ therapy may provide additional therapeutic benefit in the management of patients with severe AD.

Thymopentin

Thymopentin is a synthetic pentapeptide (Arg-Lys-Asp-Val-Tyr) corresponding to amino acids 32 to 36 of the linear 49–amino acid sequence of the human thymic hormone thymopoietin (Fig. 3) [29••]. Thymopentin has been demonstrated to enhance production of IL-2 and IFN-γ and reduce spontaneous IgE production by peripheral blood mononuclear cells from patients with AD [30]. In a recent double-blind, placebo-controlled

clinical trial, thymopentin displayed only limited efficacy in the treatment of severe AD [31]. Hsieh *et al.* [32] reported significant clinical improvement in an open clinical trial of thymopentin. Patients in this trial received three subcutaneous injections of thymopentin, 50 mg, each week for 6 weeks, after which time patients were divided into two groups: group A continued thymopentin treatment for an additional 6 weeks, and group B received normal saline. Thymopentin induces suppression of the IL-4 production and enhancement of IFN-γ production *in vitro* [32]. However, no reduction in total serum IgE levels was observed in either trial. No serious side effects are associated with thymopentin treatment, and no satisfactory management of severe AD exists at this time. Subsequently, thymopentin may be considered adjunctive therapy in the treatment of refractory AD [31,32].

Allergen-antibody complexes

Elevated levels of total serum IgE, including IgE specific for airborne and food allergens, are a feature in many patients with AD. Immunologic hyperreactivity toward allergens in the environment appears to play a significant role in the development of the immune response characteristic of AD. One of these allergens in particular, *Dermatophagoides pteronyssinus*, a common house dust mite, may play a prominent role in triggering and exacerbating symptoms in sensitive patients [33]. As a result, recent studies have investigated the potential benefit of administrating allergen-antibody complexes to patients with AD. Under some experimental circumstances, such complexes have suppressed the immune response toward allergens contained in the complexes [33,34]. Further studies need to be conducted to determine the effectiveness of this form of therapy in preventing immune hyperreactivity. A recent double-blind, placebo-controlled study reported on a group of patients with AD and hypersensitivity to *D. pteronyssinus* who were treated with intradermal injection of complexes containing autologous specific antibodies and *D. pteronyssinus* allergens [35•]. Injection with allergen-antibody complexes was effective, safe, and associated with clinical improvement [33,35•]. It is unclear whether reduction of hypersensitivity to *D. pteronyssinus* by injection of its allergen will result in skin healing and prevention of skin entry of further allergens [35•]. One limitation of this therapy is the need to obtain autologous antibodies, which in-

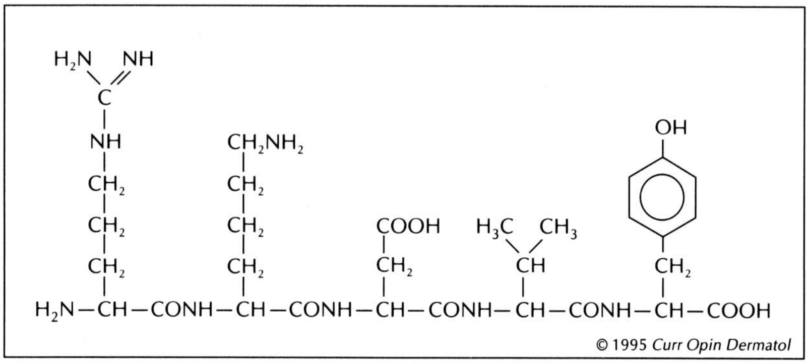

Fig. 3. The structure of thymopentin.

© 1995 *Curr Opin Dermatol*

volves a long and difficult preparation procedure. Studies are under way to simplify procedures of antibody purification and ensure safer and broader application [33].

Traditional Chinese herbal therapy

A recent 5-month controlled trial was conducted in London to assess the effectiveness of traditional Chinese herbal therapy in refractory AD [36•]. Forty adult patients with refractory AD were randomly assigned to two groups. Over 2 months, one group received a daily decoction of a formula consisting of 10 herbs, and the other group received a placebo. After a 4-week washout period, crossover to the other treatment followed for an additional 2 months. This trial resulted in significant improvement in both erythema and surface damage scores (ie, papulation, vesiculation, scaling, excoriation, and lichenification). This result is similar to that of a previous study that reported clinical improvement following traditional Chinese herbal therapy [8••,37]. Herbal treatments are potentially toxic and can specifically be associated with hepatotoxicity [36•]. In addition, the unpalatability of this mixture has limited its popularity and use. The exact mechanism of herbal therapy is unclear, although individual herbs do possess anti-inflammatory, antimicrobial, immunosuppressive, and sedative properties [36•]. Traditional Chinese herbal therapy can provide benefits for patients with refractory AD and can be introduced as a new treatment for this disease; future improvement in palatability and assurance of safety will result in wider applicability [36•].

H₁ antihistamines

Atopic dermatitis is characterized by an intense pruritus that is quite uncomfortable for the patient. Although the mechanism of itching remains unknown, several factors including dry skin and an urticarial response may be responsible [38•]. In addition, increased numbers of mast cells have been demonstrated in skin biopsy samples from chronic AD lesions [38•,39]. Sedating antihistamines have been used in the treatment of pruritus in AD for many years because the sedation produced by these antihistamines was considered instrumental in alleviating the itch.

Recent studies with nonsedating antihistamines have yielded conflicting results in alleviating pruritus. Doherty *et al.* [40] reported on 49 patients with AD who received three daily doses of either terfenadine (60 mg), acrivastine (8 mg), or placebo over 10 days. The patients also received topical steroids and emollients during this period. The patients described a significant reduction in pruritus with both terfenadine and acrivastine. Another study demonstrated the effectiveness of terfenadine over ketotifen, a mast cell stabilizer, in the treatment of pruritus in children with AD [41]. Twenty-nine children with AD received either terfenadine, 30 to 60 mg/d, or ketotifen, 1 mg twice a day. Terfenadine resulted in marked improvement in pruritus, excoriations, eczema, erythema, and sleeplessness within 2 weeks compared with ketotifen.

However, Berth-Jones and Graham-Brown [42] observed different results in a study of 24 patients with AD. They conducted a double-blind, placebo-controlled, cross-over trial with terfenadine, 120 mg twice daily for 2 weeks, on patients with AD. Treatments with topical steroids and emollients continued throughout the study. Following treatment, patients did not report a change in the degree of pruritus they experienced with terfenadine treatment compared with placebo.

So far, results of nonsedating H₁ antihistamines in the treatment of AD have been variable and inconclusive; further clinical trials are needed to determine the efficacy of H₁ antihistamines in the treatment of AD.

Conclusions

We have presented a review of the recent developments in the pathogenesis and treatment of AD. Although the pathogenesis of AD remains unknown, alterations in the immune system may be responsible. Increased IgE production and T-cell activation leading to an aggressive, late skin reaction may be factors. Recent studies have investigated the roles of both Langerhans cells and eosinophils in this inflammatory dermatosis.

There is no single effective therapy for AD. Recent therapeutic advances in the treatment of AD have introduced agents with immunosuppressive or immunomodulatory properties, or both. Phototherapy with high-dose UVA1 and IFN-γ therapy have been encouraging and may be effective in at least a subset of patients. Other agents such as thymopentin and IFN-α have more limited efficacy but may be used as adjunctive therapies in severe cases.

References and recommended reading

Papers of particular interest, published within the annual period of review, have been highlighted as:
•   Of special interest
••   Of outstanding interest

1.   Teshitani A, Ansel J, Chan S, Li S, Hanifin J: **Increased Interleukin 6 Production by T Cells Derived From Patients With Atopic Dermatitis.** *J Invest Dermatol* 1993, 100:299–304.

2.   Jujo K, Renz H, Abe J, Gelfand E, Leung D: **Decreased Interferon**
•   **Gamma and Increased Interleukin-4 Production in Atopic Dermatitis Promotes IgE Synthesis.** *J Allergy Clin Immunol* 1992, 90:323–331.
Excellent study demonstrating an imbalance of IL-4 and IFN-γ production, which may contribute to increased IgE synthesis in AD.

3.   Tang M, Kemp A, Varigos G: **IL-4 and Interferon-Gamma Production in Children With Atopic Disease.** *Clin Exp Immunol* 1993, 92:120–124.

4.   Vercelli D, Jabara H, Lauener R, Geha R: **IL-4 Inhibits the Synthesis of IFN-γ and Induces the Synthesis of IgE in Human Mixed Lymphocyte Cultures.** *J Immunol* 1990, 144:570–573.

5.   Renz H, Jujo K, Bradley K, Domenico J, Gelfand E, Leung D: **Enhanced**
•   **IL-4 Production and IL-4 Receptor Expression in Atopic Dermatitis and Their Modulation by Interferon-Gamma.** *J Invest Dermatol* 1992, 99:403–408.
A well-presented study in which higher levels of IL-4 receptor messenger RNA expression and significantly higher amounts of IL-4 production by peripheral blood mononuclear cells from AD patients were observed, as compared with normal controls.

6.   Byron K, Liberatos S, Varigos G, Wootton A: **Interferon-Gamma Production in Atopic Dermatitis: A Role for Prostaglandins?** *Int Arch Allergy Immunol* 1992, 99:50–55.

7. Fiorentino D, Bond M, Mosmann T: **Two Types of Mouse T Helper Cell: IV. Th2 Clones Secrete a Factor that Inhibits Cytokine Production by Th1 Clones.** *J Exp Med* 1989, **170**:2081–2095.

8. Cooper K: **Atopic Dermatitis: Recent Trends in Pathogenesis and Therapy.** *J Invest Dermatol* 1994, **102**:128–137.
••
Well-detailed and thorough review of the recent trends in the pathogenesis and therapy of AD.

9. Lehn M, Weiser W, Engelhorn S, Gillis S, Renold H: **IL-4 Inhibits H2O2 Production and Antileishmanial Capacity of Human Cultured Monocytes Mediated by IFN-Gamma.** *J Immunol* 1989, **143**:3020–3024.

10. Maggi E, Parronchi P, Manetti R, Simonelli C, Piccini M, Rugin F, De Carli M, Ricci M, Romagnani S: **Reciprocal Regulatory Effects of IFN-Gamma and IL-4 on the In Vitro Development of Human Th1 and Th2 Clones.** *J Immunol* 1992, **148**:2142–2147.

11. Romagnani S, Maggi E, Del Prete G, Parronchi P, Tiri A, Macchia D, Biswas P, Gallo O, Ricci M: **Regulatory Mechanism of In Vitro Human IgE Synthesis.** *Allergy* 1989, **44(suppl 9)**:9–15.

12. Bos J, Wierenga E, Smitt J, van der Heijden F, Kapsenberg M: **Immune Dysregulation in Atopic Eczema.** *Arch Dermatol* 1992, **128**:1509–1512.
•
The authors present recent findings as to the abnormal regulation of IgE synthesis in AD. Specifically, they suggest a distorted and cytokine-mediated self-perpetuating response of the skin immune system to environmental allergens in the pathogenesis of skin disease in atopy.

13. Sowden J, Powell R, Allen B: **Selective Activation of Circulating CD4+ Lymphocytes in Severe Adult Atopic Dermatitis.** *Br J Dermatol* 1992, **127**:228–232.

14. Van Bever H: **Recent Advances in the Pathogenesis of Atopic Dermatitis.** *Eur J Pediatr* 1992, **151**:870–873.
•
Well-written review focusing on the recent advances in the pathogenesis of atopic dermatitis.

15. Bruijnzeel P, Kuijper P, Kapp A, Warringa R, Betz S, Bruijnzeel-Koomen C: **The Involvement of Eosinophils in the Patch Test Reaction to Aeroallergens in Atopic Dermatitis: Its Relevance for the Pathogenesis of Atopic Dermatitis.** *Clin Exp Allergy* 1992, **23**:97–109.

16. Kapp A: **The Role of Eosinophils in the Pathogenesis of Atopic Dermatitis: Eosinophil Granule Proteins as Markers of Disease Activity.** *Allergy* 1993, **48**:1–5.
••
Excellent paper reviewing the role of eosinophils in the pathogenesis of AD. Specifically, the author states that activated eosinophils may play a major role in the allergic inflammatory process of AD.

17. Bruijnzeel P, Kuijper P, Rihs S, Betz S, Warringa R, Koenderman L: **Eosinophil Migration in Atopic Dermatitis: I. Increased Migratory Responses to N-Formyl-Methionyl-Leucyl-Phenylalanine, Neutrophil-Activating Factor, Platelet-Activating Factor, and Platelet Factor 4.** *J Invest Dermatol* 1993, **100**:137–142.

18. Sowden J, Berth-Jones J, Ross J, Motley R, Marks R, Finlay A, Salek M, Graham Brown R, Allen B, Camp R: **Double-Blind, Controlled, Crossover Study of Cyclosporin in Adults With Severe Refractory Atopic Dermatitis.** *Lancet* 1991, **338**:137–140.

19. Krutmann J, Schopf E: **High-Dose UVA1 Phototherapy: A Novel and Highly Effective Approach for the Treatment of Acute Exacerbation of Atopic Dermatitis.** *Acta Derm Venereol (Stockh)* 1992, **176(suppl)**:120–122.

20. Krutmann J, Czech W, Diepgen T, Niedner R, Kapp A, Schopf E: **High-Dose UVA1 Therapy in the Treatment of Patients With Atopic Dermatitis.** *J Am Acad Dermatol* 1992, **26**:225–230.
•
In a controlled trial comparing high-dose UVA1 irradiation with UVA-UVB therapy, high-dose UVA1 treatment was found to induce a significantly superior clinical improvement in patients with AD.

21. Baadsgaard O, Cooper K, Lisby S, Wulf H, Wantzin G: **Dose Response and Time Course for Induction of T6-DR+ Human Epidermal Antigen-Presenting Cells by In Vivo Ultraviolet A, B, and C Irradiation.** *J Am Acad Dermatol* 1987, **17**:792–800.

22. Baadsgaard O, Lisby S, Wantzin G, Wulf H, Cooper K: **Rapid Recovery of Langerhan Cell Alloreactivity, Without Induction of Autoreactivity After In Vivo Ultraviolet A, but Not Ultraviolet B Exposure of Human Skin.** *J Immunol* 1989, **142**:4213–4218.

23. Reinhold U, Kukel S, Brzoska J, Kreysel H: **Systemic Interferon Gamma Treatment in Severe Atopic Dermatitis.** *J Am Acad Dermatol* 1993, **29**:58–63.
•
Well-presented study illustrating the effects of recombinant IFN-γ treatment in severe AD. Fourteen patients with severe AD were treated with recombinant IFN-γ for 6 weeks, after which eight patients (57%) showed marked clinical improvement.

24. Hanifin J, Schneider L, Leung D, Ellis C, Jaffe H, Izu A, Bucalo L, Hirabayashi S, Tofte S, Cantu-Gonzalez G, Milgrom H, Boguniewicz
•
M, Cooper K: **Recombinant Interferon Gamma Therapy for Atopic Dermatitis.** *J Am Acad Dermatol* 1993, **28**:189–197.
A randomized, placebo-controlled, double-blind study demonstrated that recombinant IFN-γ given by daily subcutaneous injection over a 12-week period was safe, well accepted, and effective in reducing inflammation, clinical symptoms, and eosinophilia in severe AD.

25. Jullien D, Nicolas J, Frappaz A, Thivolet J: **Alpha Interferon Treatment in Atopic Dermatitis.** *Acta Derm Venereol (Stockh)* 1993, **73**:130–132.

26. Rousset F, Robert J, Andary M, Bonnin JP, Souillet G, Chretien I, Briere F, Pene J, de Vries JE: **Shifts in Interleukin-4 and Interferon-γ Production by T Cells of Patient With Elevated Serum IgE Levels and the Modulatory Effects of These Lymphokines on Spontaneous IgE Synthesis.** *J Allergy Clin Immunol* 1991, **87**:58–69.

27. Paukkonen K, Fraki J, Horsmanheimo M: **Interferon-Alpha Treatment Decreases the Number of Blood Eosinophils in Patients With Severe Atopic Dermatitis.** *Acta Derm Venereol (Stockh)* 1993, **73**:141–142.

28. Torrelo A, Harto A, Sendagorta E, Czarnetzki B, Ledo A: **Interferon-α Therapy in Atopic Dermatitis.** *Acta Derm Venereol (Stockh)* 1992, **72**:370–372.

29. Pung Y, Vetro S, Bellanti J: **Use of Interferons in Atopic (IgE-Mediated) Disease.** *Ann Allergy* 1993, **71**:234–238.
••
This interesting study introduces an innovative approach to the management of atopic dermatitis. Two patients initially treated with IFN-γ were subsequently switched to IFN-α therapy with dramatic improvement of lesions. The sequential or combined use of IFN-α and IFN-γ may offer additional therapeutic benefit in AD.

30. Leung D, Hirsh R, Schneider L, Moody C, Takaoka R, Li S, Meyerson L, Mariam S, Goldstein G, Hanifin J: **Thymopentin Therapy Reduces the Clinical Severity of Atopic Dermatitis.** *J Allergy Clin Immunol* 1990, **85**:927–933.

31. Stiller M, Shupack J, Kenny C, Jondreau L, Cohen D, Soter N: **Thymopentin in Atopic Dermatitis.** *J Am Acad Dermatol*, **30**:597–602.

32. Hsieh K, Shaio M, Liao T: **Thymopentin Treatment in Severe Atopic Dermatitis: Clinical and Immunological Evaluations.** *Arch Dis Child* 1992, **67**:1095–1102.

33. Leroy B, Lachapelle J, Jacquemin M, Saint-Remy J: **Immunotherapy of Atopic Dermatitis by Injections of Antigen-Antibody Complexes.** *Dermatology* 1993, **186**:276–277.

34. Taylor R, Tite J: **Immunoregulatory Effects of Covalent Antigen-Antibody Complex.** *Nature* 1979, **281**:488–490.

35. Leroy B, Boden G, Lachapelle J, Jacquemin M, Saint-Remy J: **A Novel Therapy for Atopic Dermatitis With Allergen-Antibody Complexes: A Double-Blind, Placebo-Controlled Study.** *J Am Acad Dermatol* 1993, **28**:232–239.
•
A double-blind, placebo-controlled study demonstrated that treatment with injections of allergen-antibody complexes is safe and effective in the majority of *D. pteronyssinus*–sensitive patients with AD.

36. Sheehan M, Rustin M, Atherton D, Buckley C, Harris D, Brostoff J, Ostlere L, Dawson A: **Efficacy of Traditional Chinese Herbal Therapy in Adult Atopic Dermatitis.** *Lancet* 1992, **340**:13–17.
•
This interesting paper presents an innovative and unusual approach to the management of AD. The authors demonstrated that traditional Chinese herbal therapy provides substantial clinical benefit in patients with refractory AD and represents a new treatment for this disease.

37. Bjorneboe A, Soyland E, Bjorneboe G, Rajka G, Drevon CA: **Effect of n-3 Fatty Acid Supplement to Patients With Atopic Dermatitis.** *J Intern Med Suppl* 1989, **225**:233–236.

38. Goldsmith P, Dowd P: **The New H1 Antihistamines: Treatment of Urticaria and Other Clinical Problems.** *Dermatol Clin* 1993, **11**:87–95.
•
Well-presented review of current H$_1$ antihistamines available for the treatment of AD.

39. Mihm M, Soter N, Dvorak H, Austen K: **The Structure of Normal Skin and the Morphology of Atopic Eczema.** *J Invest Dermatol* 1976, **67**:305–312.

40. Doherty V, Sylvester D, Kennedy C, Harvey S, Calthrop J, Gibson J: **Treatment of Itching in Atopic Eczema With Antihistamines With a Low Sedation Profile.** *BMJ* 1989, **298**:96.

41. Tholen S, Dieterich H: **Terfenadine Versus Ketotifen in Children With Atopic Dermatitis.** *Allergologie* 1989, **12**:60–63.

42. Berth-Jones J, Graham-Brown R: **Failure of Terfenadine in Relieving the Pruritus of Atopic Dermatitis.** *Br J Dermatol* 1989, **121**:635–637.

Israel Eckman, MD, and Matthew J. Stiller, MD, Department of Dermatology, Clinical Investigations Unit, Warren Building 505, Massachusetts General Hospital, Boston, MA 02114, USA.

Getting the most out of patch testing

James R. Nethercott, MD, and Jerry E. Cooley, MD

University of Maryland, Baltimore, Maryland, USA

Patch testing remains the best method of establishing that a given contact allergen is the basis for allergic contact dermatitis in a patient. Other methods such as usage trials supplement this technique and may be essential to establish the validity of a positive patch test response. The present standard method involves the application of test materials in different vehicles to the skin under a metal disk called a Finn chamber (Epitest Oy, Tuusula, Finland). A new prepackaged patch test called TRUE test (Kabi Pharmacia, Hillerod, Denmark), which will be available in the United States in 1994, will allow more consistent delivery of a specified allergen dose with less margin for error. The specificity and sensitivity of the present screening patch test panels recommended for use in the United States and Europe are comparable, and both have sensitivities and specificities of about 70%. There is thus a risk of false positive and false negative responses and a need for discretion in the evaluation of the test results. Doubtful responses may have clinical significance and should not be ignored. A second observation of the patch test sites after the initial reading is essential if true positive responses are not to be missed. The test is likely underutilized by dermatologists. Greater application of the test is warranted as a cost-effective way of managing patients who may be able to rid themselves of allergic contact dermatitis if the specific offending allergen can be identified, so that the patient can avoid it.

Current Opinion in Dermatology 1995:10–17

Although it is an old diagnostic procedure first described over one hundred years ago, the patch test still remains the best test for the confirmation of the diagnosis of allergic contact dermatitis (ACD) [1, 2]. Nevertheless, patch testing is not used as frequently as it might be by dermatologists in the management of patients with suspected ACD. In a recent survey of members of the American Academy of Dermatology, investigators found that 27% of the survey respondents did not report performing patch tests [3••]. There was only a 42% response rate to the survey, and therefore the sample may not be representative of the true prevalence of the use of the technique among all Academy members. It is possible that a larger proportion of dermatologists do use the technique. In the survey, the principle reason given for not using the patch test was the belief that the patient's history was sufficient to make a diagnosis of ACD. This belief is inconsistent with published evidence from pretest and posttest validation studies that indicate that most allergens causing ACD cannot be reliably predicted from the clinical history. Patch testing is necessary not only to confirm the presence of ACD, but also not infrequently to find the offending allergen. Patch tests of a screening nature are often required, because no clear delineation of the allergen is possible from the patient's history [4–6]. Another basis often cited for not using patch testing is that there is a risk of sensitizing patients to the test substances. In fact, the risk of this complication is quite low, and the potential is certainly not a great enough risk to the patient to justify withholding this valuable diagnostic test [7].

Many excellent reviews of patch testing have been published [7–9]. The purpose of this review is to provide a basic approach to patch testing for patients with suspected ACD. An understanding of the basic principles that underpin the technique is needed to maximize the value of this test in the clinician's hands. In addition, some recent advances in the technique are outlined.

Selection of patients

Patch testing is indicated in patients who are suspected of having ACD. The following criteria have been suggested as a basis for considering that a patient has ACD and that patch testing may be indicated to establish the specific allergen accounting for the disease [10–12]:

1) The patient has an eczematous dermatitis at the site of contact with the suspected allergen, the aller-

---

Abbreviations
ACD—allergic contact dermatitis; **NPV**—negative predictive value; **PPV**—positive predictive value.

gen is associated with an exacerbation of the dermatitis, and it has been established that the individual has had contact with the allergen.

2) The dermatitic process partially or totally resolves with avoidance of such exposure. Exposure to the allergen is considered to play a causal role when there is a recurrence of the eczema 24 to 72 hours after exposure, and other exposed individuals do not experience ACD.

Although a defect in cell-mediated immunity is thought to be one of the main characteristics of atopic dermatitis, the value of patch testing for this disease has been repeatedly confirmed [13–16]. In a prospective study of 552 patients, Fedler and Stromer [13] found that atopic patients with or without active dermatitis showed the same frequency of positive reactions to the European standard allergens as did healthy control subjects. Cronin and McFadden [14] reported that patients with atopic dermatitis frequently exhibit relevant positive patch test responses, albeit fewer than nonatopic persons.

Another population often not tested is children. Recent work indicates the usefulness of such tests in pediatric patients [17, 18].

The selection of patients for patch testing has a direct effect on the value of the results. Biostatistical considerations are as important as they are for any other diagnostic test [18–20]. A fourfold (2×2) table illustrates the relationship between patch test results and the presence of ACD in those tested (Fig. 1). Of all patients who meet the case definition of ACD, those with a positive patch test result represent the "true positives," whereas those with negative results are considered "false negatives." Of persons without disease, those with a negative patch test result would be considered "true negatives," whereas those with a positive test result would be "false positives." The proportion of true positive tests among those with disease is called the test's *sensitivity*, while the proportion of true negatives among those without disease is called its *specificity*. Sensitivity and specificity are stable characteristics of any particular test and do not vary with the prevalence of disease in a particular population.

In most published reports, patients with suspected ACD have been patch tested to identify those who do and do not have the disease. However, without having each cell of the 2×2 table filled, it is hard to interpret the results. Information about the patch test as a diagnostic tool based on these standard indices of validity is limited. More studies are needed to provide patch test results for patients who do and do not have disease, based on clear clinical criteria [21]. An example of such a study is that by Aronson *et al.* [22•], who studied 25 clay modelers at an automobile factory and divided this group into 13 with ACD and 12 without, based on a previously published standard for diagnosing occupational dermatitis according to specific clinical criteria [23]. When the investigators patch tested this group, they were able to fill in the four cells of the 2×2 table

and determine the sensitivity and specificity of patch testing. This study provided the false negative rate (*ie*, the number of patients who had ACD based on strict clinical criteria but had a negative patch test result); this is the value which is sorely missing in almost all of the patch testing literature.

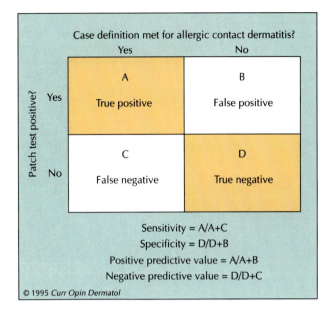

Fig. 1. The relationship between patch test response and the presence or absence of allergic contact dermatitis.

Confusion can arise in the discussion of diagnostic tests, because clinicians do not look down the 2×2 table as biostaticians do, but rather look across it. In case of a positive result, they want to know the likelihood that the patient truly has the disease. This likelihood is called the *positive predictive value* (PPV) and is equal to the proportion of all persons with a positive test result who have the disease. Clinicians also want to know, when faced with a negative test result, how likely it is that the patient does not have the disease; the proportion of all patients with a negative test result who truly do not have the disease is called the *negative predictive value* (NPV) (Fig. 1). A critical concept is that the PPV and NPV of patch testing will depend on the prevalence of ACD in those tested. As the prevalence of disease declines, so does the PPV, but the NPV increases. When the prevalence increases, so does the PPV, but the NPV declines.

This concept can be illustrated by comparing the same patch test applied to patient populations with different disease prevalences. Take the sensitivity of the test as 70% and the specificity as 80%, neither of which varies with disease prevalence (Fig. 2). If the prevalence of ACD in the tested population is only 10%, the PPV will be only 28%. The NPV, however, will be very high. Contrast this with the situation in which the prevalence of ACD in the tested population is 90%. A positive result almost certainly means the patient has ACD because the PPV is 97%. A negative result, however, is much less helpful, because the NPV is only 23%.

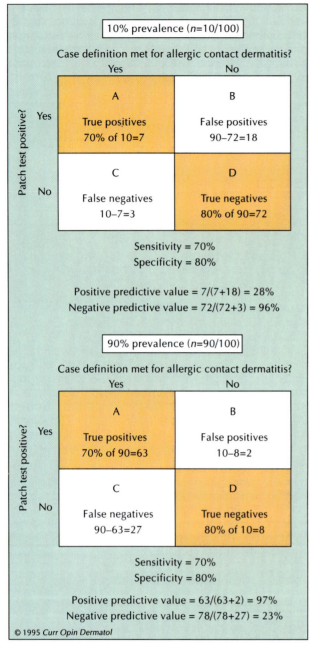

Fig. 2. Comparison of positive predictive value and negative predictive value of patch tests at different prevalence levels in a population of patients tested for allergic contact dermatitis.

Recent studies of contact nickel allergy illustrate how the prevalence of disease affects the results of patch testing. In a study of 567 people randomly selected from the Danish population, Nielsen and Menne [24] found approximately 6.7% exhibited a positive patch test response to nickel and thus were deemed to be sensitive to nickel. One can raise the prevalence of ACD in the tested population by testing only those suspected of having ACD according to clinical criteria. For example, in a study of 834 patients suspected of having ACD, Castiglioni *et al.* [25] found that 18% were al-

lergic to nickel. The prevalence of positive patch test responses to nickel increases when one selects a population of test subjects in whom the diagnosis of ACD is suspected, and the PPV of the patch test with nickel would increase in such a population.

The goal of selecting patients for patch testing should be to maximize the prevalence of ACD in tested patients by careful clinical history, thus increasing the PPV of the patch test. If one is overly selective, however, the NPV will decrease (*ie*, there will be more false negatives), and more of those with disease will be missed. Clinicians can expect to observe at least one positive patch test result in 30% to 65% of patients they test with the 20 chemicals in the American Academy of Dermatology screening tray [26]. PPV and NPV must be weighed off against one another, and in this way, the cost-effectiveness of the procedure can be maximized. If the clinician is observing fewer positive patch test responses, it may imply that the test is being applied without adequate selectivity, and thus the PPV is likely to be reduced. On the other hand, more frequent positive responses may indicate that one is being overly stringent, and that while the PPV will be high, some patients who probably should have had the benefit of the testing procedure have not been tested.

Technical considerations

After one has decided to patch test a particular patient, one has to decide which allergens to use for the test. In most instances, the standard allergen screening tray recommended by multicenter research groups such as the International Contact Dermatitis Research Group and the North American Contact Dermatitis Group should be used. The idea of using a standard screening tray for a patient with suspected ACD is based on the fact that the majority of allergic contact reactions are due to the relatively small group of allergens that are represented on the tray. Standard screening trays used in North America and Europe can be expected to identify 70% of the cases subsequently diagnosed as ACD [27, 28].

The test protocol has been standardized, and careful adherence to the recommended technique is essential if consistent results that will yield valid interpretation are to be achieved [29]. The challenge concentrations recommended are based on the use of the Finn chamber appliance (Epitest Oy, Tuusula, Finland) [30] and the application of the test material for 48 to 72 hours to the upper back (Fig. 3). A new patch test method known as the TRUE test (Kabi Pharmacia, Hillerod, Denmark) is available in Europe and will soon be available in the US (Fig. 4). In the TRUE test method, the allergens are mixed with a gel and applied to sheets of polyester film and dried to produce a thin gel film [31]. The coated water-impermeable sheets are then cut into square patches with a surface area of 0.81 cm^2 each, and the squares are mounted on pieces of tape. Each piece is placed in an airtight, light-impermeable envelope. The packages contain a desiccant to ensure minimal water absorption into the gel. The Finn chamber and the TRUE test methods yield similar results, but the TRUE test method is less cumbersome, although more expensive. The consistency and the uniform dose per unit surface area with the new test method should produce more consistent results than the older method.

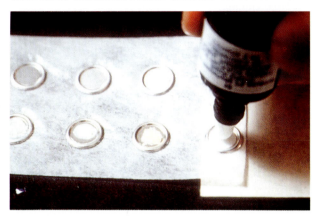

Fig. 3. Finn chamber patch test appliance (Epitest Oy, Tuusula, Finland).

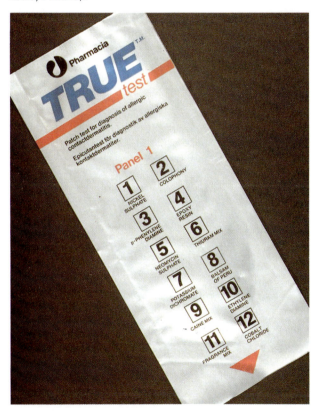

Fig. 4. TRUE test patch test appliance (Kabi Pharmacia, Hillerod, Denmark).

After the patches are removed and nonspecific irritation from the tape and from the physical effect of pressure at the patch test sites has resolved (*ie*, after 30 to 45 minutes), the test sites can be morphologically graded for intensity of response. It is essential that a second observation of the patch test sites be performed, because true positive responses may be evident only at the second observation [32]. Belsito *et al.* [33•] found that delayed readings resulted in a significant number of tests converting to positive, especially formaldehyde, quaternium-15, neomycin, and ethylenediamine. Usually, the second observation is carried out 1 to 2 days after the first reading.

Patch test responses are scored using a morphologic grading system, as shown in Table 1. Figure 5 illustrates a 2+ response to paraphenylenediamine, scored according to this method. While a number of methods have been investigated as possible ways to quantify such responses (*eg*, laser Doppler velocimeter [34]), none have been found to be useful in clinical settings.

Table 1. Morphologic grading system for patch test responses	
Response category	**Reaction and morphology**
1+	Weak reaction: erythema, infiltration, papules
2+	Strong reaction: edematous or vesicular
3+	Extreme reaction: spreading, bullous, or ulcerative
+/–	Doubtful reaction: macular erythema only
Neg	Negative reaction
IR	Irritant morphology

The issue of what to do with a responses graded as doubtful (*ie*, macular erythema only) is somewhat controversial. Some of these responses are mild irritant responses. However, some are true positives. Discarding the latter results decreases sensitivity of the test, and including those that are actually irritant responses decreases the specificity of the test. For example, in the study by Aronson *et al.* [22•] of workers who met strictly defined criteria for ACD, counting doubtful patch test reactions as positive improved the sensitivity of the test from 64% to 92% [21]. It is recommended that test substances that yield doubtful responses be retested at later date if the patient's history indicates they could be relevant. It may also be useful to retest at a higher challenge concentration to observe whether a more clearly defined positive, consistent morphologically with an allergic, rather than an irritant response, is elicited. Finally, a repeated open application test with the product or a usage trial with a substance containing the suspected allergen may be needed to establish whether the patient has ACD due to the allergen, even if only a doubtful patch test response is elicited with the allergen.

Interpretation of the positive result

An approach to the evaluation of test results and the actions that may follow from them is summarized in Figure 6. If the results is clearly positive, the clinician cannot necessarily assume that the allergen is responsible for the patient's dermatitis. One may be dealing with a false positive reaction, which is most often due to an irritant reaction. Some allergens on the screening tray, such as formalin, chromate, and nickel, have a high irritancy potential in contrast to others that have low irritancy, such as neomycin, which even when tested at a 50% concentration in petrolatum seldom causes irritation [6].

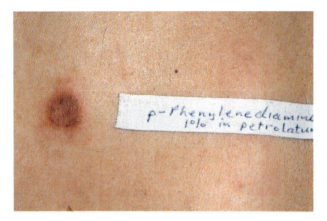

Fig. 5. A 2 + (*ie*, strong) patch test response to paraphenylene-diamine, according to morphologic grading system.

Multiple positive patch test reactions should make the clinician consider a phenomenon called the *angry back syndrome*, also known as the *excited skin syn-*

drome [35,36]. The latter may occur if a person has a strongly positive patch test response. In this instance, a state of skin hyperirritability may occur such that many other patch test sites become inflamed, but these substances do not induce a response on later, separate rechallenge. Fisher [6] notes that in his experience, nickel and chromate are the most frequent culprits, and the false positive reaction is often seen where the allergen is an irritant, such as formalin. Nethercott *et al.* [10] found a similar association between positive responses to nickel sulphate and formaldehyde. To overcome this problem, one should subsequently test each potential allergen alone (Fig. 4).

If one has determined that the patch test reaction is a real allergic response, the next step is to determine the relevance of this finding to the patient's dermatitis. It may be that the positive reaction explains the current dermatitis and is consistent with the case definition for ACD, *ie*, that the allergen causes an eczematous dermatitis at the site of cutaneous contact, with a temporal association between exposure and dermatitis at 24 to 72 hours in a usage situation, and the dermatitis partially or totally resolves with avoidance of the allergen [37]. Confirmation of ACD requires a knowledge of the particular allergen and where it is likely to be found in occupational and domestic settings. Alternatively, one may decide that the positive reaction explains a previous contact dermatitis or has no known relevance. As in the case of doubtful positive responses, usage tri-

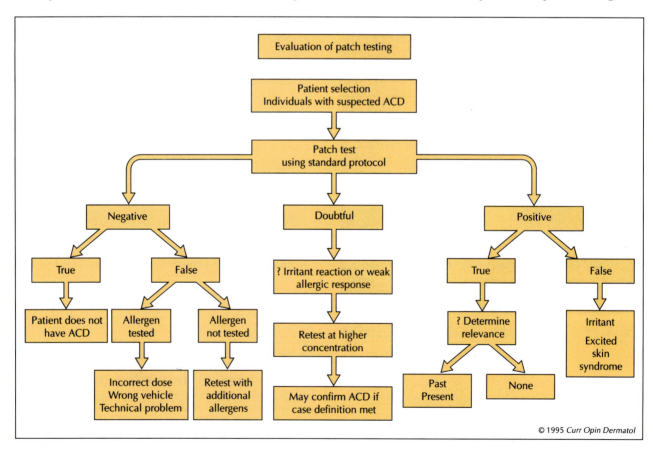

© 1995 *Curr Opin Dermatol*

Fig. 6. An approach to evaluating the performance of patch tests. ACD—allergic contact dermatitis.

als are germane in instances of more morphologically intense patch test responses and can be used to document the relevance of the response before the patient is directed to avoid a particular allergen.

Interpretation of the negative result

The interpretation of a negative patch test result requires a similar strategy. One can seldom determine with confidence that a negative reaction is a true negative. The false negative reaction can occur for several reasons. Even if the allergen causing the ACD is being tested for on the tray, there are several potential reasons why it may fail to elicit a response. The concentration of the allergen will have a profound effect on the sensitivity of the patch test [22•]. For example, in a study of patch test reactivity using nickel sulfate in aqueous solution on patients with a previously documented nickel sensitivity, Szliska *et al.* [38] demonstrated that a 5% solution produced a 96% positive response, a 1% solution produced a 58% response, a 0.1% solution produced a 6.5% response, and a 0.01% solution produced no response. Patch test concentrations are generally chosen to maximize the number of true positive reactions while minimizing irritant reactions, but there can be a significant overlap for some of the allergens; choosing a low concentration of such a substance may avoid irritant reactions but result in more false negatives.

False negative responses may occur if the correct allergen is tested but with the wrong vehicle. Some allergens are reactive in petrolatum, but not in an aqueous solution and vice versa. Whitmore described a case of scalp dermatitis to minoxidil in which patch testing to minoxidil in 10% propylene glycol caused a 2 + reaction, but negative results were obtained with minoxidil in 70% isopropyl alcohol or in petrolatum as well as with propylene glycol alone. Whitmore [39] astutely concluded that the propylene glycol vehicle was essential for sufficient penetration to cause a positive reaction, although a less likely but equally plausible explanation was that the combination of minoxidil and propylene glycol caused a compound or formulation allergy.

If the patient has any history of photosensitivity, one should consider the diagnosis of photoallergic contact dermatitis, which requires photopatch testing to diagnose. In a series of 187 patients with a history of photosensitivity, DeLeo *et al.* [40] found that 11% of the patients had clinically relevant photopatch tests confirming a diagnosis of photoallergic contact dermatitis; most of these reactions were to fragrance ingredients and sunscreen ingredients. Failure to expose such a patient to the suspected allergen and ultraviolet light would result in a false negative patch test response.

Finally, true negative responses to the test substances on the standard tray may indicate that the tray as a test has yielded a false negative result. By that we mean that the patient truly has ACD but that the test was negative. In this instance, it was falsely negative because the offending allergen was not in the series of chemicals tested. If the result with a screening tray is negative, but the clinician remains convinced that the patient has ACD and has met the case definition, and the allergen has not been identified, the clinician should search for an allergen that could be responsible for the ACD but was not tested for on the standard tray. As mentioned, the standard allergen screening trays have an estimated ability to identify 70% of ACD, which leaves 30% unidentified. For example, Kathon CG (Rohm and Haas Co., Philadelphia, PA), a biocide increasingly used in the United States for cosmetic and industrial purposes, elicits a 1.8% positive response in those suspected of having ACD, a rate higher than that of other allergens on the screening tray [41•].

Allergic contact dermatitis due to topical corticosteroid drugs is not evaluated through patch testing with routine screening trays. This problem has received increasing attention as an important cause of ACD, especially in patients with chronic eczematous dermatitis, such as atopic patients and those with hand eczema or stasis dermatitis and leg ulcers [42••,43]. In patients patch tested for suspected ACD, the positive response to corticosteroid allergens has varied from 1.5% to 4.9% [44,45]. In a recently reported study, corticosteroids were found to be the seventh most common allergens, higher than many other allergens on the routine tray [46]. Although patch testing for suspected corticosteroid allergy has demonstrated a relatively high prevalence of relevant positive reactions, some authors believe that patch testing with these drugs is not sufficiently sensitive for diagnosis and recommend intradermal challenge testing [47,48]. While the issue of which corticosteroid test substance to use to obtain the highest sensitivity is still being debated, it is likely that one or more corticosteroid allergens will soon find their way into routine screening trays in the near future.

Conclusions

Although many dermatologists do not use patch testing, it is the best method for confirming the diagnosis of ACD. It is a safe and effective test that should be considered in the evaluation of the patient with a suspected allergic contact dermatitis, including children and patients with atopic dermatitis.

Proper patient selection increases the likelihood of obtaining meaningful results. The clinical history should be used to raise the prevalence of ACD in the tested population and thereby maximize the PPV of the test results. This approach should be balanced against the need to identify as many affected patients as possible. To ensure valid results, the tests should be performed according to a standard protocol.

The positive patch test result may reflect a false positive reaction most often as the result an irritant reaction. If there are multiple, simultaneous positive reactions, one should consider the angry back syndrome and sequentially retest each allergen alone at a later date. A true positive result should be categorized as to its relevancy to the patient's current dermatitis based on the clinician's knowledge of the particular allergen.

A negative result may mean that the patient's dermatitis is not allergic in origin, but this conclusion should be reached only after other possibilities are considered. The right allergen may indeed have been tested but may not have elicited a response because the test was done under the wrong conditions (eg, inadequate concentration, or the wrong vehicle). A delayed reading should always be performed to identify late positives. Another explanation for a negative result is that the offending allergen was not tested; clinicians should be increasingly suspicious of corticosteroid allergy, especially in those who do not respond to or worsen with treatment, those with chronic hand eczema, and those with leg ulcers and stasis dermatitis.

Continuing research will help establish the validity of patch testing in the evaluation of patients with suspected ACD. More research is needed to define the role of patch testing, especially studies comparing patch test results to well-defined patient populations with and without ACD as defined by clear clinical criteria. Such information will help guide the clinician in selecting patients for patch testing and in interpreting the results.

References and recommended reading

Papers of particular interest, published within the annual period of review, have been highlighted as:
- Of special interest
- • Of outstanding interest

1. Jadassohn J: **Zur Kenntnis der Medicamentosen Dermatosen.** In *Verhandlungen der Deutschen Dermatologischen Gesellschaft, Fünfter Kongress Graz, 1885.* Edited by Jarisch A, Neisser A. Vienna: W. Braunmüller Publisher; 1896:103–129.

2. Van Arsdel P, Larson E: **Diagnostic Tests for Patients With Suspected Allergic Disease: Utility and Limitations.** *Ann Intern Med* 1989, 110:304–312.

3. James WD, Rosenthal LE, Brancaccio RR, Marks JG: **American Academy of Dermatology Patch Testing Survey: Use and Effectiveness of This Procedure.** *J Am Acad Dermatol* 1992, 26:991–994.
•• This paper provides valuable insights into the basis for patch testing and its effectiveness, based on a survey of practicing dermatologists.

4. Cronin E: **Clinical Prediction of Patch Tests.** *Trans St John's Hosp Dermatol Soc* 1972, 58:153–162.

5. Kieffer M: **Nickel Sensitivity.** *Contact Dermatitis* 1979, 5:398–401.

6. Fisher T, Maibach H: **Improved, But Not Perfect Patch Testing.** *Am J Contact Dermatitis* 1990, 1:73–90.

7. Fisher AA: *Contact Dermatitis.* Philadelphia: Lea & Febiger; 1986.

8. Hjorth N: **The Development of the Patch Testing Procedure and Working for Consistency.** *J Am Acad Dermatol* 1989, 21:855–857.

9. Sulzberger MB: **The Patch Test: Who Should and Should Not Use It and Why.** *Contact Dermatitis* 1975, 1:117.

10. Nethercott J, Holness D, Adams R, Belsito D, DeLeo V, Emmett E, Fowler J, Fisher A, Larsen W, Maibach H, *et al.*: **Patch Testing With a Routine Screening Tray in North America 1985-1989: I. Frequency of Response.** *Am J Contact Dermatitis* 1991, 2:122–129.

11. Nethercott J, Holness D, Adams R, Belsito D, DeLeo V, Emmett E, Fowler J, Fisher A, Larsen W, Maibach H, *et al.*: **Patch Testing With a Routine Screening Tray in North America 1985-1989: II. Gender and Response.** *Am J Contact Dermatitis* 1991, 2:130–134.

12. Nethercott J, Holness D, Adams R, Belsito D, DeLeo V, Emmett E, Fowler J, Fisher A, Larsen W, Maibach H, *et al.*: **Patch Testing With a Routine Screening Tray in North American 1985-1989: III. Age and response.** *Am J Contact Dermatitis* 1991, 2:198–201.

13. Fedler R, Stromer K: **Nickel Sensitivity in Atopics, Psoriatics and Healthy Subjects.** *Contact Dermatitis* 1993, 29:65–69.

14. Cronin E, McFadden JP: **Patients With Atopic Eczema Do Become Sensitized to Contact Allergens.** *Contact Dermatitis* 1993, 28:225–228.

15. Lammintausta K, Kalimo K, Fagerlund VL: **Patch Test Reactions in Atopic Patients.** *Contact Dermatitis* 1992, 26:234–240.

16. Lever R, Forsyth A: **Allergic Contact Dermatitis in Atopic Dermatitis.** *Acta Derm Vernereol (Stockh)* 1992, 176(suppl):95–98.

17. Pambor M, Kruger G, Winkler S: **Results of Patch Testing in Children.** *Contact Dermatitis* 1992, 27:326–328.

18. Ayala F, Balato N, Lembo G, Patruno C, Tosti A, Schena D, Pigatto P, Angelini G, Lisi P, Rafanelli A: **A Multicentre Study of Contact Sensitization in Children.** *Contact Dermatitis* 1992, 26:307–310.

19. Nethercott JR: **Practical Problems in the Use of Patch Testing in the Evaluation of Patients With Contact Dermatitis.** *Curr Probl Derm* 1990, 4:95–123.

20. Sackett D, Haynes R, Tugwell P: **Clinical Epidemiology-A Basic Science for Clinical Medicine.** Boston, Little Brown and Co., 1985.

21. Nethercott JR: **When is a Patch Test Positive? [Editorial].** *Am J Contact Dermatitis* 1993, 4:136–137.

22. Aronson PJ, Shettler C, Yakes B, *et al.*: **Weak Patch Test Reactions at 48 Hours Can Provide an Understanding of a Work-Related Dermatitis: A Study of Epidemic Hand Dermatitis in Industrial Clay Modellers.** *Am J Contact Dermatitis* 1993, 4:163–168.
• This paper provides insight into the validity of patch tests and, in particular, why doubtful responses should not be ignored completely.

23. Mathias CGT: **Contact Dermatitis and Workers' Compensation: Criteria for Establishing Occupational Causation and Aggravation.** *J Am Acad Dermatol* 1989, 20:842–848.

24. Nielsen NH, Menne T: **Nickel Sensitization and Ear Piercing in an Unselected Danish Population.** *Contact Dermatitis* 1993, 29:16–21.

25. Castiglioni G, Carosso A, Manzoni S, Nebiolo F, Bugiani M: **Results of Routine Patch Testing of 834 Patients in Turin.** *Contact Dermatitis* 1992, 27:182–185.

26. Rietschel RL: **Is Patch Testing Cost-Effective?** *J Am Acad Dermatol* 1989, 21:885–887.

27. Nethercott J, Holness L: **The Validity of Patch Test Screening Trays in the Evaluation of Patients With Allergic Contact Dermatitis.** *J Am Acad Dermatol* 1989, 21:568.

28. Menne T, Dooms-Goossens A, Wahlberg JE, White IR, Shaw S: **How Large a Proportion of Contact Sensitivities Are Diagnosed With the European Standard Series?** *Contact Dermatitis* 1992, 26:201–202.

29. Corey G: **Applying Patch Tests From a Technician's or Nurse's Point of View.** *Am J Contact Dermatitis* 1993, 4:175–181.

30. Fischer T, Maibach H: **Amount of Nickel Applied With a Standard Patch Test.** *Contact Dermatitis* 1984, 11:285–287.

31. TRUE© Test Study Group: **Comparative Multicenter Studies With TRUE© Test and Finn Chambers in Eight Swedish Hospitals.** *J Am Acad Dermatol* 1989, 21:846–849.

32. Nethercott J, Holness D, Adams R, Belsito D, DeLeo V, Emmett E, Fowler J, Fisher A, Larsen W, Maibach H, *et al.*: **Results of First and Second Patch Test Readings.** *Am J Contact Dermatitis* 1991, 2:255–259.

33. Belsito DV, Storrs FJ, Taylor JS, Marks J: **Reproducibility of Patch Tests: A United States Multicenter Study.** *Am J Contact Dermatitis* 1992, 3:193–200.
• This paper documents an investigation into the reproducability of patch test responses, demonstrating the robustness of the technique when it is used carefully.

34. Quinn AG, McLelland J, Essex T, Farr PM: **Quantification of Contact Allergic Inflammation: A Comparison of Existing Methods With a Scanning Laser Doppler Velocimeter.** *Acta Derm Venereol (Stockh)* 1993, 73:21–25.

35. Mitchell JC: **The Angry Back Syndrome: Eczema Creates Eczema.** *Contact Dermatitis* 1975, 1:193.

36. Mitchell JC, Maibach HI: **The Angry Back Syndrome: The Excited Skin Syndrome.** *Semin Dermatol* 1982, 1:9.

37. Nethercott JR, Holness DL: **Cutaneous Nickel Sensitivity in Toronto, Canada.** *J Am Acad Dermatol* 1990, 22:756–761.

38. Szliska C, Vocks E, Von Mayenburg J, Rakoski J: **Patch Testing With a Dilution Series of Nickel Sulfate.** *Contact Dermatitis* 1992, 27:111–112.

39. Whitmore SE: **The Importance of Proper Vehicle Selection in the Detection of Minoxidil Sensitivity.** *Arch Dermatol* 1992, 128:653–656.

40. DeLeo VA, Suarez SM, Maso MJ: **Photoallergic Contact Dermatitis.** *Arch Dermatol* 1992, **128**:1513–1518.

41. Marks JG, Moss JN, Parno JR, Adams R, Belsito D, DeLeo V, Fran-
• sway A, Fowler J, Maibach H, Mathias C, *et al.*: **Methyl-chloro-isothia-zolinone/Methylisothiazolinone (Kathon CG) Biocide: Second United States Multicenter Study of Human Skin Sensitization.** *Am J Contact Dermatitis* 1993, **4**:87–89.
This paper presents data related to the problems in the interpretation of patch test responses in terms of the predictive value of the test and the problems of usage situtations.

42. Dooms-Goossens A: **Corticosteroid Contact Allergy: A Challenge to**
•• **Patch Testing.** *Am J Contact Dermatitis* 1993, **4**:120–122.
Corticosteroid sensitivity is a practical problem that Dooms-Goosens examines in a lucid manner. This sometimes covert allergy may lead to persistent disease, which may be compounded by treatment if it remains unrecognized.

43. Wilkinson SM, English JSC: **Hydrocortisone Sensitivity: Clinical Features of Fifty-Nine Cases.** *J Am Acad Dermatol* 1992, **27**:683–687.

44. Dooms-Goossens A, Meinardi MMHM, Bos JD, Degreef H: **Contact Allergy to Corticosteroids: The Results of a Two-Centre Study.** *Br J Dermatol* 1994, **130**:42–47.

45. Burden AD, Beck MH: **Contact Hypersensitivity to Topical Corticosteroids.** *Br J Dermatol* 1992, **127**:497–500.

46. Dooms-Goossens A, Morren M: **Results of Routine Patch Testing With Corticosteroid Series in 2073 Patients.** *Contact Dermatitis* 1992, **26**:182–191.

47. Wilkinson SM, English JSC: **Patch Tests Are Poor Detectors of Corticosteroid Allergy.** *Contact Dermatitis* 1992, **26**:67–68.

48. Herbst RA, Lauerma AI, Maibach HI: **Intradermal Testing in the Diagnosis of Allergic Contact Dermatitis.** *Contact Dermatitis* 1993, **29**:1–5.

James R. Nethercott, MD, Department of Dermatology, University of Maryland, 405 West Redwood Street, 6th Floor, Baltimore, MD 21201, USA.

Classification and treatment of inflammatory diseases of pregnancy

Farah Shah, MD, and Stephanie H. Pincus, MD

State University of New York at Buffalo, Buffalo, New York, USA

Knowledge of the cutaneous changes that occur during pregnancy is of utmost importance. These changes include common skin findings not seen exclusively during pregnancy, as well as those that are specific to pregnancy. We present a review of this latter, complex group of cutaneous eruptions specific to pregnancy.

Current Opinion in Dermatology 1995:18–21

The classification of inflammatory diseases of pregnancy has become increasingly complex. Many conditions are based on isolated case reports or are poorly defined clinical entities. The following is a discussion of the current concepts pertaining to well- and poorly defined dermatoses, as well as some recently reported unique entities.

Well-defined dermatoses

Pruritic urticarial papules and plaques

Pruritic urticarial papules and plaques of pregnancy (PUPPP) is a relatively common, intensely pruritic disorder typically affecting primigravidas during the last trimester. Other names include toxemic rash of pregnancy [1] and toxic erythema of pregnancy [2]. Holmes *et al.* [3] proposed the term *polymorphic eruption of pregnancy*, because of the multiplicity of lesions, which included papules, plaques, target lesions, polycyclic wheals, and vesicles.

Pruritic urticarial papules and plaques of pregnancy is characterized by small erythematous papules beginning in abdominal striae, then gradually spreading peripherally to involve buttocks and thighs (Fig. 1). Arms may also be involved, although face, palms, and soles are usually spared. The individual papules are usually surrounded by a narrow pale halo, often coalescing into plaques and polycyclic wheals. Although vesicles may sometimes be seen, bullous lesions are rare. Excoriations are uncommon despite marked pruritus. Specific histologic findings include a perivascular lymphohistiocytic infiltrate with variable eosinophils. Edema of the papillary dermis and mild focal spongiosis may also be present.

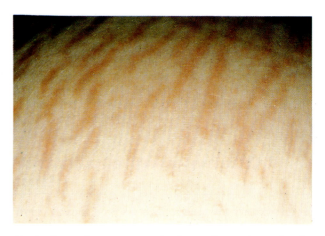

Fig. 1. The erythematous papular lesions located near the abdominal striae are characteristic of pruritic urticarial papules and plaques of pregnancy. Biopsy can be useful in excluding herpes gestationis and is often indicated in such conditions.

Most lesions, as well as the pruritus, spontaneously disappear within a few days after delivery. Postpartum exacerbations and recurrence in subsequent pregnancies are rare. There is no effect upon fetal or maternal mortality and morbidity, although there may be an associated increase in the frequency of twin pregnancies, as well as increased maternal weight gain and increased fetal weight [4].

The etiology of PUPPP is unknown. The fact that it typically begins in the abdominal striae has raised the question of whether the striae could be a "trigger factor." Some believe that excessive abdominal distention resulting from increased weight gain induces the clinical eruption [4]. There is no specific HLA haplotype associated with PUPPP. Weiss and Hull [5] recently reported on the occurrence of PUPPP in two different families,

---

Abbreviations
HG—herpes gestationis; **PUPPP**—pruritic urticarial papules and plaques of pregnancy.

both of which included sisters who were married to brothers. In one of the families, the sisters were twins married to twin brothers. Their data suggest that PUPPP is not an HLA class 1–related disease. Additionally, they raise the possibility that PUPPP may be the result of a maternal response to paternal factors.

Treatment of PUPPP depends on the severity of the symptoms. In mild cases, it is important to reassure patients that they have a self-limited condition. Potent topical corticosteroids, as well as a brief course of oral corticosteroids, may be effective in severe cases. Antihistamines are generally regarded as ineffective, and their use should be carefully considered. Beltrani and Beltrani [6] recently described a severe case of PUPPP that did not respond to conventional therapy, and in which early delivery resulted in alleviation of symptoms within 12 hours.

Herpes gestationis

Herpes gestationis (HG) is an intensely pruritic vesicobullous dermatosis that presents during pregnancy or the immediate postpartum period. Typically, pruritic urticarial lesions rapidly develop into vesicles and bullae (Fig.2). The degree of pruritus may be out of proportion to the clinical findings. Onset often occurs in the second or third trimester but is usually earlier in subsequent pregnancies. The majority of lesions begin in the periumbilical area, but atypical presentations beginning on extremities are not uncommon. Facial lesions are rare. Most women develop a flare of their disease at the time of delivery. Some women may present with explosive disease in the immediate postpartum period; it is not uncommon to have a recurrence of the disease with menstruation or with use of oral contraceptives. HG has also been associated with trophoblastic tumors [7••].

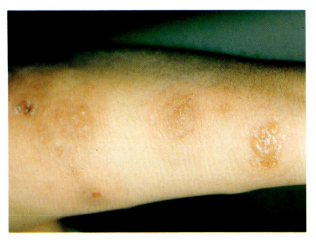

Fig. 2. These intensely vesicular bullous lesions present on the arm of a young woman are typical for herpes gestationis. The diagnosis was confirmed by routine histology and immunofluorescent testing.

Histologic findings typically reveal edema of the papillary dermis with an infiltrate of eosinophils, lympho-

cytes, and a few neutrophils. Basal cell necrosis may be seen. Subepidermal vesicle formation may result from pronounced edema. A superficial and middermal perivascular infiltrate of lymphocytes and eosinophils may be seen. Biopsy specimens taken for direct immunofluorescence from perilesional or normal skin characteristically show linear deposition of C3 along the basement membrane zone. IgG and less often IgM, IgA, Ca1, C4, C5, and factor B may be found in association with C3. Infants born to mothers with HG may also show deposits of C3. Immunoelectron microscopy has shown C3 deposits in the lamina lucida. Results of routine indirect immunofluorescence are positive in only 25% of the patients. With the indirect complement-fixation immunofluorescence technique, however, the majority of the patients will demonstrate the presence of "HG factor." This HG factor is an IgG1 antibody that avidly fixes complement. Immunochemical studies have shown that the HG factor is specific for an antigen that appears to be similar to the bullous pemphigoid antigen. However, it has preferential binding to a 180-kD protein over the 230- to 240-kD protein usually found in bullous pemphigoid. Recent evidence suggests that the 180-kD antigen and the 230- to 240-kD antigen are likely coded for by separate complimentary DNAs [8], and that the 180-kD protein likely represents a transmembrane protein [9].

Herpes gestationis is associated with an increased incidence of HLA-DR3, and -DR4, and to a lesser extent the HLA-DR3/DR4 paired haplotype [10]. Ninety percent of patients also carry a C4 null allele [11], which may be a result of linkage disequilibrium with HLA-DR3 or -DR4. Anti-HLA antibodies occur in almost all patients with a history of HG, although their exact role is unclear. Abnormal expression of class II major histocompatibility complex occurs in the chorionic villi of those with HG, leading some authors to believe that the primary immunologic event may be taking place within the placenta [12,13]. A paternally derived antigen has been postulated, because a change in paternity may result in an absence of recurrence in subsequent pregnancies [14•]. Recently, Shornick and Black [15] studied 75 patients for the frequency of other autoimmune diseases, and reported an increased frequency of Graves' disease in patients with a history of HG. In addition, they found an increased frequency of autoimmune diseases in the family members of patients with HG. Although Graves' disease was the most common disease in relatives, Hashimoto's thyroiditis and pernicious anemia were also encountered.

Controversy exists as to whether there is an increased fetal mortality or morbidity associated with HG. In a recent study in which the HG and non-HG pregnancies of 74 women were compared, no evidence for an increased rate of spontaneous abortions or fetal mortality was found [16••]. A slight increase in small-for-gestational-age and premature babies was reported, however. Additionally, treatment with systemic corticosteroids was not noted to influence these rates. Approximately 10% of neonates born to mothers with HG will develop a transient blistering disease. Neonates, even without clinical evidence of disease, usually have positive immunofluorescence findings on skin biopsies, which indicates the likelihood of subclinical disease.

Treatment of HG depends on the severity of the disease. Although topical corticosteroids and antihistamines are occasionally shown to be effective, systemic corticosteroids remain the mainstay of therapy at dosages of 0.5 mg/kg of prednisone daily.

Prurigo gravidarum

This dermatosis, also known as recurrent cholestasis of pregnancy, is characterized by intense pruritus followed within several weeks by the clinical appearance of jaundice. Typically, primary lesions are absent, although excoriations may be abundant, especially during the later stages of the disease when the pruritus becomes generalized. It characteristically appears during the third trimester, usually remits a few days after delivery, and may recur with subsequent pregnancies. Anorexia, nausea, and right upper quadrant fullness may be accompanying complaints. Although the exact pathophysiology is unknown, the condition may be hormonally related in susceptible individuals, because similar findings may occur if oral contraceptives are given after delivery.

Neonates born to mothers with prurigo gravidarum appear to be at an increased risk for prematurity and low birthweight. Additionally, the mothers themselves appear to be at increased risk for postpartum hemorrhage [17]. The pruritus may frequently be controlled with emollients, topical corticosteroids, or antihistamines. Cholestyramine has also proven to be effective.

Poorly defined eruptions

Papular dermatitis

This dermatosis of pregnancy was initially reported by Spangler et al. [18] in 1962 and has rarely been reported since. It can occur at any time during the pregnancy and is characterized by small erythematous papules with a central crust with no particular site of predilection. Recurrences in subsequent pregnancies have been reported. Although histologic findings are nonspecific, and results of immunofluorescence testing are negative, markedly elevated levels of urinary chorionic gonadotropin and low levels of urinary estriol and plasma hydrocortisone were found in the initial cases. Spangler et al. reported a 27% incidence of fetal death in untreated cases, although treated patients showed no fetal deaths. Although diethylstilbestrol was once recommended, it should not be used because of potential risks to the fetus. Treatment with systemic corticosteroids generally proves effective.

Autoimmune progesterone dermatitis

This eruption was reported in a single patient [19]. It presented early in pregnancy with papules and pustules on the extremities and buttocks. This pregnancy, as well as a previous pregnancy in which the patient experienced a similar eruption, terminated in spontaneous abortion. Oral contraceptives resulted in a flare of the disease. The result of a skin test to progesterone was positive, although the exact role of progesterone in the development of the clinical eruption is unclear.

Newly described entities

Two separate entities that differ from previously reported dermatoses have recently been described. A prospective immunofluorescence study of 111 cases of pruritic dermatoses of pregnancy by Zurn et al. [20••] revealed a subset of five patients with circulating antibasement membrane antibodies on indirect immunofluorescence with negative results on direct immunofluorescence, as well as on Western blot studies. Clinically, all the patients presented with either macular erythema or papular or urticarial lesions, mainly on the abdomen. All but one case showed rapid clearance of the lesions within a few days. Four of the patients presented in the third trimester, and one in the 11th week of pregnancy. The authors were unable to identify any external factors such as drugs, infection, or physical agents that might have been responsible for the described findings. Although deposits of IgM have been reported on direct immunofluorescence, to date this is the first report of circulating antibasement membrane zone IgM antibodies in a pruritic dermatosis of pregnancy.

A single case was reported by Ford et al. [21] in which a pustular eruption developed in abdominal striae during the third trimester in a black primigravida. This markedly pruritic dermatosis is unique not only because of the presence of pustules, but also because the eruption began abruptly between the fingers and toes and progressed rapidly to hands, feet, arms, and legs. The patient denied any exposure to scabies, as well as any personal or family history of psoriasis. Histologically, a well-defined intraepidermal pustule with neutrophils, eosinophils, and a few mononuclear cells was noted, along with papillary dermal edema and a dense cellular infiltrate of lymphocytes and eosinophils. Results of direct and indirect immunofluorescent studies were negative. The eruption resolved in a few days after treatment with oral hydroxyzine and topical triamcinolone was begun. The eruption recurred 1 month later with oral contraceptive use. The neonate appeared to be unaffected.

Conclusions

Although a concise and up-to-date description of dermatoses specific to pregnancy has been provided, we have not discussed entities for which there have been no recent developments or reports. These conditions include impetigo herpetiformis, prurigo gestationis (Besnier's prurigo), and pruritic folliculitis of pregnancy. In the dermatologic evaluation of women of childbearing age, the specific dermatoses of pregnancy should be considered, and appropriate history and laboratory evaluations should be obtained. It is important to remember, however, that common dermatologic diseases may still be present in the pregnant patient.

References and recommended reading

Papers of particular interest, published within the annual period of review, have been highlighted as:

- Of special interest
- •• Of outstanding interest

1. Bourne G: **Toxemic Rash of Pregnancy.** *J R Soc Med* 1962, **55**:462.

2. Holmes RC, Black MM, Dann J, James DCO, Bhogal: **A Comparative Study of Toxemic Erythema of Pregnancy and Herpes Gestationis.** *Br J Dermatol* 1982, **106**:499–510.

3. Holmes RC, Black MM: **The Specific Dermatoses of Pregnancy: A Reappraisal With Special Emphasis on a Proposed Simplified Classification.** *Clin Exp Dermatol* 1982, 7:65–73.

4. Cohen LM, Capeless EL, Krusinski PA, Maloney ME: **Pruritic Urticarial Papules and Plaques of Pregnancy and its Relationship to Maternal-Fetal Weight Gain and Twin Pregnancy.** *Arch Dermatol* 1989, **125**:1534–1536.

5. Weiss R, Hull P: **Familial Occurrence of Pruritic Urticarial Papules and Plaques of Pregnancy.** *J Am Acad Dermatol* 1992, **76**:715–717.

6. Beltrani VP, Beltrani VS: **Pruritic Urticarial Papules and Plaques of Pregnancy: A Severe Case Requiring Early Delivery for Relief of Symptoms.** *J Am Acad Dermatol* 1992, **26**:266–267.

7. Shornick JK: **Herpes Gestationis.** *Dermatol Clin* 1993,
•• **11**:527–533.
Comprehensive review including latest concepts.

8. Diaz LA, Ratrie H 3d, Saunders WS, Futamura S, Squiquera HL, Anhalt GJ, Giudice GJ: **Isolation of a Human Epidermal cDNA Corresponding to the 180kD Autoantigen Recognized by Bullous Pemphigoid and Herpes Gestationis Sera: Immunolocalization of this Protein to the Hemidesmosome.** *J Clin Invest* 1990, **86**:1088–1094.

9. Karpati S, Stolz W, Meurer M, Braun-Falco O, Krieg T: **Herpes Gestationis: Ultrastructural Identification of the Extracellular Antigenic Sites in Deceased Skin Using Immunogold Techniques.** *Br J Dermatol* 1991, **125**:317–325.

10. Shornick JK, Statsny P, Gillian JN: **High Frequency of Histocompatibility Antigens HLA-DR3 and DR4 in Herpes Gestationis.** *J Clin Invest* 1981, **60**:553–555.

11. Shornick JK, Artlett CM, Jenkins RE, Briggs DC, Welsh KI, Garvey MP, Kelley SE, Block MM: **Complement Polymorphism in Herpes Gestationis Association With C4 null Allele.** *J Am Acad Dermatol* 1993, **29**:545–549.

12. Borthwick GM, Holmes RC, Stirrat GM: **Abnormal Expression of Class II MHC Antigens in Placenta From Patients With Pemphigoid Gestationis: Analysis of Class II Subregion Product Expression.** *Placenta* 1988, 9:81–94.

13. Kelly SE, Black MM, Fleming S: **Hypothesis-Pemphigoid Gestationis: A Unique Mechanism of Irritation of an Autoimmune Response by MHC Class II Molecules?** *J Pathol* 1989, **158**:81–82.

14. Powell FC: **The Skin in Pregnancy: Recent Advances.** *Ir J Med Sci*
• 1992, :99–100.
Brief relevant review.

15. Shornick JK, Black MM: **Secondary Autoimmune Disease in Herpes Gestationis (Pemphigoid Gestationis).** *J Am Acad Dermatol* 1992, **26**:63–68.

16. Shornick JK, Black MM: **Fetal Risks in Herpes Gestationis (Pem-**
•• **phigoid Gestationis).** *J Am Acad Dermatol* 1992, **26**:63–68.
The latest news on the important question of fetal risk.

17. Lauley TJ, Yancey KB: **Skin Changes and Pregnancy.** In *Dermatology in General Medicine*, edn 4. Edited by Fitzpatrick TB. New York: McGraw-Hill; 1993:2105–2112.

18. Spangler AS, Reddy W, Bordaire WA, Robby CC, Emerson K: **Papular Dermatitis of Pregnancy.** *JAMA* 1962, **181**:577–581.

19. Bierman SM: **Autoimmune Progesterone Dermatitis.** *Arch Dermatol* 1973, **107**:896–901.

20. Zurn A, Celebi CR, Bernard P, Didierjean L, Saurat JH: **A Prospective**
•• **Immunofluorescence Study of 111 Cases of Pruritic Dermatoses of Pregnancy: IgM Anti-basement Membrane Zone Antibodies as a Novel Finding.** *Br J Dermatol* 1992, **26**:474–478.
May be reporting a new entity.

21. Ford MJ, Gammon WR, Kilpatrick TM: **Pustular Eruption of the Striae in a Primigravidas.** *Cutis* 1992, **50**:225–228.

Farah Shah, MD, and Stephanie H. Pincus, MD, State University of New York at Buffalo, Department of Dermatology, 100 High Street, Buffalo, NY 14203, USA.

Management of autoimmune blistering diseases

M. Joyce Rico, MD

New York University and New York Veterans
Administration Medical Center, New York, New York, USA

The purpose of this review is to highlight recent advances and controversies in the management of patients with chronic autoimmune blistering skin diseases. Corticosteroids remain the mainstay of therapy in patients with these diseases, although several anti-inflammatory agents (*eg*, dapsone, gold, antibiotics, and niacinamide) and immunosuppressants (*eg*, azathioprine, cyclophosphamide, methotrexate, and cyclosporine) are also used. Recent advances in therapy include the use of alternate protocols, plasmapheresis, and extracorporeal photopheresis in patients with severe disease.

Current Opinion in Dermatology 1995:22–26

Patients with chronic autoimmune blistering diseases present significant challenges in management for the practicing dermatologist. The goals of therapy are to control blister formation and symptoms, optimize wound healing, and prevent sequelae of the disease and the side effects of therapy. Therapy must be tailored to each patient, whose underlying health status, age, other medical problems, and prognosis should be borne in mind. Significant advances in decreasing morbidity and mortality for these diseases has been due largely to advances in managing complications both of the disease and of treatment and improvements in wound care. Corticosteroids are the mainstay of treatment for most patients with autoimmune blistering disorders. Patients with refractory disease, or those in whom steroids are not tolerable, may benefit from the addition of adjuvants, such as immunosuppressants [1•].

The purpose of this article is to review the recent literature on the treatment of autoimmune blistering diseases. For a more detailed discussion of the clinical, diagnostic, and immunophenotypic features of these diseases, the reader is referred to several detailed recent reviews [2,3•].

Pemphigus

Patients with pemphigus vulgaris (PV) limited to the oral mucosa may respond to topical corticosteroids, including a potent formulation of clobetasol in Orabase (Colgate-Hoyt Laboratories, Canton, MA) [4]. Whereas topical or intralesional steroids may be sufficient for disease control in patients with limited oral disease, in a recent retrospective review of 30 patients with oral manifestations of PV, 29 patients were treated with systemic prednisone alone or in conjunction with immunosuppressants (3 of 30 patients) or gold (2 of 30 patients) [5]. Based on the results of this study, the authors recommended long-term oral steroids as the treatment of choice in oral PV.

Similarly, patients with limited cutaneous PV or pemphigus foliaceus can be treated with topical or intralesional steroids, but the majority of these patients will require systemic steroids (Fig. 1) [1•]. Patients whose condition is not controlled with high-dose systemic steroids, or who develop significant side effects associated with steroid use, are candidates for treatment with adjuvants, including gold or immunosuppressants. Gold, in general, is well tolerated, although adverse reactions including bone marrow suppression, proteinuria, and hepatonecrosis have been reported [6••,7].

Azathioprine has been the most frequently used immunosuppressant for patients with blistering disease, followed by oral cyclophosphamide. Several reports have documented the efficacy of pulse cyclophosphamide, usually in conjunction with pulse methylprednisolone, in adults and children with pemphigus [8•,9,10]. In these protocols, cyclophosphamide is administered monthly in an intravenous injection (0.5 to 1.0 mg/m²) followed by low-dose oral cyclophosphamide (50 mg/d). One major advantage of this protocol is that a total lower dose of cyclophosphamide

Abbreviations

BP—bullous pemphigoid; **CP**—cicatricial pemphigoid; **DH**—dermatitis herpetiformis; **PV**—pemphigus vulgaris.

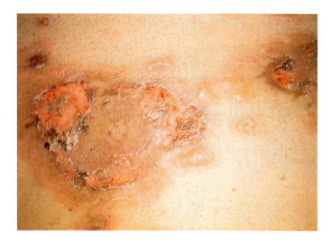

Fig. 1. Flaccid blisters and erosions in a patient with pemphigus vulgaris.

is given, which should decrease the long-term risk of malignancy. In addition, patients can be well hydrated during therapy, to minimize the risk of hemorrhagic cystitis.

In cases of severe generalized pemphigus that has not been controlled with prednisone and a single immunosuppressant agent, the addition of another immunosuppressant has been of some benefit. Citarrella *et al.* [11] reported a good response in four of five patients with refractory PV treated with prednisone, cyclophosphamide, and vincristine. Control of recalcitrant PV with extracorporeal photophoresis has been reported for a limited number of patients [12–14]. These patients received photophoresis on 2 consecutive days at 2- to 4-week intervals and responses were noted after seven treatments. The lack of availability of extracorporeal photophoresis limits its utility, but for patients with severe, refractory disease, it is an option.

Other strategies for managing pemphigus include the use of tetracycline (2 g/d) and niacinamide (1.5 g/d). In a recent series, nine of 11 patients with pemphigus, most of whom were receiving concurrent therapy with oral or topical steroids, improved [15]. Hymes *et al.* [16] reported on three patients with pemphigus foliaceus exacerbated by ultraviolet exposure who responded to adjuvant treatment with antimalarial agents.

Dapsone has been used as an adjuvant in patients with pemphigus, including children, with limited success [17]. Dapsone is the drug of choice in patients with intraepidermal neutrophilic IgA dermatosis, a newly described entity that has also been called IgA pemphigus. Approximately 50% of patients with this disorder respond to dapsone alone, and the remainder benefit from the addition of low-dose prednisone. Colchicine has recently been reported beneficial in this condition [18]. Like dapsone, colchicine is efficacious in the treatment of dermatologic conditions characterized by polymorphonuclear leukocyte predominance on histology.

Bullous pemphigoid

Like those with pemphigus, the majority of patients with bullous pemphigoid (BP) are treated with corticosteroids (Fig. 2). Patients with severe disease unresponsive to high-dose prednisone, or who develop complications associated with steroid use, are candidates for therapy with adjuvants, including immunosuppressants. There has been some debate as to whether the early use of immunosuppressants offers significant improvement in remission rates when compared with steroids alone. Guillaume *et al.* [19••] recently undertook a prospective, multicenter trial involving 100 patients with BP who received either 1) prednisolone alone, 2) prednisolone in combination with azathioprine, or 3) prednisolone in combination with plasmapheresis. There was no difference in the remission rate among the three groups, but patients who received prednisolone and azathioprine experienced more side effects from the treatment. The authors concluded that the concomitant use of azathioprine or plasmapheresis early in the course of the disease offered no significant advantages over steroids alone.

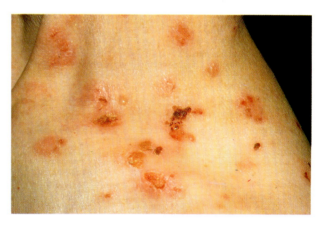

Fig. 2. Numerous tense vesicles and erosions on the upper chest and neck of a 63-year-old woman with bullous pemphigoid.

Other immunosuppressants that have been used in patients with BP include cyclophosphamide, chlorambucil, and methotrexate [1•,20]. In a retrospective review, Paul *et al.* [20] recently reported that low-dose methotrexate (< 20 mg/w) was effective as an adjuvant in suppressing blister formation and permitting tapering of steroid dosage in eight elderly patients with BP.

Other adjuvants reported effective in the management of BP include the antibiotics tetracycline and erythromycin, either alone or in conjunction with niacinamide [21,22]. Despite these published reports, my personal experience and that of others [23] are that these agents are not highly effective in patients with BP.

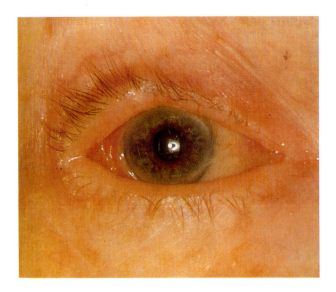

Fig. 3. This 61-year-old woman with cicatricial pemphigoid has corneal keratinization and scarring secondary to her disease.

Cicatricial pemphigoid

The term *cicatricial pemphigoid* (CP) has been used to describe patients who present with chronic, scar-ring blistering diseases involving the mucosa or skin (Fig. 3). CP tends to be recalcitrant to therapy, and patients develop progressive scarring, which may lead to blindness, or esophageal stenosis. The heterogeneity of the clinical presentation of CP may be due to the fact that different mechanisms and different antigens are targets for subsets of patients with this disorder. Chan *et al.* [24•] recently reviewed the clinical and laboratory findings of 87 patients with immune-mediated subepithelial blistering mucosal diseases and proposed a novel classification system. They identified three distinct subsets of patients with the following patterns of cutaneous and mucosal involvement: 1) skin and mucosal blistering associated with autoantibodies to BP antigens, 2) oral mucosal disease without skin disease, and 3) pure ocular CP. Patients in the latter group had a significantly lower incidence of antibody and complement deposits at the basement membrane on direct immunofluorescence. The identification of a subset of patients without evidence of autoantibody deposition supports previous investigations that suggest that some cases of ocular CP may be T-cell rather than B-cell–mediated. This observation has important ramifications for therapy, because prednisone, azathioprine, and cyclophosphamide are effective in controlling antibody-mediated autoimmune diseases, but less effective in T-cell–mediated disorders [25•]. Cyclosporine has been reported to be effective in controlling T-cell–mediated diseases, but its efficacy in randomly selected patients with CP has been disap-

Table 1. Management of chronic autoimmune blistering diseases*				
Pemphigus [2]	Bullous pemphigoid	Cicatricial pemphigoid [26••]	Epidermolysis bullosa acquisita	Dermatitis herpetiformis and linear IgA bullous disease
Localized disease 　Topical or intralesional 　　steroids [4,5] Widespread disease 　Corticosteroids (oral 　　or "pulse") 　Adjuvants 　　Gold [7] 　　Dapsone [17] 　　Azathioprine 　　Cyclophosphamide (oral 　　　or "pulse") [8•,9,10] 　　Antibiotics with or 　　　without niacin- 　　　amide [15] 　　Antimalarials [16] 　　Colchicine [18] Resistant disease 　Combination therapy 　　Azathioprine, prednisone, 　　　vincristine [11] 　　Extracorporeal 　　　photopheresis [12–14]	Corticosteroids Adjuvants 　Dapsone 　Antibiotics with or 　　without niacin- 　　amide [21–23] 　Azathioprine [19••] 　Cyclophosphamide 　Methotrexate [20] 　Chlorambucil [1•] 　Plasmapharesis [19••]	Prednisone Dapsone Azathioprine Cyclophosphamide Cyclosporine	Prednisone Dapsone Azathioprine Cyclophosphamide Cyclosporine Intravenous immuno- 　globulins [30]	Dapsone Sulfapyridine Gluten-free diet [33] Elemental diet [34•] Cyclosporine [36] Antibiotics with or 　without niacin- 　amide [15]

*Numbers in *brackets* indicate references in which treatments are discussed.

pointing [26••,27]. Topical cyclosporine (5mL of 100 mg/mL cyclosporine oral solution, three times daily, swish and spit) has been reported effective in one patient with oral CP unresponsive to oral steroids and dapsone [28]. Further studies in the management of patients with CP, classifying patients is the manner detailed by Chan *et al.* [24•], may identify subgroups of patients with enhanced responses to specific therapeutic agents.

Foster *et al.* [26••] recently published a retrospective analysis of treatment outcome in 200 patients with ocular involvement and CP with and without concomitant skin disease [26••]. In this series, the cure rate was 35%, and the relapse rate was 27%, underscoring the need for long-term follow-up in these patients. The drugs most commonly used were dapsone, azathioprine, cyclophosphamide, and prednisone; however, no one agent was associated with a better response rate.

The surgical management of complications of ocular CP has been improved with the evolution of buccal mucosal and split-thickness dermal grafts in patients with medically controlled CP [29,30].

Epidermolysis bullosa acquisita

Like those with CP, patients with the classic form of epidermolysis bullosa acquisita tend to have chronic, scarring blistering that responds poorly to therapy. Agents reported to be effective in some patients include dapsone, prednisone, azathioprine, cyclophosphamide, and cyclosporine. Recently, high-dose intravenous immunoglobulins in combination with cyclosporine and prednisolone were effective in controlling blistering in a 16-year-old boy with resistant epidermolysis bullosa acquisita [31].

Dermatitis herpetiformis and linear IgA bullous disease

Dapsone remains the drug of choice for patients with dermatitis herpetiformis (DH) and linear IgA bullous disease, including chronic bullous disease of childhood. Side effects associated with dapsone therapy include anemia and methemoglobinemia. In patients who do not tolerate these side effects, the ingestion of vitamin E (400 IU twice daily) has been reported to decrease the hemolysis associated with dapsone, while coadministration of cimetidine (400 mg three times daily) has reduced methemoglobinemia in patients on high dose dapsone [32,33].

Although most cases of DH are controlled with dapsone, a gluten-free diet is beneficial in patients with recalcitrant disease or in those who are unable to tolerate dapsone. A recent report on the role of a gluten-free diet in the management of patients with DH underscored the need for a skilled nutritionist in assisting with dietary management for these patients [34•]. Because dietary antigens other than gluten have been postulated to be relevant in the pathogenesis of DH, an elemental diet has also been shown to be effective in patients with recalcitrant DH [35]. In patients with severe, recalcitrant DH, the administration of cyclosporine (3 mg/kg/d) has demonstrated significant clinical improvement in a series of two patients [36].

Conclusions

A variety of therapeutic agents, including anti-inflammatory drugs (eg, prednisone, gold, antibiotics, and niacinamide) and immunosuppressants (eg, azathioprine, cyclophosphamide, methotrexate, and cyclosporine) have been used in the management of chronic autoimmune blistering diseases (Table 1). These agents all act nonspecifically to decrease the inflammatory or the immune response of the host. The future goals of therapy are to devise less toxic, selective agents to specifically abrogate the host's immune response to the specific antigenic target. Advances in our understanding of the target antigens in these diseases and in the regulation of autoimmune responses suggest that such treatment options are possible.

Acknowledgment

Supported in part by a Clinical Investigator Award from the National Institutes of Arthritis, Musculoskeletal and Skin Diseases (KO-8 AR01808).

References and recommended reading

Papers of particular interest, published within the annual period of review, have been highlighted as:
• Of special interest
•• Of outstanding interest

1. Rico MJ: **Treatment of Autoimmune Blistering Diseases.** *Cutis* 1993,
• 52:357–361.
A clinically oriented review of the major drugs used in managing blistering diseases, with discussion of the usual doses, side effects, and complications of therapy.

2. Hall RP, Rico MJ: **Autoimmune Skin Diseases.** In *Clinical Immunology: Principles and Practice.* Edited by Rich RR, Fleisher TA, Schwartz BD, Shearer WT, Strober W. St. Louis: Mosby Year Book; 1994: in press.

3. Stanley JR: **Cell Adhesion Molecules as Targets of Autoantibodies**
• **in Pemphigus and Pemphigoid: Bullous Diseases Due to Defective Epidermal Cell Adhesion.** *Adv Immunol* 1993, 53:291–325.
A comprehensive overview of advances in understanding the molecular targets of autoimmune blistering diseases by one of the major contributors to the field.

4. Lozada-Nur F, Huang MZ, Zhou GA: **Open Preliminary Clinical Trial of Clobetasol Propionate Ointment in Adhesive Paste for Treatment of Chronic Oral Vesiculoerosive Diseases.** *Oral Surg Oral Med Oral Pathol* 1991, 71:283–287.

5. Lamey P, Rees TD, Binnie WH, Wright JM, Rankin K, Simpson NB: **Oral Presentation of Pemphigus Vulgaris and Its Response to Systemic Steroid Therapy.** *Oral Surg Oral Med Oral Pathol* 1992, 74:54–57.

6. Wolverton SE: **Monitoring for Adverse Effects From Systemic Drugs**
•• **Used in Dermatology.** *J Am Acad Dermatol* 1992, 26:661–679.
An extensive review of the adverse reactions and complications associated with a number of the therapeutic agents used in treating patients with blistering diseases.

7. Rye B, Krusinski PA: **Hepatonecrosis Resulting From Parenteral Gold Therapy in Pemphigus Vulgaris.** *J Am Acad Dermatol* 1993, 28:99–101.

8. Pandya AG, Sontheimer RD: **Treatment of Pemphigus Vulgaris**
•   **With Pulse Intravenous Cyclophosphamide.** *Arch Dermatol* 1992,
    128:1626–1630.
Discusses the rationale and use of pulse cyclophosphamide.

9. Pasricha JS, Das SS: **Curative Effect of Dexamethasone-Cyclophos-
    phamide Pulse Therapy for the Treatment of Pemphigus Vulgaris.**
    Int J Dermatol 1992, **31**:875–877.

10. Kanwar AJ, Dhar S, Kaur S: **Further Experience With Pemphigus in
    Children.** *Pediat Dermatol* 1994, in press.

11. Citarrella P, Gebbia V, DeMarco P, Tambone-Reyes M, Noto G, Arico
    M: **Cyclophosphamide Plus Vincristine and Prednisone in the Treat-
    ment of Severe Pemphigus Vulgaris Refractory to Conventional Ther-
    apy.** *J Chemother* 1992, **4**:56–58.

12. Rook AH, Jegasothy BV, Heald P, Nahass GT, Ditre C, Wit-
    mer WK, Lazarus GS, Edelson RL: **Extracorporeal Photochemother-
    apy for Drug-Resistant Pemphigus Vulgaris.** *Ann Intern Med* 1990,
    112:303–305.

13. Liang G, Nahass G, Kerdel FA: **Pemphigus Vulgaris Treated With
    Photopheresis.** *J Am Acad Dermatol* 1992, **26**:779–780.

14. Gollnick HPM, Owsianowski M, Taube KM, Orfanos CE: **Unre-
    sponsive Severe Generalized Pemphigus Vulgaris Successfully Con-
    trolled by Extracorporeal Photophoresis.** *J Am Acad Dermatol* 1993,
    28:121–124.

15. Chaffins ML, Collison D, Fivenson DP: **Treatment of Pemphigus and
    IgA Dermatosis With Nicotinamide and Tetracycline: A Review of
    13 Cases.** *J Am Acad Dermatol* 1993, **28**:998–1000.

16. Hymes SH, Jordon RE: **Pemphigus Foliaceus: Use of Antimalarial
    Agents as Adjuvant Therapy.** *Arch Dermatol* 1992, **128**:1462–1464.

17. Leibowitz MR, Voss SP: **Juvenile Pemphigus Foliaceus: Response to
    Dapsone [Letter].** *Arch Dermatol* 1993, **129**:910.

18. Gengoux P, Tennstedt D, Lachapelle JM: **Intraepidermal Neutrophilic
    IgA Dermatosis: Pemphigus-Like IgA Deposits.** *Dermatology* 1992,
    185:311–313.

19. Guillaume J, Vaillant L, Bernard P, Picard C, Prost C, Labeille B, Guil-
•• lot B, Goldes-Pauwels C, Prigent F, Joly P, *et al.*: **Controlled Trial of
    Azathioprine and Plasma Exchange in Addition to Prednisolone in the
    Treatment of Bullous Pemphigoid.** *Arch Dermatol* 1993, **129**:49–53.
A multicenter, prospective, randomized trial comparing three different treatment regimens in patients with BP. This study demonstrates no significant benefit in patients treated with azathioprine or azathioprine in combination with
plasmapheresis versus corticosteroids alone.

20. Paul M, Jorrizzo J, Fleischer A: **Low-Dose Methotrexate in Elderly
    Patients With Bullous Pemphigoid.** *J Am Acad Dermatol* 1994, in
    press.

21. Thomas I, Khorenian S, Arbesfeld DM: **Treatment of Generalized
    Bullous Pemphigoid With Oral Tetracycline.** *J Am Acad Dermatol*
    1993, **28**:74–77.

22. Oranje AP, Vuzevski VD, van Joost T, ten Kate F, Naafs B: **Bul-
    lous Pemphigoid in Children: Report of Three Cases With Special
    Emphasis on Therapy.** *Int J Dermatol* 1991, **30**:339–342.

23. Miralles ES, Cabezon MN, Pozueta AL: **Treatment of Generalized Bul-
    lous Pemphigoid With Oral Tetracycline [Letter].** *J Am Acad Der-
    matol* 1994, **30**:291.

24. Chan LS, Yancey KB, Hammerberg C, Soong HK, Regezi JA, Johnson
•   K, Cooper KD: **Immune-Mediated Subepithelial Blistering Diseases of
    Mucous Membranes: Pure Ocular Cicatricial Pemphigoid Is a Unique
    Clinical and Immunopathological Entity Distinct From Bullous Pem-
    phigoid and Other Subsets Identified by Antigenic Specificity of Au-
    toantibodies.** *Arch Dermatol* 1993, **129**:448–455.
This article proposes a novel classification system for mucosal blistering diseases based on a retrospective analysis of 87 patients that suggests that patients
with pure ocular involvement form a distinct subset.

25. Bach J: **Immunosuppressive Therapy of Autoimmune Diseases.** *Im-
•   munol Today* 1993, **14**:322–326.
A general overview of immunosuppressant therapy in B-cell– and T-
cell–mediated autoimmune diseases.

26. Foster CS, Neumann R, Tauber J: **Long Term Results of Systemic
•• Chemotherapy for Ocular Cicatricial Pemphigoid.** *Doc Ophthalmol*
    1992, **82**:223–229.
In this retrospective analysis of 104 consecutive patients with ocular involvement and cicatricial pemphigoid, approximately one third of the patients
achieved a remission, one third were free of disease activity, and the final
third failed to respond to treatment. The most commonly used agents were
dapsone, azathioprine, and cyclophosphamide; a few patients received long-
term treatment with prednisone.

27. Hess AD: **Mechanisms of Action of Cyclosporine: Considerations for
    the Treatment of Autoimmune Diseases.** *Clin Immunol Immunopath*
    1993, **68**:220–228.

28. Azana JM, de Misa RF, Boixeda JP, Ledo A: **Topical Cyclosporine
    for Cicatricial Pemphigoid.** *J Am Acad Dermatol* 1993, **28**:134–135.

29. Shore JW, Foster CS, Westfall CT, Rubin PAD: **Results of Buccal
    Mucosal Grafting for Patients With Medically Controlled Ocular Ci-
    catricial Pemphigoid.** *Ophthalmology* 1992, **99**:383–395.

30. Mauriello JA, Pokorny K: **Use of Split-Thickness Dermal Grafts to
    Repair Corneal and Scleral Defects: A Study of 10 Patients.** *Br J
    Ophthalmol* 1993, **77**:327–331.

31. Meier F, Sonnichsen K, Schaumburg-Lever G, Dopfer R, Rassner G:
    **Epidermolysis Bullosa Acquisita: Efficacy of High-Dose Intravenous
    Immunoglobulins.** *J Am Acad Dermatol* 1993, **29**:334–337.

32. Prussick R, Ali MA, Rosenthal D, Guyatt G: **The Protective Effect
    of Vitamin E on the Hemolysis Associated With Dapsone Treat-
    ment in Patients With Dermatitis Herpetiformis.** *Arch Dermatol* 1992,
    128:210–213.

33. Coleman MD, Rhodes LE, Scott AK, Verbov JL, Friedman PS, Breck-
    enridge AM: **The Use of Cimetidine to Reduce Dapsone-Dependent
    Methaemoglobinaemia in Dermatitis Herpetiformis Patients.** *Br J Clin
    Pharmacol* 1993, **34**:244–249.

34. Andersson H, Mobacken H: **Dietary Treatment of Dermatitis Her-
•   petiformis.** *Eur J Clin Nutr* 1992, **46**:309–315.
A review of the role of gluten in pathogenesis of DH, including a discussion
of the nutritional consequences of a gluten-free diet.

35. Kadunce DP, McMurry MP, Avots-Avotins A, Chandler JP, Meyer LJ,
    Zone JJ: **The Effect of an Elemental Diet With and Without Gluten
    on Disease Activity in Dermatitis Herpetiformis.** *J Invest Dermatol*
    1991, **97**:175–182.

36. Stenveld HJ, Starink TM, van Joost T, Stoof TJ: **Efficacy of Cy-
    closporine in Two Patients With Dermatitis Herpetiformis Resistant
    to Conventional Therapy.** *J Am Acad Dermatol* 1993, **28**:1014–1015.

M. Joyce Rico, MD, Chief, Dermatology Service, New York VA Medical Center, 423 East 23rd Street, New York, NY 10010, USA.

Controversies in the management of erythema multiforme and toxic epidermal necrolysis

Philip Barton, MD, and Franklin Flowers, MD

University of Florida College of Medicine, Gainesville, Florida, USA

Controversy and confusion surround the classification and management of erythema multiforme (EM) and toxic epidermal necrolysis (TEN). A poor understanding of the pathophysiology of these entities and the lack of prospective, well-controlled clinical trials have compounded the problem. Treatment is frequently based on personal experience, clinical intuition, or case reports. In this article, we describe the two major forms of EM (ie, minor and major) and TEN and review the current literature on their management. In particular, we focus on the treatment of recurrent EM minor and the role of corticosteroids in the management of EM and TEN.

Current Opinion in Dermatology 1995:27–31

Erythema multiforme (EM) and toxic epidermal necrolysis (TEN) are acute mucocutaneous reactions to infections, drugs, and other agents. EM is a heterogeneous syndrome characterized clinically by symmetrically distributed, round, fixed skin lesions and mucosal injury [1]. Current classifications divide EM into two distinct, though overlapping, subgroups [1,2•]. EM minor is the mild mucocutaneous form. EM major (ie, Stevens-Johnson syndrome) is the more severe form with marked mucosal involvement. TEN is characterized by the acute onset of widespread bullae and epidermal sloughing with tender, confluent erythema and marked mucosal injury and is associated with considerable morbidity and mortality [3]. In this article, we discuss the manifestations, causes, and treatment of EM minor, EM major, and TEN.

Erythema multiforme minor

Erythema multiforme minor is an acute, self-limited mucocutaneous eruption characterized by a dull red macule or plaque with concentric color changes and, often, central epidermal necrosis or blister formation that forms the classic target lesion (Fig. 1) [1,2•,4]. EM minor is a common and frequently recurrent condition with minimal or no mucosal involvement [2•,5]. The lesions are typically located on the extremities with frequent palm and sole involvement [5]. Patients may occasionally have mild nonspecific prodromal symptoms of cough, rhinitis, and low-grade fever [2•]. Approximately one third of cases are recurrent, which can cause significant morbidity when mucous membranes are involved [5,6,7•,8].

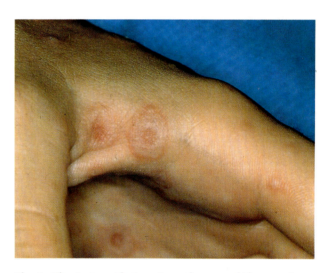

Fig. 1. Classic target lesions in erythema multiforme minor.

Infectious agents and drugs are the most frequently implicated causes of EM minor. In particular, herpes simplex virus (HSV) is the most common precipitating factor [4,7•,9]. Other well-documented associated infections include those with *Mycoplasma pneumoniae or Yersinia organisms*, infectious mononucleosis, tuberculosis, and histoplasmosis [1,2•]. Anticonvulsants (eg, phenytoin, carbamazepine, and phenobarbital), nonsteroidals anti-inflammatory drugs (NSAIDs), sulfonamides, and allopurinol are the most commonly implicated drugs [1,10].

Given the self-limited and typically benign course of episodic EM minor, conservative, supportive care is

---

Abbreviations
EM—erythema multiforme; HSV—herpes simplex virus; NSAID—nonsteroidal anti-inflammatory drug; TEN—toxic epidermal necrolysis.

the major treatment [4,5]. Initially, identification of underlying causes should be sought. Suspected and nonessential drugs should be discontinued and infections treated, if possible. Supportive measures include cool water compresses, acetaminophen [5], and antihistamines [2•,10]. These measures may be helpful in relieving symptoms, but they have little impact on the course of EM minor. Secondary infections of lesions should be treated as indicated with debridement, compresses, and topical or systemic antibiotics or both [5]. The use of corticosteroids in the treatment of EM minor is controversial. Although the benefits of corticosteroids are supported by many anecdotal reports [11], controlled clinical trials have yet to prove the effectiveness of these drugs.

Corticosteroids have the potential to worsen infection-triggered cases of EM minor. Because of this and other well-known adverse effects of corticosteroids and the typically benign course of EM minor, corticosteroids are considered unnecessary and are generally not recommended [2•].

Acyclovir has been shown to be effective in the treatment of HSV-associated recurrent EM minor [6,7•,12]. Schofield *et al.* [7•] recommended that acyclovir, 200 mg five times a day for 5 days, be given in the very early stage of HSV infection. This regimen is most effective when there is a clearly defined association and interval between HSV infection and EM. Otherwise, attack-initiated acyclovir therapy tends to be disappointing [2•,4,12]. Long-term prophylactic use of acyclovir in recurrent HSV-associated EM minor is effective in preventing both HSV recurrence and EM [2•,4]. Reported effective dosages are 200 to 800 mg/d [2•,4,7•]. Surprisingly, prophylactic acyclovir has been proven beneficial in recurrent EM minor without overt herpes infection [4]. This result coincides with the finding of HSV DNA by polymerase chain reaction in cutaneous lesions of EM in patients without clinical HSV-associated disease [13], implying that subclinical HSV infections may be responsible for some cases of recurrent EM minor [4,10,14].

Not all cases of recurrent EM minor are responsive to acyclovir, however [12]. Several studies [7•,15] have shown that dapsone may be effective in these cases. Varied beneficial responses have also been noted with levamisole [8], cimetidine [12,16], potassium iodide [6,17], colchicine [6], antimalarials [6,7•], cyclosporine [18], and thalidomide [6,19]. Azathioprine has demonstrated to be consistently effective in patients resistant to other therapies [7•]. Because of its potential serious adverse effects, however, it is considered by some to be the final treatment choice [7•].

Erythema multiforme major

Erythema multiforme major, the more severe form of EM, is characterized by erythema, edema, and superficial erosions of at least two mucous membranes [1,20•]. Skin findings may include fixed macules, atypical targetoid lesions, widespread erythema and necrosis, and large hemorrhagic bullae (Fig. 2) [1,5]. These lesions are nontender, and the Nikolsky sign is negative. A prodrome of headache, fever, malaise, sore throat, myalgia and arthralgia may be observed in patients with EM major [1].

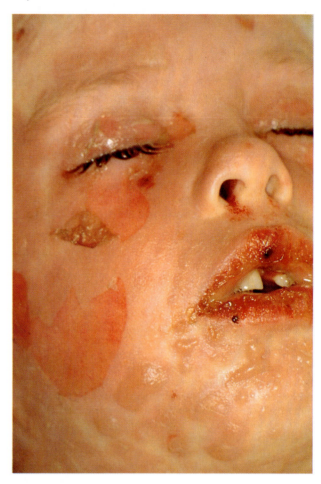

Fig. 2. Vesicles, erythema, necrosis, and mucosal erosions in erythema multiforme major.

Drugs are the most common cause of EM major [1]. As in EM minor, sulfonamides, NSAID, and anticonvulsants are the three groups most commonly implicated [1,2•,10]. HSV and *M. pneumoniae* are less frequent causes of EM major [2•,21]. Other suspected etiologic agents include neoplasia [2•,5], deep radiation therapy [5,22], connective tissue diseases [2•,5], and contactants [2•,5,22].

As in EM minor, the mainstay of treatment of EM major, is supportive care and withdrawal or treatment of the inciting agent. Because of more extensive mucosal involvement, patients may be very symptomatic. Oropharyngeal lesions are frequently painful and may restrict oral intake. Therefore, the patient's fluid status needs to be evaluated. Viscous lidocaine may be applied topically to lessen pain [23]. Conjunctival involvement can occasionally lead to problematic scarring upon healing, and an ophthalmologist should be consulted to prevent these complications [5]. The administration of corticosteroids in EM major, as well as in TEN, is disputed. This controversy is examined in the following discussion of TEN.

Toxic epidermal erythema

Toxic epidermal necrolysis is a severe cutaneous and systemic reaction with significant morbidity and mortality. We define TEN as the acute onset (usually within 24 to 48 hours) of widespread erythema and bullae with involvement of at least 70% of total body surface area, exquisite skin tenderness of involved areas, the absence of target lesions, a positive Nikolsky sign, and a histologic finding of full-thickness epidermal confluent necrosis and a minimal to absent dermal infiltrate (Fig. 3), all in conjunction with the criteria proposed by Goldstein *et al.* [24].

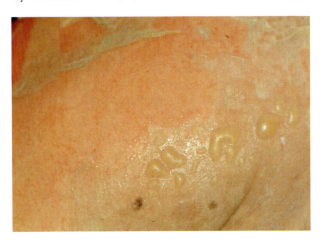

Fig. 3. Epidermal sloughing, erythema, and vesicles in toxic epidermal necrolysis.

Superficial hemorrhagic ulcerations of the conjunctival, nasal, oral, and urogenital mucous membranes occur frequently [3,20•], A prodrome of fever, malaise, rhinitis, and anorexia usually precedes TEN [25]. Fever is extremely common, and a patient's temperature may reach a peak of 40.5° to 41°C (105° to 106°F) [26••,27].

Of the various causes of TEN, drugs are the most common. Anticonvulsants (*eg*, phenytoin, phenobarbital and carbamazepine) [5,25,26••], antibiotics (*eg*, amoxicillin, sulfamethoxazole, trimethoprim, and other sulfonamides) [25,26••,28], NSAID [5,25,26••] and allopurinol [5,25,26••] are among the most frequently implicated drugs. HSV and *M. pneumoniae* have rarely been associated with TEN [9,25,26••]. Confirmation of suspected agents is difficult, however, because the patients often have complicated medical problems and are taking numerous medications. The absence of definitive skin and laboratory tests and the risks associated with provocative testing further complicates this problem.

An understanding of the complications of TEN is essential when constructing treatment strategies for these patients. Oculocutaneous complications are frequently

the most devastating sequelae in patients surviving TEN. These complications include symblepharon, entropion, ectropion, trichiasis, corneal opacities, inadequate tearing, and permanent visual impairment including blindness [20•]. An ophthalmologist should be consulted to help prevent these complications [25,26••,29].

Potentially fatal complications of TEN include fluid and electrolyte imbalance [25,29], leukopenia [3,25], pneumonitis [25], pneumonia [25], pulmonary embolus [3], gastrointestinal hemorrhage [3], and infection [3,25,29]. Sepsis is the most common cause of death in TEN patients [29,30]. The most frequently involved organisms are *Pseudomonas aeruginosa* and other gram-negative bacteria [25,31,32], *Staphylococcus aureus* [3,25,31,32], and *Candida albicans* [31]. Common sources of these organisms are skin, lung, urinary catheters, and intravenous lines [25,30].

Care of patients with TEN is complex and demands a multidisciplinary approach. Because the treatment requirements exceed the capacity of general medical wards or intensive care units, many authorities recommend treatment in a burn unit [3,25,26••,30].

The most important aspect of treatment is supportive care and diligent prevention and treatment of infection. Supportive care consists of careful fluid and electrolyte monitoring [25,33], nutritional support [25,26••,30], physical therapy [25], pain control [25], emotional support [26••,31], and an air-fluidized bed to minimize shearing forces [25,26••,29,33]. Skin, mucous membrane, urine, blood, and sputum cultures should be obtained daily [25]. Intravenous and urinary catheters should be used prudently with subsequent removal and obtaining culture whenever possible [3,25].

Wound care is a vital aspect of the treatment of TEN. Most authorities recommend painstaking debridement of necrotic tissue, which can harbor bacteria [3,25,26••,30,33]. Because of the associated exquisite skin tenderness and the extensive body surface area involved, this procedure often requires general anesthesia with careful monitoring of the patient's temperature [3,26••,30]. Debridement is then followed by the application of biologic or synthetic dressings. Both types of dressings have been demonstrated to decrease pain, inhibit fluid loss, improve thermal regulation, reduce the risk of sepsis, and possibly enhance reepithelialization [26••,29,30]. Halebian *et al.* [3] suggest, however, that these skin substitutes are not necessary for healing or survival.

Various topical antimicrobial agents have been used. Traditionally, silver sulfadiazine was the drug of choice, but it has fallen out of favor because of reports of associated leukopenia and the frequent implication of sulfonamides as etiologic agents of TEN [25,26••,29–31]. Probably the most commonly used local therapy is silver nitrate 0.5% solution applied to the potential dressing every 2 to 4 hours with complete changing of the dressing every 12 to 24 hours [3,31].

Concentrations of silver nitrate less than 1% minimize the complications of hyponatremia, hypochloremia, argyria, and occasional methemoglobinemia [26••]. Two opposing views exist concerning systemic antibiotic usage in TEN. Under the first theory, broad spectrum antibiotics are administered prophylactically upon diagnosis of TEN [2•], because the most common cause of death is infection. The disadvantage of this approach, however, is the development of resistant organisms and superinfections. The other strategy is to withhold antibiotics until documented infection exists [29]. This approach decreases the likelihood of complications of prophylactic antibiotics but has the obvious disadvantage of delaying treatment of potentially lethal infections. We, along with others [25,26••,29], recommend systemic antibiotics only for documented infections, signs of sepsis (eg, hypotension, mental status changes, persistent fever, or sudden, unexplained change in the patient's condition), or increased risk of sepsis (eg, neutropenia or heavy single-strain bacterial colonization of the skin) [25,26••,29].

The major controversy in the treatment of TEN (and EM major) is the use of systemic corticosteroids. Although they were once the recommended treatment, several articles have questioned their use and safety [3,27,29–31]. Several arguments can be raised in favor of corticosteroid use. First, the presumed pathogenesis of TEN is immunologically mediated cell damage [26••], and corticosteroids could inhibit this process. Second, numerous reports have attributed positive outcomes to the administration of corticosteroids [34–36]. Last, although corticosteroids may promote the likelihood of infection, this disadvantage is treatable and should not prohibit the administration of an agent that can arrest the progression of the disease [2•].

Numerous concerns exist, however, that discourage the use of corticosteroids. Importantly, no controlled study has convincingly proved their efficacy in the treatment of TEN. Halebian et al. [31] reported that moderate to high dose corticosteroids were ineffective in preventing progression of necrolysis, and several patients showed no extension of skin loss despite lowering of the steroid doses. In a nonrandomized, retrospective study, Halebian et al. [3] later demonstrated a 66% mortality rate with corticosteroid use and a 33% mortality rate without corticosteroids. Although infections were documented in two thirds of patients in each group, infections caused death in more patients treated with corticosteroids compared with patients not treated with them [3]. In addition, TEN has been documented to develop in patients already receiving corticosteroids for a different, preexisting condition [3,29,30]. Furthermore, corticosteroids have potentially harmful side effects. They impair the immune response of patients with defective skin and mucosal barrier, rendering them even more vulnerable to infection. They can also suppress the clinical signs of sepsis [3,29]. Some authors [31] report an increased incidence of gastrointestinal hemorrhage in patients treated with corticosteroids. Therefore, because of the lack of proven effectiveness and numerous adverse effects, we, along with others [7•,25,26••,29–31],

do not advocate corticosteroids for the treatment of TEN.

Other immunosuppressive agents, including cyclosporine [26••,37] and cyclophosphamide [38], have been used in the treatment of TEN. Documentation has been limited to small case reports, however, and well-controlled trials are needed to confirm their efficacy.

Plasmapheresis has also been used in the treatment of TEN [39]. Obtaining vascular access in the presence of large areas of denuded skin, however, may be difficult, and the access site is a potential source of infection [26••]. In addition, controlled studies have yet to be done [29]. Therefore, plasmapheresis should be used with considerable caution.

Conclusions

Erythema multiforme and TEN are well-known mucocutaneous reactions to infections, drugs, and other stimuli. The classification of these diseases remains a matter of debate and confusion. Whether EM and TEN are different diseases or variants along a continuous spectrum remains to be determined. Nonetheless, supportive care and withdrawal or treatment of the inciting agent are the most crucial elements of treatment. Corticosteroids have no proven efficacy in EM and TEN. The role of other agents has yet to be elucidated. Further improvement in treatment of EM and TEN will require a better understanding of the pathogenesis of these diseases and universal criteria for their classification.

References and recommended reading

Papers of particular interest, published within the annual period of review, have been highlighted as:
•   Of special interest
••   Of outstanding interest

1.   Huff JC, Weston WL, Tonnesen MG: **Erythema Multiforme: A Critical Review of Characteristics, Diagnostic Criteria, and Causes.** *J Am Acad Dermatol* 1983, **8**:763–775.

2.   Fritsch PO, Elias PM: **Erythema Multiforme and Toxic Epidermal**
•   **Necrolysis.** In *Dermatology in General Medicine*, edn 4. Edited by Fitzpatrick TB, Eisen AZ, Wolff K, Freedburg IM, Austen KF. New York: McGraw-Hill; 1993:585–600.
Comprehensive review of EM and TEN with emphasis on corticosteroid therapy.

3.   Halebian PH, Madden MR, Finklestein JL, Corder VJ, Shires GT: **Improved Burn Center Survival of Patients With Toxic Epidermal Necrolysis Managed Without Corticosteroids.** *Ann Surg* 1986, **204**:503–512.

4.   Champion RH: **Disorders of Blood Vessels.** In *Textbook of Dermatology*, edn 5. Edited by Champion RH, Burton JL, Ebling FJG. Cambridge: Blackwell Scientific Publications; 1992:1834–1838.

5.   Jorizzo JL: **Blood Vessel-Based Inflammatory Disorders.** In *Dermatology*, edn 3. Edited by Moschella SL, Hurley HJ. Philadelphia: WB Saunders Co.; 1992:580–584.

6.   Moisson YF, Janier M, Civatte J: **Thalidomide for Recurrent Erythema Multiforme.** *Br J Dermatol* 1992, **126**:92–93.

7.   Schofield JK, Tatnall FM, Leigh IM: **Recurrent Erythema Multiforme:**
•   **Clinical Features and Treatment in a Large Series of Patients of Patients.** *Br J Dermatol* 1993, **128**:542–545.
Reviews the clinical feature of recurrent EM and responses to various treatment modalities in a large series of patients.

8. Lozada-Nur F, Cram D, Gorsky M: **Clinical Response to Levamisole in Thirty-Nine Patients With Erythema Multiforme.** *Oral Surg Oral Med Oral Pathol* 1992, 74:294–298.

9. Bastuji-Garin S, Rzany B, Stern RS, Shear NH, Naldi L, Roujeau JC: **Clinical Classification of Cases of Toxic Epidermal Necrolysis, Stevens-Johnson Syndrome, and Erythema Multiforme.** *Arch Dermatol* 1993, 129:92–96.

10. Feldman SR: **Bullous Dermatoses Associated With Systemic Disease.** *Dermatol Clin* 1993, 11:597–609.

11. Rasmussen JE: **Special Symposium: Corticosteroids for Erythema Multiforme?** *Pediatr Dermatol* 1989, 6:231–233.

12. Kurkcuoglu N, Tuglular T, Oz G: **Cimetidine Prevents Erythema Multiforme.** *Ann Allergy* 1993, 70:180.

13. Darragh TM, Egbert BM, Berger TG, Yen TSB: **Identification of Herpes Simplex Virus DNA in Lesions of Erythema Multiforme by the Polymerase Chain Reaction.** *J Am Acad Dermatol* 1991, 24:23–26.

14. Leigh IM, Mowbray JF, Leven GM, Sutherland S: **Recurrent and Continuous Erythema Multiforme: A Clinical and Immunological Study.** *Clin Exp Dermatol* 1985, 10:58–67.

15. Duhra P, Paul CJ: **Continuous Erythema Multiforme Clearing on Dapsone.** *Br J Dermatol* 1988, 118:731.

16. Kurkcuoglu N, Alli N: **Cimetidine Prevents Recurrent Erythema Multiforme Major Resulting From Herpes Simplex Virus Infection.** *J Am Acad Dermatol* 1989, 21:814–815.

17. Horio T, Danno K, Okamoto H, Miyachi Y, Imamura S: **Potassium Iodide in Erythema Nodosum and Other Erythematous Dermatoses.** *J Am Acad Dermatol* 1983, 9:77–81.

18. Wilkel CS, McDonald CJ: **Glyclosporine Therapy for Bullous Erythema Multiforme.** *Arch Dermatol* 1990, 126:397–398.

19. Naafs B, Faber WR: **Thalidomide Therapy.** *Int J Dermatol* 1985, 24:131–134.

20. Wilkins J, Morrison L, White CR: **Oculocutaneous Manifestations of the Erythema Multiforme/Stevens-Johnson Syndrome/Toxic Epidermal Necrolysis Spectrum.** *Dermatol Clin* 1992, 10:571–582.
   • Detailed description of the ocular manifestations and treatment, both medical and surgical, of EM and TEN.

21. Detjen PF, Patterson R, Noskin GA, Phair JP, Loyd SO: **Herpes Simplex Virus Associated With Recurrent Stevens-Johnson Syndrome.** *Arch Intern Med* 1992, 152:1513–1516.

22. Ridgway HB, Miech DJ: **Erythema Multiforme (Stevens-Johnson Syndrome) Following Deep Radiation Therapy.** *Cutis* 1993, 51:463–464.

23. Barone CM, Bianch MA, Lee B, Mitra A: **Treatment of Toxic Epidermal Necrolysis and Stevens-Johnson Syndrome in Children.** *J Oral Maxillofac Surg* 1993, 51:264–268.

24. Goldstein SM, Wintroub BW, Elias PM: **Toxic Epidermal Necrolysis: Unmuddying the Waters.** *Arch Dermatol* 1987, 123:1153–1155.

25. Avakian R, Flowers FP, Araujo OE, Ramos-Caro F: **Toxic Epidermal Necrolysis: A Review.** *J Am Acad Dermatol* 1991, 25:69–79.

26. Parsons JM: **Toxic Epidermal Necrolysis.** *Int J Dermatol* 1992,
   •• 31:749–768.
   Comprehensive and well-referenced review of toxic epidermal necrolysis with detailed discussion of recommended supportive care.

27. Ruiz-Maldonado R: **Acute Disseminated Epidermal Necrosis Types 1, 2, and 3: Study of Sixty Cases.** *J Am Acad Dermatol* 1985, 13:623–635.

28. Chan HL, Stern RS, Arndt KA, Langlois J, Jick SS, Jick H, Walker AM: **The Incidence of Erythema Multiforme, Stevens-Johnson Syndrome, and Toxic Epidermal Necrolysis.** *Arch Dermatol* 1990, 126:43–47.

29. Revuz J, Roujeau JC, Guillaume JC, Penso D, Touraine R: **Treatment of Toxic Epidermal Necrolysis: Creteil's Experience.** *Arch Dermatol* 1987, 123:1156–1158.

30. Heimbach DM, Engrav LH, Marvin JA, Harnar TJ, Grube BJ: **Toxic Epidermal Necrolysis: A Step Forward in Treatment.** *JAMA* 1987, 257:2171–2175.

31. Halebian P, Corder V, Herndon D, Shires GT: **A Burn Center Experience With Toxic Epidermal Necrolysis.** *J Burn Care Rehabil* 1983, 4:176–182.

32. Revuz J, Penso D, Roujeau JC, Guillaume JC, Payne CR, Wechsler J, Touraine R: **Toxic Epidermal Necrolysis: Clinical Findings and Prognosis Factors in 87 Patients.** *Arch Dermatol* 1987, 123:1160–1165.

33. Pye RJ: **Bullous Eruptions.** In *Textbook of Dermatology*, edn 5. Edited by Champion RH, Burton JL, Ebling FJG. Cambridge: Blackwell Scientific Publications; 1992:1667–1668.

34. Bjornberg A: **Fifteen Cases of Toxic Epidermal Necrolysis (Lyell).** *Acta Derm Venereol (Stockh)* 1973, 53:149–152.

35. Beare M: **Toxic Epidermal Necrolysis.** *Arch Dermatol* 1962, 86:118–133.

36. Esterly N: **Special Symposium: Corticosteroids for Erythema Multiforme?** *Pediatr Dermatol* 1989, 6:229.

37. Hewitt J, Ormerod AD: **Toxic Epidermal Necrolysis Treated With Cyclosporin.** *Clin Exp Dermatol* 1992, 17:264–265.

38. Heng MCY, Allen SG: **Efficacy of Cyclophosphamide in Toxic Epidermal Necrolysis: Clinical and Pathophysiological Aspects.** *J Am Acad Dermatol* 1991, 25:778–786.

39. Kamanabroo D, Schmitz-Landgraf W, Czarnetzki BM: **Plasmapheresis in Severe Drug-Induced Toxic Epidermal Necrolysis.** *Arch Dermatol* 1985, 121:1548–1549.

Franklin Flowers, MD, Division of Dermatology and Cutaneous Surgery, University of Florida College of Medicine, P. O. Box 100277, Gainesville, FL 32610-0277, USA.

Neoplasms

Edited by

Pearon G. Lang, Jr.
Medical University of South Carolina
Charleston, South Carolina, USA

CURRENT SCIENCE

Precursors of cutaneous T-cell lymphoma

Rein Willemze, MD

Free University Hospital, Amsterdam, the Netherlands

The term *precursor of cutaneous T-cell lymphoma* (CTCL) refers to a heterogeneous group of skin disorders that may precede the histologic diagnosis of CTCL, in particular mycosis fungoides, the most common type of CTCL. Conditions generally included in this group are large plaque parapsoriasis, alopecia mucinosa, and lymphomatoid papulosis. In this article, clinical and histological characteristics and differential diagnostic aspects of these precursors as well as potential risk factors for the development of mycosis fungoides are discussed. It is emphasized that the development of a CTCL is a multistep phenomenon, and that controversy about whether these conditions should be considered as precursors or as early-stage CTCL cannot be solved as long as the molecular mechanisms underlying the steps of tumor progression have not been clarified.

Current Opinion in Dermatology 1995:33–37

Cutaneous T-cell lymphomas (CTCLs) represent a heterogeneous group of neoplasms of skin-homing T cells that clinically originate in the skin [1]. Patients with mycosis fungoides (MF), the most common type of CTCL, and Sézary's syndrome may have skin lesions for several years before a definitive diagnosis of CTCL can be made. These skin disorders are designated as precursors of CTCL, or more often, because of the frequent association with MF, as premycotic eruptions [2]. Roughly, two groups can be distinguished. The first and larger group includes skin lesions that are neither clinically nor histologically diagnostic. They may resemble psoriasis or several types of eczema, such as contact dermatitis, seborrheic dermatitis, atopic dermatitis, or nummular eczema, but they nearly always lack the clinical and histologic features characteristic of these diseases [2,3]. The second group contains some rather well-defined entities that are considered more likely to progress to genuine CTCL. These entities include various types of parapsoriasis, alopecia mucinosa (also called follicular mucinosis), and lymphomatoid papulosis (LyP). It should be emphasized, however, that there is no agreement as to whether these conditions should be considered as precursors of CTCL or as an early stage of CTCL.

In this article, the clinical and histologic characteristics of the conditions in this second category are presented. Differential diagnostic aspects and potential risk factors predictive of the development of genuine MF are discussed. Finally, because of the ongoing controversy as to the exact nature of these conditions—benign, premalignant, or malignant—the concept of precursors of CTCL will be critically evaluated.

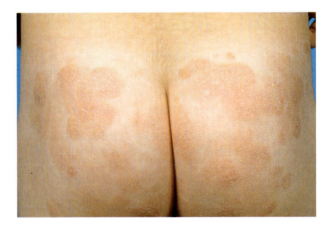

Fig. 1. Slightly scaling erythematous patches characteristic of large plaque parapsoriasis appear on the buttocks.

Parapsoriasis

Small plaque and pityriasis lichenoides

The term parapsoriasis refers to a heterogeneous group of disorders, in which three major entities have been recognized: 1) large plaque parapsoriasis, 2) small plaque parapsoriasis, and 3) pityriasis lichenoides [4]. Large plaque parapsoriasis can be considered prototypic for the group of precursors of MF and is therefore treated in more detail below. With respect to small plaque parapsoriasis, there is almost universal agreement that although this condition may persist for years to decades, it lacks the potential to develop into CTCL [2,4]. In a recent study, clinical and histologic similari-

Abbreviations
CTCL—cutaneous T-cell lymphoma; **LCL**—large cell lymphoma; **LyP**—lymphomatoid papulosis; **MF**—mycosis fungoides; **PCR**—polymerase chain reaction.

ties between small plaque parapsoriasis and MF were emphasized, but clinical evidence that patients can develop frank malignancy was not provided [5]. Pityriasis lichenoides is a distinct inflammatory disease that includes acute and chronic variants. Association with poikiloderma and development of MF has occasionally been reported [6–8]. Moreover, clonal T-cell populations have been detected in some patients with pityriasis lichenoides [9]. In two large studies including 128 and 82 patients with pityriasis lichenoides, respectively, however, no association with or progression into MF was noted [10,11]. At present, most investigators agree that pityriasis lichenoides should be considered a distinct entity that is not associated with large plaque parapsoriasis, MF, or LyP, and that it should not be included in the parapsoriasis group [2,4,5,11].

Large plaque

Clinically, large plaque parapsoriasis is recognized by large, ill-defined, irregularly shaped erythematous to brown patches or plaques that show a fine scaling (Fig. 1). Lesions showing mottled hyper- and hypopigmentation, marked atrophy, and telangiectasia are commonly designated poikiloderma vasculare atrophicans. Sites of predilection are the buttocks, trunk, proximal extremities, and in women, the breasts. Progression of large plaque parapsoriasis into genuine MF is reported to occur in 10% to 30% of patients [4,12]. Histologically, large plaque parapsoriasis is characterized by the presence of sparse perivascular infiltrates of lymphocytes and histiocytes in the upper dermis. Lymphocytes may be observed occasionally in the epidermis, but there is no cellular atypia. In poikiloderma vasculare atrophicans, there is epidermal atrophy and more often a bandlike lymphohistiocytic infiltrate that may obscure the dermal-epidermal junction. Both clinically and histologically, differentiation between large plaque parapsoriasis and early patch-stage MF may be difficult. The presence of small or medium-sized hyperchromatic lymphoid cells in the epidermis, either as single cells often surrounded by a halo, or in a linear configuration at the dermal-epidermal junction, is considered highly suggestive of patch-stage MF [13,14]. However, similar histologic features have also been described in cases of large plaque parapsoriasis [4].

Because of such overlapping clinical and histologic features, some investigators have concluded that large plaque parapsoriasis should be considered early-stage MF [13,15]. Because of the benign clinical course in most patients with the clinical appearance of large plaque parapsoriasis, however, other investigators still believe that these patients have a benign or, at most, premalignant condition. Irrespective of which concept one adheres to, there has been a continued search for criteria that may be helpful in the diagnosis of early malignant disease. DNA cytometry and quantitative electron microscopy (ie, nuclear contour indexing) have been considered valuable adjuncts in early diagnosis, but these techniques are not widely used [16]. Immunophenotypical studies using monoclonal antibodies are not very helpful in differentiating between early stage MF and benign inflammatory dermatoses [17], except in those rare cases of MF in which a clonal T-cell population can be demonstrated through the use of antibodies against the variable regions of the T-cell receptor [18]. Clonal T-cell populations can also be detected at the DNA level by T-cell receptor gene rearrangement studies, ie, either by Southern blot hybridization or by polymerase chain reaction (PCR) amplification [19•]. With Southern blot hybridization, clonal T-cell populations can easily be detected in skin lesions of advanced plaque- or tumor-stage MF, but only rarely in early patch-stage MF or large plaque parapsoriasis (Table 1) [19•,20–23]. Preliminary results of PCR studies indicate that clonal T-cell populations are already present in most patients with early patch-stage disease [19•,24,25•], and also in a proportion of benign inflammatory dermatoses not suspected of being CTCL and therefore designated "clonal dermatitis" [25•]. These data indicate that the proportion of clonal T cells in these early patch-stage lesions is below the detection level of Southern blot hybridization (1% to 3% of the total number of cells). Further studies are necessary to determine the frequency of clonal T-cell populations in patients with large plaque parapsoriasis and to establish whether such patients have an increased risk of developing genuine MF.

Alopecia mucinosa

Alopecia mucinosa is clinically characterized by the presence of grouped follicular papules, scaling erythematous patches and plaques, and alopecia (Fig. 2). His-

Table 1. Cellular atypia, aberrant phenotype, and clonality in cutaneous stages of mycosis fungoides

	Precusor of MF	Patch stage	Plaque stage	Tumor stage
Cellular atypia*	None	Few	Some	Many
Aberrant phenotype†	No	No	Sometimes	Almost always
Clonality				
Southern blot	No	Sometimes	Often	Almost always
Polymerase chain reaction	Sometimes	Often	Almost always	Almost always

*Refers to the number of atypical cells.
†Defined as absence of pan–T cell markers CD2, CD3, and CD5 or absence of both CD4 and CD8.
MF—mycosis fungoides.

tologic features include perifollicular lymphocytic infiltrates and mucinous degeneration of the follicular epithelium (*ie,* follicular mucinosis). In addition to being the hallmark of alopecia mucinosa, which is also referred to as the primary or idiopathic form of follicular mucinosis, follicular mucinosis has been found in association with a variety of other skin diseases. The association of follicular mucinosis and MF in particular has been well documented [26–36]. Several studies have described the gradual progression from alopecia mucinosa to MF, suggesting that in at least some patients, alopecia mucinosa may be regarded as a precursor of MF [26–29,31,32,34]. It has been suggested that in particular, patients with alopecia mucinosa who develop a generalized skin eruption when they are past their 30s are at risk [31,32]. Other investigators do not concur with this view, however, and have suggested that patients in whom progression from alopecia mucinosa to MF has been reported have had MF from the very beginning [30,37]. These conflicting views clearly illustrate that differentiation between alopecia mucinosa and follicular mucinosis associated with early MF may be extremely difficult [35]. Recent studies suggest that the development of more infiltrated skin lesions, in particular in the head and neck region, and histologically, the development of more diffuse and cellular infiltrates and a gradual increase of atypical cells and eosinophils are highly suggestive of early or impending MF [33,34]. Clonal T-cell populations have been detected by Southern blot hybridization not only in patients with an unequivocal diagnosis of MF-associated follicular mucinosis [38], but also in skin samples of some patients with alopecia mucinosa without evidence for CTCL [36,39]. These conflicting results indicate that further studies are necessary to determine which patients with the clinical appearance of alopecia mucinosa already have or are at risk for developing genuine MF.

Lymphomatoid papulosis

Lymphomatoid papulosis is defined as a chronic, recurrent, self-healing papulonecrotic or nodular skin disease with histologic features suggestive of a malignant lymphoma [39] (Fig. 3). Histologically, two major types of LyP can be distinguished: LyP type A, with large, atypical, sometimes Reed-Sternberg–like CD30+ cells showing morphological and immunophenotypical characteristics similar to those of the tumor cells in CD30+ large cell lymphomas (LCLs); and LyP type B, with atypical CD30− T cells similar to those observed in MF [40–42]. Mixed types with histologic features of both type A and B are regularly found, suggesting that these histologic types must be regarded as different expressions of a single disease.

In most patients, LyP has a protracted but benign clinical course. However, in 10% to 20% of patients, LyP is preceded by, associated with, or followed by another type of malignant lymphoma, in particular MF, Hodgkin's disease, or a CD30+ LCL [43,44•,45–47]. The prognosis for these LyP-associated malignancies is generally favorable, except for those LyP patients developing a systemic CD30+ LCL [44•,45]. In contrast to MF and Hodgkin's disease, which may develop several years before or after the diagnosis of LyP is made, CD30+ LCLs generally develop in patients with well-established LyP and may be considered a further step in tumor progression. Patients who develop more persistent nodular lesions or have recurrent, self-healing skin lesions that at histologic examination show cohesive sheets of CD30+ cells and relatively few inflammatory cells may have an increased risk of progressing to a CD30+ LCL [43,44•]. Clonal T-cell receptor gene rearrangements have been found in the majority of the LyP patients studied and cannot therefore be considered a risk factor [48–51]. Although some LyP patients may develop MF or a CD30+ LCL in the course of their disease, LyP should not be designated as a precursor of CTCL. Previous studies have already suggested a close relationship between LyP, MF, CD30+ LCL, and some types of Hodgkin's disease. In a recent study of an LyP patient who subsequently developed Hodgkin's disease and an erythrodermic CTCL, it was found that these different entities were derived from a common T-cell clone [52••]. Because of the frequent association with other types of malignant lymphomas, the histologic appearance, the presence of clonal T-cell populations in the majority of patients, and in particular the overlapping clinical and histologic features of LyP and the primary cutaneous CD30+ LCL [53•], LyP would better be regarded as a low-grade malignant CTCL that, at least in most patients, is still controlled effectively by the host immune response.

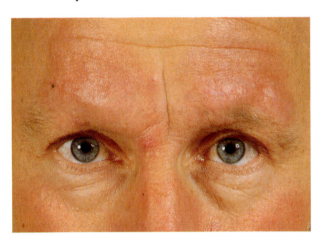

Fig. 2. Infiltrated erythematous plaques with characteristic loss of eyebrows are seen in a patient with alopecia mucinosa.

The development of mycosis fungoides as a multistep phenomenon

There is an ongoing discussion about whether the conditions described must be considered benign, premalignant (*ie,* precursors of MF), or an early stage of MF. Numerous studies have attempted to solve this problem by defining clinical, histologic, or other criteria to

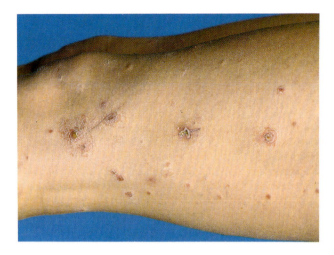

Fig. 3. In a patient with lymphomatoid papulosis, recurrent, self-healing papular and papulonecrotic lesions are seen in various stages of development.

distinguish between benign and malignant cutaneous lymphoid infiltrates. It should be noted, however, that the development of a malignant lymphoma is a multistep phenomenon, and that the distinction between benign and malignant is not always clear-cut. The description of the three successive stages of classic MF (*ie*, patch stage, plaque stage, and tumor stage), which were recognized in 1870 by Bazin, is in line with this concept (Table 1). Although the initiating factor is unknown, chronic stimulation by viral or environmental antigens is supposed to play a key role in the development of MF. The development of skin lesions without the histologic changes diagnostic of MF, including some of the conditions described in this review, may be regarded as a first step in lymphomagenesis. In most patients, these initial skin lesions may resolve or persist for years or even decades. In some patients, however, continued stimulation may result in cellular atypia and clonal expansion, clinically and histologically manifesting as patch- or early plaque-stage MF. Further steps in tumor progression include the development of infiltrated plaques and tumors, involvement of peripheral lymph nodes, and finally in some patients the development of biologically aggressive disease (Table 1). This final step, clinically manifesting as visceral involvement or transformation of MF into a high-grade malignant lymphoma, is generally associated with rapidly fatal disease.

The question of the stage at which this continuous disease process should be considered malignant cannot be answered easily. It should be noted that not only in patients with a so-called premycotic eruption, but also in many patients with patch-stage MF, further progression to plaque- or tumor-stage disease may take years or decades or may not occur at all. As noted before, the proportion of clonal T cells in these early stages is relatively low. These observations suggest that the early clonal expansion can be controlled effectively for a long time by the host immune response. Further progression will occur only if the neoplastic cells gain a growth advantage either by additional chromosomal al-

terations or if the immune response becomes deficient. The question of whether or which patients with a so-called precursor of CTCL, or with patch-stage CTCL, already have malignant disease cannot be answered as long as the initiating events and the molecular mechanisms underlying the subsequent steps of tumor progression in MF are largely unknown. As long as this information is not available, studies should continue to define clinical, histologic, immunohistochemical, and other criteria (*eg*, clonality) that in well-defined patient groups may identify patients who have already developed or are at risk of developing frank malignancy.

References and recommended reading

Papers of particular interest, published within the annual period of review, have been highlighted as:
- • Of special interest
- •• Of outstanding interest

1. Willemze R, Beljaards RC, Meijer CJLM: **Classification of Primary Cutaneous T-Cell Lymphoma.** *Histopathology* 1994, in press.

2. Lambert WC: **Premycotic Eruptions.** *Dermatol Clin* 1985, 3:629–645.

3. Abel EA: **Clinical Features of Cutaneous T-Cell Lymphoma.** *Dermatol Clin* 1985, 3:647–664.

4. Lambert WC, Everett MA: **The Nosology of Parapsoriasis.** *J Am Acad Dermatol* 1981, 6:373–395.

5. King-Ismael D, Ackerman AB: **Guttate Parapsoriasis/Digitate Dermatosis (Small Plaque Parapsoriasis) Is Mycosis Fungoides.** *Am J Dermatopathol* 1992, 14:518–530.

6. Samman PD: **Poikiloderma With Pityriasis Lichenoides.** *Trans St John's Hosp Dermatol Soc* 1971, 57:143–147.

7. Grice K, Smith N: **Pityriasis Lichenoides With Poikiloderma Atrophicans Vasculare.** *Br J Dermatol* 1980, 103(suppl 18):66–67.

8. Bleehan, Slater DN: **Pityriasis Lichenoides Developing Into Mycosis Fungoides.** *Br J Dermatol* 1986, 115(suppl 30):69–70.

9. Weiss LM, Wood GS, Ellison LW, Reynolds TC, Sklar J: **Clonal T-Cell Populations in Pityriasis Lichenoides et Varioliformis Acuta (Mucha-Habermann Disease).** *Am J Pathol* 1987, 126:417–421.

10. Marks R, Black M, Wilson Jones E: **Pityriasis Lichenoides: A Reappraisal.** *Br J Dermatol* 1972, 86:215–225.

11. Willemze R, Scheffer E: **Clinical and Histologic Differentiation Between Lymphomatoid Papulosis and Pityriasis Lichenoides.** *J Am Acad Dermatol* 1985, 13:418–428.

12. Lazar AP, Caro WA, Roenigk HH, Pinski KS: **Parapsoriasis and Mycosis Fungoides: The Northwestern University Experience, 1970 to 1985.** *J Am Acad Dermatol* 1989, 21:919–923.

13. Sanchez A, Ackerman AB: **The Patch Stage of Mycosis Fungoides: Criteria for Histologic Diagnosis.** *Am J Dermatopathol* 1979, 1:5–26.

14. Nickoloff BJ: **Light-Microscopic Assessment of 100 Patients With Patch/Plaque Stage Mycosis Fungoides.** *Am J Dermatopathol* 1988, 10:469–477.

15. Samman PD: **Mycosis Fungoides and Other Cutaneous Reticuloses.** *Clin Exp Dermatol* 1976, 1:197–214.

16. van Vloten WA, Willemze R: **New Techniques in the Evaluation of Cutaneous T-Cell Lymphoma.** *Dermatol Clin* 1985, 3:665–672.

17. Ralfkiaer E: **Immunohistochemical Markers for the Diagnosis of Cutaneous Lymphoma.** *Semin Diagn Pathol* 1991, 8:62–72.

18. Boehncke WH, Krettek S, Parwaresh MR, Sterry W: **Demonstration of Clonal Disease in Early Mycosis Fungoides.** *Am J Dermatopathol* 1992, 14:95–99.

19. Weinberg JM, Rook AH, Lessin SR: **Molecular Diagnosis of Lymphocytic**
• **Infiltrates in the Skin.** *Arch Dermatol* 1993, 129:1491–1500.
This article reviews the results of T-cell receptor and immunoglobulin gene rearrangement studies by Southern blot hybridization and PCR amplification in a large variety of cutaneous lymphoproliferative disorders, including potential precursors of CTCL.

20. Ralfkiaer E: **Genotypic Analyses of Cutaneous T-Cell Lymphomas.** *J Invest Dermatol* 1987, 88:762–765.

21. Dosaka N, Tanaka T, Fujita M, Miyachi Y, Horio T, Imamura S: **Southern Blot Analysis of Clonal Rearrangements of T-Cell Receptor**

Gene in Plaque Lesion of Mycosis Fungoides. *J Invest Dermatol* 1989, 93:626–629.

22. Zelickson BD, Peters MS, Muller SA, Thibodeau SN, Lust JA, Quam LM, Pittelkow MR: T-Cell Receptor Gene Rearrangement Analysis: Cutaneous T-Cell Lymphoma, Peripheral T-Cell Lymphoma, and Premalignant and Benign Cutaneous Lymphoproliferative Disorders. *J Am Acad Dermatol* 1991, 25:787–796.

23. Kikuchi A, Naka W, Harada T, Sakuraoka K, Harada R, Nishikawa T: Parapsoriasis en Plaques: Its Potential for Progression to Malignant Lymphoma. *J Am Acad Dermatol* 1993, 29:419–422.

24. Volkenandt M, Soyer HP, Cerroni L, Koch OM, Atzpodien J, Kerl H: Molecular Detection of Clone-Specific DNA in Hypopigmented Lesions of a Patient With Early Evolving Mycosis Fungoides. *Br J Dermatol* 1993, 128:423–428.

25. Wood GS, Tung RM, Haeffner AC, Crooks CF, Liao S, Orozco R,
• Veelken H, Kadin ME, Koh H, Heald P, Barnhill RL, Sklar J: Cutaneous Lymphoid Infiltrates: Analysis of T Cell Receptor γ Gene Rearrangements by Polymerase Chain Reaction and Denaturing Gradient Gel Electrophoresis (PCR/DGGE). *J Invest Dermatol* 1994, in press.
This report describes the results of T-cell receptor-γ gene rearrangement analysis by PCR amplification in combination with denaturing gradient gel electrophoresis in 80 patients with CTCL and 105 patients with unrelated skin disorders. The authors find clonal T-cell populations not only in most patients with early CTCL, but also in some patients with histologically nonspecific dermatitis, for which they introduce the term *clonal dermatitis*.

26. Kim R, Winkelmann RK: Follicular Mucinosis (Alopecia Mucinosa). *Arch Dermatol* 1962, 85:490–498.

27. Brunstring LA: Alopecia Mucinosa With Transition to Mycosis Fungoides. *Arch Dermatol* 1962, 85:683–684.

28. Pinkus H: The Relationship of Alopecia Mucinosa to Malignant Lymphoma. *Dermatologica* 1964, 129:266–270.

29. Plotnick H, Abbrecht M: Alopecia Mucinosa and Lymphoma. *Arch Dermatol* 1965, 92:137–141.

30. Emmerson RW: Follicular Mucinosis: A Study of 47 Patients. *Br J Dermatol* 1969, 81:395–413.

31. Coskey RJ, Mehregan AH: Alopecia Mucinosa: A Follow-Up Study. *Arch Dermatol* 1970, 102:193–194.

32. Kanno S, Niizuma K, Machida S, Mori T: Follicular Mucinosis Developing Into Cutaneous Lymphoma: Report of Two Cases and Review of Literature and 64 Cases in Japan. *Acta Derm Venereol (Stockh)* 1984, 64:86–88.

33. Nickoloff BJ, Wood C: Benign Idiopathic Versus Mycosis Fungoides-Associated Follicular Mucinosis. *Pediatr Dermatol* 1985, 2:201–206.

34. Sentis HJ, Willemze R, Scheffer E: Alopecia Mucinosa Progressing Into Mycosis Fungoides: A Long-Term Follow-Up Study of Two Patients. *Am J Dermatopathol* 1988, 10:478–486.

35. Gibson LE, Muller SA, Leiferman KM, Peters MS: Follicular Mucinosis: Clinical and Histopathologic Study. *J Am Acad Dermatol* 1989, 20:441–446.

36. Mehregan DA, Gibson LE, Muller SA: Follicular Mucinosis: Histopathologic Review of 33 Cases. *Mayo Clin Proc* 1991, 66:387–390.

37. Hempstead RW, Ackerman AB: Follicular Mucinosis: A Reaction Pattern in Follicular Epithelium. *Am J Dermatopathol* 1985, 7:245–257.

38. LeBoit PE, Abel EA, Cleary ML: Clonal Rearrangement of the T-Cell Receptor Beta Gene in the Circulating Lymphocytes of Erythrodermic Follicular Mucinosis. *Blood* 1988, 71:1329–1333.

39. McCaulay WL: Lymphomatoid Papulosis, a Self Healing Eruption, Clinically Benign, Histologically Malignant. *Arch Dermatol* 1968, 97:23–30.

40. Willemze R, Meijer CJLM, Scheffer E, van Vloten WA: The Clinical and Histologic Spectrum of Lymphomatoid Papulosis. *Br J Dermatol* 1982, 107:131–144.

41. Kadin M, Nasu K, Sako D, Said J, Vonderheid E: Lymphomatoid Papulosis: A Cutaneous Proliferation of Activated Helper T Cells Expressing Hodgkin's Disease Associated Antigens. *Am J Pathol* 1985, 119:315–325.

42. Kaudewitz P, Stein H, Burg G, Mason DY, Braun-Falco O: Atypical Cells in Lymphomatoid Papulosis Express the Hodgkin Cell Associated Antigen Ki-1. *J Invest Dermatol* 1986, 86:350–354.

43. Willemze R: Lymphomatoid Papulosis. *Dermatol Clin* 1985, 3:735–747.

44. Beljaards RC, Willemze R: The Prognosis of Patients With Lymphoma-
• toid Papulosis Associated With Other Types of Malignancies. *Br J Dermatol* 1992, 126:596–602.
This paper reviews the clinical data of 50 malignant lymphomas associated with LyP, including 19 patients with MF, 12 with Hodgkin's disease, and 16 with a CD30+ LCL. Evaluation of follow-up data in 70 LyP patients suggests that the risk of an individual LyP patient to develop a systemic lymphoma is less than 5%.

45. Harabuchi Y, Kataura A, Kobayashi K, Yamamoto T, Yamanaka N, Hirao M, Onodera K, Kon S: Lethal Midline Granuloma (Peripheral T-Cell Lymphoma) After Lymphomatoid Papulosis. *Cancer* 1992, 70:835–839.

46. Wang HH, Lach L, Kadin ME: Epidemiology of Lymphomatoid Papulosis. *Cancer* 1992, 70:2951–2957.

47. Zackheim HS, LeBoit PE, Gordon BI, Glassberg AB: Lymphomatoid Papulosis Followed by Hodgkin's Lymphoma. *Arch Dermatol* 1993, 129:86–91.

48. Weiss L, Wood G, Trela M, Warnke R, Sklar J: Clonal T-Cell Populations in Lymphomatoid Papulosis. *N Engl J Med* 1986, 315:475–479.

49. Kadin M, Vonderheid E, Sako D, Clayton L, Olbricht S: Clonal Composition of T-Cells in Lymphomatoid Papulosis. *Am J Pathol* 1987, 126:13–17.

50. Whittaker S, Smith N, Jones RR, Luzzatto L: Analysis of β, γ, and δ T-Cell Receptor Genes in Lymphomatoid Papulosis: Cellular Basis of Two Distinct Histologic Subsets. *J Invest Dermatol* 1991, 96:786–791.

51. Parks JD, Synovec MS, Mash AS, Braddock SW, Nakamine H, Sanger WG, Harrington DS, Weisenburger DD: Immunophenotypic and Genotypic Characterization of Lymphomatoid Papulosis. *J Am Acad Dermatol* 1992, 26:968–975.

52. Davis TH, Morton CC, Miller-Cassman R, Balk SP, Kadin M: Hodgkin's
•• Disease, Lymphomatoid Papulosis and Cutaneous T-Cell Lymphoma Derived From a Common T-Cell Clone. *N Engl J Med* 1992, 326:1115–1122.
The authors describe a patient in whom LyP developed in 1971, Hodgkin's disease in 1975, and an erythrodermic CTCL in 1985. Using PCR with "tumor-specific primers," they demonstrated that all three conditions were derived from a common T cell clone. Cytogenetic studies revealed a translocation, t(8;9)(p22;p24), in the CTCL.

53. Willemze R, Beljaards RC: Spectrum of Primary Cutaneous CD30 (Ki-
• 1) Positive Lymphoproliferative Disorders: A Proposal for Classification and Guidelines for Management and Treatment. *J Am Acad Dermatol* 1993, 28:973–980.
This review emphasizes the intimate relationship between primary cutaneous CD30+ LCL and other CD30+ disorders that may occur in the skin. A working classification with practical guidelines for the management and treatment of patients with primary cutaneous CD30+ lymphoproliferative disorders is presented.

Rein Willemze, MD, Department of Dermatology, Free University Hospital, De Boelelaan 1117, 1081 HV Amsterdam, the Netherlands.

Medical management of squamous cell carcinoma of the skin

Hubert T. Greenway, MD, Matthew K. Abele, MD, and Dwight L. McKee, MD

Scripps Clinic and Research Foundation, La Jolla, California, USA

The incidence of advanced and metastatic squamous cell carcinoma continues to increase along with the need for successful therapies. Combination modalities appear to offer enhanced results. Intralesional therapy of primary squamous cell carcinoma may be advantageous in certain cases. Prevention of premalignant lesions is appropriate in high-risk individuals.

Current Opinion in Dermatology 1995:38–43

Epidemiology

Squamous cell carcinoma (SCC) is the second most common cutaneous malignancy, and its frequency is increasing. There are an increasing number of advanced and metastatic cases related to a number of underlying factors. At our institution, the number one cause of metastatic neck disease is SCC of the skin. Currently, metastatic SCC contributes to over 2000 deaths per year in this country; the 5-year survival rate is 35%, with 90% of the metastases occurring by 3 years. Metastasis almost always occurs at the first lymphatic drainage station. The need for medical therapy for advanced cases is clear, a medical approach to early primary lesions may be advantageous in certain cases.

Medical therapy for primary carcinoma

A successful medical therapy for primary SCC of the skin would obviate the need for surgical excision with its potential for scarring and other side effects. This development might be desirable especially for facial lesions. The evaluation of the lymphatics prior to treatment for metastatic disease would be indicated just as it is prior to surgical removal.

Interferons
Interferons are a group of glycoproteins that exhibit antitumor effects in addition to antiviral and immune properties. Currently, interferons are divided into three types: alfa or leukocyte interferon, beta or fibroblast interferon, and gamma or immune interferon. Interferon alfa appears to have the most promise in cutaneous neoplasms, including SCC.

Edwards et al. [1••] evaluated the effect of intralesional interferon alfa-2b on primary SCC. This study was a natural step after they had demonstrated the effectiveness of interferon in basal cell carcinomas and actinic keratosis. A total of 36 SCCs were treated (28 invasive and eight in situ lesions with no evidence of metastasis) with interferon alfa-2b, 1.5 MU (0.15 mL) injected intralesionally three times per week for 3 weeks (nine injections; total dose 13.5 MU). Eighteen weeks after completion of therapy, the treated areas were totally excised and examined histologically for remaining SCC. The overall response rate was excellent, with 26 of 27 invasive SCCs cured, and seven of seven in situ lesions cured. Four cases did reveal residual actinic keratosis at the site, which may or may not be significant, resulting in an overall complete response rate of 88.2%. Figure 1 demonstrates the clinical histologic pre- and posttreatment evaluation of our patient with an invasive SCC of the left prelobular cheek, which was completely cured with interferon in this study. Side effects were mild; flulike symptoms well known to occur with interferon therapy and at the doses used were well tolerated in all but one patient. Cosmetic results were very good or excellent in over 90% of the cases. The cure rate with interferon alfa-2b was a significant improvement over previous results with other interferons, notably alfa 2c and human natural leukocyte interferon.

Lebbe et al. [2] have described a patient with hairy cell leukemia treated with interferon alfa-2a for 3 months who in addition to hematologic remission also demonstrated partial remission (>50%) of vulvar and perianal intraepithelial squamous cell carcinomas with localized microinvasive areas.

Photodynamic therapy
Photodynamic therapy is a medical technique for treating SCC and other tumors with a photosensitizing drug followed by exposure to an intense visible light. Many trials using photodynamic therapy in the treatment of

---

Abbreviation
SCC—squamous cell carcinoma.

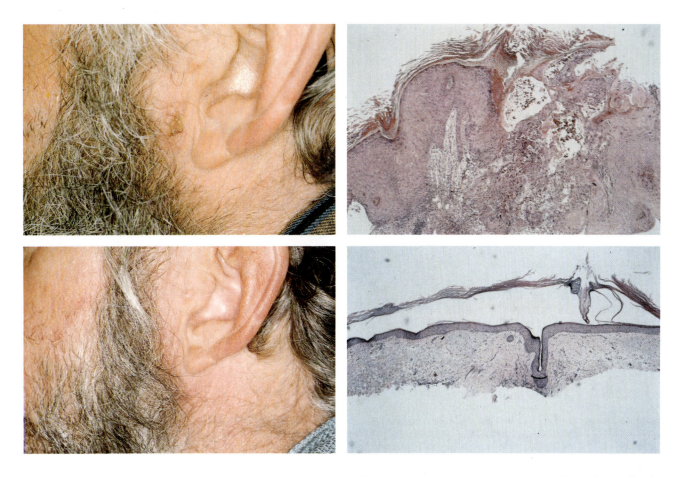

Fig. 1. Upper left, Invasive squamous cell carcinoma (SCC) of left prelobular cheek prior to intralesional interferon alfa-2b therapy was clinically palpable and indurated with crust. There was no evidence of lymphadenopathy or metastatic disease. **Upper right**, Pretreatment punch biopsy of the lesion, which removed less than 25% of the total lesion, demonstrates invasive SCC. **Lower left**, Posttreatment (nine intralesional injections) clinical evaluation just prior to total excision of the treated site at week 18 found no evidence of residual SCC. There was no lymphadenopathy or metastatic disease. **Lower right**, Histologic evaluation reveals no residual SCC from the excision of the site. Note preservation of appendages.

nonmelanoma skin malignancies have been completed at several institutions, although this modality is still in the investigational stage. McCaughan *et al.* [3] treated multiple types of cutaneous and subcutaneous tumors, including three patients with a total of five SCCs and one patient with two lesions of Bowen's disease. Of the five SCCs, three had complete responses at 1 month, one had a partial response (>50% reduction in size), and one had some response (20% to 50% reduction in size). Two of the three complete responders showed no local recurrence in a 1-year follow-up. The hematoporphyrin derivatives used in this study were administered intravenously 2 to 6 days before treatment with an argon pumped tunable dye laser. Photosensitivity was a problem for up to 6 months in some patients, even after a single dose of hematoporphyrin derivative, and all patients were instructed to limit sun exposure for 1 month.

Jones *et al.* [4] treated six patients with eight Bowen's disease lesions using intravenous Photofrin (Ortho Diagnostics, Raritan, NJ), 1 mg/kg, followed by argon pumped dye laser (Coherent Inova 100+ Dye Laser; Coherent, Palo Alto, CA) treatment (630 nm) of the

lesions 48 hours later. Some of these lesions were in anatomic sites that were difficult to treat, and one was large (7.5×6.0 cm), but all lesions responded and remained recurrence-free for at least 1 year. Wolf *et al.* [5] treated nine solar keratoses on the face or scalp in three patients and six early invasive SCCs (three of them on the face) in three patients. A 20% 5-aminolevulinic acid preparation was applied topically to the lesion and 1 cm of surrounding normal skin under occlusion for 4 to 8 hours, followed by photoactive irradiation. 5-Aminolevulinic acid is absorbed preferentially into cancer cells and other abnormal fast-growing cells, and it is converted to protoporphyrin IX, a natural, potent photosensitizing agent. All of the actinic keratoses responded, and, five of the six SCCs responded, but follow-up was only 3 to 12 months. One of the patients treated had an SCC of the dorsal hand and xeroderma pigmentosum and responded without any systemic photosensitivity. These results indicate that superficial SCC tumors may respond to photodynamic therapy, and treatment may be indicated in patients with large superficial tumors, tumors in difficult-to-treat locations, or multiple tumors. Topical application of hematoporphyrin would be preferred, but further studies with longer follow-up times are indicated. The concerns about topical application of hematoporphyrin include poor penetration into the deeper dermis and subcutaneous tissues, which detracts from the effectiveness of photodynamic therapy. Similarly, superficial laser therapy may not penetrate deep enough to treat other than superficial tumors. Interstitial therapy allows laser fibers to be inserted directly into the tissue, so that more intense laser energy may be delivered. Investigations using interstitial photodynamic therapy for cutaneous malignancies have been completed, and a study by Lowdell *et al.* [6] shows this method results in less cutaneous necrosis than superficial therapy and is able to treat deeper tumors in addition to cutaneous and subcutaneous metastases.

5-Fluorouracil implants

Orenberg *et al.* [7] investigated the use of intralesional therapeutic implants to deliver 5-fluorouracil and cisplatin to treat 185 primary SCCs in horses, cats, and dogs. A response rate of 82% was obtained with 62% having complete responses. Further human studies were done with our participation [8] in evaluating basal cell carcinomas with 5-fluorouracil implants, achieving results equaling our finds with interferon alfa-2b (80% range). SCC in humans should be the next step for evaluation of 5-fluorouracil implant therapy. The implant is a viscous injectable gel consisting of a protein carrier matrix (purified bovine collagen), epinephrine (0.1 mg/mL), and 5-fluorouracil (30 mg/mL) prepared just prior to injection, and it should offer the advantage of optimizing the retention and release of the drug in the SCC.

Therapy for advanced and metastatic disease

Chemotherapy

Chemotherapy is not a first-line treatment for the large majority of cutaneous SCCs owing to the side effects of treatment and the good results and ease of other treatment methods. For advanced or metastatic disease, however, it is a viable option.

Guthrie *et al.* [9] treated seven patients with advanced SCC (two had had prior surgery, and four had had prior surgery and radiation) with chemotherapy alone consisting of cisplatin and doxorubicin. A 57% response rate was achieved, with two complete responses and two partial responses in patients who had no evidence of metastasis at onset of therapy. Of the three nonresponders, two had metastatic disease at the onset of therapy.

Sadek *et al.* [10] treated 14 patients with advanced SCC of the lip and skin (all with locally recurrent disease and nine with nodal involvement) with combination chemotherapy consisting of cisplatin, 5-fluorouracil, and bleomycin. The overall response rate was 79%. Four had complete responses; all four received

further therapy, and three obtained prolonged remissions. Seven had partial responses, and of these seven, three received further therapy resulting in remissions. Four died from their disease, despite further therapy in two patients.

Khansur and Kennedy [11] treated seven patients with advanced SCC of the skin (six with nodal involvement, two with lung metastases) with cisplatin and 5-fluorouracil. The overall response rate was 86%. Three patients had complete responses and three had partial responses.

Tantranond *et al.* [12] published a case report of the combination of cisplatin and 5-fluorouracil in the successful treatment of a large, advanced primary SCC involving the right cheek and right ear with erosion into the temporal bone. The patient was also taking isotretinoin concurrently at a dosage of 50 mg orally twice a day for two months; a complete response was obtained at a 2.5-year follow-up.

Chang *et al.* [13] reported on three elderly patients with advanced SCC who were treated with iontophoretic cisplatin to decrease the systemic side effects. Only partial responses were obtained.

Isotretinoin was used by Lippman *et al.* [14] to treat four patients with advanced SCC. Two responded completely, and two responded partially. Patients experienced mild, reversible side effects with isotretinoin at 1 mg/kg divided into a twice-daily dosage. Hu *et al.* [15] discovered that abnormally low expression of retinoic receptor B in certain SCC cell lines may determine the responsiveness of SCC to retinoids.

According to these studies, cisplatin-based chemotherapy in combination with 5-fluorouracil, doxorubicin, bleomycin, or even retinoids provides good results, and combination chemotherapy for advanced or metastatic cutaneous SCC may offer advantages over a single-drug regimen.

Retinoids and interferon in combination therapy

Lippman *et al.* [16••] completed the first clinical trial of 13-*cis*-retinoic acid and interferon alfa-2a in the treatment of advanced SCC of the skin. Recombinant interferon alfa-2a was given subcutaneously at 3 MU/d, and 13-*cis*-retinoic acid was given orally at 1 mg/kg per day for at least 2 months. The overall response rate was 68%. Among 14 patients with locally advanced disease, the response rate was 93% (6 with complete response, 7 with partial). Four (67%) of six patients with regional disease had a partial response. Of those with distant metastasis, there was one complete and one partial response for an overall response rate of 25% (2/8). These patients experienced multiple side effects including fatigue (78%), flulike symptoms (25%), and granulocytopenia (22%) from the interferon and dry skin (86%), cheilitis (75%), hypertriglyceridemia (50%), conjunctivitis (33%), and epistaxis (10%) from the retinoid. The use of combination therapy with interferon and retinoids may be advantageous in selected patients; side effects are clearly related to the dosages of each drug.

Prevention of squamous cell carcinoma and therapy and prevention of premalignant lesions

Sunscreens

Stern *et al.* [17] estimated that the regular use of a sunscreen with a sun protection factor of 15 during the first 18 years of life could reduce the incidence of nonmelanoma skin cancers by 78%. Thompson *et al.* [18••] performed a randomized, blinded, controlled trial of a broad-spectrum sunscreen (sun protection factor 17) to determine its effect on premalignant actinic keratoses in 588 patients during a summer in Australia. The group of patients using the sunscreen had fewer total lesions, fewer new lesions, and more remissions of lesions than the control patients. A dose-response relationship was found between the amount of sunscreen used to the remission of existing lesions. The use of sunscreens should be an important part of the prophylactic requirements for nonmelanoma skin cancer. However, the avoidance of high-intensity sun exposures, the use of wide brim hats (*ie*, ≥ 10 cm brim size), and other protective measures must also be included.

Retinoids

Because of their success in the treatment of SCCs, retinoids have been actively investigated for their possible role in prevention of new SCCs and premalignant lesions. Kraemer *et al.* [19•] conducted a 3-year controlled prospective study of the use of high-dose oral isotretinoin (2 mg/kg) in patients with xeroderma pigmentosum and found a 63% reduction in new skin cancer development. All patients experienced significant side effects. This same group was the subject of a follow-up study on the use of isotretinoin, 0.5 mg/kg, to decrease side effects [20]. Five of seven patients showed a reduction of skin tumors, and four showed a dose-response relationship. Berth-Jones and Graham-Brown [21] published a case report on the use of low-dose etretinate (25 mg/d orally for 22 months) to repress skin tumor development in a single patient with xeroderma pigmentosum. This treatment was well tolerated.

Transplantation patients have higher incidences of SCC. Kelly *et al.* [22] reported on four renal transplantation patients with significant reduction in SCC during 1-year of treatment with oral etretinate, 50 mg/d. Side effects were mild. Vandeghinste *et al.* [23] used oral acitretin at 0.5 mg/kg/d to suppress SCC and Bowen's disease for 15 months in one renal transplantation patient. Shuttleworth *et al.* [24] also used etretinate, 1 mg/kg for 6 months, in patients with a history of SCC or current actinic keratoses and found regression of the keratoses, with only one patient developing SCC. Four remained free of tumors for 6 months after treatment.

Other therapies

Greenberg *et al.* [25•] conducted a randomized, double-blind, controlled study of oral β-carotene, 50 mg/d, in 1805 patients and found no reduction in the occurrence of SCC. Al-Saleem [26] examined the treatment of cutaneous tumors including SCC with indomethacin and concluded that there is a role for nonsteroidal anti-inflammatory drugs in reducing the incidence of skin cancer.

Topical treatments

In a controlled, double-blind randomized study, Euvrard *et al.* [27•] found topical 0.05% tretinoin (all-*trans* retinoic acid) cream to be effective in treating actinic keratoses in transplantation patients. Twenty-five patients were enrolled and for 3 months used the active cream on one arm and the control cream on the other. The response was maintained 3 months after the treatment was discontinued.

Alirezai *et al.* [28•] performed a randomized, double-blind, placebo-controlled study in 79 patients using topical 0.1% isotretinoin cream. Significant clinical clearance of actinic keratoses on the face was found in the isotretinoin group compared with the control patients, but the difference was only apparent at the 16-week point and thereafter. There was an improvement in the treatment groups on the scalp, forearms and dorsal hands, but it was not significant. No histologic confirmation of clearance of individual lesions was obtained.

Misiewicz *et al.* [29] completed a randomized, double-blind study comparing topical tretinoin to Ro 14-9706, an arotinoid methylsulfone at 0.05%. The 26 patients used each agent on opposite sides of their faces for 16 weeks. The decrease in keratosis on the tretinoin side was 30.3% compared with 37.8% for the side treated with the Ro 14-9706. There was no significant difference between the two, although the side effects with the Ro 14-9706 cream were milder.

Olsen *et al.* [30•] performed a double-blind, vehicle-controlled study of topical 10% masoprocol (Actinex; Reed & Carnrick, Jersey City, NJ) in 113 patients, who used the cream twice daily for 2 to 4 weeks. There was a 71.4% decrease in the number of actinic keratoses in the treatment group compared with 4.3% in the control group; 61.5% of the treated patients developed irritation, which was significant enough in 24% to cause discontinuation of treatment.

Griffen and Van Scott [31] found the combination of pyruvic acid and 5-fluorouracil effective in treating actinic keratoses. Pearlman [32] found that pulse dosing of 5-fluorouracil (twice daily 1 to 2 days per week) cleared 98% of the keratoses in 10 patients with many fewer side effects than continual treatment with 5-fluorouracil. The average duration of treatment necessary to achieve significant clearing was 6.7 weeks.

Edwards *et al.* [33] evaluated topical interferon alfa-2b gel on actinic keratosis. It had previously been shown that intralesional interferon alfa-2b was effective in the treatment of actinic keratosis but not a practical modality owing to the number of injections required and their cost. With topical interferon alfa-2b gel for actinic keratosis applied four times per day for 4 weeks, there was clinical improvement, but the improvement was equal only to that obtained with the placebo preparation. Many treatments for actinic keratosis are available and effective, and retinoids may also have a role in chemoprevention of SCC. However, sunscreens, sun avoidance, and sun protection should be used by all patients at risk for SCC or actinic keratosis.

Conclusions

Medical management of primary SCC of the skin has advanced significantly in the past few years with new methods for treatment including photodynamic, intralesional interferon, and retinoid therapy. Longer follow-up times and further studies will be required to determine whether these approaches will have more than selected applications in certain cases. Chemotherapy continues to be a mainstay for the treatment of metastatic disease, especially as part of a combination regimen. Medical therapy and prophylaxis for premalignant lesions are exciting concepts that promise to decrease the ever-increasing incidence of this skin cancer.

References and recommended reading

Papers of particular interest, published within the annual period of review, have been highlighted as:
•   Of special interest
•• Of outstanding interest

1. Edwards L, Berman B, Rapini RP, Whiting DA, Tyring S, Greenway
•• HT, Eyre SP, Tanner DJ, Taylor EL, Peets E, Smiles, KA: **Treatment of Cutaneous Squamous Cell Carcinomas by Intralesional Interferon Alfa-2b Therapy.** *Arch Dermatol* 1992, 128:1486–1489.
Thirty-six cutaneous squamous cell carcinomas were treated with interferon alfa-2b, 1.5 MU intralesionally three times per week for 3 weeks. Eighteen weeks after completion of therapy, the lesions were excised and evaluated histologically. Overall complete response rate was 88.2%.

2. Lebbe C, Rybojad M, Miclea J, Verola O, Cordoliani F, Ablon G, Morel P: **Extensive Human Papillomavirus-Related Disease (Bowenoid Papulosis, Bowen's Disease and Squamous Cell Carcinoma) in a Patient With Hairy Cell Leukemia: Clinical and Immunological Evaluation After an Interferon Alfa Trial.** *J Am Acad Dermatol* 1993, 29:644–645.

3. McCaughan JS, Guy JT, Hicks W, Laufman L, Nims TA, Walker J: **Photodynamic Therapy for Cutaneous and Subcutaneous Malignant Neoplasms.** *Arch Surg* 1989, 124:211–216.

4. Jones CM, Mang T, Cooper M, Wilson BD, Stoll HL: **Photodynamic Therapy in the Treatment of Bowen's Disease.** *J Am Acad Dermatol* 1992, 27:979–982.

5. Wolf P, Rieger E, Kerl H: **Topical Photodynamic Therapy With Endogenous Porphyrins After Application of 5-Aminolevulinic Acid.** *J Am Acad Dermatol* 1993, 28:17–21.

6. Lowdell CP, Ash DV, Driver I, Brown SB: **Interstitial Photodynamic Therapy: Clinical Experience With Diffusing Fibres in the Treatment of Cutaneous and Subcutaneous Tumors.** *Br J Cancer* 1993, 67:1398–1403.

7. Orenberg EK, Luck EE, Brown DM, Kitchell BE: **Implant Delivery System: Intralesional Delivery of Chemotherapeutic Agents for Treatment of Spontaneous Skin Tumors in Veterinary Patients.** *Clin Dermatol* 1992, 9:561–568.

8. Orenberg EK, Miller BH, Greenway HT, Koperski JA, Lowe N, Rosen T, Brown DM, Inui M, Korey AG, Luck EE: **The Effect of Intralesional 5-Fluorouracil Therapeutic Implant (MPI 5003) for Treatment of Basal Cell Carcinoma.** *J Am Acad Dermatol* 1992, 27:723–728.

9. Guthrie TH, Porubsky ES, Luxenberg MN, Shah KJ, Wurtz KL, Watson PR: **Cisplatin-Based Chemotherapy in Advanced Basal and Squa-**

mous Cell Carcinomas of the Skin: Results in 28 Patients Including 13 Patients Receiving Multimodality Therapy. *J Clin Oncol* 1990, 8:342–346.

10. Sadek H, Azli N, Wendling JL: **Treatment of Advanced Squamous Cell Carcinoma of the Skin With Cisplatin, 5-Fluorouracil, and Bleomycin.** *Cancer* 1990, 66:1692–1696.

11. Khansur T, Kennedy A: **Cisplatin and 5-Fluorouracil for Advanced Locoregional and Metastatic Squamous Cell of the Skin (Clinical Trials).** *Cancer* 1991, 67:2030–2032.

12. Tantranond P, Balducci L, Karam F, Wang TY, Parker M, Hescock H, Cherryholmes D: **Alternative Management of Cutaneous Squamous Cell Carcinoma in an Elderly Man: Report of a Case and Review of the Literature.** *J Geriatr Soc* 1992, 40:510–512.

13. Chang B, Guthrie TH, Hayakawa K, Gangarosa LP: **A Pilot Study of Iontophoretic Cisplatin Chemotherapy of Basal and Squamous Cell Carcinomas of the Skin (The Cutting Edge).** *Arch Dermatol* 1993, 129:425–427.

14. Lippman SM, Meyskens FL: **Treatment of Advanced Squamous Cell Carcinoma of the Skin With Isotretinoin.** *Ann Intern Med* 1987, 107:499–501.

15. Hu L, Crowe DL, Rheinwald JG, Chambon P, Gudas LJ: **Abnormal Expression of Retinoic Acid Receptors and Keratin 19 by Human Oral and Epidermal Squamous Cell Carcinoma Cell Lines.** *Cancer Res* 1991, 51:3972–3981.

16. Lippman SM, Parkinson DR, Itri LM, Weber RS, Schantz SP, Ota
•• DM, Schusterman MA, Krakoff IH, Gutterman JU, Hong WK: **13-cis-Retinoic Acid and Interferon Alfa 2a: Effective Combination Therapy for Advanced Squamous Cell Carcinoma of the Skin.** *J Natl Cancer Inst* 1992, 84:235–241.
Twenty-eight patients with advanced cutaneous SCC were treated for at least 2 months with interferon alfa-2a given at 3 MU/d simultaneously with 13-cis-retinoic acid at 1 mg/kg. The overall response rate was 68%; the response rate for locally advanced disease was 93%. Side effects from both drugs were significant.

17. Stern RS, Weinstein MC, Baker SG: **Risk Reduction for Non-melanoma Skin Cancer With Childhood Sunscreen Use.** *Arch Dermatol* 1986, 122:537–545.

18. Thompson SC, Jolley D, Marks R: **Reduction of Solar Keratoses by**
•• **Regular Sunscreen Use.** *N Engl J Med* 1993, 329:1147–1151.
A randomized blinded, controlled trial of a broad-spectrum sunscreen (sun protection factor 17) was conducted to determine the effectiveness of a sunscreen in treating and preventing actinic keratoses in 588 patients. The treatment group had fewer actinic keratosis, and a dose-response relationship was found.

19. Kraemer KH, DiGiovanna JJ, Moshell AN, Tarone RE, Peck GL: **Pre-**
•   **vention of Skin Cancer in Xeroderma Pigmentosum With the Use of Oral Isotretinoin.** *N Engl J Med* 1988, 318:1633–1637.
Five xeroderma pigmentosum patients completed a 3-year prospective study of high-dose oral isotretinoin (2 mg/kg), and the incidence of new cancer development among them decreased 63%.

20. Kraemer KH, DiGiovanna JJ, Peck GL: **Oral Isotretinoin Prevention of Skin Cancer in Xeroderma Pigmentosum: Individual Variation in Dose Response [Abstract].** *J Invest Dermatol* 1990, 94:544.

21. Berth-Jones J, Graham-Brown RAC: **Xeroderma Pigmentosum Variant: Response to Etretinate.** *Br J Dermatol* 1990, 122:559–561.

22. Kelly JW, Sabto J, Gurr FW, Bruce F: **Retinoids to Prevent Skin Cancer in Organ Transplant Recipients.** *Lancet* 1991, 338:1407.

23. Vandeghinste N, De Bersaques J, Geerts ML, Kint A: **Acitretin as Cancer Chemoprophylaxis in a Renal Transplant Recipient.** *Dermatology* 1992, 185:307–308.

24. Shuttleworth D, Marks R, Griffin PJA, Salaman JR: **Treatment of Cutaneous Neoplasia With Etretinate in Renal Transplant Recipients.** *Q J Med* 1988, 257:717–725.

25. Greenberg ER, Baron JA, Stukel TA, Stevens MM, Mandel JS, Spencer
•   SK, Elias PM, Lowe N, Nierenberg DW, Bayrd G, Vance JC, Freeman DH, Clendenning WE, Kwan T: **A Clinical Trial of Beta Carotene to Prevent Basal Cell and Squamous Cell Cancers of the Skin.** *N Engl J Med* 1990, 323:789–795.
A randomized, double-blind controlled study using SCC oral β-carotene, 50 mg/d, was conducted in 1805 patients. No significant reduction of SCC was found.

26. Al-Saleem T: **Nonsteroidal Anti-inflammatory Drugs in Skin Cancer: Revisited.** *J Natl Cancer Inst* 1993, 85:581.

27. Euvrard S, Verschoore M, Touraine J, Dureau G, Cochat P,
•   Czernielewski J, Thivolet J: **Topical Retinoids for Warts and Keratoses in Transplant Recipients.** *Lancet* 1992, 340:48–49.

Twenty-five transplantation patients were studied in a controlled, double-blind, randomized study. Topical 0.05% tretinoin cream was found to be effective in treating keratoses.

28. Alirezai M, Dupuy P, Amblard P, Kalis B, Souteyrand P, Frappaz A,
• Sendagorta E: **Clinical Evaluation of Topical Isotretinoin in the Treatment of Actinic Keratosis.** *J Am Acad Dermatol* 1994, **30**:447–451.
Seventy-nine patients were studied in a randomized, double-blind, controlled study of topical isotretinoin cream, which was found to be significantly effective in treating actinic keratoses on the face. Results were evident after 16 weeks of therapy.

29. Misiewicz J, Sendagorta E, Golebiowska A, Lorenc B, Czarnetzki BM, Jablonska S: **Topical Treatment of Multiple Actinic Keratoses of the Face with Arotinoid Methyl Sulfone (Ro 14-9706) Cream Versus Tretinoin Cream: A Double-Blind, Comparative Study.** *J Am Acad Dermatol* 1991, **24**:448–451.

30. Olsen EA, Abernethy ML, Kulp-Shorten C, Callen JP, Glazer SD,
• Huntley A, McCray M, Monroe AB, Tschen E, Wolf JE: **A Double-Blind, Vehicle-Controlled Study Evaluating Masoprocol Cream in the Treatment of Actinic Keratoses on the Head and Neck.** *J Am Acad Dermatol* 1991, **24**:738–743.

One hundred thirteen patients were studied in a double-blind controlled trial of topical masoprocal cream used twice daily. The cream produced a 71.4% decrease in the number of actinic keratosis.

31. Griffin TD, Van Scott EJ: **Use of Pyruvic Acid in the Treatment of Actinic Keratoses: A Clinic and Histopathologic Study.** *Cutis* 1991, **47**:325–329.

32. Pearlman DL: **Weekly Pulse Dosing: Effective and Comfortable Topical 5-Fluorouracil Treatment of Multiple Facial Actinic Keratoses.** *J Am Acad Dermatol* 1991, **25**:665–667.

33. Edwards L, Levine N, Smiles KA: **The Effect of Topical Interferon Alfa-2b on Actinic Keratosis.** *J Dermatol Surg Oncol* 1990, **16**:446–449.

Hubert T. Greenway, MD, Matthew K. Abele, MD, Department of Dermatology and Cutaneous Surgery, and Dwight L. McKee, MD, Department of Hematology and Oncology, Scripps Clinic and Research Foundation, 10666 North Torrey Pines Road, La Jolla, CA 92037, USA.

Potential precursors to malignant melanoma

Rona M. MacKie, MD

University of Glasgow, Glasgow, Scotland

A number of conditions are considered possible precursors to melanoma, but there are few if any obligate precursors. Very limited data are available on the quantitative risk of melanomas' developing in any of these situations, which makes logical management plans impossible; at present, therefore, clinicians vary in their approaches. The current situation is reviewed with regard to xeroderma pigmentosum, *in situ* melanoma, lentigo maligna, congenital nevi, nevus spilus, Spitz nevus, and dysplastic nevi. It is stressed that further accurate documentation of the prevalence of these putative precursors is needed, so that logical treatment plans can be developed.

Current Opinion in Dermatology 1995:44–50

Cutaneous malignant melanoma arises in stepwise progression from the epidermal melanocyte. At present there is great interest in the molecular events in this stepwise progression from the benign melanocyte to the fully established malignant melanocytic cell with the capacity to invade and metastasize. It has been suggested that there are several steps that can be identified at the pathological level: 1) melanocyte, 2) benign nevus cell, 3) *in situ* malignancy, 4) radial growth phase malignant melanoma, 5) vertical growth phase malignant melanoma, 6) malignant melanoma that has spread into vascular channels, and 7) malignant melanoma established at distant sites, causing distant metastases. There is currently much interest in the search for molecular markers of cells in these stages of tumor progression. It is likely that there will be markers associated with the growth or expansion capacity of the relevant cell, and the invasive capacity of the cell, and acquisition of the metastatic phenotype. At the clinical level it would be of great value to identify at an early stage those lesions containing cells that have the capacity to complete the path to invasive malignancy. If precursors to melanoma could be accurately identified at the clinical level, then appropriate management plans could be devised at an early stage when the prospects of success are reasonable.

Precursor lesions of any condition can be divided into obligate or facultative precursors. In the obligate situation, all lesions identified are inexorably set on a pathway of transformation to malignancy. In the facultative situation, a proportion of the lesions identified may progress to malignancy, and they are more likely to do so than cells associated with normal skin or other banal lesions, but the development of invasive malignancy is not inevitable.

In the melanocytic situation at the present time, there are no definitely known obligate precursor lesions. Lesions that might be considered obligate would be radial growth phase melanomas or lentigo maligna melanomas. It is clearly impossible, however, to follow one individual lesion to establish its potential for transformation from the *in situ* or radial growth phase to frank invasive malignancy; clearly, an excision biopsy is needed to establish the diagnosis, and data in this area must therefore be drawn from circumstantial evidence.

It would seem from such studies that a relatively small proportion of lentigo malignas progress over a fixed period of time to frank invasive lentigo maligna melanoma, and that an unknown proportion of radial growth phase melanomas progress to the vertical growth phase and thence to metastatic lesions in a proportion of cases. Table 1 lists possible facultative precursors of malignant melanoma.

Table 1. Possible facultative precursors of invasive malignant melanoma

Xeroderma pigmentosum
Level 1 or *in situ* malignant melanoma
Lentigo maligna
Congenital nevi (giant, small, and intermediate sizes)
Nevus spilus
Spitz nevus
Dysplastic or atypical nevus
Banal acquired nevus

Xeroderma pigmentosum

It is well established that patients with xeroderma pigmentosum (Fig. 1) are at increased risk of developing malignant melanoma. The risk relative to the rest of the population is of the order of ×1000 to ×2000 [1], and therefore lifetime surveillance is necessary. The risk of developing nonmelanoma skin cancer is even higher. The mechanisms associated with increased risk in xeroderma pigmentosum patients appear to be associated with inadequate, unscheduled DNA repair following exposure to natural sunlight. Although patients with sporadic malignant melanoma have been well studied and do not appear to have a defect in unscheduled DNA repair, as identified by currently available techniques, after exposure to ultraviolet radiation, it would appear that in the xeroderma pigmentosum situation, faulty DNA repair may directly or indirectly contribute to increased risk of malignant melanoma [2•].

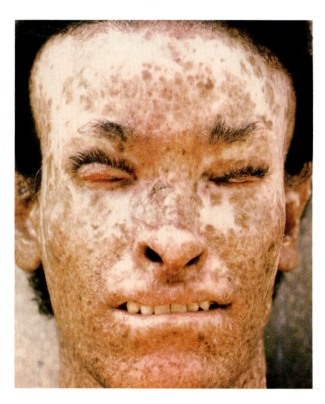

Fig. 1. Young boy aged 16 years with xeroderma pigmentosum. Note the gross actinic damage.

Successful management of patients with xeroderma pigmentosum depends on rapid diagnosis as shortly after birth as possible. Diagnosis will be relatively easy if the child is born into a family at known increased risk, but less so in children with apparently sporadic xeroderma pigmentosum. The usual early warning signs are severe sunburn of the infant when he or she is first exposed to sunlight and delayed clearing of the ultraviolet-associated erythema. Once the diagnosis of xeroderma pigmentosum is made, affected individuals must be protected from all direct sunlight. A combination of appropriate housing, appropriate clothing, and total ultraviolet blocks is associated with a decreased risk of malignant change in these children. Although the decreased risk of malignant change with ultraviolet avoidance is at present observed more with basal

and squamous cell carcinomas than with melanoma, the melanoma-associated mortality is high in these children, and therefore a regimen of sun avoidance is essential. Because of the rarity of xeroderma pigmentosum, there are no studies recording the relationship between the number of malignancies and degree of protection offered by total sunscreening in these children.

Level 1 or *in situ* malignant melanoma

At the present time, results of population education and melanoma screening programs indicate that an increasingly high proportion of individuals are presenting for treatment with pigmented lesions that have the histologic features of *in situ* or level 1 cutaneous malignant melanoma (Fig. 2). Clinically, these lesions do not appear to have any features that consistently distinguish them from thin or early level 2 malignant melanomas. The majority are irregularly outlined, irregularly pigmented lesions with a diameter of 3 to 8 mm. The histologic appearance is that of atypical and cytologically malignant melanocytes all confined to the epidermis, with no apparent breach of the basement membrane zone. The number of lesions reported, particularly in Australia, does suggest that not all of the lesions would have been obligate precursors to invasive malignant melanoma. This conclusion, which is drawn from inferential study of the number of *in situ* melanomas in, for example, the Hunter Valley in New South Wales [3••], in comparison with anticipated invasive melanomas, is strengthened by observations from the West Coast of the United States [4••], where the Lawrence Livermore Laboratory has for some years now carried out a screening program of its employees. Both the invasive and *in situ* melanomas have been identified, and a small case control study has suggested that the risk factors for *in situ* melanomas differ from those associated with invasive melanomas [5]. If confirmed, this observation would be further important evidence to suggest that in cancer registries and other studies that register level 1 melanomas, there may be a subset of melanocytic lesions that do not have the capacity for completion of the metastatic cascade. In the light of our present knowledge, however, the treatment of lesions with clinical features suggestive of cutaneous level 1 melanoma must continue to be excision with a narrow 1- to 2-mm margin of normal skin around the lesion.

Good guidelines are urgently needed for the pathological reporting of *in situ* or level 1 malignant melanomas. There is considerable controversy in this area, with expert melanoma pathologists disagreeing on the criteria used to differentiate early level 1 melanoma from a severely dysplastic nevus with striking cytologic atypia. Guidelines for the nonspecializing pathologist would greatly improve the degree of comparison possible between centers.

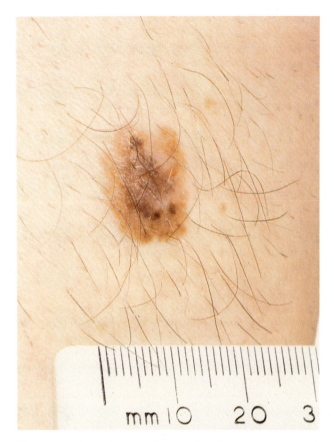

Fig. 2. Level 1 melanoma that has developed over a period of 6 months on the thigh of a woman aged 23 years.

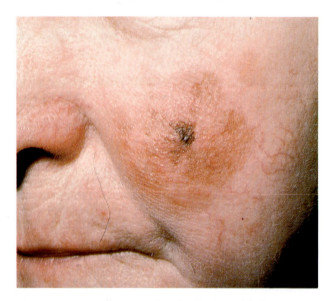

Fig. 3. Lentigo maligna on the cheek of an elderly patient.

Lentigo maligna

Lentigo maligna is the *in situ* lesion associated with lentigo maligna melanoma (Fig. 3). Alternative names for this *in situ* or level 1 phase are Hutchinson's melan-

otic freckle or premalignant melanosis of Dubreuilh. These terms are used to describe an irregularly pigmented lesion seen most often on facial skin and associated with no obvious central palpable area. Lentigo maligna may expand slowly and laterally for many years. In the course of lateral extension, there may be central clearance or depigmentation, which suggests that a degree of partial regression is taking place within the lentigo maligna. If lentigo malignas are left untreated, a proportion, after a variable period of time, progress to invasive lentigo maligna melanoma. The proportion and the time frame are not well established. Weinstock and Sober [6] have suggested on the basis of the prevalence of lentigo maligna in the elderly population and the number of lentigo maligna melanomas diagnosed that the risk of malignant progression to frank lentigo maligna melanoma is relatively small, with a lifetime risk of 4.7, or 2.2%. Thus, the suggestion is that lentigo maligna is rarely a precursor to lentigo maligna melanoma. It is important, however, to remember that the age at which patients present with lentigo maligna is falling steadily and that Weinstock and Sober's study concerned an elderly population with facial lentigo maligna on the Eastern Seaboard of the United States. In countries with high solar exposure, such as Australia, lentigo maligna is being diagnosed in the 3rd and 4th decades of life, and there is no established study reporting on the risk of malignant change in this setting. It is likely that over time, the risk will be considerably higher than that quoted for elderly individuals.

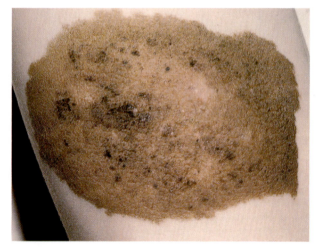

Fig. 4. Giant congenital pigmented nevus.

At the present time, there are no clear guidelines for the management of lentigo maligna. It is important to establish the diagnosis by biopsy, and this is one of the few situations in which a punch biopsy into a melanocytic lesion is, in my opinion, permissible. The two commonest differential diagnoses are invasive lentigo maligna and the flat type of seborrheic keratosis. If a biopsy is done, the sample should be taken from the most likely area of invasion, *eg*, the area that is most deeply pigmented or the area with any evi-

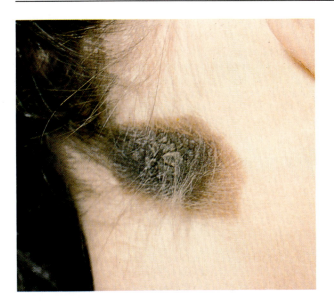

Fig. 5. Smaller congenital pigmented nevus.

dence of a palpable lesion within the main body of the lentigo maligna. If the pathology shows that the diagnosis of lentigo maligna without invasion is correct, there are various treatment options available. In the very elderly and otherwise unfit a "no treatment" policy with careful observation would not be unreasonable, and in practice it is carried out for many old people. In younger individuals, cryotherapy can be extremely effective in removing all visible trace of pigmentation. It is important to remember, however, that there may be a few residual lentigo maligna cells remaining following cryotherapy, and careful follow-up is mandatory even if there has been complete clinical clearance of the lesion.

Some centers have reported success with the use of topical azaleic acid in the treatment of lentigo maligna, but others have urged caution with reports of progression from lentigo maligna to lentigo maligna melanoma during azaleic acid treatment [7]. Excision of the area of lentigo maligna is also a treatment option and is perhaps the current standard therapy. The problem with excision is that many lentigo malignas are large lesions, and the majority are on facial skin. The excision may therefore be relatively large, and there may be problems with closure of wounds adjacent to the eyes and nose. Thus, it will be seen that there is at present no one gold standard for the management of lentigo malignas, and large prospective studies are needed to establish recurrence rates in patients treated by any of the modalities mentioned here.

Congenital melanocytic nevi

Traditionally, congenital melanocytic nevi are divided into 3 groups according to size: 1) the giant garment or bathing suit nevi (Fig. 4), 2) the intermediate sized nevi, and 3) the small congenital nevi. There are vary-

ing definitions of these different groups, some based on surface area and some on maximum diameter. A more sensible working approach to definition would be to divide congenital nevi into large lesions in which complete excision is difficult if not impossible, and smaller lesions that with the introduction of new techniques such as tissue expanders can be completely excised.

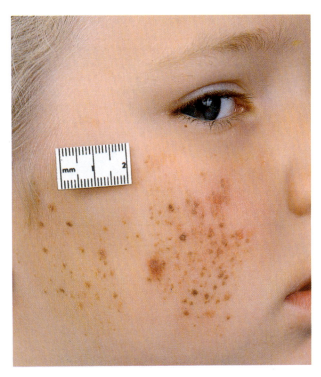

Fig. 6. Speckled and lentiginous nevus on the cheek of a young girl.

The risk of malignant change in congenital nevi is a subject of ongoing study and some degree of controversy. The literature pertaining to the risk of malignant change in congenital nevi relates mainly to giant garment or bathing trunk nevi. Many of the papers describe isolated case reports from centers with a particular interest in the management of these lesions. These reports tend to give a falsely high impression of the risk of malignant change in giant congenital nevi. One of the more reliable studies comes from Scandinavia and is the result of a prospective follow-up study of a population of individuals identified with congenital nevi and followed up without therapy for many years [8]. The data obtained from this study suggest that the risk of malignant change in these patients over a lifetime is between 3% and 5%. The risk is therefore relatively high, and any management approach that reduces this risk is entirely justified. Current approaches to the management of congenital nevi of the giant type are varied. Among plastic surgeons, there has been a vogue in the past decade for early dermabrasion of these lesions within the first 48 hours of life [9]. The rationale is that treatment at such an early age will significantly reduce the cosmetic sequelae of these giant lesions, and because of the early removal of large numbers of nevomelanocytes, may also reduce the risk of malignancy. There is yet no long-term study validating the second part of this hypothesis. The main problem with early dermabrasion relates to speed of referral and practicability. When a child is born with a giant nevus, the parents are naturally distressed, and a rush to immediate surgery is not always feasible. Nevertheless, the short-term cosmetic results do appear to show significant improvement, and follow-up studies are required to establish whether or not the risk of malignant change is reduced. It is therefore suggested that a neonate with a giant congenital nevus be referred as a matter of urgency and with all possible speed to an appropriate center equipped to counsel the parents and carry out the dermabrasion procedure if warranted. Data on malignant change within giant nevi indicate that this risk is present from birth and that a high proportion of reported melanomas arise in these lesions in prepubertal children.

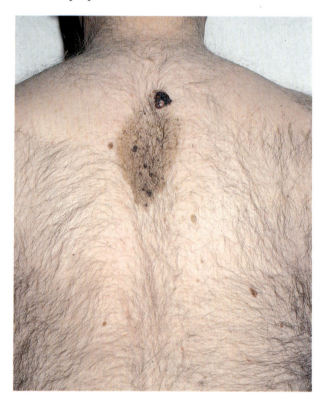

Fig. 7. Malignant change in nevus spilus on the back of a man aged 43 years.

In the case of smaller congenital nevi (Fig. 5), the risk of malignant change is poorly established. A study by Rhodes *et al.* [10] suggested that a risk does exist, and that the risk is higher for small congenital nevi than for acquired nevi. In a study carried out in Glasgow of patients who presented with melanoma before their 30th birthday, it was found that an unexpectedly high proportion of these patients had melanomas that had developed on a preexisting small congenital or early-onset nevus [11]. These two studies suggest that there is an increased risk of malignant change in smaller con-

genital nevi, but the degree of risk is not yet established. A study by Osburn *et al.* [12] indicated that 1% of neonates have a congenital nevus. Removing these lesions to prevent development of an unknown proportion of melanomas is not at present considered justified. The current policy in most centers is to observe children who are referred with small congenital nevi and remove lesions showing any signs of growth or change. My own personal experience is that around puberty many patients request removal of such congenital nevi on cosmetic grounds, and this would appear to be a reasonable procedure. In contrast with the giant nevi and the age at which malignant change has been recorded, melanomas developing in small congenital nevi have in the great majority of cases been recorded after puberty.

The ideal theoretic study to compute accurately the risk of malignant change in small congenital nevi would involve screening a very large population of around 500,000 to identify individuals with congenital nevi and then observing that population for many years to find the incidence of malignant change. The ethics of such a study are clearly questionable, and it is doubtful if patients or parents would give informed consent for such a procedure. Thus, it seems unlikely that the true risk of malignant change within small congenital nevi will ever be established. A molecular marker of congenital nevi containing cells with the capacity for malignant change and metastases would be extremely valuable, but it is not yet available.

Nevus spilus (lentiginous and speckled nevus)

These lesions are clinically recognized as areas of deeply pigmented and palpable nodules situated in an area of pale macular pigmentation (Fig. 6). Thus, the appearance is that of multiple pigmented nevi set in an area of lentiginous change. Until the late 1980s, there was no suggestion that these lesions were precursors to melanoma. Over the past 5 years, however, the development of malignant melanoma within a nevus spilus has been noted in a number of case reports (Fig. 7) [13,14•]. Epidemiological data are need first to establish the incidence and prevalence of nevus spilus within the population at large, and second to quantitate the risk of malignant change within these lesions. At present, it is clear that if nevus spilus is diagnosed, the patient must be followed up for any change that might be associated with the development of malignant melanoma. There is not yet any convincing quantitative evidence to justify excision of all nevi spili.

Spitz nevus

Spitz nevus (*ie*, spindle and epithelioid cell nevus) was identified by Spitz [15] as a lesion in children that was previously considered to be malignant melanoma. On the basis of clinicopathologic data, Spitz sug-

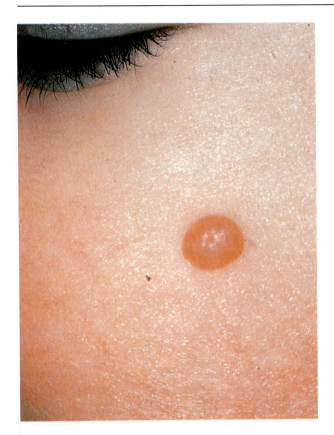

Fig. 8. Spitz nevus on the cheek of a girl aged 6 years.

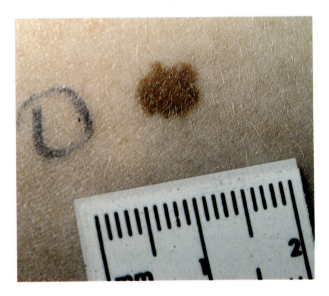

Fig. 9. So called dysplastic nevus on the trunk of a girl whose father and grandfather both died of melanoma. This girl has more than 60 similar lesions on her trunk.

gested that they were in fact a variant of benign compound nevi, and the natural history of these lesions would justify this conclusion in the great majority of cases. These nevi are commonest on the face, are usually red or brown (Fig. 8), and may be found at any age, although they are commoner in children. There is a subset of melanomas, however, that have pathologic features similar to those found in Spitz nevus but with additional signs of malignant change. It has not yet been established whether or not these Spitzoid melanomas develop from Spitz nevi, or if they have a separate pathway of development [16•]. At the present time, and in the light of current knowledge, it is recommended that lesions clinically recognized as Spitz nevi should be excised.

Dysplastic or atypical nevi

Much controversy has raged over the true role of both familial and acquired clinically atypical or dysplastic nevi (Fig. 9) and their potential as precursors to malignant melanoma. As defined by Elder [17], atypical nevi with pathological features of dysplasia require both architectural atypia and clear cytological atypia of melanocytes within the lesion. Some authors have allowed the diagnosis of dysplastic nevus to be made in the presence only of architectural atypia and have thus given rise to much confusion and controversy. At the present time, it would appear that at least in the familial setting, patients with atypical nevi are at significantly increased risk of developing malignant melanoma. Our own data [18••] suggest that this risk is of the order of ×400 in the familial setting, and ×90 in the sporadic setting. It is not established, however, that all melanomas in patients with atypical nevi develop within preexisting nevi, and there is clear evidence of melanomas developing on clinically normal skin in some patients with dysplastic nevi.

In the light of our present knowledge, it would appear that wholesale excision of all dysplastic nevi on the basis that some may be precursors to melanoma is unjustified. Our own policy is to carefully photograph and map nevi of patients who present with atypical nevi and then follow-up all these patients at intervals of 3 to 6 months, depending on the degree of concern. Nevi are excised only if they show photographic evidence of growth or change between visits. In over 10 years of carrying out this practice, no melanomas have progressed in these patients.

Banal or acquired nevi

Banal or acquired nevi are extremely common. The average young adult in the West of Scotland has between 20 and 50 such lesions, the majority of which develop around puberty. The current incidence of malignant melanoma is around 10 new cases annually per 100,000 persons. On this basis there is no evidence whatever to suggest that prophylactic removal of acquired nevi is justified. One must not neglect, however, to give good advice on sensible sun exposure and on detection of early melanoma to those members of the population who have an above average number of nevi [19], because large numbers of clinically banal nevi constitute the strongest risk yet identified for malignant melanoma.

Conclusions

At present, a large number of apparently benign melanocytic lesions can be considered potential precursors to melanoma. There is an urgent need for cell or preferably molecular markers to identify at an early stage lesions of this type, which have the potential to evolve into invasive malignant lesions. Until such markers are available, a wide range of nevoid melanocytic lesions require clinical examination and in many cases surgical excision for accurate pathologic diagnosis.

References and recommended reading

Papers of particular interest, published within the annual period of review, have been highlighted as:
- •   Of special interest
- ••   Of outstanding interest

1.   Kraemer KH, Slor H: **Xeroderma Pigmentosum.** *Clin Dermatol* 1984, 2:33–69.

2.   Brodkin RH, Altman EM: **Controlling Malignant Melanoma: A Focus**
•   **on Pediatricians.** *Am J Dis Child* 1993, 147:875–881.
A useful review on melanoma control aimed at those who care for children.

3.   Burton RC, Coates MS, Hersey P, Roberts G, Chetty MP, Chen S,
••   Hayes MH, Howe CG, Armstrong BK: **An Analysis of a Melanoma Epidemic.** *Int J Cancer* 1993, 55:765–770.
An extremely interesting and thought-provoking account of a public education campaign and the resultant increase in workload.

4.   Gong G, Whittemore AS, West D, Moore DH II: **Cutaneous Melanoma**
••   **at Lawrence Livermore National Laboratory: Comparison With Rates in Two San Francisco Bay Area Counties.** *Cancer Causes Control* 1992, 3:191–197.
Further intriguing data from the Lawrence Livermore laboratory emphasizing the observed increase in incidence only in thin melanomas.

5.   Moore DH, Schneider JS, Sagebiel RW: **Discordance of Risk Factors for Invasive and Non-invasive Melanoma.** *Lancet* 1990, 335:1523–1524.

6.   Weinstock MA, Sober AJ: **The Risk of Progression of Lentigo Maligna to Lentigo Maligna Melanoma.** *Br J Dermatol* 1987, 116:303–310.

7.   Mclean DI, Peter KK: **Apparent Progression of Lentigo Maligna to Invasive Melanoma During Treatment With Topical Azaleic Acid.** *Br J Dermatol* 1986 114:685–689.

8.   Lorentzen M, Pers M, Brettville Jensen G: **The Incidence of Malignant Transformation in Giant Pigmented Nevi.** *Scand J Plast Reconstr Surg* 1977, 11:163–167.

9.   Johnson HA. **Permanent Removal of Pigmentation From Giant Hairy Naevi by Dermabrasion Early in Life.** *Br J Plast Surg* 1977, 30:321–323.

10.   Rhodes AR, Sober AJ, Day CL, Melski JW, Harrist J, Mihm MC, Fitzpatrick TB: **The Malignant Potential of Small Congenital Naevo Cellular Naevi.** *J Amer Acad Dermatol* 1982, 6:230–241.

11.   MacKie RM, Watt D, Doherty V, Aitchison T: **Malignant Melanoma occurring in Those Aged Under 30 in the West of Scotland, 1979–1986: A Study of Incidence, Clinical Features, Pathological Features and Survival.** *Br J Dermatol* 1991, 124:560–564.

12.   Osbum K, Schosser RH, Everett MA: **Congenital Pigmented and Vascular Lesions in Newborn Infants.** *J Amer Acad Dermatol* 1987, 16:788–792.

13.   Wagner RF, Cottel WI: **In Situ Malignant Melanoma Arising in a Speckled Lentiginous Naevus.** *J Amer Acad Dermatol* 1989, 20:125–126.

14.   Guillot B, Bessis D, Barneon G, Monpoint S, Guilhou JJ: **Malignant**
•   **Melanoma Occurring on a Naevus on Naevus.** *Br J Dermatol* 1991, 124:610–611.
Another case report emphasizing that nevus spilus is a precursor to melanoma.

15.   Spitz S: **Melanomas of Childhood.** *Amer J Pathol* 1948, 24:591–609.

16.   Tai-Yuen W, Duncan LM, Mihm MC Jr: **Melanoma Mimicking Dermal**
•   **and Spitz's Nevus ("Nevoid" Melanoma).** *Semin Surg Oncol* 1993, 9:188–193.
A good review of a pathologically difficult area.

17.   Elder DE: **The Dysplastic Naevus.** *Pathology* 1985, 17:291–297.

18.   MacKie RM, McHenry P, Hole D: **Accelerated Detection With**
••   **Prospective Surveillance for Cutaneous Malignant Melanoma in High-Risk Groups.** *Lancet* 1993, 341:1618–1620.
A 10-year prospective study quantitating the melanoma risk in both the familial and sporadic setting of dysplastic nevus.

19.   Sverdlow AJ, English JSC, MacKie RM, O'Docherty CJ, Hunter JAA, Clark J, Hole DJ: **Benign Melanocytic Naevi as a Risk Factor for Melanoma.** *BMJ* 1986, 292:987–989.

Rona M. MacKie, MD, Department of Dermatology, University of Glasgow, 56 Dumbarton Road, Glasgow G11 6NU, Scotland.

Advances in research on the histiocytic syndromes X and non-X

Ruggero Caputo, MD, and Ramon Grimalt, MD

University of Milan, Milan, Italy

The main advances in the field of Langerhans cell histiocytosis during 1993 are reviewed, among them the observation that human herpesvirus 6 may represent the triggering factor for the proliferating cells, the possible usefulness of an antibody against a protein found in most proliferating cells as a prognostic index to evaluate the aggressiveness of the histiocytic disease, and the successful result obtained with thalidomide in the treatment of Langerhans cell histiocytosis skin lesions. In non–Langerhans cell histiocytosis, a histologic study on a large number of cases confirmed that many forms of the syndrome with peculiar clinical features are in fact closely related. All the data in this field point to a future unification of some of these diseases into a more realistic and useful classification.

Current Opinion in Dermatology 1995:51–54

Histiocytic syndromes represent a puzzling and poorly understood group of diseases, and something new is offered to our attention every year. In this review, we focus on the most interesting clinical, therapeutic, and investigative observations made in recent studies.

Langerhans cell histiocytosis (histiocytosis X)

In a review on Langerhans cell histiocytosis (LCH) in childhood, Bonifazi [1] distinguished 5 forms of LCH according to their predominant cutaneous manifestations: 1) Self-healing solitary nodular histiocytosis, which is most frequently congenital; 2) self-healing congenital papulonodular histiocytosis, which corresponds to Hashimoto-Pritzker histiocytosis; 3) self-healing acquired histiocytosis, which corresponds to Illig-Fanconi disease and is characterized by the monomorphous papular eruption of a small number of lesions that appear during the first few months of life and regress within the 1st year; 4) the disseminated form with benign evolution, which corresponds to Letterer-Siwe disease without organ dysfunction; and 5) the disseminated form with malignant evolution, which corresponds to Letterer-Siwe disease with organ dysfunction and growth cessation. This last form requires immediate therapeutic measures.

Enjolras et al. [2] described the notorious polymorphism of LCH at birth. They indicated that the main problem in these cases is the lack of prognostic criteria and the consequent difficulty of management. They concluded that ultrastructural findings of dense, laminated bodies in the cytoplasm of cells with Birbeck granules indicate a self-healing, benign form of LCH.

In regard to prognostic criteria, a very interesting observation, which may still need further confirmation, was made by Helm et al. [3••], who detected an immunostaining of the histiocytes with an antibody against the proliferating cell nuclear antigen, a protein found in most proliferating cells. Their study showed that this protein was present in patients with more aggressive disease. As demonstrated in some lymphomas, a relationship might exist between a higher percentage of proliferating cell nuclear antigen–positive histiocytes and progressive skin disease or systemic manifestations. These data suggest that a strong positivity for this antibody could be a useful prognostic marker.

In a literature review, Maarten Egeler et al. [4•] reported a possible association between LCH and malignant neoplasms, particularly lymphomas, leukemias, and lung tumors. The intimate and simultaneous association of LCH with lymphomas or with solid tumors would appear to be the result of a specific dendritic reaction. In patients with lymphomas or solid tumors, however, the latency of the malignant neoplasm after the diagnosis of LCH suggests a therapy-related process. Therefore, chemotherapy used in the treatment of LCH may increase the risk of secondary leukemia or solid tumors.

Abbreviations

BCH—benign cephalic histiocytosis; GEH—generalized eruptive histiocytosis; JXG—juvenile xanthogranuloma; LCH—Langerhans cell histiocytosis; NLCH—non–Langerhans cell histiocytosis; PNH—progressive nodular histiocytosis.

© 1995 Current Science ISBN 1-85922-686-8 ISSN 1068–381X

It is well known that the management of LCH depends on the organ involved and the extent and severity of the disease. In cases of aggressive disease with organ dysfunction, monochemotherapy with vinblastine or more recently with etoposide [5] is the treatment of choice. Both in children and adults, etoposide may be used at the dosage of 100 to 200 mg/m² daily for 3 days, repeated every 3 to 4 weeks for four to eight cycles.

Thomas *et al.* [6•] reported the successful treatment of adult LCH with thalidomide. Two patients with papular manifestations associated with diabetes insipidus and involving the perianal region, axilla, and groin were treated with thalidomide (100 mg/d for 1 month). Improvement of the cutaneous manifestations was dramatic, and there were no side effects. Dosages can be reduced to 50 mg/d after 1 month, and treatment can be stopped after 1 or 2 additional months. The mechanism by which thalidomide acts is not known; it is believed, however, that thalidomide has not only an immunomodulatory action, but also an anti-inflammatory function. The skin would therefore be the main target of the drug. In fact, in both patients, the diabetes insipidus itself and associated visceral lesions were not modified by this therapy.

Last, an important report concerning the pathogenesis of LCH was published by Leahy *et al.* [7••], who demonstrated that human herpesvirus 6 DNA was present in the lesions of 14 (47%) of 30 patients with LCH. They also found the virus in 10 (63%) of 16 patients with extracutaneous disease and in 4 of 14 patients with disease limited to the bone. Although the presence of a virus alone does not establish a causal role in the disease, it supports a possible etiologic relationship. Human herpesvirus 6 may be an agent in the initiation of LCH-activating histiocytes or in the modification of the immunoregulation of histiocytic proliferation.

Non–Langerhans cell histiocytosis (non-X histiocytosis)

Juvenile xanthogranuloma

Juvenile xanthogranuloma (JXG) is the most common non–Langerhans cell histiocytosis (NLCH) in childhood. Two main clinical forms have been described: a small nodular form and a large nodular form. Caputo *et al.* [8•] reported on a few variants of the disease, which are unique for the type, distribution, location, and course of the lesions.

The mixed form of JXG is characterized by the simultaneous presence of both small and large nodules (Fig. 1). Because the small nodular form of JXG may be associated in 20% of patients with a family history of neurofibromatosis, it is important when dealing with the mixed form of JXG to determine that the large nodular lesions are not neurofibromas.

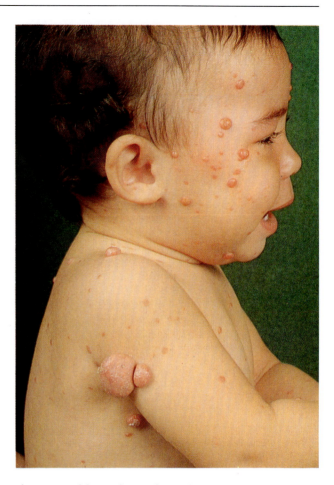

Fig. 1. Mixed form of juvenile xanthogranuloma. Both nodular and popular variants are present.

It is well known that the lesions of JXG, when multiple, are irregularly scattered on the skin, without the tendency to cluster. The term *JXG en plaque* is used to define a group of JXG lesions as the only expression of the disease (Fig. 2). Up to now, only two such cases have been described.

The large nodular form of JXG is marked by one or a few lesions. In the same report, Caputo *et al.* provided the first description of "Cyrano nose" in JXG, which they named for the giant, congenital JXG located on the nose (Fig. 3). At birth, the tumor was firm, purple-red in color, centrally ulcerated, and covered by a hematic crust. During the next 3 years, the tumor became softer and more xanthomatous and developed evident telangiectases.

Botella-Estrada *et al.* [9] reported on JXG lesions with central nervous system involvement in a 10-year-old child. The lesions were clinically manifested by a significant loss of memory in the patient and instrumentally demonstrated through computed tomography and magnetic resonance imaging. Such cases may be fatal or remain totally asymptomatic throughout the patient's life.

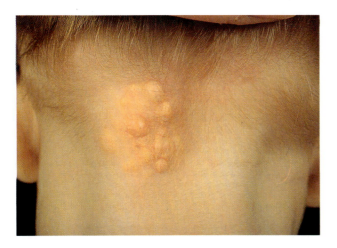

Fig. 2. Clustered juvenile xanthogranuloma, or juvenile xanthogranuloma *en plaque*.

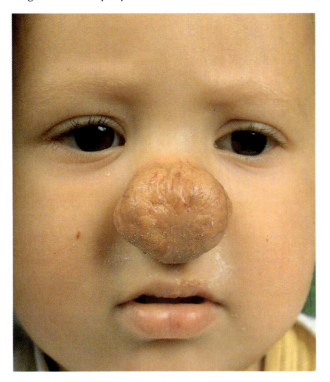

Fig. 3. "Cyrano nose" due to juvenile xanthogranuloma.

Xanthogranuloma in adults is very rare. It usually appears in the macronodular form with one or few lesions, and it almost never shows any extracutaneous involvement. Konohana *et al.* [10] provided the first description of multiple adult xanthogranuloma with lesions involving the conjunctiva, oral mucosa, and genitalia.

The question of why the foamy cells that constitute the main part of the xanthogranuloma accumulate lipids despite normal levels of plasma lipids has been addressed by Bergman *et al.* [11•]. These authors studied the degradation rates of ^{125}I-labeled low-density lipoprotein and the rate of intracellular cholesterol synthesis in human monocyte-derived macrophages of

adult patients with xanthogranuloma. The uptake of low-density lipoprotein cholesterol and the biosynthesis of intracellular cholesterol were both enhanced. Such enhancement might play a role in the process of accumulation of cholesterol esters in the macrophages that form the xanthogranuloma lesions.

Benign cephalic histiocytosis

Benign cephalic histiocytosis (BCH) (Fig. 4) is a maculopapular, benign, nonlipid NLCH characterized by 1) onset during the first three years of life, 2) location principally on the head without lesions on the mucous membranes, the palmoplantar surface or the viscera, and 3) spontaneous regression during childhood without sequelae. Two cases of BCH were reported in 1993 [12,13] bringing the number of cases described to approximately 30.

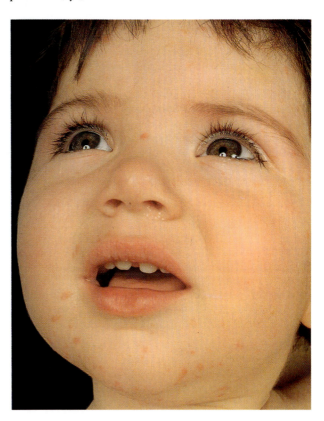

Fig. 4. A typical case of benign cephalic histiocytosis.

Benign cephalic histiocytosis versus generalized eruptive histiocytosis

Some cases initially diagnosed as BCH subsequently develop the diffuse papular lesions associated with generalized eruptive histiocytosis (GEH), and histopathologic findings in both forms are very similar. Some authors therefore believe that BCH is a localized form of GEH. In an attempt to clarify this problem, Gianotti *et al.* [14•] performed a blind histologic study with 18 biopsy specimens obtained from 14 patients affected by BCH in comparison with four biopsies of GEH, 11 of papular xanthoma, and 25 of JXG. A close histologic relationship was observed among

BCH, GEH, and JXG in their early, nonxanthomatous stages. These data suggest that BCH might be a localized form of GEH or an aborted phase of JXG. It is still to be determined why BCH has so far been reported only in children and why GEH occurs mostly in adults, and the mucous membranes are involved in adults only.

Progressive nodular histiocytosis

Progressive nodular histiocytosis (PNH) is a very rare histiocytosis (approximately 10 cases have been reported) characterized by the progressive appearance of widespread papules and nodules that on the face tend to merge, causing a leonine appearance. The disease is disfiguring, but the general health of the patient remains good. Histologically, the histiocytes forming the infiltrate show abundant, vacuolated, clear eosinophilic cytoplasm and irregular nuclei; multinucleated giant cells may be present.

Torres *et al.* [15] confirmed the close relationship from a histologic and ultrastructural point of view between multicentric reticulohistiocytosis and PNH. From their point of view, PNH could represent a clinical variant of multicentric reticulohistiocytosis. This observation is supported by the work of Flaming and Weigand [16] in which a patient with multicentric reticulohistiocytosis was reported to show a leonine face.

Conclusions

There were three main advances in the field of LCH during 1993: 1) the observation that human herpesvirus 6 may represent the triggering factor for the proliferating cells, 2) the possible discovery of a prognostic index to evaluate the aggressiveness of histiocytic disease by cell positivity to an antibody against the proliferating cell nuclear antigen, and 3) the discovery that thalidomide is useful in treating the cutaneous lesions of LCH.

Non–Langerhans cell histiocytosis remains a fascinating, astonishing, and relatively unknown field. Every year, new varieties of NLCH are described as the mixed form or the *en plaque* form of JXG. Nevertheless, histologic findings from a large number of cases have confirmed that many forms of NLCH with peculiar clinical features are in fact closely related.

From our point of view, NLCH with prevalent cutaneous involvement can be divided into three groups: 1) benign, commonly self-healing diseases including JXG, BCH, GEH, papular xanthoma, and xanthoma disseminatum, all of which might represent a wide spectrum of clinical features for a single entity; 2) reticulohistiocytosis (progressive nodular histiocytosis is a possible clinical aspect) with a typical clinical course and histologic and ultrastructural aspects; 3) sinus histiocytosis marked by peculiar symptomatology, clinical features, histologic appearance, and immunohistochemical features, *ie*, S100 positivity and CD1a negativity.

References and recommended reading

Papers of particular interest, published within the annual period of review, have been highlighted as:
- •   Of special interest
- ••   Of outstanding interest

1. Bonifazi E: **Place des Histiocytoses auto-involutives au Sein des Histiocytoses Langerhansienses.** *Ann Dermatol Venereol* 1992, 119:397–402.
2. Enjolras O, Leibowitch M, Bonacini F, Vacher-Lavenu MC, Escande JP: **Histiocytoses Langerhansiennes congenitales cutanées: à propos de 7 Cas.** *Ann Dermatol Venereol* 1992, 119:111–117.
3. •• Helm KF, Lookingbill DP, Marks JG Jr: **A Clinical and Pathologic Study of Histiocytosis X in Adults.** *J Am Acad Dermatol* 1993, 29:166–170.
An antibody against a protein found in most proliferating cells (proliferating cell nuclear antigen) might provide an index of aggressiveness of the disease. A relationship might exist between a higher percentage of proliferating cell nuclear antigen–positive histiocytes and progressive skin disease or systemic manifestations. A strong positivity for this antibody could be a useful prognostic marker.
4. • Maarten Egeler R, Neglia JP, Puccetti DM, Brennan CA, Nesbit ME: **Association of Langerhans Cell Histiocytosis With Malignant Neoplasms.** *Cancer* 1993, 71:865–873.
This literature review demonstrates that an association between LCH and malignant neoplasms could exist, particularly with lymphomas, leukemias, and lung tumors. However, the latency of the malignant neoplasm after the diagnosis of LCH suggests a therapy-related process.
5. Tsele E, Thomas M, Chu AC: **Treatment of Adult Langerhans Cell Histiocytosis With Etoposide.** *J Am Acad Dermatol* 1992, 27:61–64.
6. • Thomas L, Ducros B, Secchi T, Balme B, Moulin G: **Successful Treatment of Adult's Langerhans Cell Histiocytosis With Thalidomide.** *Arch Dermatol* 1993, 129:1261–1264.
A successful treatment of adult LCH with thalidomide is reported. Improvement of the cutaneous manifestations was dramatic, and there were no side effects.
7. •• Leahy MA, Krejci SM, Friednash M, Stockert SS, Wilson H, Huff JC, Weston WL, Brice SL: **Human Herpesvirus 6 Is Present in Lesions of Langerhans Cell Histiocytosis.** *J Invest Dermatol* 1993, 101:642–645.
Demonstrates that human herpesvirus 6 DNA may be present in lesions of patients with LCH. The virus may be involved in initiating LCH by activating histiocytes or modifying immunoregulation of histiocytic proliferation.
8. • Caputo R, Grimalt R, Gelmetti C, Cottoni F: **Unusual Aspects of Juvenile Xanthogranuloma.** *J Am Acad Dermatol* 1993, 29:868–870.
Three clinical variants of JXG, unique for the type, distribution, location, and course of the lesions are described: a mixed form of JXG, JXG *en plaque*, and Cyrano nose.
9. Botella-Estrada R, Sanmartin O, Grau M, Alegre V, Mas C, Aliaga A: **Juvenile Xanthogranuloma With Central Nervous System Involvement.** *Pediatr Dermatol* 1993, 10:64–68.
10. Konohana A, Noda J, Koimuzi M: **Multiple Xanthogranulomas in an Adult.** *Clin Exp Dermatol* 1993, 18:462–463.
11. • Bergman R, Aviram M, Shemer A, Oikine Y, Vardi DA, Friedman-Birnbaum R: **Enhanced Low-Density Lipoprotein Degradation and Cholesterol Synthesis in Monocyte-Derived Macrophages of Patients With Adult Xanthogranulomatosis.** *J Invest Dermatol* 1993, 101:880–882.
The uptake of low-density lipoprotein cholesterol and the biosynthesis of intracellular cholesterol were both enhanced in human monocyte-derived macrophages of patients with adult xanthogranuloma. Such enhancement might play a role in the process of accumulation of cholesterol esters in the macrophages that form the xanthogranuloma lesions.
12. Goday JJ, Raton JA, Landa N, Eizaguirre X, Dial-Perez JL: **Benign Cephalic Histiocytosis: Study of a Case.** *Clin Exp Dermatol* 1993, 18:280–282.
13. Hogan PA, Morelli JG, Weston WL: **An 18-Month-Old Boy With a Persistent Popular Eruption.** *Pediatr Dermatol* 1993, 10:195–197.
14. • Gianotti R, Alessi E, Caputo R: **Benign Cephalic Histiocytosis: A Distinct Entity or a Part of a Wide Spectrum of Histiocytic Proliferative Disorders of Children?** *Am J Dermatopathol* 1993, 15:315–319.
A blind histological study of BCH in comparison with GEH, papular xanthoma, and JXG suggests that BCH might be a localized form of GEH or an aborted phase of JXG.
15. Torres L, Sanchez JL, Ribera A, Gonzalez A: **Progressive Nodular Histiocytosis.** *J Am Acad Dermatol* 1993, 29:278–280.
16. Flaming JA, Weigand DA: **Unusual Case of Multicentric Reticulohistiocytosis.** *Int J Dermatol* 1993, 32:125–127.

Ruggero Caputo, MD, Prima Clinica Dermatologica, Via Pace 9, 20122 Milano, Italy.

Pigmented and adnexal disorders

Edited by

Jean L. Bolognia
Yale University School of Medicine
New Haven, Connecticut, USA

CURRENT SCIENCE

Update on incontinentia pigmenti

Julie S. Francis, MD, and Virginia P. Sybert, MD

University of Washington School of Medicine and Children's Hospital and Medical Center, Seattle, Washington, USA

This article reviews the recent literature and updates the reader on the current concepts concerning incontinentia pigmenti. Cutaneous manifestations and histopathologic findings are reviewed. Extracutaneous findings are summarized, and emphasis is placed on those in which timely intervention is important. The genetics of incontinentia pigmenti are reviewed, including the mode of inheritance and recent advances in genetic mapping. The differential diagnosis and appropriate management strategies are also discussed.

Current Opinion in Dermatology 1995:55–60

Incontinentia pigmenti (Bloch-Sulzberger syndrome) is an inherited multisystem disorder with a constellation of unique cutaneous findings (Table 1) [1,2,3••]. Described by Bloch [4] and Sulzberger [5] in the 1920s, incontinentia pigmenti remains a fascinating and complex disorder whose underlying basic defect is unknown. The recent literature on incontinentia pigmenti is reviewed for the dermatologist, who plays a pivotal role in the diagnosis and appropriate management of patients with this disorder.

Cutaneous findings

Incontinentia pigmenti classically presents with blisters in the first few weeks of life. The blisters can occur in crops, are grouped on an erythematous base, and are scattered over the body in swirls and patches along the lines of Blaschko (Fig. 1) [6]. This first stage resolves over a period of several weeks to months, and then begins the second phase, which consists of warty, hyperkeratotic plaques on an erythematous base that can also erupt in patches and swirls (Fig. 2). The distribution can be similar to that seen in the first stage but is not necessarily identical. This stage also resolves over time. The third stage of incontinentia pigmenti is characterized by streaks and whorls of brown, tan, or slate-gray pigmentation distributed along the lines of Blaschko (Fig. 3). It can occur in areas unaffected by previous stages. This macular pigmentation often fades and is replaced by the fourth stage of incontinentia pigmenti, hypopigmented atrophic areas in which hair follicles and eccrine glands may be absent (Fig. 4). All four cutaneous phases may occur simultaneously or overlap, and patients may first present with any stage.

Table 1. Cutaneous manifestations of incontinentia pigmenti

Stage	Clinical features	Histopathologic features
I	Erythema, papules, vesicles in swirls and patches	Intercellular edema, intraepidermal vesicles with numerous eosinophils, scattered dyskeratotic keratinocytes, whorls of abnormal keratinization
II	Warty, hyperkeratotic erythematous plaques in patches and lines	Acanthosis and hyperkeratosis, whorls of abnormal epidermal keratinization, dyskeratotic cells
III	Streaks and whorls of brown, tan, or slate-gray pigmentation	Basal layer degeneration, dermal macrophages loaded with melanin
IV	Hypopigmented atrophic streaks devoid of appendages	Thinned, effaced epidermis, absence of epidermal appendages

Other cutaneous features seen in some, but not all, patients with incontinentia pigmenti include a diffuse alopecia, primarily of the vertex of the scalp, often associated with scarring (Fig. 5); and nail dystrophy. The nail dystrophy is variable and ranges from mild ridging or pitting of the nail plate to thickened, dystrophic nails involving most of the nails on the hands and feet [2,3••].

Extracutaneous findings

Although the diagnosis of incontinentia pigmenti is based on the unique constellation of cutaneous findings, it is the extracutaneous manifestations that are most problematic to the patients, and they are important considerations in patient management and genetic counseling.

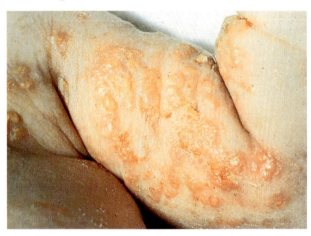

Fig. 1. Stage I incontinentia pigmenti is characterized by erythema and vesicles along the lines of Blaschko. (*From* Sybert and Holbrook [43]; with permission.)

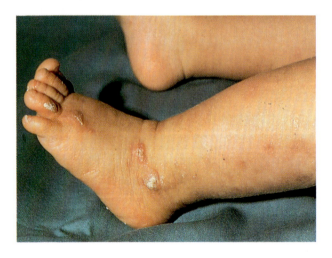

Fig. 2. Stage II incontinentia pigmenti is characterized by linear verrucous plaques.

Dental

Dental abnormalities have been described in almost 70% of patients with incontinentia pigmenti and can involve both deciduous and permanent teeth [1]. The abnormalities include hypodontia or anodontia, peg or conical deformities of the teeth, delayed eruption, and enamel disorders (Fig. 6). The enamel abnormalities

may predispose these individuals to multiple caries [7]. Dermatologists should become familiar with these dental abnormalities, because they may be the only residual clinical finding of incontinentia pigmenti in adult life.

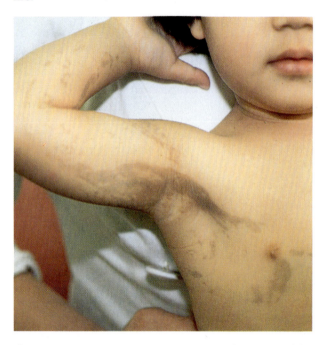

Fig. 3. Stage III incontinentia pigmenti is characterized by linear, brown-gray, streaky pigmentation.

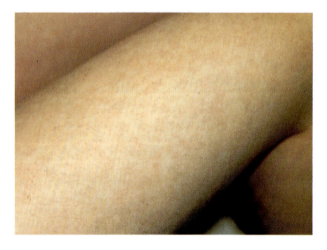

Fig. 4. Stage IV incontinentia pigmenti is characterized by hypopigmentation with atrophy.

Ophthalmologic

The ophthalmologic findings in incontinentia pigmenti are significant and occur in over one third of patients. There are both retinal and nonretinal findings, and involvement can be strikingly asymmetric [8••]. The retinal findings are the most important and specific of the ophthalmologic findings. Dysplasia of the neurosensory retina and retinal vessels results in areas of avas-

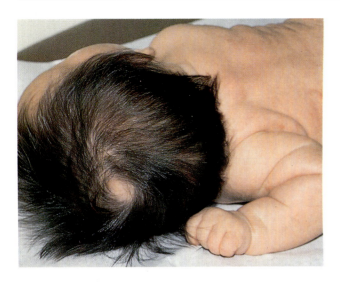

Fig. 5. Scarring alopecia of vertex of scalp occurs in some patients with incontinentia pigmenti.

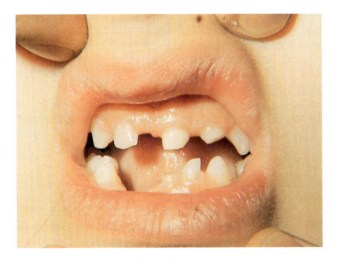

Fig. 6. Dental abnormalities (*eg*, hypodontia and peg and conical deformities) may be the only residual clinical finding of incontinentia pigmenti in adults.

cular retina. A reactive fibrovascular proliferation can ensue, and this can lead to scar formation, tractional retinal detachments, and loss of vision [9]. If the retinal vascular abnormalities are detected early, patients can be observed closely for the appearance of the abnormal fibrovascular proliferation, which, if found, may be treated with photocoagulation [10]. If fibrovascular proliferation is severe enough to cause retinal detachment, vitreoretinal surgery may successfully reattach the retina and restore vision [11•].

Other retinal abnormalities include foveal hypoplasia and abnormalities of the retinal pigment epithelium. Foveal hypoplasia (*ie*, hypoplasia of the central portion of the retina) is a newly recognized feature described in a recent series of patients with incontinentia pigmenti [8••], and its specificity to incontinentia pigmenti has yet to be determined. Alterations of the retinal pigment epithelium can vary from diffuse mottling to localized

areas of hypopigmentation. Histologic studies of the abnormal retinal pigment epithelium have shown accumulations of melanin-containing macrophages reminiscent of the cutaneous pigmentary stage of incontinentia pigmenti [6].

It requires an ophthalmologist comfortable with retinal pathology to detect and follow these ocular abnormalities in patients. Dermatologists should be aware that the presence of a large retinal detachment can be heralded by the finding of a white pupil (leukocoria) or strabismus, and in a patient with incontinentia pigmenti, these findings should be thoroughly evaluated.

Central nervous system

Mental retardation, seizures, hemiparesis, and spasticity can be devastating neurologic consequences of incontinentia pigmenti, and they have been reported in up to a third of patients [1]. In a recent series of 100 patients, fewer than 10% had neurologic deficits [3••]. In our clinical experience of 30 patients with incontinentia pigmenti, most of whom were referred because of skin findings and not because of developmental problems, 20% had neurologic impairment.

The pathogenesis of these central nervous system abnormalities is unknown. A current hypothesis suggests that a progressive destructive encephalopathy causes acute hemorrhagic necrosis, brain edema, and subsequent cerebral atrophy [12,13]. The encephalopathy appears to occur in the neonatal period, and those patients who do not develop seizures or abnormalities on imaging studies in infancy appear to have a good neurologic prognosis [2,3••]. Characteristic magnetic resonance imaging findings of acute hemorrhagic necrosis appear to correlate with the few reported neuropathologic findings in patients with incontinentia pigmenti [12]. A number of other magnetic resonance imaging and computed tomography findings have been reported [14•], but none appear to be specific.

Other abnormalities

There are occasional reports of a variety of structural malformations associated with incontinentia pigmenti, including skull deformities, short stature, cleft palate, and club foot [2]. These may be incidental findings and not part of the syndrome.

Histopathology

The histopathology depends on the stage of the cutaneous lesions [15]. In the inflammatory, blistering stage, there are intercellular edema and intraepidermal vesicles. Eosinophils are prominent in the vesicles and throughout the epidermis and dermis. Dyskeratotic keratinocytes are scattered throughout the epidermis, individually or in clusters, and small whorls of abnormal keratinization are seen. In the second cutaneous stage of incontinentia pigmenti, the epidermis is thickened and hyperkeratotic. The whorls of abnormal keratinization and dyskeratotic cells can be quite prominent in this stage. The pigmentary or third stage shows degeneration of the basal keratinocytes and melanin-loaded macrophages in the dermis, hence the condition's name. The fourth, atrophic stage shows a thinned, effaced epidermis and absence of epidermal appendages. Melanocytes are reduced in number in some patients. Round homogeneous eosinophilic bodies in the upper dermis have been described in this stage and are believed to represent degenerated basal keratinocytes [16,17].

Risk of malignancy

Laboratory studies of a small number of patients with incontinentia pigmenti have yielded conflicting results pertaining to an increased number of chromosome breaks in cultured cells. Some have demonstrated such an increase; others have failed to do so. Based on these reports and anecdotal reports of various malignancies in a few patients, one paper has suggested that there is an increased risk for malignancy in incontinentia pigmenti [18], but there is little evidence to support this contention.

Genetics

Mode of inheritance
Incontinentia pigmenti is an X-linked dominant disorder that is lethal in males. When the disorder occurs in a live-born male, it is thought to be due to a postzygotic mutation or the result of a half-chromatid mutation such that some of the cells have a normal gene on the X chromosome allowing survival [3••, 19]. Affected males with 47,XXY karyotype have been reported [20]. Carrier females usually express the disorder clinically, although their clinical features may be subtle. Pedigrees are characterized by an increased incidence of miscarriages (presumably of affected males), and a female-to-male ratio of 2 to 1 for offspring of carriers. The patchy distribution of the skin lesions is thought to result from tissue mosaicism secondary to random X inactivation. The X chromosome with the normal gene and one X chromosome with the incontinentia pigmenti gene are active in uninvolved and involved skin, respectively [6].

Studies have been done of patterns of X inactivation to determine if preferential cell selection exists against those cells expressing the defective incontinentia pigmenti gene. The studies are few in number, and the results are inconclusive [21–23].

Genetic mapping
The gene for incontinentia pigmenti has been mapped to the long arm of the X chromosome (Xq28) by linkage studies [24–27]. The recent literature is confusing, because chromosomal analyses of sporadic cases of females with pigment changes similar to those found in incontinentia pigmenti have shown X-autosome translocations with break points at Xp11 [28–30]. This observation has resulted in a nomenclature designation of incontinentia pigmenti 1 (IP-1), associated with Xp11 break points, and incontinentia pigmenti 2 (IP-

2), which is linked to Xq28. These new incontinentia pigmenti designations [25, 26, 31, 32] have been questioned because of the confusion they generate [33,34]. Of all the patients with "incontinentia pigmenti" characterized by X autosome translocations, only one had skin changes typical of incontinentia pigmenti. None of the others had blisters or verrucous changes, and their pigmentary abnormalities were consistent with those associated with chromosomal mosaicism. We believe the terms *incontinentia pigmenti 1* and *incontinentia pigmenti 2* should be withdrawn from the medical literature. The term *incontinentia pigmenti* should be reserved for the classic disorder described in this review, also known as the Bloch-Sulzberger syndrome, which has been mapped to Xq28. The multisystem conditions with pigmentary abnormalities that map to the Xp11 region await further investigation [35,36].

Diagnosis

Prenatal
Prenatal diagnosis is unreliable; the inconsistent distribution of skin lesions does not allow accurate diagnosis by fetal skin biopsy. In some families, linkage studies may be informative.

Differential
Each cutaneous stage of incontinentia pigmenti engenders a number of distinct differential diagnoses. Taken as a whole, there are few disorders that need to be considered in the differential diagnosis of incontinentia pigmenti:

1) Focal dermal hypoplasia of Goltz is an X-linked dominant disorder whose associated malformations are similar to incontinentia pigmenti [37]. The skin findings are distinct and consist of discrete linear areas of atrophic scarring with superimposed telangiectasias, perioral papillomas, and yellow-brown, soft nodules that represent areas of marked dermal hypoplasia and herniation of the subcutaneous fat. The linear streaks may also have areas of hypo- and hyperpigmentation.

2) Hypomelanosis of Ito is the term given to a heterogeneous group of disorders with pigmentary disturbances consisting of whorls and streaks of hypopigmentation or depigmentation following Blaschko's lines [30,38,39]. Approximately half of these individuals have multisystem involvement including ocular, skeletal, or neurologic abnormalities. A significant number of patients are mosaic for chromosomal abnormalities including trisomy 18, tetrasomy 12p, X-chromosome abnormalities, triploidy, and others. This disorder may be confused with incontinentia pigmenti by the uninformed because of its original name incontinentia pigmenti achromians. The skin pigmentation is not proceeded by blisters, inflammation, or verrucous plaques, and the family history is negative for other affected individuals.

3) Naegeli-Franceschetti-Jadassohn syndrome and dermatopathia pigmentosa reticularis are two pigmen-

tary disorders consisting of reticulate hyperpigmentation often associated with other cutaneous abnormalities such as alopecia, onychodystrophy, and dental malformations [40]. These conditions may be confused with incontinentia pigmenti, but they both have palmar-plantar hyperkeratosis, and both are autosomal dominant in inheritance. Neither has the cutaneous findings of the first, second or fourth stage of incontinentia pigmenti.

4) Linear and whorled nevoid hypermelanosis is characterized by reticulate hyperpigmentation that forms whorls and streaks that follow the lines of Blaschko [41]. This disorder is not inherited and differs histologically from the third stage of incontinentia pigmenti, and the skin pigmentation is not proceeded by blisters or verrucous plaques. Some patients with chromosomal mosaicism will have swirly hyperpigmentation [42] rather than hypopigmentation, but these patients should not be classified as having linear and whorled nevoid hypermelanosis. This is a benign disorder without multisystem involvement, and in an otherwise normal child, swirled hyperpigmentation is not an indication for chromosomal studies.

Management

Once the diagnosis of incontinentia pigmenti is made, dermatologists should be aware of management issues that can maximize quality of life in their patients:

1) Treatment of skin vesicles is usually not required, but the skin should be kept clean to prevent bacterial infection. Heat may exacerbate blistering in some patients.

2) Meticulous oral hygiene, preventative dental care, and dental restoration may be indicated. Parents should be informed that delayed eruption of teeth is common.

3) Complete ophthalmologic evaluation including indirect ophthalmoloscopy by an ophthalmologist familiar with incontinentia pigmenti should be performed at the time of diagnosis and regularly for the first few years of life. In our experience, infants with neurologic involvement are very likely to have ocular involvement.

4) A complete neurologic examination should be performed. If abnormalities are found, imaging studies and referral to a neurologist familiar with incontinentia pigmenti is recommended. Parents should be reassured if there is no evidence of central nervous system involvement or seizures in infancy.

5) Genetic counseling is invaluable in families in which the diagnosis of incontinentia pigmenti has been made. A woman with an affected child should be examined closely for clinical features of incontinentia pigmenti, especially stage IV changes, to determine if she is a carrier. Male infants with incontinentia pigmenti should be karyotyped for Klinefelter syndrome (47,XXY).

References and recommended reading

Papers of particular interest, published within the annual period of review, have been highlighted as:
- • Of special interest
- •• Of outstanding interest

1. Carney RG: **Incontinentia Pigmenti; A world Statistical Analysis.** *Arch Dermatol* 1976, 112:535–542.

2. Cohen BA: **Incontinentia Pigmenti.** *Neurol Clin* 1987, 5:361–377.

3. Landy SJ, Donnai D: **Incontinentia Pigmenti (Bloch-Sulzberger Syndrome).** *J Med Genet* 1993, 30: 53–59.
•• Concise review of the literature draws the experience of the authors, who have seen over 100 patients with incontinentia pigmenti.

4. Bloch B: **Eigentümliche bisher nicht beschriebene Pigmentakkektion (Incontinentia Pigmenti).** *Schweiz Med Wochenschr* 1926, 7:404.

5. Sulzberger MB: **Über eine bisher nicht beschriebene congenitale Pigmentanomalie (Incontinentia Pigmenti).** *Arch Dermatol Syphilol* 1927, 154:19–32.

6 Happle R: **The Lines of Blaschko: A Developmental Pattern Visualizing Functional X-Chromosome Mosaicism.** *Curr Probl Dermatol* 1987, 17:5–18.

7. Himelhoch DA, Scott BJ, Olsen RA: **Dental Defects in Incontinentia Pigmenti: Case Report.** *Pediatr Dent* 1987, 9:236–239.

8. Goldberg MF, Custis PH: **Retinal and Other Manifestations of Incontinentia Pigmenti (Bloch-Sulzberger Syndrome).** *Ophthalmology* 1993, 100:1645–1654.
•• Reports on the findings in a series of 13 patients with incontinentia pigmenti who underwent detailed ophthalmologic examinations.

9. Catalano RA: **Incontinentia Pigmenti.** *Am J Ophthalmol* 1990, 110:696–700.

10. Catalano RA, Lopatynsky M, Tasman WS: **Treatment of Proliferative Retinopathy Associated With Incontinentia Pigmenti.** *Am J Ophthalmol* 1990, 110: 701–702.

11. Wald KJ, Mehta MC, Katsumi O, Sabates NR, Hirose T: **Retinal Detachments in Incontinentia Pigmenti.** *Arch Ophthalmol* 1993, 111:614–617.
• Reports on the first successful surgical interventions for retinal detachment in patients with incontinentia pigmenti.

12. Chatkupt S, Gozo AO, Wolansky LJ, Sun S: **Characteristic MR Findings in a Neonate with Incontinentia Pigmenti.** *AJR Am J Roentgenol* 1993, 160:372–374.

13. Shuper A, Bruan RN, Singer HS: **Destructive Encephalopathy in Incontinentia Pigmenti: A Primary Disorder?** *Pediatr Neurol* 1990, 6:137–140.

14. Pont MS, Elster AD: **Lesions of Skin and Brain: Midern Imaging of the Neurocutaneous Syndromes.** *AJR Am J Roentgenol* 1992, 158:1193–1203.
• A general review which highlights the roles of some of the newer imaging techniques in the more common neurocutaneous syndromes.

15. Lever W, Schaumburg-Lever G: **Incontinentia Pigmenti.** In *Histopathology of the Skin*, edn 7. Edited by Morris A. Philadelphia: JB Lippincott Co.; 1990:93–95.

16. Nazzaro V, Brusasco A, Gelmetti C, Ermacora E, Caputo R: **Hypochromic Reticulated Streaks in Incontinentia Pigmenti: An Immunohistochemical and Ultrastructural Study.** *Pediatr Dermatol* 1990, 7:174–178.

17. Zillkens D, Mehringer A, Lechner W, Burg G: **Hypo- and Hyperpigmented Areas in Incontinentia Pigmenti: Light and Electron Microscopic Studies.** *Am J Dermatopathol* 1991, 13:57–62.

18. Roberts WM, Jenkins JJ, Moorhead EL II, Douglass EC: **Incontinentia Pigmenti, A Chromosomal Instability Syndrome, Is Associated With Childhood Malignancy.** *Cancer* 1988, 62:2370–2372.

19. Emery MM, Siegfried EC, Stone MS, Stone EM, Patil SR: **Incontinentia Pigmenti: Transmission From Father to Daughter.** *J Am Acad Dermatol* 1993, 29:368–372.

20. García-Dorado J, de Unamuno P, Fernàndez-Lòpez E, Veloz JS, Armijo M: Incontinentia Pigmenti: XXY Male With a Family History. *Clin Genet* 1990, **38**:128–138.

21. Migeon BR, Axelman J, Jan de Beur S, Valle D, Mitchell GA, Rosenbaum KN: Selection Against Lethal Alleles in Females Heterozygous for Incontinentia Pigmenti. *Am J Hum Genet* 1989, **44**:100–106.

22. Harris A, Collins J, Vetrie D, Cole C, Bobrow M: X Inactivation as a Mechanism of Selection Against Lethal Alleles: Further Investigation of Incontinentia Pigmenti and X Linked Lymphoproliferative Disease. *J Med Genet* 1992, **29**:608–614.

23. Coleman R, Genet SA, Harper JI, Wilkie AOM: Interaction of Incontinentia Pigmenti and Factor VIII Mutations in a Female With Biased X Inactivation, Resulting in Haemophilia. *J Med Genet* 1993, **30**:497–500.

24. Sefiani A, Abel L, Heuertz S, Sinnett D, Lavergne L, Labuda D, Hors-Cayla M: The Gene for Incontinentia Pigmenti Is Assigned to Xq28. *Genomics* 1989, **4**:427–429.

25. Sefiani A M'rad R, Simard L, Vincent A, Julier C, Holvoet-Vermaut L, Heuertz S, Dahl N, Stalder JF, Peter MO, Moraine C, Maleville J, Boyer J, Oberlè I, Labuda D, Hors Cayla MC: Linkage Relationship Between Incontinentia Pigmenti (IP2) and Nine Terminal X Long Arm Markers. *Hum Genet* 1991, **86**:297–299.

26. Scheuerle AE, Lewis RA, Levy ML, Nelson DL: Incontinentia Pigmenti Type 2: Confirmation of Linkage to Xq28 and Demonstration of a New Mutation [Abstract]. *Am J Hum Genet* 1993, **53**:1756.

27. Hydèn-Granskog C. Salonen R, von Koskull H: Three Finnish Incontinentia Pigmenti (IP) Families With Recombinations With the IP Loci at Xq28 and Xp11. *Hum Genet* 1993, **91**:185–189.

28. Hodgson SV, Neville B, Jones RWA, Fear C, Bobrow M: Two Cases of X/Autosome Translocation in Females With Incontinentia Pigmenti. *Hum Genet* 1985, **71**:231.

29. Cannizzaro LA, Hecht F: Gene for Incontinentia Pigmenti Maps to Band Xp11 with an (X;10) (p11;q22) Translocation. *Clin Genet* 1987, **32**:66–69.

30. Koiffmann CP, de Souza DH, Diament A, Ventura HB, Alves RS, Kihara S, Wajntal A: Incontinentia Pigmenti Achromians (Hypomelanosis of ITO, MIM 146150) Further Evidence of Localization at Xp11. *Am J Med Genet* 1993, **46**:529–533.

31. Tommerup N: Mendelian Cytogenetics: Chromosome Rearrangements Associated With Mendelian Disorders. *J Med Genet* 1993, **30**:713–727.

32. Bitoun P, Philippe C, Cherif M, Mulcahy M-T, Gilgenkrantz S: Incontinentia Pigmenti (Type I) and X;5 Translocation. *Ann Genet* 1992, **35**:51–54.

33. Happle R. Tentative Assignment of Hypomelanosis of Ito to 9q33→qer. *Hum Genet* 1987 **75**:98–99.

34. Sybert VP: Incontinentia Pigmenti Nomenclature. *Am J Hum Genet* 1994, in press.

35. Gorski JL, Boehnke M, Reyner EL, Burright EN: A Radiation Hybrid Map of the Proximal Short Arm of the Human X Chromosome Spanning Incontinentia Pigmenti 1 (IP1) Translocation Breakpoints. *Genomics* 1992, **14**:657–665.

36. Gorski JL, Burright EN, Reyner EL, Goodfellow PN, Burgess DL: Isolation of DNA Markers From a Region Between Incontinentia Pigmenti 1 (IP1) X-Chromosomal Translocation Breakpoints by a Comparative PCR Analysis of a Radiation Hybrid Subclone Mapping Panel. *Genomics* 1992, **14**:649–656.

37. Kegel MF: Dominant Disorders With Multiple Organ Involvement. *Dermatol Clin* 1987, **5**:205–219.

38. Sybert VP, Pagon RA, Donlan M, Bradley CM: Pigmentary Abnormalities and Mosaicism for Chromosomal Aberration: Association With Clinical Features Similar to Hypomelanosis of Ito. *J Pediatr* 1990, **116**:581–586

39. Sybert VP: Hypomelanosis of Ito. *Pediatr Dermatol* 1990, **7**:74–76.

40. Heimer II, WL, Brauner G, James WD: Dermatopathia Pigmentosa Reticularis: A Report of a Family Demonstrating Autosomal Dominant Inheritance. *J Am Acad Dermatol* 1992, **26**:298–301.

41. Alvarez J, Peteiro C, Toribio J: Linear and Whorled Nevoid Hypermelanosis. *Pediatr Dermatol* 1993, **10**:156–158.

42. Kubota Y, Shimura Y, Shimada S, Tamaki K, Amamiya S: Linear and Whorled Nevoid Hypermelanosis in a Child with Chromosomal Mosaicism. *Int J Dermatol* 1992, **31**:345–347.

43. Sybert VP, Holbrook KA: Prenatal Diagnosis and Screening *Dermatol Clin* 1987 **5**:17–41.

Julie S. Francis, MD, and Virginia P. Sybert, MD, Division of Dermatology, Children's Hospital and Medical Center, 4800 Sand Point Way NE, Ch-25, Seattle, WA 98105-0371, USA.

New treatment options for the patient with facial hyperpigmentation

Thomas G. Salopek, MD, and Kowichi Jimbow, MD, PhD

University of Alberta, Edmonton, Alberta, Canada

Facial hyperpigmentation is a common disorder, particularly in dark-colored individuals. There are a multitude of etiologic factors for facial hyperpigmentation, which clinically may be either circumscribed or a feature of a generalized disorder of hyperpigmentation. Histologically, pigmentation is the result of either an increased number of melanocytes or increased melanin, and it may be of either the epidermal or dermal type. Treatment options include management of the underlying dermatoses, as well as more specific therapies aimed at the increased skin pigmentation, such as camouflage, depigmenting creams, and various surgical procedures (ie, lasers, chemical peels, dermabrasion, and cryosurgery). The success of these different modalities depends on the underlying skin disorder, constitutive skin color, and various external factors (eg, sun exposure). The most recent advances in the treatment of facial hyperpigmentation are presented.

Current Opinion in Dermatology 1995:61–68

Facial hyperpigmentation is not uncommon, particularly in darkly pigmented individuals, and it can be a complex diagnostic problem. The factors responsible for facial hyperpigmentation are myriad. Facial hypermelanosis may represent a localized phenomenon, or it may be a manifestation of a generalized disorder of hyperpigmentation. In addition, it may be either acquired, hereditary, or developmental. Histologically, the hypermelanosis may be the result of increased pigment within the epidermis, dermis, or both. These findings in turn may be secondary to an increased number of melanocytes, an increased amount of melanin, or the presence of nonmelanin pigments (eg, tattoo pigment) [1•].

A classification system for facial hyperpigmentation that incorporates these features is presented in Table 1. Clinically, this approach is relevant in that it is often possible to distinguish epidermal from dermal hyperpigmentation after clinical examination and inspection with a Wood's lamp. Epidermal pigmentation is usually dark brown or black (Fig. 1), and it is accentuated under Wood's lamp examination. In contrast, dermal pigmentation is often slate-gray or blue (Fig. 2) and becomes less prominent after Wood's lamp examination. This distinction has therapeutic implications in that most medical treatment modalities are best suited to treat epidermal causes of hyperpigmentation, whereas surgical options may be effective for both epidermal and dermal types of hyperpigmentation. The most re-

cent advances in the treatment of benign pigmented lesions (Table 2) are reviewed in this paper.

General measures

Because hyperpigmentation is often aggravated by sun exposure, the need for photoprotection in the treatment of facial hypermelanosis should be emphasized. Use of a broad-spectrum sunscreen with a sun-protection factor greater than or equal to 15 should be started before the initiation of any specific treatment and continued indefinitely thereafter. Patients should be advised not to rely solely on sunscreens, particularly in light of recent concerns about their safety [2••,3•,4,5], and therefore they should be encouraged to minimize their exposure to the sun and to wear protective clothing such as a wide-brimmed hats when outdoors.

The importance of camouflage in the treatment of facial hyperpigmentation should not be forgotten [6]. Consultation with a cosmetician trained in dealing with medical disfigurement is a valuable adjuvant to the overall treatment regimen.

Medical treatment

Azelaic acid
Azelaic acid is a dicarboxylic acid originally isolated from *Pityrosporum ovale*, the organism responsible for

---

Abbreviations

MBEH—monobenzyl ether of hydroquinone; Nd:YAG—neodymium:yttrium-aluminum-garnet.

Table 1. Pathophysiology and clinical features of facial hyperpigmentation*

Pathophysiology		Clinical features	
Level of pigmentation	Histogenesis	Limited†	Widespread‡
Epidermal	Melanocytotic (increase in number of of melanocytes)	Lentigines syndromes (Peutz-Jeghers,§ and centrofacial) Lentigo maligna Lentigo maligna melanoma	Suntan Lentigines, simple and solar Lentigines syndromes (eg, LEOPARD syndrome, Carney's [NAME/LAMB] complex) Atypical mole syndrome
	Melanotic (increase in melanin)	Melasma (epidermal form) Periorbital hyperpigmentation (familial,** atopic dermatitis–related, associated with hyperthyroidism, idiopathic) Erythromelanosis follicularis facei et colli Postinflammatory hyperpigmentation Drugs (eg, phenytoin, oral contraceptives, estrogens)	Ephelides Café au lait macule¶ Cronkite-Canada syndrome Urticaria pigmentosa Porphyria cutanea tarda Drugs (eg, AZT, 5-fluorouracil, topical mechlorethamine, busulfan, topical carmustine, bleomycin)†† Addison's disease and Addison-like conditions†† Systemic diseases (hyperthyroidism, renal insufficiency, biliary cirrhosis) Hemochromatosis Pellagra Postinflammatory hyperpigmentation POEMS syndrome Scleroderma
Dermal	Melanocytic (increase in number of melanocytes) Melanotic (increase in melanin)	Nevus of Ota and its clinical variants Melasma (dermal form) Poikiloderma of Civatte Actinic lichen planus Lupus erythematosus Riehl's melanosis	Metastatic melanoma (cellular deposits) Fixed drug eruption Metastatic melanoma with melanogenuria Erythema dyschromicum perstans Pinta Postinflammatory hyperpigmentation Actinic lichen planus
	Nonmelanotic (melanin absent or minor component)	Tattoos Ochronosis (hydroquinone-induced) Apocrine chromhidrosis Drugs (eg, mercury-containing cosmetics)	Drugs (eg, amiodarone, phenothiazine,‡‡ minocycline,‡‡ antimalarials) Heavy metal (eg, bismuth, chrysiasis, argyria) Alkaptonuria (hereditary ochronosis) Hemosiderin§§

*Adapted from Mosher et al. [1•]; with permission.
†Generally limited to the head and neck region.
‡Generalized disorder with possible or frequent involvement of the face.
§Not all cases; some patients have normal number of melanocytes.
¶Also increase in number of melanocytes in some cases.
**Dermal melanin also seen.
††Often accentuated in sun-exposed areas.
‡‡Melanin or melanin-drug complex can play a significant role.
§§Seen in patients with hemochromatosis.
AZT—azidothymidine; POEMS—polyneuropathy, organomegaly, endocrinopathy, M protein, and skin.

pityriasis versicolor. It has been shown to be a competitive inhibitor of tyrosinase *in vitro*. Anecdotal evidence suggests it can be used successfully in the treatment of melasma and lentigo maligna [7]. Its precise mechanism of action in these conditions has yet to be elucidated.

In a randomized, double-blind study of 155 patients of Indo-Malay-Hispanic origin who suffered from melasma, those who were treated with 20% azelaic acid cream did markedly better than those treated with

2% hydroquinone cream [8]. After 24 weeks of treatment, 74% of the azelaic acid–treated patients showed good to excellent results; in contrast, only 19% of hydroquinone-treated patients had a similar response. Patients with both epidermal and mixed (*ie*, epidermal plus dermal) types of melasma responded to treatment with azelaic acid.

A second study comparing the efficacy of 20% azelaic acid cream with 4% hydroquinone cream for the treat-

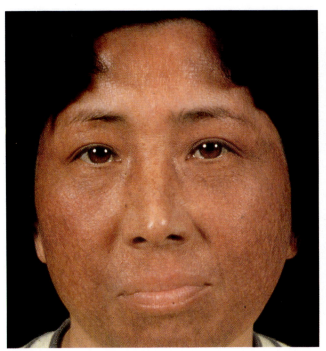 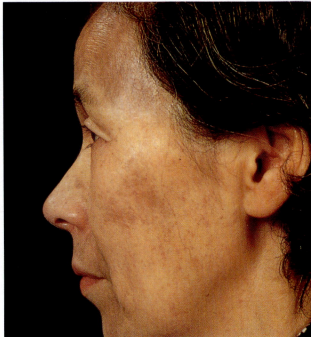

Fig. 1. Frontal (*left panel*) and lateral (*right panel*) views of facial pigmentation of melasma, which derives primarily from epidermal pigmentation and is therefore dark brown.

ment of melasma failed to demonstrate the superiority of azelaic acid [9]. In a 24-week double-blind study of 329 women, 65% of the azelaic acid–treated patients showed good to excellent results, and 73% of the hydroquinone group had similar results; the difference was not statistically significant. Azelaic acid was associated with fewer side-effects, however, which suggested that its use may be beneficial if prolonged treatment is necessary.

Retinoic acid

Tretinoin has been shown to lighten hyperpigmented macules associated with photoaging [10] and to inhibit melanogenesis *in vitro* [11]. Bulengo-Ransby *et al.* [12•] investigated the efficacy of topical tretinoin 0.1% cream in a 40-week randomized, double-blind, vehicle-controlled study in 54 black patients with postinflammatory facial hyperpigmentation of various etiologies. There was significant lightening of the pigmented lesions toward normal skin color in the treated patients, as judged by clinical evaluation and colorimetry. Histologically, there was a corresponding reduction in the epidermal melanin content in the lesions. Fifty percent of tretinoin-treated patients developed contact dermatitis, which did not alter the efficacy of the treatment and gradually diminished as the study progressed.

Phenolic thioethers

Phenolic thioethers represent a new family of depigmenting compounds related to catechols and phenols. These melanocytotoxic agents are derived from the sulfation of phenols and catechols to produce cysteinylphenol and cysteaminylphenol. A preliminary study of a 4% preparation of *N*-acetyl-4-*S*-cys-

teaminylphenol was conducted on 12 Japanese patients with melasma [13]. Marked to moderate improvement was seen in 11 patients after 2 to 4 weeks of topical application of the depigmenting agent. One patient showed complete clearance. The beneficial effects were still present after a mean follow-up period of 8.4 months. The compound appeared to be less irritating to the skin than hydroquinone.

Lasers

In that the treatment of pigmented lesions on the face is often done for cosmetic reasons, it is important that the treatment be the most effective, with the fewest complications. The treatment should therefore be directed toward selective destruction of pigment or pigment-containing cells, and it should produce the least amount of collateral damage [14•]. The selective photothermolysis of melanosomes and other pigments that is possible with lasers (Table 3) greatly minimizes the complications seen with other treatment modalities. As a result, lasers are quickly becoming the treatment of choice for many of the conditions responsible for facial hypermelanosis. Unfortunately, there is no one laser that will suffice in the treatment of all pigmented lesions [15••,16•,17,18].

Argon laser

The argon laser was one of the first lasers to be used for the treatment of benign pigmented lesions, and although satisfactory results have been obtained, its usefulness has been limited by problems with homogenous energy delivery and its inability to treat extensive areas rapidly [19•]. These shortcomings have been

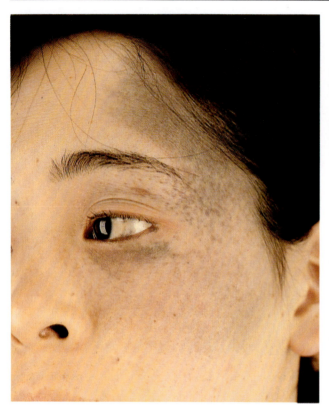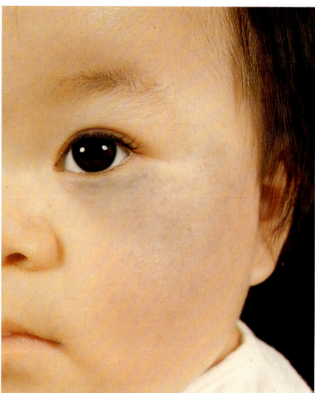

Fig. 2. Nevus of Ota in a young woman (*left panel*) and a child (*right panel*) shows bluish discoloration of the face (skin) and eye (conjunctiva), which derives primarily from dermal pigmentation.

remedied with the Hexascan (Lihtan Technologies, San Rafael, CA), an automated, hand-held scanning laser that allows for rapid, reproducible, homogenous treatment of large surface areas. Several pigmented lesions have improved dramatically after treatment with the Hexascan argon laser, including lentigines, ephelides, nevus spilus, Becker's nevus, and café au lait macules. Melasma responds somewhat inconsistently to the laser [20•]. Although the laser's pulse width (30 to 50 ms) is considerably longer than the thermal relaxation time of melanosomes (20 to 40 ns), it is thought that the microprocessor placement of treatment spots into larger and larger hexagonal grids allows for heat diffusion such that "pseudoselective" photothermolysis of pigment cells can occur. Heavily pigmented skin does not appear to be a contraindication, as long as lower fluences are used.

A recent modification of the argon laser that incorporates a dichroic filter into the unit allows for the use of the green line of the laser. Trelles *et al.* [21] used a monoline argon laser with a pulse width of 200 to 300 ms to treat 620 benign pigmented lesions (*eg*, solar lentigines, nevus spilus, ephelides, and café au lait macules). Satisfactory results were obtained with few complications despite the fact that the pulse width was significantly longer than the thermal relaxation time of melanosomes.

Q-switched ruby laser

The Q-switched ruby laser emits a red light at a wavelength of 694 nm for a pulse duration of 20 to 60 ns,

which is similar to the theoretic thermal relaxation time of melanosomes. Its long wavelength makes it well suited for the treatment of disorders associated with deep dermal pigmentation [22]. In addition, it has been used effectively in the treatment of epidermal hyperpigmentation seen in lesions such as ephelides and lentigines [23,24•,25•]. The removal of these pigmented lesions appears to be secondary to an injury to pigmented epidermal cells, which are then sloughed, and followed by reepithelialization. Other epidermal pigmentary anomalies, such as Becker's nevus and café au lait macules, also respond well to the Q-switched ruby laser [24•], although the results with the latter two conditions tend to be more unpredictable than those seen with ephelides and lentigines [25•]. Frequently, a second treatment is required to clear residual pigmentation at the border, presumably due to pigment that was inadvertently missed at the first treatment session [23]. In addition, hypopigmentation, hyperpigmentation, and repigmentation are not uncommon 6 to 12 months after the treatment. Melasma and nevus spilus respond erratically to the Q-switched ruby laser, with the best results in individuals with a fair complexion [23,25•].

The Q-switched ruby laser has proven itself effective in the treatment of various conditions associated with dermal pigment, such as tattoos [22] and nevus of Ota [26,27,28•]. In the latter condition, it has now become the treatment of choice [27,28•]. Because of the laser's long wavelength, pigmented melanocytes lying deep within the dermis are selectively destroyed by

Table 2. Treatment options for facial hyperpigmentation	
General measures	Cosmetic camouflage
	Sunscreens, sunblocks, sun avoidance
	Removal of precipitating or aggravating factors (*eg*, estrogens, photosensitizers)
Medical	Hydroquinone
	Salicylic acid
	Topical corticosteroids
	Retinoic acid
	Glycolic acid lotion, 10%
	Azelaic acid
	Phenolic thioethers
Surgical	Cryosurgery
	Chemical peels
	Resorcinol
	Trichloroacetic acid
	Phenol
	α-Hydoxy acids (*eg*, glycolic acid)
	Jessner's solution
	Lasers
	Candela* (510-nm pigmented lesion dye laser)
	Copper vapor
	Q-switched ruby
	Q-switched Nd:YAG (1064 nm; frequency-doubled 532 nm)
	Argon (Hexascan† and monoline)
	Dermabrasion
	Cold-steel surgery

*Candela Laser Corp., Wayland, MA.
†Lihtan Technologies, San Rafael, CA.
Nd:YAG—neodymium:yttrium-aluminum-garnet.

the laser, with no injury to the overlying epidermis. Generally, several treatments (average number approximately four) are required to produce satisfactory results.

Q-switched neodymium: yttrium-aluminum-garnet laser

The Q-switched neodymium:yttrium-aluminum-garnet (Nd:YAG) laser emits a light within the infrared spectrum at a wavelength of 1064 nm, which allows for the treatment of lesions with pigment located deep within the dermis [29]. Several studies have shown that the Nd:YAG laser works as well as if not better than the Q-switched ruby laser in the treatment of tattoos, with fewer complications [29,30•]. In addition, tattoos that were resistant to Q-switched ruby laser treatment have improved with the Q-switched Nd:YAG laser [30•,31•].

Frequency-doubled Q-switched neodymium: yttrium-aluminum-garnet laser

The frequency-doubled Q-switched Nd:YAG laser, in which a frequency-doubling crystal halves the wavelength from 1064 to 532 nm, is a recent addition to the laser surgeon's armamentarium [30•]. The light emitted falls within the green portion of visible light spectrum and is well absorbed by red pigment, which has been difficult to treat with other lasers, particularly the Q-switched ruby laser [16•]. In addition, melanin absorbs

well in this region of the visible spectrum, which permits the treatment of epidermal pigmented lesions. The frequency-doubled Q-switched Nd:YAG laser is, however, less effective for blue-black tattoos than either the Q-switched Nd:YAG or Q-switched ruby laser.

Candela laser (pigmented lesion dye laser)

The Candela pigmented lesion dye laser (Candela Laser Corp., Wayland, MA) emits green light at a wavelength of 510 nm for a pulse width of 300 to 400 ns. The wavelength and pulse duration allow for selective photothermolysis of melanosomes within superficial pigmented lesions [32,33•].

Fitzpatrick *et al.* [34•] treated 65 patients with various benign pigmented lesions using the Candela laser. Lesions included café au lait macules, lentigines, and postinflammatory hyperpigmentation. Ten (63%) of 16 patients with café au lait spots had 75% to 100% clearing after one to three treatments. Lentigines were somewhat more sensitive in that 81% of lesions showed 75% to 100% clearing. Postinflammatory hyperpigmentation also improved after the Candela laser treatment, although in general more treatments were required to obtain 100% clearing.

Other lesions that have improved following the use of the Candela laser include ephelides and red tattoo pigment [33•,35]. Melasma responded inconsistently to the laser treatments, which often resulted in postinflammatory hyperpigmentation [33•]. Hemosiderin deposition has been reported to clear with the Candela laser treatment [36].

Copper vapor laser

The copper vapor laser emits simultaneously at two wavelengths of equal intensity, 511 nm (green light) and 578 nm (yellow light). The desired wavelength can be selected using a filter that enables one to change from yellow light for vascular lesions to green light for epidermal pigmented lesions. The copper vapor laser is effective in the treatment of various disorders associated with epidermal pigment including ephelides, lentigines, and café au lait macules. The results are generally no better than those obtained with more cost-effective modalities such as liquid nitrogen cryosurgery or other lasers [37•]. Hyperpigmentation secondary to hemosiderin deposition may benefit from the copper vapor laser [38].

Chemical peels

The area of chemexfoliation has seen marked growth in recent times in response to the public's demand for improved facial esthetics. This increased interest has resulted in improved methodology, making chemexfoliation a safe and efficient means to correct textural and pigmentary changes of the skin [39,40•].

Glycolic acid peels

α-Hydroxy acids are a group of organic acids that include compounds such as lactic acid and glycolic acid.

Table 3. Lasers useful in the treatment of facial hyperpigmentation

Laser type*	Wavelength, nm	Beam features	Indications

Hexascan† argon [19•,20•]	514	Continuous wave, pulse width of 30–50 ms at fluence of 10–12 J/cm²	Epidermal
			  Ephelides
			  Café au lait macules
			  Lentigines
			  Nevus spilus
			  Becker's nevus
			  Melasma (variable)
			  (Heavily pigmented patients may be treated)

Monoline argon [21]	514	Continuous wave, pulse width of 200–300 ns	Epidermal
			  Solar or senile lentigines
			  Ephelides
			  Café au lait macules
			  Nevus spilus

Q-switched ruby [22,23,24•,25•, 26,27,28•]	694	Q-switched, pulse width 20–60 ns	Epidermal
			  Ephelides
			  Café au lait macules
			  Lentigines
			  Nevus spilus
			  Becker's nevus
			  Melasma (variable)
			Dermal
			  Tattoos, particularly with blue, black, and green pigment (amateur tattoos respond better than professional tattoos)
			  Nevus of Ota

Q-switched Nd:YAG [29,30•,31•]	1064	Q-switched, pulse width of 10 ns	Dermal
			  Tattoos (blue and black pigment)
			  Nevus of Ota

Frequency doubled Q-switched Nd:YAG [16•,30•]	532	Q-switched, pulse width of 10 ns	Epidermal
			  Solar or senile lentigines
			  Ephelides
			  Café au lait macules
			  Nevus spilus
			Dermal
			  Red pigment tattoos

Candela‡ (flash-lamp pulsed tunable dye) [32,33•,34•,35,36]	510	Pulse width of 300–400 ns, fluence of 2–4 J/cm²	Epidermal
			  Ephelides
			  Café au lait macules
			  Lentigines
			  Melasma
			  Nevus spilus
			  Becker's nevus
			Dermal
			  Red tattoo pigment
			  Hemosiderin deposition

Copper vapor [37•,38]	511	Continuous pulse width 20 ns with 67-μs intervals between pulses	Epidermal
			  Ephelides
			  Café au lait macules
			  Lentigines
			  Nevus spilus
			Dermal
			  Hemosiderin deposition

*Numbers in *brackets* indicate references in which individual lasers are discussed.
†Lihtan Technologies, San Rafael, CA.
‡Candela Laser Corp., Wayland, MA.
Nd:YAG—neodymium:yttrium-aluminum-garnet.

Their specific mode of action has yet to be elucidated, but it has been shown that they can induce the discohesion of keratinocytes.

Glycolic acid peels at concentrations of 50% to 70% are a safe and effective method for treating facial pigmen-tary disorders such as melasma and lentigines [41]. Both conditions respond well to the peel, although lentig-ines generally require higher concentration and longer application times. The effectiveness of the peel can be enhanced by the use of 10% to 15% glycolic acid lotion with or without hydroquinone (2%) in the pretreatment period. Dark-colored skin does not appear to be a contraindication to the use of glycolic acid peels.

Resorcinol

Resorcinol (*m*-dihydroxybenzene), an isomer of catechol and hydroquinone, was one of the first chemical peels to be used. It is usually compounded with zinc oxide and ceyssatite in benzoinated axungia at a 50% concentration. At this strength, it results in medium-depth peel. In contrast to other peels, it can be used safely in skin types I to V. It has been useful in the treatment of postinflammatory pigmentary changes due to acne, as well as melasma, freckles, and solar lentigines [42].

Dermabrasion

Seventeen Japanese patients with nonhairy melanocytic macules (thought to represent nevus spilus in Asians) were treated with dermabrasion followed by 5% monobenzyl ether of hydroquinone (MBEH) cream and sunscreen [43]. Fifteen of the dermabraded patients who used MBEH cream and sunscreens postoperatively showed good to excellent cosmesis (82%). In contrast, 40% of patients treated with dermabrasion alone had fair results, and 50% of those treated with MBEH cream and sunscreen had good results. The only complication was hypopigmentation, which occurred in one patient. It is important to remember that MBEH is currently recommended only for the treatment of widespread vitiligo, given the risk of permanent depigmentation at the site of application, as well as at distant sites.

Conclusions

Facial hyperpigmentation is a common problem for which, until recently, there have been few effective treatment options available. Improvements in laser technology and chemexfoliaton methodology represent substantial therapeutic advances in the management of facial hypermelanosis.

References and recommended reading

Papers of particular interest, published within the annual period of review, have been highlighted as:
- Of special interest
- Of outstanding interest

1. Mosher DB, Fitzpatrick TB, Hori Y, Ortonne J-P: **Disorders of Pigmentation**. In *Dermatology in General Medicine*, edn. 4. Edited by Fitzpatrick TB, Eisen AZ, Wolff K, Freedberg IM, Austen KF. New York: McGraw-Hill; 1993:903–995.
Well-written, comprehensive review of disorders of pigmentation. A logical approach to such conditions is presented early in the discussion.

2. Wolf P, Donawho CK, Kripke ML: **Effect of Sunscreens on UV Radiation–Induced Enhancement of Melanoma Growth in Mice**. *J Natl Cancer Inst* 1994, 86:99–105.
Sunscreens have been shown to protect against nonmelanoma skin cancers in rodents. It is generally thought that they also protect against melanoma by preventing sunburns. A murine model is used to show that protection against sunburn does not necessarily confer protection against ultraviolet radiation–induced enhancement of melanoma growth. In fact, sunscreen protection against sunburns may encourage prolonged exposure to ultraviolet radiation and thus increase the risk for developing melanoma.

3. Garland CF, Garland FC, Gorham ED: **Rising Trends in Melanoma: An Hypothesis Concerning Sunscreen Effectiveness**. *Ann Epidemiol* 1993, 3:103–110.
The effectiveness of sunscreens in preventing skin cancers is questioned. The authors suggest that traditional methods of minimizing sun exposure may be more prudent than relying on sunscreens.

4. Knowland J, McKenzie EA, McHugh PJ, Cridland NA: **Sunlight-Induced Mutagenicity of a Common Sunscreen Ingredient**. *FEBS Lett* 1993, 324:309–313.

5. Setlow RB, Grist E, Thompson K, Woodhead AD: **Wavelengths Effective in the Induction of Malignant Melanoma**. *Proc Natl Acad Sci U S A* 1993, 90:6666–6670.

6. Westmore MG: **Make-Up as an Adjunct and Aid to the Practice of Dermatology**. *Dermatol Clin* 1991, 9:81–88.

7. Nazzaro-Porro M, Passi S, Zina G, Breathnach AS: **Ten Years' Experience of Treating Lentigo Maligna With Topical Azelaic Acid**. *Acta Derm Venereol (Stockh)* 1989, 143(suppl):49–57.

8. Verallo-Rowell VM, Verallo V, Graupe K, Lopez-Villafuerte L, Garcia-Lopez M: **Double-Blind Comparison of Azelaic Acid and Hydroquinone in the Treatment of Melasma**. *Acta Derm Venereol (Stockh)* 1989, 143(suppl):58–61.

9. Balina LM, Graupe K: **The Treatment of Melasma: 20% Azelaic Acid Versus 4% Hydroquinone Cream**. *Int J Dermatol* 1991, 30:893–895.

10. Weinstein GD, Nigra TP, Pochi PE, Savin RC, Allan A, Benik K, Jeffes E, Lufrano L, Thorne EG: **Topical Tretinoin for Treatment of Photodamaged Skin: A Multicenter Study**. *Arch Dermatol* 1991, 127:659–665.

11. Orlow SJ, Chakraborty A, Pawelek JM: **Retinoic Acid Is a Potent Inhibitor of Inducible Pigmentation in Murine and Hamster Melanoma Cell Lines**. *J Invest Dermatol* 1990, 94:461–464.

12. Bulengo-Ransby SM, Griffiths CEM, Kimbrough-Green CK, Kinkel LJ, Hamilton TA, Ellis CN, Voorhees JJ: **Topical Tretinoin (Retinoic Acid) Therapy for Hyperpigmented Lesions Caused by Inflammation of the Skin in Black Patients**. *N Engl J Med* 1993, 328:1438–1443.
Postinflammatory hyperpigmentation is a common and often severely disfiguring problem in highly pigmented individuals. Therapy has generally been unsatisfactory. This well-conducted, randomized, double-blind, vehicle-controlled study in 54 black patients with postinflammatory hyperpigmentation showed that tretinoin could significantly lighten lesions after 40 weeks of therapy ($P < 0.001$).

13. Jimbow K: **N-Acetyl-4-S-Cysteaminylphenol as a New Type of Depigmenting Agent for the Melanoderma of Patients With Melasma**. *Arch Dermatol* 1991, 127:1528–1534.

14. Hruza GJ, Geronemus RG, Dover JS, Arndt KA: **Lasers in Dermatology: 1993**. *Arch Dermatol* 1993, 129:1026–1035.
This is an excellent review article of the use of lasers in dermatology as of 1993.

15. Dover JS, Kilmer SL, Anderson RR: **What's New in Cutaneous Laser Surgery**. *J Dermatol Surg Oncol* 1993, 19:295–298.
With an ever increasing number of lasers available to the clinician, confusion abounds as to which laser is best suited for a particular problem. This timely review discusses the use of pulsed lasers for the treatment of benign pigmented epidermal and dermal lesions, as well as the treatment of vascular anomalies, photodynamic therapy, diode laser technology, and laser diagnostics.

16. Nelson JS: **Lasers: State of the Art in Dermatology**. *Dermatol Clin* 1993, 11:15–26.
An excellent review article that discusses laser-tissue interactions, the various types of lasers that are available, and the indications for their use.

17. Weber LA, Vidimos AT, McGillis ST, Bailin PL: **Laser Surgery**. *Clin Dermatol* 1992, 10:291–303.

18. Sheehan-Dare RA, Cotterill JA: **Lasers in Dermatology**. *Br J Dermatol* 1993, 129:1–8.

19. McBurney EI: **Clinical Usefulness of the Argon Laser for the 1990s**. *J Dermatol Surg Oncol* 1993, 19:358–362.
Despite the appearance of numerous lasers on the market in recent years, the argon laser continues to play an important role in the treatment of vascular and superficial pigmented lesions.

20. McDaniel DH: **Clinical Usefulness of the Hexascan: Treatment of Cutaneous Vascular and Melanocytic Disorders**. *J Dermatol Surg Oncol* 1993, 19:312–319.
Illustrates how the Hexascan argon laser is able to achieve "pseudoselective" photothermolysis. The laser delivers 1-mm circular treatment spots in a nonadjacent manner, assembling the spots into an enlarging hexagonal grid up to 13 mm in diameter.

21. Trelles MA, Verkruysse W, Pickering JW, Velez M, Sanchez J, Sala P: **Monoline Argon Laser (514 nm) Treatment of Benign Pigmented Lesions With Long Pulse Lengths.** *J Photochem Photobiol B* 1992, 16:357–65.

22. Reid WH, Miller ID, Murphy MJ, Paul JP, Evans JH: **Q-switched Ruby Laser Treatment of Tattoos: A 9-Year Experience.** *Br J Plast Surg* 1990, 43:663–669.

23. Taylor CR, Anderson RR: **Treatment of Benign Pigmented Epidermal Lesions by Q-switched Ruby Laser.** *Int J Dermatol* 1993, 32:908–912.

24. Nelson JS, Applebaum J: **Treatment of Superficial Cutaneous Pig-**
• **mented Lesions by Melanin-Specific Selective Photothermolysis Using the Q-switched Ruby Laser.** *Ann Plast Surg* 1992, 29:231–237.
The Q-switched ruby laser was an effective method of treating various benign pigmented lesions (*eg*, lentigines, café au lait macules, nevi spili, Becker's nevi, and ephelides). Scarring, textural, or pigmentary changes were not seen.

25. Goldberg DJ: **Benign Pigmented Lesions of the Skin: Treatment With**
• **the Q-switched Ruby Laser.** *J Dermatol Surg Oncol* 1993, 19:376–379.
Review article on the use of the Q-switched ruby laser in the treatment of epidermal and dermal causes of hypermelanosis.

26. Geronemus R: **Q-switched Ruby Laser Therapy of Nevus of Ota.** *Arch Dermatol* 1992, 128:1618–1622.

27. Goldberg D, Nychay S: **Q-switched Ruby Laser Treatment of Nevus of Ota.** *J Dermatol Surg Oncol* 1992, 18:817–821.

28. Lowe NJ, Wieder JM, Sawcer D, Burrows P, Chalet M: **Nevus of**
• **Ota: Treatment With High Energy Fluences of the Q-switched Ruby Laser.** *J Am Acad Dermatol* 1993, 29:997–1001.
Sixteen patients with nevus of Ota were treated with the Q-switched ruby laser at high energy fluences and short pulse width (28 ns). All patients showed 50% or greater improvement after an average of four treatments with no adverse sequelae noted. It as concluded that the Q-switched ruby laser is the treatment of choice for nevus of Ota.

29. DeCoste SD, Anderson RR: **Comparison of Q-switched Ruby and Q-switched Nd:YAG Laser Treatment of Tattoos.** *Lasers Surg Med* 1991, 3(suppl): 64.

30. Kilmer SL, Anderson RR: **Clinical Use of the Q-switched Ruby and the**
• **Q-switched Nd:YAG (1064 nm and 532 nm) Lasers for the Treatment of Tattoos.** *J Dermatol Surg Oncol* 1993, 19:330–338.
Excellent review article on the principles and indications for use of the Q-switched Nd:YAG (1064 and 532 nm) lasers.

31. Kilmer SL, Lee MS, Grevelink JM, Flotte TJ, Anderson RR: **The**
• **Q-switched Nd:YAG Laser Effectively Treats Tattoos: A Controlled, Dose-Response Study.** *Arch Dermatol* 1993, 129:971–978.
In a controlled, dose-response study, the Q-switched Nd:YAG laser was shown to remove black tattoos effectively. Multicolored tattoos responded minimally to treatment.

32. Tan OT, Morelli JG, Kurban AK: **Pulsed Dye Laser Treatment of Benign Cutaneous Pigmented Lesions.** *Lasers Surg Med* 1992, 12:538–542.

33. Grekin RC, Shelton RM, Geisse, Frieden I: **510-nm Pigmented Lesion**
• **Dye Laser: Its Characteristics and Clinical Uses.** *J Dermatol Surg Oncol* 1993, 19:380–387.
Excellent review article on the Candela laser, which discusses the principles of the laser and its clinical uses.

34. Fitzpatrick RE, Goldman MP, Ruiz-Esparaza J: **Laser Treatment of**
• **Benign Pigmented Epidermal Lesions Using a 300 Nsecond Pulse and 510 nm Wavelength.** *J Dermatol Surg Oncol* 1993, 19:341–347.
Sixty-five patients with 492 benign pigmented epidermal lesions were treated with the Candela 510-nm pigmented lesion dye laser. Over 70% of patients showed 75% to 100% clearing after one treatment.

35. Alster TS: **Treatment of Benign Epidermal Pigmented Lesions With the 510nm Pulsed Dye Laser: Further Clinical Experience and Treatment Parameters.** *Lasers Surg Med* 1993, 5(suppl):55.

36. Goldman MP: **Postsclerotherapy Hyperpigmentation: Treatment With a Flashlamp-Excited Pulsed Dye Laser.** *J Dermatol Surg Oncol* 1992, 18:417–422.

37. Dinehart SM, Wanter M, Flock S: **The Copper Vapor Laser for the**
• **Treatment of Cutaneous Vascular and Pigmented Lesions.** *J Dermatol Surg Oncol* 1993, 19:370–375.
Discusses the effectiveness of the copper laser in the treatment of benign pigmented lesions.

38. Thibault P, Wlodarczyk J: **Postsclerotherapy Hyperpigmentation: The Role Serum Ferritin Levels and the Effectiveness of Treatment With the Copper Vapor Laser.** *J Dermatol Surg Oncol* 1992, 18:47–52.

39. Matarasso SL, Glogau RG. **Chemical Face Peels.** *Dermatol Clin* 1991, 9:131–149.

40. Brody HJ: **Update on Chemical Peels.** *Adv Dermatol* 1992,
• 7:275–288.
Presents a succinct and up-to-date review on chemexfoliation.

41. Moy LS, Murad H, Moy RL: **Glycolic Acid Peels for the Treatment of Wrinkles and Photoaging.** *J Dermatol Surg Oncol* 1993, 19:243–246.

42. Karam PG: **50% Resorcinol Peel.** *Int J Dermatol* 1993, 32:569–5573.

43. Tezuka T, Saheki M, Kusuda S, Umemoto K: **Treatment of Non-hairy Melanocytic Macules by Dermabrasion and Topical Application of 5% Hydroquinone Monobenzyl Ether Cream.** *J Am Acad Dermatol* 1993, 28:771–772.

Thomas G. Salopek, MD, and Kowichi Jimbow, MD, PhD, Department of Dermatology, 260G Heritage Medical Research Centre, University of Alberta, Edmonton, Alberta T6G 2S2, Canada.

Therapeutic options for the follicular occlusion tetrad

Andrew C. Reis, MD, and Zeno Chicarilli, MD, DMD

Yale University School of Medicine, New Haven, Connecticut, USA

Acne conglobata, hidradenitis suppurativa, dissecting cellulitis or folliculitis decalvans, and pilonidal sinus have in common the occlusion of sebaceous or apocrine glands, with subsequent inflammation and scarring. These disorders may be seen in isolation or in various combinations, and their treatment is often challenging for both the patient and the physician. Medical and surgical therapies for each disease are reviewed with an emphasis on recent developments and trends in the care of patients.

Current Opinion in Dermatology 1995:69–74

The follicular occlusion tetrad comprises four clinical entities: dissecting cellulitis of the scalp, acne conglobata, hidradenitis suppurativa, and pilonidal sinus. The similarity of their etiopathogeneses was first suggested by Goeckerman [1], and Brunsting [2] described the anatomic, pathophysiologic, and clinical similarities of the first three disorders (the follicular occlusion triad), stating that they appeared to be fulminant forms of acne vulgaris. He pointed out that they had features in common, including 1) glandular hyperplasia of the pilosebaceous apparatus or apocrine gland with hyperactivity; 2) follicular orifice occlusion and double comedo formation; 3) bacterial invasion with suppuration and undermining of loose areolar tissue; and 4) cicatricial healing (Fig. 1). The subsequent inclusion of pilonidal sinus led to the designation follicular occlusion tetrad [3]. The clinical characteristics of these four entities have been previously well described and are outlined in Table 1.

Treatment options have traditionally involved the use of topical and systemic antibiotics and retinoids, ei-ther alone or in concert with surgical therapy. Other less commonly employed treatment modalities such as orthovoltage radiation, ultraviolet irradiation, and hormonal manipulation have also been used, but with varying degrees of success.

With so many options available, no one modality has demonstrated clear superiority. This article attempts to summarize the current trends, both medical and surgical, in the approach to these rather difficult-to-treat disorders.

Folliculitis decalvans or dissecting cellulitis of the scalp

Folliculitis decalvans, or dissecting cellulitis, is an unusual, chronic, and progressive purulent folliculitis that leads to follicular atrophy, alopecia [4,5], and scarring. It occurs primarily in adult men and African Americans, and it initially affects the vertex and occiput of

Table 1. Clinicopathologic differentiating features of the follicular occlusion tetrad*

Feature	Acne vulgaris	Acne conglobata	Dissecting cellulitis	Hidradenitis suppurativa
Site (gland)	Sebaceous	Sebaceous	Sebaceous	Apocrine
Sex	Equal	Male	Male	Female ≥ male
Age	Adolescence	Postadolescence	Postadolescence	Postadolescence
Epidermoid inclusion cysts	+	+	−	−
Comedones				
Single	+	+	−	−
Double	−	+	+	+
Abscesses				
Discrete	+	+	±	+
Dissecting	−	+	+	+
Scar bridges	−	+	+	+

*From Brunsting [2]; with permission.
+, present; −, absent; ±, may be present.

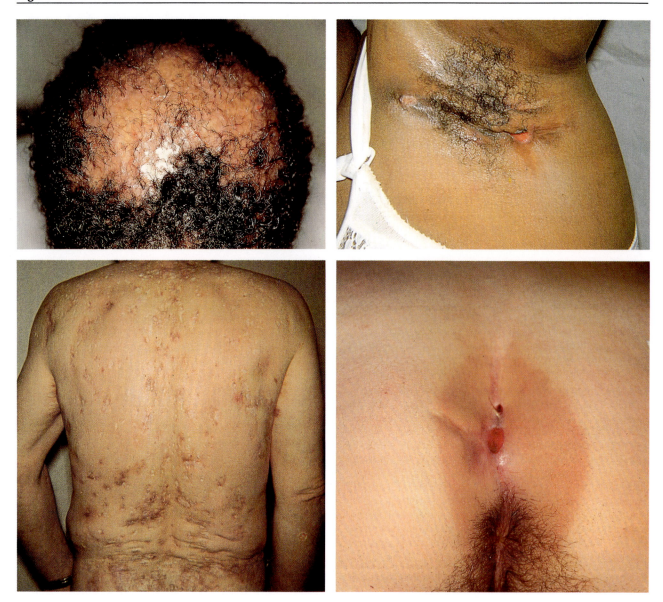

Fig. 1. Components of the follicular occlusion tetrad. **Upper left**, Folliculitis decalvans with scarring alopecia. (*Courtesy of* J. L. Bolognia, New Haven, CT.) **Upper right**, Hidradenitis suppurativa of the axilla. **Lower left**, Acne conglobata of the back. **Lower right**, Pilonidal cyst.

the scalp [6]. Cystic papules or discrete abscesses are less common than a diffuse phlegmon or abscess that forms from the coalescence of multiple nodules. Sinuses discharging seropurulent material may be found at the base of individual nodules or within collections of nodules. Alopecia occurs over the nodular swellings, and following "burnout" of the disease, atrophic scarring and convoluted ridges can be seen. The latter is similar in appearance to cutis verticis gyrata.

The treatment of folliculitis decalvans or dissecting cellulitis has encompassed radiation therapy, incision and drainage, excision and grafting, antibiotic use, and cauterization. The acute suppurative phase is often treated with topical and systemic antibiotics and local cleansing, but this practice may not halt the progression of the disease process.

Efforts have recently focused on retinoids and anti-inflammatory agents in an attempt to induce longer lasting remissions. A good response to isotretinoin (0.5 to 2 mg/kg/d) alone has been recently reported [7•,8,9]; however, the long-term clinical response needs to be confirmed.

Both the combination of isotretinoin with radical excision and tissue expansion [10•] and the combination of isotretinoin with intralesional triamcinolone acetate (40 to 80 mg) [11•] have also been recommended as therapeutic options in dissecting folliculitis. The anti-inflammatory effects of isotretinoin have been touted as being of benefit in the treatment of this disorder. Oral zinc therapy (400 mg/d), either alone [12] or in combination with oral (1500 mg/d) and topical (1.5%) fusidic acid [13•], has also been reported as a therapeutic option with good results observed after follow-ups of up to 2 years. Zinc presumably has an anti-inflammatory effect, whereas fusidic acid is an effective antimicrobial.

Surgical excision with or without grafting is reserved for recalcitrant cases that are unresponsive to medical management. Reconstructive options for the resultant alopecia are difficult if the disease process remains active. Hair transplantation, grafting, or local flap operations, with or without tissue expansion, and fractional excision are available if the chronic, progressive nature of the disease can be suppressed.

Acne conglobata

Spitzer [14] is credited with giving the first description of acne conglobata, and other authors have added to its clinical [15,16] and histologic description [17,18]. Histologically, involvement of the pilosebaceous apparatus is observed, differentiating acne conglobata from hidradenitis suppurativa. In addition, it was noted that all hair-bearing areas, including the entire trunk, the buttocks, and the extremities, were susceptible to this eruption. Florid acne conglobata does not occur until the late teens or early twenties, and it is almost exclusively limited to men. The age of onset has been at-

tributed to a postadolescent functional hyperplasia of sebaceous glands incited by hormonal influences.

Tropical acne, described by Sulzberger *et al.* [19] during World War II in military personnel stationed in the Pacific, closely resembles acne conglobata. However, its rapid onset and resolution, dependent on tropical climatic exposure, led Novy [20] and others to disclaim it as a variant of acne conglobata.

The pathogenesis of acne conglobata is similar to that of hidradenitis suppurativa, except that in the former follicular occlusion causes rupture of the pilosebaceous unit. In acne conglobata, in contrast to hidradenitis suppurativa, single comedones, inflammatory papules, and cystic lesions are frequently found. However, double comedones can occur, and clusters of 10 to 20 or more comedones may be observed [18]. Abscesses, communicating fistulas, and discharging sinuses are also characteristic findings. Brunsting [2] stated that acne conglobata, more than hidradenitis and dissecting cellulitis, resembled a severe form of acne with superimposed pyogenic infection. He regarded hidradenitis and dissecting cellulitis as primarily pyogenic diseases that have little resemblance to acne and occur in structurally predisposed anatomic areas.

The association of acne conglobata, as well as the other members of the follicular occlusion tetrad, with mus-

Table 2. Options for surgical treatment of hidradenitis suppurativa[*]

Study	Method	Procedures, *n*	Hospital stay after operation, *d*	Time to healing, *wk*	Recurrences, *n*
Morgan *et al.* [40]	Excision of axillary and perineal skin; silicone foam	17	5–30 (mean, 15)	6–14 (mean, 8)	1 at 1 y (perineal)
Tasche *et al.* [41], Bell and Ellis [42]	Primary closure	24	7–20	6–12	1 at 2 y (in 11 patients followed up for 1 y or more)
Hartwell [43], Harrison [44]	Split skin grafting	41	7–14	6–8	6 at 1 y
Paletta [45]	Skin grafting and stapling	30	7 after grafting (but grafts were multiple and staged)	4	2 at 1 y
Paletta [45]	Staged resection and skin grafting	35	28–42 (staged)	4–6	5 at 1 y
O'Brien *et al.* [46], Masson [47]	Flap grafting	27	16–30	5–8	3 at 1 y
Blanc *et al.* [48]	Pedicle grafting	18	14	4–8	3 at 1 y (data unclear)
Knaysi *et al.* [49]	Excision and skin grafting Superficial axilla	23	7–14	6–8	0 at 2 y
Knaysi *et al.* [49]	Deep axilla	9	14–21	6–8	2 at 2 y
Anderson and Dockerty [50]	Perineum	38	21	6–8	29 at 8 y (45% needed a further operation)
Harrison *et al.* [51]	Excision and silicone foam Axillary	56	NA	7–30 (mean, 11)	3 at 6 y
	Perineal	15	NA	NA	0 at 6 y
	Inguinoperineal	41	NA	8–30 (mean, 16)	15 at 6 y
	Mammary	6	NA	12–30 (mean, 17.5)	3 at 6 y

[*]*From* Banerjee [34••]; with permission.
NA—not available.

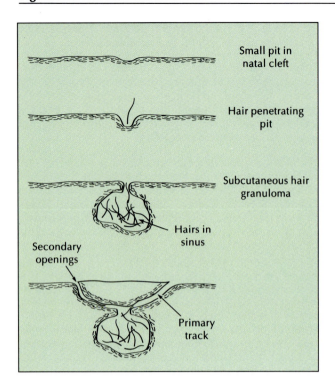

Fig. 2. Pathogenesis of a pilonidal sinus. (*From* Jones [36••]; with permission.)

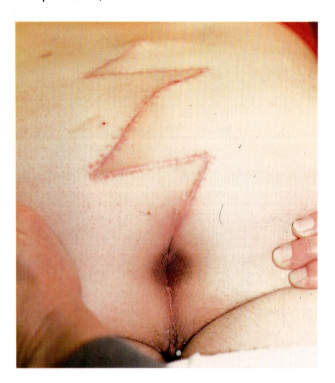

Fig. 3. Z-plasty for excision of pilonidal sinus.

culoskeletal manifestations such as arthritis, myalgias, muscle weakness, and enthesopathies has led investigators to propose a genetic or an immune system basis for the disorder [21••,22••].

Surgical treatment of acne conglobata is not practical as the sole modality because of the widespread distribution of involved skin. Medical management has been used more frequently for this reason [23]. The results were generally poor until the recent release and use of isotretinoin (Accutane; Hoffmann-LaRoche, Nutley, NJ). This agent is presumed to have a direct inhibitory effect on the sebaceous glands. The side effects are common and vary from dryness of the skin and mucous membranes to osteophyte formation [24]. When medical management fails, surgical extirpation has provided significant alleviation of problematic regions. Skin grafting has been the most common method for resurfacing these areas. Finding donor sites free of disease can, however, be difficult [25,26].

Hidradenitis suppurativa

Hidradenitis suppurativa is believed to be caused by the occlusion of the follicular orifice of an overactive apocrine gland, resulting in periglandular inflammation. When two adjacent follicles are obstructed and their respective glands coalesce, a double comedo is formed [27]. Retrograde infection produces suppuration, which invades the loose subcutaneous areolar plane, producing a phlegmon. Healing occurs with substantial scarring [2].

The axillary, inguinocrural, and anogenital regions are the primary sites of involvement. There is a slight female predominance, and the disease process does not occur before puberty and is rare in the postmenopausal patient. An increased incidence is observed in obese patients and those with a family history. Recently, *Chlamydia trachomatis* has been implicated in perineal hidradenitis suppurativa [28•].

Bacterial invasion of the obstructed gland is common and must be treated appropriately with local care and systemic antibiotic therapy. The mildest forms of the disease process are often palliated with local care, adequate hygiene, and avoidance of irritating agents. Retinoid therapy, either alone [29] or in combination with erythromycin (1 g/d) [30•], has shown promise in moderate cases of hidradenitis. Controlled studies are needed to confirm the effectiveness of these agents, however.

The recent work implicating hidradenitis suppurativa as an androgen-dependent disorder [31•] has led to attempts at hormonal therapy. Treatment using gonadotropin-releasing hormone agonists in combination with dexamethasone [32] or total abdominal hysterectomy and bilateral salpingo-oophorectomy [33•] have been shown to eradicate persistent hidradenitis suppurativa in case reports. The theoretical basis for these treatments as well as others for antiandrogens, *eg*, flutamide, makes this an interesting future field of investigation.

Surgical excision of established hidradenitis suppurativa, in conjunction with local medical therapy, remains a mainstay of therapy. Various surgical techniques have been employed for treating hidradenitis suppurativa. The complete excision of all involved skin and tissues is necessary to ensure eradication of the condition. A comparison of techniques is difficult because of the variations in the methods of excision and reconstruction used by different authors. Banerjee [34••] however, attempted to compare various methods of excision and reconstruction (Table 2). It appears from his data that inadequate excision is the main reason for recurrence and that radical excision with healing by secondary intention is the "best" treatment in most cases.

Skin graft failure remains significant in the convoluted areas involved with hidradenitis suppurativa, and in many instances the use of skin grafts adds little benefit over healing by secondary intention. Our experience has been that patients who have skin grafting heal more quickly and comfortably than those who do not. If purulent discharge is copious, a two-stage procedure can be done, with excision followed by the use of local dressings. When the infection has resolved, grafting can be performed. The time interval is usually 5 to 10 days after excision. Advancement, local, and fasciocutaneous flap coverage are alternative options for difficult cases and produce excellent results in the proper hands [35•].

Pilonidal sinus

Pilonidal sinus is a common disease process of young adults in which persistence and recurrence are significant problems. Pilonidal sinus is now thought to be due to an acquired hair-containing deformity, as seen in Figure 2. The etiopathogenesis of pilonidal sinus is therefore somewhat different from that of the other disorders of this tetrad. Pilonidal sinuses usually present from the time of puberty (when androgens begin to act on the pilosebaceous glands) to middle age. Cavities become secondarily infected; this process may result in the formation of multiple subcutaneous sinus tracts [36••], which can require immediate drainage.

Therapeutic options for pilonidal sinuses remain mostly in the surgical realm. Any therapy that does not include excision of the involved areas results in a very high recurrence rate. A recent comparison of open versus closed treatment of chronic pilonidal sinuses [37••] supported excision and primary closure, citing the lower morbidity and improved cost-effectiveness of this method. The economic benefit of primary closure was confirmed by Khawaja *et al.* [38••] in their prospective study of the economic and clinical outcomes with primary closure. The authors cited a lower complication rate and a more rapid return to normal activities in the group with primary closure. A follow-up longer than the 1-year follow-up provided in this study is necessary to evaluate recurrence rates fully.

Advancement flap operations [39••], which address and eliminate the causative process of hair insertion, have also shown excellent results. Karydakis's series of 6545 cases, which had 95% follow-up rate and only a 1% recurrence rate, is to be commended. The concept of

addressing the underlying cause rather than just treating the problem is the basis for this preferred treatment modality and success. In our hands, complete excision with Z-plasty closure to eliminate the deep cleft has provided the most successful result in eradicating disease and minimizing recurrence (Fig. 3).

Conclusions

The disorders of the follicular occlusion tetrad—folliculitis decalvans or dissecting cellulitis, acne conglobata, hidradenitis suppurativa, and pilonidal sinus—may be seen singly or in various combinations. The medical and surgical options for these disorders remain rather limited in their effectiveness. Aside from the treatment of secondary infections with topical and systemic antibiotics, the use of isotretinoin and judicious surgical intervention remain the mainstays of treatment. Recent hormonal and immunologic studies may contribute to the management of these disorders.

Acknowledgments

We wish to thank Anne M. P. Reis, Elena Barbard, and Helen Roginel for their contributions to this text.

References and recommended reading

Papers of particular interest, published within the annual period of review, have been highlighted as:
- Of special interest
•• Of outstanding interest

1. Goeckerman WJ: **A Case of Perifolliculitis Capitis Abscedens et Suffodiens, Cutis Verticis Gyrata, Hydradenitis [Discussion].** *Plast Reconstr Surg* 1951, 7:143.

2. Brunsting HA: **Hidradenitis and Other Variants of Acne.** *Arch Dermatol Syphilol* 1952, 65:303–315.

3. Plewig G, Kligman AM: *Acne and Rosacea,* edn 2. New York: Springer-Verlag; 1993.

4. Bogg A: **Folliculitis Decalvans.** *Acta Derm Venereol (Stockb)* 1963, 43:14–24.

5. Suter L: **Folliculitis Decalvans.** *Hautarzt* 1983, 32:429–431.

6. McMullen FM, Zeligman I: **Peri-folliculitis Capitis Abscedens et Suffodiens.** *Arch Dermatol* 1956, 73:256–263.

7. Benvenuto ME. Reboza A: **Fluctuant Nodules and Alopecia of the**
• **Scalp.** *Arch Dermatol* 1992, 128:1115–1119.
A brief discussion of a case report in which perifolliculitis abscedens et suffodiens was treated successfully with isotretinoin. The authors point out that the short-term follow-up should lead to skepticism and that further work is needed.

8. Schewach-Millet M, Ziv R, Shapira D: **Perifolliculitis Capitis Abscedens et Suffodiens Treated With Isotretinoin (13 Cisretinoic Acid).** *J Am Acad Dermatol* 1986, 6:1291–1292.

9. Taylor AEM: **Dissecting Cellulitis of the Scalp: Response to Isotretinoin.** *Lancet* 1987, ii:225.

10. Bachginsky T, Antonyshon OM: **Dissecting Cellulitis of the Scalp:**
• **A Case Report of Combined Treatment Using Tissue Expansion, Radical Excision, and ISO Tretinoin.** *J Dermatol Surg Oncol* 1992, 28:877–880.
The authors point out that the difficult nature of the problem and set out to prove that combined therapy may offer the best solution. They illustrate this with their case report and experience.

11. Shaffer N, Billick R, Scolovitz M: **Perifolliculitis Capitis Abscedens et**
• **Suffodiens: Resolution With Combination Therapy.** *Arch Dermatol* 1992, 182:1329–1331.

Good summary of the history and difficult nature of the disease process. This case report demonstrates resolution with the use of isotretinoin and triamcinolone along with surgical debridement.

12.   Berne B, Verge P, Olamn S: **Perifolliculitis Capitis Abscedens et Suffodiens**. *Arch Dermatol* 1985, 121:1028–1030.

13.   Abeck D, Korting HC, Braun-Falco O: **Folliculitis Decalvans: Long
 •   Lasting Response to Combined Therapy With Fusidic Acid and Zinc**. *Acta Derm Venereol (Stockh)* 1992, 22:143–145.
Demonstration of the response of folliculitis decalvans to the combination of fusidic acid and zinc in three patients with follow-up of more than 1 year. The possible mechanisms of action of the authors' chosen regimen are also discussed.

14.   Spitzer L: **Dermatitis Follicularis et Perifollicularis Conglobata**. *Dermatol Z* 1901, 10:8.

15.   Lang E: *Hautkrankheiten*. Wiesbaden: JF Bergmann; 1902.

16.   Reitman K: **Acne Aggregata sev Conglobata**. *Arch Dermatol Syphilol* 1908, 90:249.

17.   Belote GH: **Acne Conglobata: An Experimental Study**. *Arch Dermatol Syphilol* 1933, 27:302–311.

18.   Michelson HE, Allen PK: **Acne Conglobata**. *Arch Dermatol Syphilol* 1931, 23:49–67.

19.   Sulzberger MB, *et al.*: **Tropical Acne**. *Med Bull US Navy* 1946, 46:1178.

20.   Novy FG Jr: **Tropical Acne**. *Calif Med* 1946, 65:1.

21.   Rosner I, Burg C, Wisnieski J, Schacter B, Richter D: **The Clinical
 ••   Spectrum of the Arthropathy Associated With Hidradenitis Suppurativa and Acne Conglobata**. *J Rheumatol* 1993, 20:684–687.
A fairly large series demonstrating some of the systemic arthropathies associated with acne conglobata and hidradenitis suppurativa. The clinical, laboratory, and principal findings are outlined.

22.   Olafsson S, Khan MA: **Musculoskeletal Features of Acne, Hidradenitis
 ••   Suppurativa and Dissecting Cellulitis of the Scalp**. *Rheum Dis Clin North Am* 1992, 18:215–224.
A good overview of the follicular occlusion triad of hidradenitis suppurativa, acne, and dissecting cellulitis of the scalp and of the relationship of these conditions to musculoskeletal manifestations. Information on the treatment course, prognosis, and evaluation is included. The etiology is also discussed.

23.   Berge T, Gunduren J: **Acne Conglobata**. *Acta Derm Venereol (Stockh)* 1967, 97:41–49.

24.   Peck GL, Olsen T, Toder F, Strauus J, Downing D, Pandya M, Butkus D, Arnaud-Battner J: **Prolonged Remissions of Cystic and Conglobata Acne With 13-Cisretinoic Acid**. *N Engl J Med* 1979, 7:329–333.

25.   Grosser A: **Surgical Treatment of Chronic Axillary and Genitocrural Acne Conglobata by Split Thickness Skin Grafting**. *J Dermatol Surg Oncol* 1982, 8:391–398.

26.   Weinrauch L, Peled I, Hacham-Zadeh S, Wexler M: **Surgical Treatment of Severe Acne Conglobata**. *J Dermatol Surg Oncol* 1981, 7:492–493.

27.   Ornsby OS, Montgomery H: **Acne**. In *Disease of the Skin*, edn 6. Philadelphia: Lea & Febiger; 1943:1216–1233.

28.   Bendahan J, Pacan H, Kolman S, Neufeld DM, Freund U: **The
 •   Possible Role of *Chlamydia trachomatis* in Perineal Suppurativa Hidradenitis**. *Eur J Surg* 1992, 158:213–215.
The authors follow up seven consecutive patients who have perineal hidradenitis suppurativa and compare them with 10 control patients who have cryptogenic perianal abscesses. They show that six of seven in the hidradenitis group and none in the control group demonstrate IgA antibodies to *C. trachomatis*. A possible link, but not proof of *Chlamydia*'s role in hidradenitis.

29.   Vahlquist A, Griffiths WAD: **Retinoid Therapy in Hidradenitis Suppurativa: A Report of a Case**. *Retinoids Today Tomorrow* 18:28–30.

30.   Chow ETY, Motimer PS: **Successful Treatment of Hidradenitis Sup-
 •   purativa and Retroauricular Acne With Etretinate**. *Brit J Dermatol* 1992, 126:415.
A correspondence outlining the possible usefulness of etretinate in the treatment of hidradenitis suppurativa. A case report demonstrates the success of the authors' treatment regimen.

31.   Lewis F, Messenger AG, Wales JK: **Hidradenitis Suppurativa as a
 •   Presenting Feature of Premature Adrenarche**. *Br J Dermatol* 1993, 129:447–448.
Brief discussion proposing a link between hidradenitis suppurativa and adrenarche and the support it lends to the supposition that hidradenitis is an androgen-dependent disorder.

32.   Camisa C, Sexton C, Friedman C: **Treatment of Hidradenitis Suppurativa With Combination Hypothalmic-Pituitary-Ovarian and Adrenal Suppression: A Case Report**. *J Reprod Med* 1989, 34:543–546.

33.   Bogus JW, Minderhoud-Bassie W, Huikesnoven FJM: **A Case of
 •   Hidradenitis Suppurativa Treated With Gonadotropin-Releasing Hormone Agonist and by Total Abdominal Hysterectomy With Bilateral Salpingo-Oophorectomy**. *Am J Obstet Gynecol* 1992, 167:517–518.
A startlingly radical concept of treating hidradenitis suppurativa with combined surgery and estrogen therapy. The theory and the results are presented briefly.

34.   Banerjee AK: **Surgical Treatment of Hidradenitis Suppurativa**. *Br J
 ••   Surg* 1992, 79:863–866.
An excellent review of the surgical options available for hidradenitis suppurativa. The author outlines the pathogenesis, complications, management, and outcome of various options from multiple authors. This article is an excellent reference guide.

35.   Elliot D, Kangesu L, Bainbridge C, Venkataramakrishnan V: **Recon-
 •   struction of the Axilla With a Posterior Arm Fasciocutaneous Flap**. *Br J Plast Surg* 1992, 45:101–104.
The authors present their series of axillary reconstructions with posterior arm fasciocutaneous flaps and outline how even extremely radical excisions may be covered with properly designed local flaps.

36.   Jones DJ: **A B C of Colorectal Diseases: Pilonidal Sinus**. *BMJ* 1992,
 ••   305:410–412.
An excellent quick reference guide to pilonidal sinus. A great deal of information is packed into only three pages.

37.   Sondenaa K, Anderson E, Soreide JA: **Morbidity and Short-Term Re-
 ••   sults in a Randomized Trial of Open Compared With Closed Treatment of Chronic Pilonidal Sinus**. *Eur J Surg* 1992, 158:351–355.
This excellent randomized study of open versus closed treatment of pilonidal sinus shows better outcome with closed treatment in terms of cost-effectiveness and morbidity than with the traditional open method.

38.   Khawaja HT, Bryan S, Weaver PC: **Treatment of Natal Cleft Si-
 ••   nus: A Prospective Clinical and Economic Evaluation**. *BMJ* 1992, 304:1282–1283.
A brief outline of the cost-effectiveness of closed treatment of natal cleft sinus. The authors conclude that primary closure should be widely used.

39.   Karydakis GE: **Easy and Successful Treatment of Pilonidal Sinus Af-
 ••   ter Explanation of Its Causative Process**. *Aust N Z J Surg* 1992, 62:385–389.
Tremendous series of 6545 cases of advancement flap surgery to eradicate the process of hair insertion into the natal cleft. This huge experience and outline of the procedure and its results should be in every dermatologist's reference section.

40.   Morgan WP, Harding KG, Richardson G, Hughes LE: **The Use of Silastic Foam Dressing in the Treatment of Advanced Hidradenitis Suppurativa**. *Br J Surg* 1980, 67:277–280.

41.   Tasche C, Angelats J, Jayaram B: **Surgical Treatment of Hidradenitis Suppurativa of the Axilla**. *Plast Reconstr Surg* 1975, 55:559–562.

42.   Bell BA, Ellis H: **Hidradenitis Suppurativa**. *J R Soc Med* 1978, 71:511–515.

43.   Hartwell SW: **Surgical Treatment of Hidradenitis Suppurativa**. *Surg Clin North Am* 1975, 55:1107–1109.

44.   Harrison SH: **Axillary Hidradenitis**. *Br J Plast Surg* 1964, 17:95–98.

45.   Paletta FX: **Hidradenitis Suppurativa: Pathologic Study and Use of Skin Flaps**. *Plast Reconstr Surg* 1963, 31:307–315.

46.   O'Brien J, Wysocki J, Anastasi G: **Limberg Flap Coverage for Axillary Defects Resulting From Excision of Hidradenitis Suppurativa**. *Plast Reconstr Surg* 1976, 58:354–358.

47.   Masson JK: **Surgical Treatment of Hidradenitis Suppurativa**. *Surg Clin North Am* 1969, 49:1043–1052.

48.   Blanc D, Tropet Y, Balmat P: **Surgical Treatment of Suppurative Axillary Hidradenitis: Value of a Musculocutaneous Island Flap of the Latissimus Dorsi**. *Ann Dermatol Venereol* 1990, 117:277–281.

49.   Knaysi GA, Cosman B, Crikelair GF: **Hidradenitis Suppurativa**. *JAMA* 1968, 203:19–22.

50.   Anderson MJ, Dockerty MB: **Perianal Hidradenitis Suppurativa: A Clinical and Pathological Study**. *Dis Colon Rectum* 1958, 1:23–31.

51.   Harrison BJ, Mudge M, Hughes LE: **Recurrence After Surgical Treatment of Hidradenitis Suppurativa**. *BMJ* 1987, 294:487–489.

Zeno Chicarilli, MD, DMD, 40 Temple Street, New Haven, CT 06510, USA.

Systemic diseases

Edited by

Warren W. Piette

University of Iowa College of Medicine
Iowa City, Iowa, USA

CURRENT SCIENCE

Antineutrophil cytoplasmic and anti–endothelial cell antibodies: new mechanisms for vasculitis

James A. Goeken, MD

University of Iowa College of Medicine, Iowa City, Iowa, USA

Two new groups of autoantibodies have recently been undergoing intensive study because they have been associated with a group of necrotizing vasculitic diseases for which previously no diagnostic laboratory test was available and no pathogenetic mechanism was delineated. Accumulated evidence has indicated that antineutrophil cytoplasmic antibody (ANCA) is a sensitive and specific serologic marker for a spectrum of these diseases. The contribution of ANCA to the pathogenesis of these diseases is being explored, and several pieces of evidence suggest that ANCA may be more than an epiphenomenon. Anti–endothelial cell antibodies have started to be studied even more recently than ANCA, but they have been identified in several forms of vasculitis. Less information on their pathogenetic significance is currently known, but recent studies of these antibodies, together with those of ANCA, have significantly enhanced our understanding of the mechanisms of the systemic necrotizing vasculitides.

Current Opinion in Dermatology 1995:75–82

Vasculitis has been a topic of medical interest since the first description, by Kussmaul and Maier [1] in 1866, of periarteritis nodosa, which has subsequently come to be known as polyarteritis nodosa. Since that initial description, many other vasculitic syndromes have been clinically and pathologically described, classification systems advanced, and pathophysiologic mechanisms proposed. Although immune complex–mediated injury is well established as a mechanism in certain forms of vasculitis, in both Wegener's granulomatosis (WG) and most cases of polyarteritis nodosa, evidence of immune complex deposits is lacking on immunopathologic examination [2]. A different mechanism is therefore likely in these diseases.

The systemic necrotizing vasculitides include a number of diseases that were previously classified separately or only loosely grouped together. As studies of these entities have accumulated, it has become increasingly clear that these conditions are part of a disease continuum characterized by 1) necrotizing vasculitis (either systemic or localized) and 2) frequent involvement of the renal glomeruli with a characteristic necrotizing segmental and crescentic glomerulonephritis with few or no immune deposits [3,4]. These diseases include WG, polyarteritis nodosa and microscopic polyarteritis, Churg-Strauss syndrome, "overlap" vasculitis, and "idiopathic" pauci-immune crescentic glomerulonephritis. Various percentages of all of these diseases have been demonstrated in studies around the world to be associated with the group of autoantibodies collectively known as antineutrophil cytoplasmic antibodies (ANCA).

Antineutrophil cytoplasmic antibodies

The autoantibodies directed at lysosomal enzymes of neutrophils and monocytes were initially reported in 1982 by Davies et al. [5], who described eight patients with focal, segmental immune deposit–negative crescentic glomerulonephritis, arthralgias, and myalgias whose sera contained an autoantibody that stained the cytoplasm of neutrophils in an indirect immunofluorescence assay. Half of these patients also had dyspnea, hemoptysis, or both. ANCA was the name given to these autoantibodies. Although it was suggested that ANCA was an epiphenomenon in these Southern Australian patients who had been exposed to an arbovirus infection, it now seems probable that these patients had some form of systemic necrotizing vasculitis, which is associated with ANCA. Two years later, ANCA was linked to vasculitis in an additional four cases and was suggested as a possible diagnostic test

Abbreviations

AECA—anti–endothelial cell antibody; ANCA—antineutrophil cytoplasmic antibody; C-ANCA—cytoplasmic staining ANCA; LF—lactoferrin; MPO—myeloperoxidase; P-ANCA—perinuclear/nuclear staining ANCA; PR-3—proteinase 3; WG—Wegener's granulomatosis.

for it [6]. In 1985, van der Woude *et al.* [7] first linked ANCA to WG, and in the next few years, this association was rapidly confirmed by other authors [8–10]. A large study involving both US and European patients demonstrated ANCA in more than 90% of patients with active, systemic WG, in 65% to 70% of patients with active, limited WG, and in approximately 35% of patients in remission [9]. ANCA was subsequently reported in microscopic polyarteritis, Churg-Strauss syndrome, and some cases of polyarteritis nodosa [11–14]. In 1988, a second form of ANCA was described in patients with pauci-immune crescentic glomerulonephritis by Jennette and Falk [3]. They demonstrated that this autoantibody, which they called P-ANCA (for perinuclear/nuclear staining), had specificity for myeloperoxidase (MPO). This was the first proof that ANCA was directed against lysosomal enzymes of neutrophils and monocytes.

Patterns and specificities

Antineutrophil cytoplasmic antibodies have been named according to the three microscopic patterns detected by immunofluorescence assay on ethanol-fixed human neutrophils (Table 1).

Two of these patterns, C-ANCA (for cytoplasmic staining) and P-ANCA, are associated with systemic necrotizing vasculitides. C-ANCA, the type associated with approximately 90% of WG cases, produces a finely granular cytoplasmic staining pattern with perinuclear accentuation on ethanol-fixed neutrophil substrate (Fig. 1), whereas vasculitis-associated P-ANCA produces a nuclear staining pattern that becomes perinuclear with increasing dilution (Fig. 2). Both C-ANCA and vasculitis-associated P-ANCA produce the granular cytoplasmic pattern on formalin-fixed neutrophils, indicating that the cytoplasm is the true location of the antigen [3]. The nuclear and perinuclear staining caused by P-ANCA is caused by an artifactual translocation of the antigen from the lysosomes to the nucleus following ethanolic permeabilization of the nuclear and lysosomal membranes and charge-based redistribution of the negatively charged (cationic) antigen to the positively charged (anionic) nucleus [3,4,15•]. P-ANCA is technically more difficult to identify than C-

ANCA because antinuclear antibodies are readily confused with them [16••]. This confusion is evident from the widely divergent fraction of P-ANCA, ranging from as many as 90% to as few as 24%, reported to be associated with vasculitis, glomerulonephritis, or both [16••,17•]. Ulmer *et al.* [17•] noted that antinuclear antibodies were present in a large number of the "P-ANCA–positive" (but anti-MPO–negative) specimens, suggesting that in many cases antinuclear antibodies may have been misinterpreted as P-ANCA.

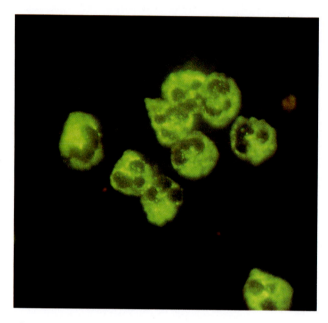

Fig. 1. Cytoplasmic staining antineutrophil cytoplasmic antibody from a patient with Wegener's granulomatosis, as shown by an indirect immunofluorescence assay on an ethanol-fixed neutrophil substrate (original magnification, ×500).

The third ANCA pattern, which was designated atypical ANCA at the Fourth International Workshop on ANCA (Lübeck, Germany, 1992) but is sometimes referred to as X-ANCA or atypical P-ANCA, has been associated mainly with inflammatory bowel and liver diseases, especially ulcerative colitis, primary sclerosing cholangi-

Table 1. Immunofluorescence pattern and neutrophil fixation of the three antineutrophil cytoplasmic antibodies and of antinuclear antibody

Pattern	Ethanol-fixed	Formalin-fixed
C-ANCA	Granular, cytoplasmic	Granular, cytoplasmic
P-ANCA (MPO-positive)	Nuclear pattern that becomes perinuclear with increasing dilution of serum	Granular, cytoplasmic
ANA*	Nuclear	Negative or nuclear
Atypical ANCA	"Very perinuclear," center of nucleus unstained	Negative or diffuse cytoplasmic

*Reactive on HEp-2 cells.
ANA—antinuclear antibody; ANCA—antineutrophil cytoplasmic antibody; C-ANCA—cytoplasmic staining ANCA; MPO—myeloperoxidase; P-ANCA—perinuclear/nuclear staining ANCA.

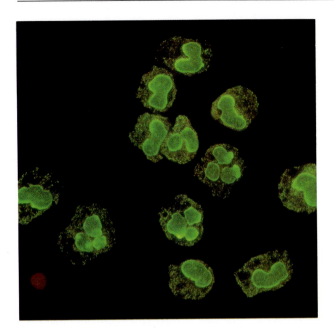

Fig. 2. Perinuclear/nuclear staining antineutrophil cytoplasmic antibody with antimyeloperoxidase specificity from a patient with pauci-immune crescentic glomerulonephritis, as shown by an indirect immunofluorescence assay on an ethanol-fixed neutrophil substrate (original magnification, ×500).

tis, and autoimmune hepatitis [15•,16••,18–22,23•,24•]. Atypical ANCA is often confused with P-ANCA because it also produces a perinuclear staining pattern on ethanol-fixed neutrophils (Fig. 3). It can be distinguished because it does not produce the granular cytoplasmic staining pattern on formalin-fixed neutrophils that vasculitis-related P-ANCA does. Atypical ANCA–positive sera may produce a diffuse (rather than a granular) cytoplasmic staining of formalin-fixed neutrophils and does not stain the majority of monocytes [15•,16••,18,22,23•].

The immunofluorescence assay patterns and associated antigenic specificities of ANCA are summarized in Table 2. The specificity of 80% to 90% of C-ANCA has been determined to be proteinase 3 (PR-3), an elastinolytic serine proteinase of the primary granules of neutrophils and monocytes [8,15•,16••,25]. PR-3 has subsequently been proven to be identical to azurophilic granule proteinase 7 and myeloblastin [25]. The specificity of the remaining 10% to 20% of C-ANCA includes cationic antimicrobial protein 57, which was described by Falk *et al.* [26] but has not thus far been sufficiently explored by other investigators to establish its frequency. Evidence from the EEC-BCR (European Economic Community–British Commonwealth Research) Study Group for ANCA Assay Standardization indicated that one of 12 examples of C-ANCA from patients with confirmed vasculitis does not have anti–PR-3 specificity [15•], and this is generally the experience of most investigators. Occasional examples of C-ANCA are reported to demonstrate anti-MPO specificity [27••]. Anti-MPO more frequently causes the nuclear and perinuclear immunofluorescence assay pattern and has been shown to account for 80% to 90% of vasculitis- or glomerulonephritis-associated P-ANCA [4,14]. If preselection of patients for vasculitis or glomerulonephritis is not done, the fraction of all "P-ANCA" (as detected by immunofluorescence assay on ethanol-fixed neutrophils) that have anti-MPO specificity decreases to approximately 40% [28••]. Other, less common specificities of P-ANCA include human leukocyte elastase, cathepsin G, lysozyme, and lactoferrin (LF) [28••]. Cohen Tervaert *et al.* [29] studied a large number of patients with vasculitis and determined that human leukocyte elastase was a rare P-ANCA–associated specificity. Mulder *et al.* [30] found that anti-LF antibodies were present in 22% of 94 rheumatoid arthritis patients' sera analyzed. Of these, most demonstrated a typical P-ANCA pattern. Mulder *et al.* [31] also found anti-LF in patients with inflammatory bowel and autoimmune liver diseases. Anti-LF, unlike anti-MPO, does not seem to be associated with vasculitis.

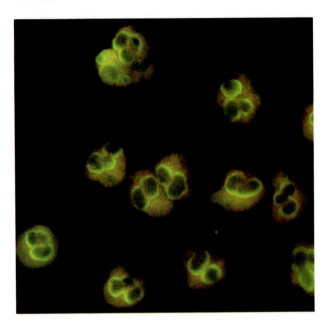

Fig. 3. Atypical antineutrophil cytoplasmic antibody from a patient with ulcerative colitis, as shown by an indirect immunofluorescence assay on an ethanol-fixed neutrophil substrate (original magnification, ×500).

Disease associations and clinical significance

The disease associations of ANCA have been recently reviewed [4,9,15•,16••,27••,28••,32]. The major disease associations of C-ANCA and P-ANCA are summarized in Table 3. ANCA has been shown to be a very sensitive marker for active, generalized WG (>90%). ANCA has a lower sensitivity for limited, locoregional WG. C-ANCA predominates in WG, but it is also expressed in about 40% to 45% of patients with microscopic polyarteritis and overlap vasculitis and in approximately one third of patients with pauci-immune crescent glomerulonephritis. Some patients with pauci-immune crescentic glomerulonephritis have progression to active generalized WG or microscopic polyarteri-

Table 2. Immunofluorescence patterns and antigenic specifications of antineutrophil cytoplasmic antibodies

Pattern	Antigenic specificities
C-ANCA	85%–90% proteinase 3 10%–15% cationic antimicrobial protein 57 and others
P-ANCA	90% myeloperoxidase 10% others (cathepsin G, elastase, lactoferrin, and others)
Atypical ANCA	Undefined (lactoferrin, cathepsin G, or other?)

ANCA—antineutrophil cytoplasmic antibody; C-ANCA—cytoplasmic staining ANCA; P-ANCA—perinuclear/nuclear staining ANCA.

tis, demonstrating the connection between the various diseases of the spectrum of systemic necrotizing vasculitis. Anti-MPO–specific P-ANCA is found most frequently in association with pauci-immune crescentic glomerulonephritis, microscopic polyarteritis, polyarteritis nodosa, overlap vasculitis, and Churg-Strauss syndrome. Although its reported frequency varies, essentially all investigators now agree that some patients with WG have anti-MPO (P-ANCA) rather than anti–PR-3 (C-ANCA) [15•,16••,27••,28••,32,33].

The predictive value of a positive or negative test results for ANCA in patients with suspected systemic necrotizing vasculitis was calculated in my laboratory. A positive test result for C-ANCA or P-ANCA predicted a 96% likelihood that the patient had, or was developing, systemic necrotizing vasculitis (of any variant), whereas a negative test result predicted a 93% likelihood that the patient did not have systemic necrotizing vasculitis [32].

The significance of ANCA titers remains under discussion. Several authors have presented data indicating that titer was of significance in monitoring patients with ANCA. The majority agree that a stable or falling titer is correlated with remission; some have also stated that a rising titer predicts relapse [9,10,27••,34•]. Oth-

ers caution that such increases in ANCA titer were accompanied by clinical relapse in approximately only half of the cases and recommend careful clinical monitoring rather than prophylactic treatment of such patients [15•,35].

Indirect immunofluorescence assay remains the gold standard for ANCA screening and titration, but confirmatory testing by another method is recommended in patients whose clinical signs or symptoms do not definitely indicate the diagnosis of systemic necrotizing vasculitis. Enzyme-linked immunosorbent assays for anti-MPO and anti–PR-3 have become widely available; however, these assays are still not completely standardized, and some discrepancies between laboratories exist. ANCA titers determined by enzyme-linked immunosorbent assay have not correlated with disease activity as well as those determined by immunofluorescence assay [15•,27••,36].

Pathogenetic role

The question of the pathogenetic role of ANCA in vasculitis is still unanswered; however, several pieces of experimental evidence points toward their involvement (Fig. 4). The following sequence of events is suggested to occur:

1. Bacterial or viral infections stimulate leukocytes to release cytokines, including interleukin-1 and tumor necrosis factor-α. Many patients with WG and other systemic necrotizing vasculitides give a history of a "flu-like illness" just preceding the onset of vasculitic signs and symptoms, so there are clinical reasons to suspect that infections may be involved in activation events preceding vasculitis [37].

2. Although ANCA is not displayed on resting neutrophil or monocyte cell membranes, activation by tumor necrosis factor-α or interleukin-1 causes lysosomes to move to the cell membrane, and their contents become accessible to circulating ANCA [38].

3. Tumor necrosis factor-α–primed neutrophils can be induced to undergo a respiratory burst and degranulation by ANCA [37,39]. This generates reactive oxygen species, which could damage endothelial cells.

Table 3. Disease associations and antigenic specificities of antineutrophil cytoplasmic antibodies

Disease	Specificity, % Anti–PR-3	Anti-MPO	Other
Wegener's granulomatosis	80–85	10	5–10 (other)
Microscopic polyarteritis	45	45	5–10 (other)
Churg-Strauss syndrome	10	70	20 (negative)
Classic polyarteritis nodosa	10	20	70 (negative)
Overlap vasculitis	40	20	40 (other)
Pauci-immune crescentic glomerulonephritis	30	65	5 (other)

MPO—myeloperoxidase; PR-3—proteinase 3.

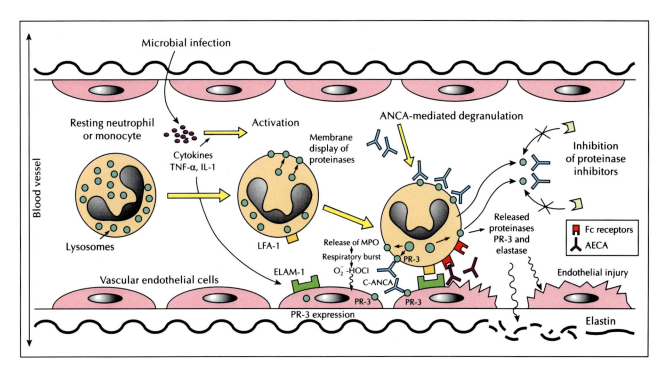

Fig. 4. Proposed roles of antineutrophil cytoplasmic antibody (ANCA) and anti–endothelial cell antibody (AECA) in the pathogenesis of vasculitis. Initially resting neutrophils or monocytes and endothelial cells (ECs) are activated by cytokines elaborated by inflammatory cells in response to infections. ANCA antigens come to the cell membranes and interact with ANCA, causing degranulation and release of proteinase 3 (PR-3) and myeloperoxidase (MPO). Activated ECs and leukocytes increase adhesion molecule expression, bringing these cells into contact, whereupon PR-3 and reactive oxygen species (O_2^--HOCl) generated by the enzymatic action of MPO can damage ECs. PR-3 expression by ECs or AECA reacting with Fc receptors for immunoglobulin on leukocytes may also bring ECs and leukocytes into contact. C-ANCA *ie*, ANCA with cytoplasmic staining pattern, may inhibit proteinase inhibitors, allowing PR-3 to do more extensive damage to vessel walls. ELAM-1—endothelial leukocyte cell adhesion molecule-1; IL-1—interleukin-1; LFA-1—lymphocyte function–associated antigen-1; TNF-α—tumor necrosis factor-α. (*From* Goeken [64]; with permission.)

4. Increased binding of neutrophils and monocytes to endothelial cells can be demonstrated in association with the activation of these cells by tumor necrosis factor-α. Adhesion molecules on leukocytes (intercellular adhesion molecule-1) and endothelial cells (endothelial leukocyte cell adhesion molecule-1) are upregulated. These leukocytes can then kill endothelial cells by antibody-dependent cell cytotoxicity [40,41••,42]. C-ANCA has been shown to upregulate endothelial leukocyte cell adhesion molecule-1 on endothelial cells directly [43].

5. Antineutrophil cytoplasmic antibodies can become bound to endothelial cells. Varagunam *et al.* [44] demonstrated that MPO, which has a cationic charge (pI > 10), can bind directly to endothelial cells, which have an anionic charge. Thus, MPO, anti-MPO, and endothelial cells may be brought into direct contact, so reactive oxygen species produced by the enzymatic action of MPO could cause endothelial cell injury.

6. Proteinase 3 has been reported to be present in the cytoplasm of endothelial cells by Mayet *et al.* [43,45•], who also found that interleukin-1 activation of endothelial cells increased PR-3 expression. This finding is extremely interesting because it would allow C-ANCA to target both endothelial cells and neutrophils directly. The lack of evidence of immunoglobulin bound to endothelial cells in most patients with systemic necrotizing vasculitis seems to conflict with this finding, and confirmation by other investigators is awaited [2]. PR-3, as an elastinolytic proteinase, would be capable of digesting both endothelial cells and the elastin of the blood vessel walls.

7. C-ANCA may further exacerbate endothelial cell injury by interfering with the function of α_1-antitrypsin, the normal inhibitor of PR-3. Dolman *et al.* [46] reported that C-ANCA inhibited the action of α_1-antitrypsin on PR-3. ANCA also interfered with, but did not completely block, the proteinase activity of PR-3. Thus, C-ANCA may allow PR-3 to circulate and damage endothelial cells. Esnault *et al.* [47] recently reported that patients lacking α_1-antitrypsin activity have an increased frequency of developing C-ANCA–associated vasculitis, and they proposed that proteinase inhibitor deficiency could allow the immune system greater opportunity to make an autoimmune response to PR-3 than it would if rapidly complexed with its inhibitor.

8. A last piece of evidence relating the immunologic response to PR-3 to WG is the discovery that

the T cells of patients with WG proliferate in response to PR-3, whereas the T cells of normal individuals do not [48,49]. Although it is poorly defined at this time, the cellular immune system's involvement in systemic necrotizing vasculitis is likely to be significant, and further investigation is needed.

Anti–endothelial cell antibodies

Endothelial cells, as the lining cells of the blood vessels, occupy an important location involved in controlling the escape of plasma proteins into the extracellular space and permitting transport of many critical metabolites while maintaining an antithrombotic environment. Damage to the endothelium may clearly have serious consequences, including vasculitis. Possible scenarios by which ANCA might damage endothelial cells have been described previously. Antibodies directed primarily at the endothelial cells, the anti–endothelial cell antibodies (AECA), are another potential cause of immune–mediated vasculitis.

Anti–endothelial cell antibodies have been reported in several primary vasculitides including WG, microscopic polyarteritis, and Kawasaki disease [50–54,55••]. Their significance has been uncertain because of their presence in secondary vasculitides as well as a number of other inflammatory diseases and conditions, including systemic lupus erythematosus [53,56], systemic sclerosis [57], HLA-matched graft rejection [58], IgA nephropathy [56,59], hemolytic-uremic syndrome [60], thrombotic thrombocytopenic purpura [61], and preeclampsia [62]. Studies of AECA in the primary vasculitides have demonstrated that these antibodies can be coexpressed with ANCA and may contribute to the development of pathology, perhaps by providing an additional means of bringing the neutrophils and monocytes into contact with endothelial cells (Fig. 4) [50]. Frampton *et al.* [53] suggested that AECA titer correlated with disease activity in WG, supporting the involvement of AECA in the pathogenesis of vasculitis. Chan *et al.* [63•] also found coexpression of AECA and ANCA in patients with WG or microscopic polyarteritis and followed titers of both over time. They found that increases in ANCA titer were associated with relapses in all cases studied, and decreases were associated with remissions in 89%. AECA titer rises accompanied ANCA titer increases in 82% of cases, but this finding was not statistically significant. Patients who became ANCA-negative but remained AECA-positive were at greater risk for relapse than were those who became negative for both.

Conclusions

Antineutrophil cytoplasmic antibodies are now well established as serologic markers for a spectrum of systemic necrotizing vasculitides, and substantial evidence indicates that they may play a pathogenetic role in these diseases. ANCA assays have become widely available and merit use whenever the question of systemic necrotizing vasculitis arises. Assays for AECA are not yet as widely available as those for ANCA, and they are not standardized sufficiently to compare results between laboratories, but continued investigation may change this in the near future. The discoveries of ANCA and AECA have improved our understanding of the pathogenesis of the systemic vasculitides. The complexities of these illnesses, involving many factors beyond the autoantibodies, have begun to be revealed. The importance of the cytokine-mediated activation of both the leukocytes and the endothelial cells and the subsequent increased expression of adhesion molecules is now evident. Yet to be clearly defined is the role of the cellular immune system. Improved understanding of the pathogenesis of the systemic vasculitides, as well as the ready availability of useful serologic markers for their diagnosis and monitoring, will probably lead to better therapy and potentially new therapeutic strategies.

Acknowledgment

I thank Ruth Kjaer for her secretarial assistance.

References and recommended reading

Papers of particular interest, published within the annual period of review, have been highlighted as:
•   Of special interest
••   Of outstanding interest

1. Kussmaul A, Maier R: Ueber eine bisher nicht beschriebene eigentümliche Arterienerkrankung (Periarteritis nodosa), die mit Morbus Brightii und rapid fort schreitender allgemeiner Muskellähmung einhergeht. *Dtsch Arch Klin Med* 1866, 1:484–518.

2. Ronco P, Verroust P, Mifnon F, Kourilsky O, Vanhille P, Meyrier A, Maerz JP, Morel-Maroger L: Immunopathological Studies of Polyarteritis Nodosa and Wegener's Granulomatosis: A Report of 43 Patients With 51 Renal Biopsies. *Q J Med* 1983, 52:212–223.

3. Jennette JC, Falk RJ: Anti-neutrophil Cytoplasmic Autoantibodies With Specificity for Myeloperoxidase in Patients With Systemic Vasculitis and Idiopathic Necrotizing and Crescentic Glomerulonephritis. *N Engl J Med* 1988, 318:1651–1657.

4. Jennette JC, Wilkman AS, Falk RJ: Anti-neutrophil Cytoplasmic Antibody-Associated Glomerulonephritis and Vasculitis. *Am J Pathol* 1989, 135:921–930.

5. Davies D, Moran ME, Niall JF, Ryan GB: Segmental Glomerulonephritis With Anti-neutrophil Antibody: Possible Arbovirus Aetiology. *BMJ* 1982, 285:606.

6. Hall JB, Wadham B, Wood CJ, Ashton V, Adam WR: Vasculitis and Glomerulonephritis: A Subgroup With Anti-neutrophil Cytoplasmic Antibody. *Aust N Z J Med* 1984, 14:277–278.

7. van der Woude FJ, Rasmussen N, Lobatto S, Wiik A, Permin H, van Es LA: Autoantibodies Against Neutrophils and Monocytes: Tool for Diagnosis and Marker of Disease Activity in Wegener's Granulomatosis. *Lancet* 1985, i:425–429.

8. Lüdemann G, Gross W: Autoantibodies Against Cytoplasmic Structures of Neutrophil Granulocytes in Wegener's Granulomatosis. *Clin Exp Immunol* 1987, 69:350–357.

9. Nölle B, Specks U, Lüdemann J, Rohrbach MS, DeRemee RA, Gross WL: Anticytoplasmic Antibodies: Their Immunodiagnostic Value in Wegener's Granulomatosis. *Ann Intern Med* 1989, 111:28–40.

10. Cohen Tervaert JW, van der Woude FJ, Fauci AS, Ambrus JL, Velosa J, Keane WF, Meijer S, van der Giessen M, The TH, van der Hem GK, Kallenberg CGM: Association Between Active Wegener's Granulomatosis and Anticytoplasmic Antibodies. *Arch Intern Med* 1989, 149:2461–2465.

11. Venning M, Arfeen S, Bird A: **Antibodies to Neutrophil Cytoplasmic Antigen in Systemic Vasculitis.** *Lancet* 1987, i:850.

12. Feehally J, Wheeler DC, Walls J, Jones S, Lockwood CM, Savage COS: **A Case of Microscopic Polyarteritis Associated With Antineutrophil Cytoplasmic Antibodies.** *Clin Nephrol* 1987, 27:214–215.

13. Wathen CW, Harrison DJ: **Circulating Antineutrophil Antibodies in Systemic Vasculitis.** *Lancet* 1987, i:1037.

14. Cohen Tervaert JW, Goldschmeding R, Elema JD, Limburg PC, van der Giessen M, Huitema MG, Koolen MI, Hene RJ, The TH, van der Hem GK, von dem Borne AEGKr, Kallenberg CGM: **Association of Autoantibodies to Myeloperoxidase With Different Forms of Vasculitis.** *Arthritis Rheum* 1990, 33:1264–1272.

15. Hagen EC, Ballieux BEPB, van Es LA, Daha MR, van der Woude
   • FJ: **Antineutrophil Cytoplasmic Autoantibodies: A Review of the Antigens Involved, the Assays, and the Clinical and Possible Pathogenetic Consequences.** *Blood* 1993, 81:1996–2002.
   A review of ANCA and its possible role in the pathogenesis of vasculitis.

16. Kallenberg CGM, Mulder AHL, Cohen Tervaert JW: **Antineutrophil
   •• Cytoplasmic Antibodies: A Still-Growing Class of Autoantibodies in Inflammatory Disorders.** *Am J Med* 1992, 93:675–682.
   A very good review of ANCA and ANCA-associated diseases. This article has more discussion of non–vasculitis-related atypical ANCA than do other reviews.

17. Ulmer M, Rautmann A, Gross WL: **Immunodiagnostic Aspects
   • of Autoantibodies Against Myeloperoxidase.** *Clin Nephrol* 1992, 37:161–168.
   A discussion of P-ANCA, its disease associations and difficulty in distinguishing it from antinuclear antibodies.

18. Saxon A, Shanahan F, Landers C, Ganz T, Targan S: **A Distinct Subset of Anti-neutrophil Cytoplasmic Antibodies Is Associated With Inflammatory Bowel Disease.** *J Allergy Clin Immunol* 1990, 86:202–210.

19. Duerr RH, Targan SR, Landers CJ, Sutherland LR, Shanahan F: **Antineutrophil Cytoplasmic Antibodies in Ulcerative Colitis: Comparison With Other Colitides/Diarrheal Illness.** *Gastroenterology* 1991, 100:1590–1596.

20. Duerr RH, Targan SR, Landers CJ, La Russo NF, Lindsay KL, Wiesner RH, Shanahan F: **Neutrophil Cytoplasmic Antibodies: A Link Between Primary Sclerosing Cholangitis and Ulcerative Colitis.** *Gastroenterology* 1991, 100:1385–1391.

21. Seibold F, Weber P, Klein R, Berg PA, Wiedmann KH: **Clinical Significance of Antibodies Against Neutrophils in Patients With Inflammatory Bowel Disease and Primary Sclerosing Cholangitis.** *Gut* 1992, 33:657–662.

22. Cambridge G, Rampton DS, Stevens TRJ, McCarthy DA, Kamm M, Leaker B: **Anti-neutrophil Antibodies in Inflammatory Bowel Disease: Prevalence and Diagnostic Role.** *Gut* 1992, 33:668–674.

23. Hardarson S, LaBrecque D, Mitros F, Neil G, Goeken J: **Anti-neu-
   • trophil Cytoplasmic Antibody in Inflammatory Bowel and Hepatobiliary Diseases.** *Am J Clin Pathol* 1993, 99:277–281.
   A discussion of the association of atypical P-ANCA with inflammatory bowel and liver diseases.

24. Oudkerk Pool M, Ellerbroek PM, Ridivan BU, Goldschmeding R, von
   • Blomberg BME, Pena AS, Dolman KM, Bril H, Dekker W, Nauta JJ, Gans ROB, Breed H, Meuwissen SGM: **Serum Antineutrophil Cytoplasmic Autoantibodies in Inflammatory Bowel Disease Are Mainly Associated With Ulcerative Colitis: A Correlation Study Between Perinuclear Antineutrophil Cytoplasmic Autoantibodies and Clinical Parameters, Medical and Surgical Treatment.** *Gut* 1993, 34:46–50.
   A discussion of atypical P-ANCA, its disease associations, and proof of test reproducibility in two different European laboratories.

25. Gross WL, Csernok E, Flesch BK: **"Classic Antineutrophil Cytoplasmic Autoantibodies (cANCA), "Wegener's Autoantigen" and Their Immunopathogenic Role in Wegener's Granulomatosis.** *J Autoimmun* 1993, 6:171–184.

26. Falk RJ, Becker B, Terrell R, Jennette JC: **Antigen Specificity of P-ANCA and of C-ANCA.** *Am J Kidney Dis* 1991, 18:197.

27. Geffriaud-Ricouard C, Noel LH, Chauveau D, Houhou S, Grunfeld
   •• JP, Lesavre P: **Clinical Spectrum Associated With ANCA of Defined Antigen Specificities in 98 Selected Patients.** *Clin Nephrol* 1993, 39:125–136.
   A careful analysis of the clinical spectrum of diseases associated with ANCA of defined antigenic specificity.

28. Gross WL, Schmitt WH, Csernok E: **ANCA and Associated Diseases:
   •• Immunodiagnostic and Pathogenetic Aspects.** *Clin Exp Immunol* 1993, 91:1–12.
   A review of ANCA detection, specificity, and pathogenetic role in vasculitis. This article briefly mentions ANCA in inflammatory bowel and liver diseases.

29. Cohen Tervaert JW, Mulder AHL, Stegeman C, Elema J, Huitema M, The H, Kallenberg C: **Occurrence of Autoantibodies to Human Leucocyte Elastase in Wegener's Granulomatosis and Other Inflammatory Disorders.** *Ann Rheum Dis* 1993, 52:115–120.

30. Mulder AHL, Horst G, van Leeuwen MA, Limburg PC, Kallenberg CGM: **Antineutrophil Cytoplasmic Antibodies in Rheumatoid Arthritis.** *Arthritis Rheum* 1993, 36:1054–1060.

31. Mulder AHL, Horst G, Haagsma E, Limburg P, Kleibeuker J, Kallenberg C: **Prevalence and Characterization of Antineutrophil Cytoplasmic Antibodies in Autoimmune Liver Diseases.** *Hepatology* 1993, 17:411–417.

32. Goeken JA: **Anti-neutrophil Cytoplasmic Antibody: A Useful Serological Marker for Vasculitis.** *J Clin Immunol* 1991, 11:161–174.

33. Mulder AHL, Horst G, Broekroelofs J, Nelis G, Kallenberg C: **ANCA in Inflammatory Bowel Disease Recognize Several Antigens.** *Adv Exp Med Biol* 1993, 336:519–522.

34. Pettersson E, Heigl A: **Antineutrophil Cytoplasmic Antibody (cANCA
   • and pANCA) Titer in Relation to Disease Activity in Patients With Necrotizing Vasculitis: A Longitudinal Study.** *Clin Nephrol* 1992, 37:219–228.
   A study following ANCA titers and vasculitic disease activity.

35. Hoffman GS, Kerr GS, Leavitt RY, Hallahan CW, Lebovics RS, Travis WD, Rottem M, Fauci AS: **Wegener's Granulomatosis: An Analysis of 158 Patients.** *Ann Intern Med* 1992, 116:488–498.

36. Hagen EC, Andrassy K, Chernok E, Daha MR, Gaskin G, Gross W, Lesavre P, Lüdemann J, Pusey CD, Rasmussen N, Savage COS, Sinico A, Wiik A, van der Woude FJ: **The Value of Indirect Immunofluorescence and Solid Phase Techniques for ANCA Detection.** *J Immunol Methods* 1993, 159:1–16.

37. Falk RJ, Hogan S, Carey TS, Jennette JC: **Clinical Course of Antineutrophil Cytoplasmic Autoantibody-Associated Glomerulonephritis and Systemic Vasculitis.** *Ann Intern Med* 1990, 113:656–663.

38. Charles LA, Caldas MLR, Falk RJ, Terrell RS, Jennette JC: **Antibodies Against Granule Proteins Activate Neutrophils In Vitro.** *J Leukoc Biol* 1991, 50:539–546.

39. Falk RJ, Terrell R, Charles LA, Jennette JC: **Antineutrophil Cytoplasmic Autoantibodies Induce Neutrophils to Degranulate and Produce Oxygen Radicals In Vitro.** *Proc Natl Acad Sci U S A* 1990, 87:4115–4119.

40. Ewert BH, Jennette JC, Falk RJ: **Antibodies Against Myeloperoxidase Stimulate Primed Neutrophils to Damage Human Endothelial Cells In Vitro.** *Kidney Int* 1992, 41:375–383.

41. Jennette JC, Ewert BH, Falk RJ: **Do Antineutrophil Cytoplasmic Au-
   •• toantibodies Cause Wegener's Granulomatosis and Other Forms of Necrotizing Vasculitis?** *Rheum Dis Clin North Am* 1993, 19:1–14.
   A review of ANCA and its role in the pathogenesis of vasculitis.

42. Savage OS, Pottinger BE, Gaskin G, Pusey CD, Pearson JD: **Autoantibodies Developing to Myeloperoxidase and Proteinase-3 in Systemic Vasculitis Stimulate Neutrophil Cytotoxicity Toward Cultured Endothelial Cells.** *Am J Pathol* 1992, 141:335–342.

43. Mayet WJ, Meyer zum Büschenfelde KH: **Antibodies to Proteinase-3 Increase Neutrophil Adhesion to Endothelial Cells.** *Clin Exp Immunol* 1993, 94:440–446.

44. Varagunam M, Adu D, Taylor CM, Michael J, Richards N, Neuberger J, Thompson RA: **Endothelium, Myeloperoxidase, Anti-myeloperoxidase Interaction in Vasculitis.** *Adv Exp Med Biol* 1993, 336:129–132.

45. Mayet WJ, Csernok E, Symkowiak C, Gross WL, Meyer zum
   • Büschenfelde KH: **Human Endothelial Cells Express Proteinase-3, the Target Antigen of Anticytoplasmic Antibodies in Wegener's Granulomatosis.** *Blood* 1993, 82:1221–1229.
   An interesting study demonstrating PR-3 in endothelial cells.

46. Dolman KM, Stegeman CA, van de Wiel BA, Hack CE, von dem Bourne AE, Kallenberg CG, Goldschmeding R: **Relevance of Classic Anti-neutrophil Cytoplasmic Autoantibody (C-ANCA)-Mediated Inhibition of Proteinase-3-α-1-Antitrypsin Complexation to Disease Activity in Wegener's Granulomatosis.** *Clin Exp Immunol* 1993, 91:405–410.

47. Esnault VLM, Testa A, Audraine M, Rogé C, Hamidou M, Barrier JH, Sesboüé R, Martin J-P, Lesavre P: **Alpha-1-Antitrypsin Genetic Polymorphism in ANCA-Positive Systemic Vasculitis.** *Kidney Int* 1993, 43:1329–1332.

48. van der Woude FJ, van Es LA, Daha MR: **The Role of C-ANCA Antigen in the Pathogenesis of Wegener's Granulomatosis Based on Both Humoral and Cellular Mechanisms.** *Neth J Med* 1990, 36:169–171.

49. Peterson J, Rasmussen N: **Cellular Immune Responses and Pathogenesis in C-ANCA Positive Vasculitides.** *J Autoimmun* 1993, 6:227–236.

50. Savage COS, Pottinger BE, Gaskin G, Lockwood CM, Pusey CD: **Vascular Damage in Wegener's Granulomatosis and Microscopic Pol-**

yarteritis: Presence of Anti-endothelial Cell Antibodies and Their Relationship to Anti-neutrophil Cytoplasm Antibodies. *Clin Exp Immunol* 1991, **85**:14–19.

51. Ferraro G, Meroni PL, Tincani A, Sinico A, Barcelleni W, Radice A, Gregorini G, Froldi M, Borghini MO, Balestrieri G: **Anti-endothelial Cell Antibodies in Patients With Wegener's Granulomatosis and Micropolyarteritis.** *Clin Exp Immunol* 1990, **79**:47–53.

52. Brasile L, Kremer JM, Clarke JL, Cerelli J: **Identification of an Autoantibody to Vascular Endothelial Cell-Specific Antigens in Patients With Systemic Vasculitis.** *Am J Med* 1989, **87**:74–80.

53. Frampton G, Jaynes DRW, Perry GJ, Lockwood CM, Cameron JS: **Autoantibodies to Endothelial Cells and Neutrophil Cytoplasmic Antigens in Systemic Vasculitis.** *Clin Exp Immunol* 1990, **82**:227–232.

54. D'Cruz DP, Houssiau FA, Ramirez G, Baguley E, McCutcheon J, Vianna J, Haga HJ, Swana GT, Khamashta MA, Taylor JC, Davies DR, Hughes GVR: **Antibodies to Endothelial Cells in Systemic Lupus Erythematosus: A Potential Marker for Nephritis and Vasculitis.** *Clin Exp Immunol* 1991, **85**:254–261.

55. Savage COS, Cooke SP: **The Role of the Endothelium in Systemic**
•• **Vasculitis.** *J Autoimmun* 1993, **6**:237–249.
An excellent overview of endothelial cell–leukocyte interaction and the role of the endothelial cell in vasculitis.

56. Wang MX, Walker RG, Kincaid-Smith P: **Clinicopathologic Associations of Anti-endothelial Cell Antibodies in Immunoglobulin A Nephropathy and Lupus Nephritis.** *Am J Kidney Dis* 1993, **22**:378–386.

57. Penning CA, Cunningham J, French MAH, Harrison G, Rowell NR, Hughes P: **Antibody-Dependent Cytotoxicity of Human Vascular Endothelium in Systemic Sclerosis.** *Clin Exp Immunol* 1984, **57**:548–556.

58. Cerilli J, Holliday JE, Fesperman DP, Folger MA: **Antivascular Endothelial Cell Antibody: Its Role in Transplantation.** *Surgery* 1977, **81**:132–138.

59. Yap HK, Sakai RS, Bahn L, Rappaport V, Woo KT, Ananthuraman V, Lim CH, Chiang GSC, Jordan SC: **Antivascular Endothelial Cell Antibodies in Patients With IgA Nephropathy: Frequency and Clinical Significance.** *Clin Immunol Immunopathol* 1988, **49**:450–453.

60. Leung DYM, Moake JL, Havens PL, Kim M, Prober JS: **Lytic Antiendothelial Cell Antibodies in Haemolytic Uraemic Syndrome.** *Lancet* 1988, **ii**:183–186.

61. Burns ER, Zucker-Franklin D: **Pathologic Effects of Plasma From Patients With Thrombotic Thrombocytopenic Purpura on Platelets and Cultured Vascular Endothelial Cells.** *Blood* 1982, **60**:1030–1037.

62. Rappaport VJ, Hirata G, Yap HK, Jordan SC: **Antivascular Endothelial Cell Antibodies in Severe Preeclampsia.** *Am J Obstet Gynecol* 1990, **162**:138–146.

63. Chan TM, Frampton G, Jayne DRW, Perry GI, Lockwood CM,
• Cameron JS: **Clinical Significance of Anti-endothelial Cell Antibodies in Systemic Vasculitis: A Longitudinal Study Comparing Anti-endothelial Cell Antibodies and Anti-neutrophil Cytoplasmic Antibodies.** *Am J Kidney Dis* 1993, **22**:387–392.
A good study of the clinical significance of ANCA and AECA in systemic vasculitis.

64. Goeken JA: **Using ANCA Tests in Vasculitis Diagnosis.** *Clin Immunol Spectrum* 1992, **4**:4–5.

James A. Goeken, MD, Professor of Pathology, Immunopathology Laboratory, 5238 RCP, University of Iowa College of Medicine, Iowa City, IA 52242-1009, USA.

Psychopharmacologic approaches to the difficult dermatologic patient

John Koo, MD, and Jaeho Lee, MD

University of California, San Francisco Medical Center, San Francisco, California, USA

A significant proportion of dermatologic patients present with underlying psychologic factors associated with their skin complaints. Most psychodermatologic cases that are blatant enough in their clinical presentations to catch the attention of the dermatologist fall into four categories, namely anxiety, psychosis, depression, and obsessive-compulsive disorder. This article discusses developments in psychopharmacology that are relevant to the treatment of such patients.

Current Opinion in Dermatology 1995:83–86

It is well known among dermatologists that a significant proportion of their patients present with underlying psychologic factors associated with their chief complaint (Table 1). For example, there are patients with real skin disorders such as eczema or psoriasis who report that emotional stress is frequently responsible for the flare of their skin disease. A different kind of patient has no real skin problems whatsoever but presents with self-induced lesions, as in trichotillomania, delusions of parasitosis, or neurotic excoriations. Another group of patients experiences significant psychiatric morbidity owing to disfigurement from skin disease. Lastly, there are patients who present mainly with chronic cutaneous sensory complaints such as itching, burning, or stinging sensations with no visible rash and no apparent medical or neurologic explanation for their symptoms; for some of these patients, underlying anxiety or depression may play a causative or exacerbating role in their perception of the cutaneous sensory complaints. If the number of dermatologists trained in the United States diminishes, and primary care physicians take over the care of simpler cases of acne, psoriasis, eczema, and warts, dermatologists may end up with a different composition of patient population, many of whom their primary care physicians consider difficult either to diagnose or to manage; it is entirely conceivable that many of these difficult-to-diagnose or difficult-to-manage cases will turn out to have more psychologic undercurrents.

Many people with psychodermatologic complaints often refuse to see a psychiatrist or any other mental health professional. On the other hand, dermatologists generally have neither the time nor the training to conduct psychotherapy or behavioral therapy. If a dermatologist addressed the psychologic component of the chief complaint, the most feasible method would still be the judicious use of psychopharmacologic agents. However, there are at least two major obstacles to dermatologists' adding psychopharmacologic agents to their therapeutic options, namely a doubt as to whether it is appropriate for a dermatologist to use psychopharmacologic agents, and second, the fear of certain side effects associated with each class of agents.

Table 1. Categories of psychodermatologic problems

Primary psychiatric disorders
    Delusions of parasitosis
    Tricotillomania
    Neurotic excoriations
Psychophysiologic disorders
    Psoriasis
    Atopic dermatitis
    Urticaria
Cutaneous sensory disorders
    Pruritis sine materia
    Pruritis ani
    Glossodynia
Secondary psychiatric disorders
    Any disfiguring skin disease
        Vitiligo
        Alopecia areata

Whether it is appropriate to use psychopharmacologic agents is a concern unique to dermatologists. Nonpsychiatric physicians in other fields such as medicine and family practice have long used psychopharmacologic agents, and thus, it would not be an issue for them. For years, in fact, nonpsychiatric physicians have prescribed more psychopharmacologic agents than psychiatrists have, except in the categories of antipsychotic and anti–manic-depressive agents such as lithium, because most patients with depression or anxiety disorders prefer to be treated by their primary care physician rather than by a psychiatrist. Thus, a dermatologist who learns to use psychopharmacologic agents may be a pioneer in the field but presents no anomaly in the wider context of medical practice.

The other concern that prevents dermatologists from utilizing psychopharmacologic options is the fear of side effects. Each category of agent has certain characteristic, troublesome side-effect profiles. For example, antianxiety agents may cause sedation and pose a risk of addiction. Antipsychotic agents are associated with extrapyramidal side effects such as tardive dyskinesia. Antidepressants can be associated with cardiac side effects as well as with orthostatic hypotension, sedation, and anticholinergic side effects. Lastly, anti–obsessive-compulsive agents, which are also antidepressants, share the same risks of side effects as the antidepressants. Therefore, what is truly exciting is the recent development of new agents that are designed to eliminate those stereotypical side effects. This article discusses the new developments in each class of psychopharmacologic agents. It will become clear that in the foreseeable future, psychopharmacologic agents may be free of many of their traditional side effects. To use psychopharmacologic agents appropriately, the clinician must first determine the nature of the underlying psychopathology involved. Although any of the myriad psychopathologies can conceivably be involved, most of psychodermatologic cases that are blatant enough in their clinical presentations to catch the attention of the dermatologist fall into four categories, namely anxiety, psychosis, depression, and obsessive-compulsive disorder (Fig. 1).

Antianxiety agents

The traditional benzodiazepine-type antianxiety agents such as diazepam (Valium; Roche Products, Manati, PR) or chlordiazepoxide hydrochloride (Librium; Roche Products, Manati, PR) have three major drawbacks, namely the risks of sedation, addiction, and accumulation after prolonged use. Because these agents have so many active metabolites with a long half-life, their chronic use may result in a build-up in the body, leading to what has been described as a "zombie-like appearance" in some patients. When a new type of benzodiazepine, alprazolam (Xanax; Upjohn Co., Kalamazoo, MI), became available, it was initially seen as a great advance, because it had a more predictable half-life, and most of the medication was excreted out of the system by the time the next dose was taken. Over time, however, the initial enthusiasm for alprazolam was dampened when many patients who had abruptly discontinued its use reported a quick recurrence of the symptoms of their anxiety disorders. Many of these cases were initially misjudged as manifestations of physical addiction. In retrospect, however, many of these cases appear to represent a simple recurrence of anxiety following an abrupt fall in the level of alprazolam in the blood as one would expect from its short half-life. One analogy would be the difference between oral prednisone and intramuscular triamcinolone acetonide in treating severe inflammatory conditions such as poison oak contact dermatitis. If a patient who is on prednisone forgets to take his or her dose, it is not unusual for the contact dermatitis to reflare in 1 or 2 days, whereas if the same patient is treated with an intramuscular triamcinolone injection, such a quick recurrence would be unlikely, because triamcinolone acetonide tapers itself off. Alprazolam extended release (Xanax XR; Upjohn Co., Kalamazoo, MI), which will be available, has been developed to overcome the shortfalls of alprazolam. A single dose of alprazolam extended release is adequate to give relatively stable coverage for an entire day.

The goal of new developments in antianxiety agents is to eliminate the risk of sedation and addiction typically associated with traditional benzodiazepine-class antianxiety agents. Buspirone (BuSpar; Meade Johnson Pharmaceuticals, Evansville, IN) is the first of the nonsedating, nonaddictive antianxiety agents to come on the market. Unlike benzodiazepines, which can be used as needed, buspirone must be used on a regular basis to be effective, and the onset of therapeutic effect may not occur until at least 2 weeks after the initiation of therapy. One of the biggest complaints among clinicians has been that a significant proportion of the patients treated with buspirone appear to experience no therapeutic benefit whatsoever. Obviously, a nonsedating, nonaddictive, and efficacious antianxiety agent would be ideal. Such agents are being developed, one of which is a β-carboline type of antianxiety agent named abecarnil. Abecarnil has a high affinity for benzodiazepine receptors [1•] and decreases γ-aminobutyric acid conduction to the same degree as some benzodiazepines do. Despite the apparent similarity of their mechanisms, abecarnil is known to be nonsedating and nonaddictive [1•,2]. So far, side effects are relatively rare and usually consist of dizziness, unsteady gait, and di-

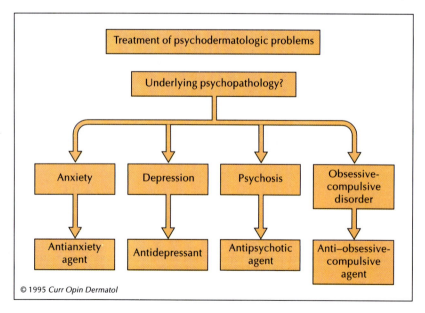

Fig. 1. Treatment options for psychodermatologic problems, based on underlying psychopathology.

© 1995 *Curr Opin Dermatol*

minished concentration. There are reasons to believe that abecarnil may fulfill the expectations of high efficacy without the side effects typically associated with the traditional antianxiety agents.

Antipsychotic agents

In the dermatologic community, pimozide (Orap; Gate Pharmaceuticals, Sellersville, PA) is well known as the treatment of choice for delusions of parasitosis, which is one subtype of encapsulated delusional disorders called monosymptomatic hypochondriacal psychosis [3]. However, the use of pimozide and other traditional antipsychotic agents has been complicated by the extrapyramidal (*ie*, pseudoparkinsonian) side effects such as stiffness, restlessness, acute dystonic reaction, and tardive dyskinesia. Recent developments in psychopharmacology have led to the understanding that there are different subsets of dopamine receptors in the brain, each of which is responsible for different effects of these medications. Dopamine D_2 receptors in the mesolimbic area of the brain mediate the antipsychotic effect, whereas the dopamine D_1 receptors in the nigrostriatal pathway mediate extrapyramidal side effects [4•,5,6]. Recently, an antipsychotic agent called clozapine (Clozaril; Sandoz Pharmaceuticals Corp., East Hanover, NJ) became available in the United States. This is the first agent that selectively blocks dopamine D_2 receptors with almost no effect on the dopamine D_1 receptors. With this antipsychotic agent, therefore, there is essentially no risk of extrapyramidal side effects, including tardive dyskinesia. In fact, in the worldwide literature, there are no reported cases of tardive dyskinesia associated with this agent, even though clozapine has been used extensively in Europe and China. However, the most serious drawback of this medication is the risk of agranulocytosis, which may occur at a frequency of as much as 1% to 2% [7,8].

New medications are therefore being developed, such as sulpiride and risperidone. Sulpiride, a selective D_2 antagonist, has an antipsychotic efficacy comparable to that of haloperidol (Haldol; McNeil Pharmaceutical, Spring House, PA) and produces fewer and less intense extrapyramidal side effects [6], and yet this agent has not been associated with agranulocytosis. Another new antipsychotic, risperidone, has recently received the approval of the Food and Drug Administration. Risperidone is a benzisoxazole derivative and has antagonistic properties toward both D_2 and serotonin receptors. It is a potent antipsychotic medication with fewer extrapyramidal side effects than traditional neuroleptics [4•,5,6]. Without losing efficacy, these and other medications with similar profiles are likely to eliminate much of the concern about the most troublesome side effects associated with the use of antipsychotic agents.

Antidepressants

The traditional antidepressants such as amitriptyline (Elavil; Merck & Co., West Point, PA) or doxepin (Sinequan; Pfitzer, New York, NY) have been associated with many anticholinergic side effects such as dry mouth, constipation, exacerbation of narrow angle glaucoma, blurred vision, and urinary retention; these effects are mediated through the blocking of muscarinic cholinergic receptors. Moreover, α_1-noradrenergic receptor blockade by these agents results in orthostatic hypotension, and histamine$_1$ receptor blockade results in sedation. Finally, these agents are also associated with an increased QT interval in the cardiac cycle that can lead to fatal arrhythmia. The initial goal of antidepressant research was to develop secondary tricyclic antidepressants such as desipramine (Norpramin; Marion Merrill Dow Pharmaceuticals, Cincinnati, OH) and nortriptyline (Pamelor; Sandoz Pharmaceuticals Corp., East Hanover, NJ), which possess far fewer anticholinergic, sedative, or arrhythmogenic properties. The other approach to eliminating these side effects was to develop nontricyclic "second generation" antidepressants such as trazodone (Desyrel; Meade Johnson Pharmaceuticals, Evansville, IN), bupropion (Wellbutrin; Burroughs Wellcome Co., Research Triangle Park, NC), and fluoxetine (Prozac; Lilly, Eli, and Co., Indianapolis, IN). These nontricyclic agents generally have better side-effect profiles than the tricyclics because they tend to have no effect on muscarinic cholinergic receptors, α_1-noradrenergic receptors, or histaminic receptors. They generally do not interfere with myocardial conduction. Many of these agents selectively block the reuptake of serotonin in the brain. It has been recognized for many years that most antidepressants are either potent reuptake blocking agents for noradrenergic or serotonergic receptors. In clinical practice, when a particular case of depression proves unresponsive to a norepinephrine reuptake inhibitor, the patient is tried on medications that preferentially block the reuptake of neurotransmitters in the serotonergic system.

Among the latest development in the evolution of antidepressants is venlafaxine. This agent has no affinity for α_1-adrenergic, dopaminergic, cholinergic, or histaminergic receptors, and generally, therefore, it has not been associated with the side effects of the traditional tricyclic antidepressants [9••]. Moreover, it does inhibit the reuptake of both norepinephrine and serotonin. This agent has been tested in more than 2500 patients and has been found to have superior efficacy and early onset of action as compared with the antidepressants currently in use. The introduction of such an agent is expected to ease the anxiety related to the use of antidepressants, especially for nonpsychiatric physicians.

Anti–obsessive-compulsive agents

In the United States, the only agent that is currently approved by the Food and Drug Administration for use as an anti–obsessive-compulsive agent is clomipramine (Anafranil; Ciba-Geigy Corp., Summit, NJ), a tertiary tricyclic antidepressant with a side effect profile similar to those of amitriptyline and doxepin. Currently, there is growing evidence that fluoxetine is just as effective as clomipramine in treating obsessive-compulsive disorders (Fig. 2) [10,11,12], and there is a possibility that this agent may also be approved by the Food and Drug Administration for use in obsessive-compulsive patients. As stated in the section on antidepressants, fluoxetine is free of most of the side effects associated with traditional tricyclic antidepressants. Although it does have a unique side-effect profile of its own—a relatively high frequency of drug eruption and a propensity to increase agitation and anxiety in some patients, especially in the first 2 to 3 weeks of use—it is generally easier to use than clomipramine for most practitioners.

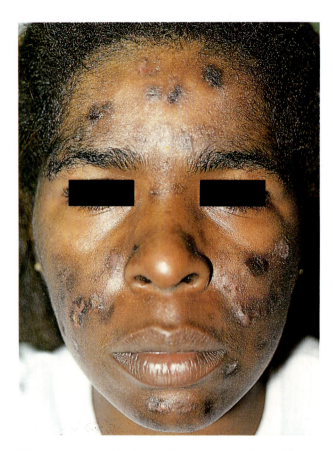

Fig. 2. Acne excoriée due to obsessive-compulsive disorder.

Conclusions

In this article, new developments in psychopharmacology that are relevant to the treatment of psychodermatologic cases have been discussed in detail. The unmistakable trend is toward the development of psychopharmacologic agents that have fewer and fewer side effects and are therefore easier to use. An antianxiety agent without risk of sedation or addiction and an antipsychotic agent without risk of dyskinesia are already on the market. Overall, psychopharmacologic agents are generally associated with less risk for serious side effects than many of the agents that dermatologists already use routinely, such as methotrexate, systemic steroids, and cyclosporine. As psychopharmacologic agents be-

come more and more "user-friendly," it will become easier for a dermatologist to incorporate these important therapeutic options into his or her therapeutic armamentarium.

References and recommended reading

Papers of particular interest, published within the annual period of review, have been highlighted as:
•   Of special interest
•• Of outstanding interest

1.   Duka T, Schutt B, Krause W, Dorow R, McDonald S, Fichte F: **Human**
•   **Studies on Abecarnil, a New Beta-Carboline Anxiolytic: Safety, Tolerability and Preliminary Pharmacological Profile.** *Br J Clin Pharmacol* 1993, **35**:386–394.
Single- and multiple-dose abecarnil administration to normal subjects resulted in effects in high doses (20 or 40 mg single administration, or 20 or 30 mg three times daily) that resembled those of other similarly acting antianxiety compounds with the exception of a lack of marked sedation or drowsiness.

2.   Steppuhn KG, Schneider HH, Turski L, Stephens DN: **Long-Term Treatment With Abecarnil Does Not Induce Diazepam-like Dependence in Mice.** *J Pharmacol Exp Ther* 1993, **264**:1395–1400.

3.   Koo JYM, Pham CT: **Psychodermatology.** *Arch Dermatol* 1992, **128**:381–388.

4.   Meltzer HY: **New Drugs for the Treatment of Schizophrenia.** *Psychiatr*
•   *Clin North Am* 1993, **16**:365–385.
This article reviews four classes of newly established and potential antipsychotics: 1) selective D_2/D_3 receptor antagonists and D_1 antagonists, 2) partial D_2 receptor agonists, 3) nondopaminergic antipsychotics, and 4) antagonists of D_2 and other receptors.

5.   Deutch AY, Moghaddam B, Innis RB, Krystal JH, Aghajanian GK, Bunney BS, Charney DS: **Mechanisms of Action of Atypical Antipsychotic Drugs: Implications for Novel Therapeutic Strategies for Schizophrenia.** *Schizophr Res* 1991, **4**:121–156.

6.   Gerlach J: **New Antipsychotics: Classifications, Efficacy and Adverse Effects.** *Schizophr Bull* 1991, **17**:289–309.

7.   Claas FHJ: **Drug Induced Agranulocytosis: Review of Possible Mechanisms, and Prospects for Clozapine Studies.** *Psychopharmacology* 1989, **99**:5113–5117.

8.   Krupp P, Barnes P: **Leponex-Associated Granulocytopenia: A Review of the Situation.** *Psychopharmacology* 1989, **99**:5118–5121.

9.   Montgomery SA: **Venlafaxine: A New Dimension in Antidepressant**
•• **Pharmacotherapy.** *J Clin Psychiatry* 1993, **54**:119–126.
This is an excellent review of the evolution of currently used antidepressants as wells as venlafaxine, the first of a new class of antidepressants that selectively inhibit the uptake of both norepinephrine and serotonin. The excellent safety profile of venlafaxine during long-term treatment is superior to that of the standard antidepressants.

10. Pigott TA, Pato MT, Bernstein SE, Grover GN, Hill JL, Tolliver TJ, Murphy DL: **Controlled Comparisons of Clomipramine and Fluoxetine in the Treatment of Obsessive-Compulsive Disorder: Behavioral and Biological Results.** *Arch Gen Psychiatry* 1990, **47**:926–932.

11. Liebowitz MR, Hollander E, Fairbanks J, Campeas R: **Fluoxetine for Adolescents With Obsessive-Compulsive Disorder.** *Am J Psychiatry* 1990, **147**:370–371.

12. Turner SM, Jacob RG, Beidel DC, Himmelhoch J: **Fluoxetine Treatment of Obsessive-Compulsive Disorder.** *J Clin Psychopharmacol* 1985, **5**:207–212.

John Koo, MD, and Jaeho Lee, MD, University of California, San Francisco Medical Center, Suite A-135, 400 Parnassus Avenue, San Francisco, CA 94143, USA.

The multisyndrome spectrum of necrolytic migratory erythema

Cherylyn K. Black, MD, and Warren W. Piette, MD

University of Iowa, Iowa City, Iowa, USA

While the term *necrolytic migratory erythema* implies an associated glucagonoma, in fact many other eruptions occurring in separate and distinctive clinical settings may present with very similar clinical and pathologic cutaneous findings. These syndromes include in part such apparently disparate metabolic settings as zinc deficiency, essential fatty acid deficiency, maple syrup urine disease and other aminoacidurias, niacin deficiency, cystic fibrosis, kwashiorkor, nephrotic syndrome, biotin disorders, and pyridoxine deficiency. This paper first presents the typical manifestations of necrolytic migratory erythema and then explores what is known concerning the metabolic alterations that might explain the cutaneous findings in each of the syndromes. Finally, possible common metabolic links between these seemingly distinct metabolic syndromes are considered.

Current Opinion in Dermatology 1995:87–93

The cutaneous eruption associated with a pancreatic islet cell tumor, first described in 1942 [1], was subsequently named necrolytic migratory erythema (NME) on the basis of distinctive clinical and histologic features [2,3]. There followed reports of this eruption in patients without islet cell tumors, both with and without hyperglucagonemia [3–5]. In fact, multiple clinical settings appear capable of producing NME-like eruptions. Each of these clinical settings is described briefly, and possible common links between these different metabolic alterations and the production of NME-like eruptions are explored.

Glucagonoma and hyperglucagonemia syndromes

Glucagon is stored in pancreatic α-islet cells and released in response to hypoglycemia or stress, stimulating gluconeogenesis. Glucagonoma is a rare tumor of the α-islet cells of the pancreas resulting in excess production of glucagon, with compensatory insulin secretion adequate to suppress lipolysis and keto acid production [6••,7••]. Hypoaminoacidemia is characteristic of glucagonoma syndrome; serum amino acid levels are usually less than 50% of normal [7••,8–10].

The glucagonoma syndrome is characterized by NME (68% to 90% of cases), mild glucose intolerance (83%), hypoaminoaciduria (100%), anemia (85%), weight loss (66%), stomatitis, glossitis, diffuse alopecia, brittle nails,

diarrhea, and thromboembolic events [2,6••,7••]. NME may precede other signs of a pancreatic tumor by several years. Most typically, it involves the perineum, buttocks, and lower abdomen, and frequently, the periorificial and mucosal areas, although lesions may develop anywhere. The lesions begin as erythematous patches, then develop epidermal separation centrally (sometimes producing vesicles or bullae), followed by scaling and crusting. Annular or gyrate morphologies are characteristic (Fig. 1). Lesions heal over a period of 7 days to 3 weeks, leaving hyperpigmented areas.

Typical cutaneous pathologic features of the eruption include epidermal necrosis, subcorneal pustules, confluent parakeratosis, epidermal hyperplasia, papillary dermal angiodysplasia, and suppurative folliculitis, although these features may be lacking in early cutaneous disease [2,11].

The actual cause of NME is not clear. Despite the histologic and clinical similarity of NME to that of acrodermatitis enteropathica, zinc levels in glucagonoma syndrome are normal. Hyperglucagonemia alone, independent of a glucagonoma, can produce this eruption [2]. Hyperglucagonemia does not directly cause NME, however, because resolution of the eruption occurs with the administration of amino acids despite unchanged plasma glucagon levels [10,12].

The diagnosis of glucagonoma with NME depends on a high index of suspicion in evaluating unusual periorificial, annular, or bullous eruptions, a compatible clin-

---

Abbreviations
EFA—essential fatty acid; **MSUD**—maple syrup urine disease; **NME**—necrolytic migratory erythema.

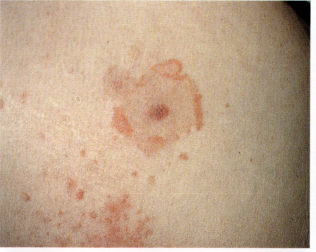

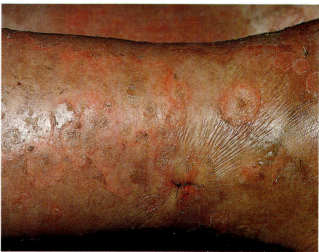

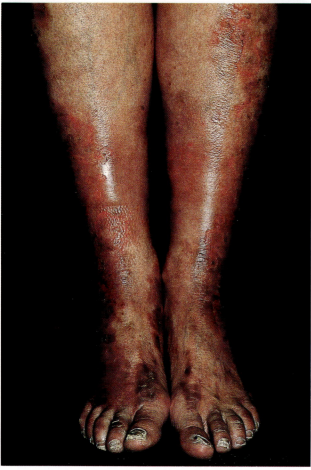

Fig 1. Upper left, Lesion with central vesicle and annular and gyrate erythematous borders in a patient with glucagonoma syndrome. **Upper right**, Annular and erosive necrolytic migratory erythema (NME) in the same patient, with early hyperpigmentation. **Bottom**, Later, prior to curative surgery, NME in the same patient evolves to very hyperpigmented lesions.

ical syndrome and histopathology, and confirmation of highly elevated serum glucagon levels (usually above 1000 pg/mL) [6••].

The mainstay of treatment for glucagonoma is surgical removal of the tumor [7••]. Somatostatin analogues may decrease glucagon secretion with clinical improvement and may be useful when complete removal of the tumor mass is not possible. Intravenous administration of amino acids has been shown to clear the rash without the addition of zinc or essential fatty acids (EFAs) [10,12].

Acrodermatitis enteropathica and zinc deficiency

Acrodermatitis enteropathica is a rare autosomal recessive disorder resulting from an inherited malabsorption of zinc. It was first described in 1936 and in 1973 was shown to resolve with zinc supplements alone [13,14]. Acquired zinc deficiency has been reported with malabsorption and malnutrition from alcoholic liver cirrhosis and alcoholic pancreatitis, malabsorption from short bowel or bowel bypass syndrome, inadequate dietary intake, parenteral hyperalimentation without adequate replacement, cancer chemotherapy, and progressive HIV infection [14,15,16•]. Cirrhosis and alcoholism are known to cause zinc deficiency in part by increasing the urinary loss of zinc [4]. In both hereditary acrodermatitis enteropathica and acquired zinc depletion syndrome, the clinical and systemic manifestations are similar although somewhat age-dependent.

Zinc deficiency is characterized by acrodermatitis, alopecia, nail dystrophy, gastrointestinal disturbances, impaired cellular immunity, recurrent infections, poor wound healing, and growth failure [13,14,16•,17]. Symptoms prominent in infancy include diarrhea, mood changes, anorexia, and neurological disturbances; in toddlers, growth retardation, alopecia, weight loss, and recurrent infections predominate.

The dermatitis develops in an acral and periorificial pattern, then extends to the trunk and extremities. The skin lesions begin as small, moist, erythematous patches and papules and progress to vesicles, bullae, or moist, fissured, crusted erosions or psoriasiform plaques over bony prominences. They quickly cover large areas.

The histopathologies of hereditary and acquired zinc depletion are indifferentiable [15,17]. Cutaneous pathologic features are also very similar to those described in NME, pellagra, and Hartnup disease [18–20].

Zinc absorption in acrodermatitis enteropathica is abnormal, but the mechanism of malabsorption remains uncertain [13,21]. Zinc deficiency results in inactivity of zinc-dependent enzymes, less stable cell membranes, and secondary gastrointestinal abnormalities leading to additional nutritional deficiencies [13,21]. One aspect of this altered metabolism and malabsorption is a change in the plasma levels of EFAs, due both to decreased enteral absorption of unsaturated fatty acids and to impaired desaturation of linoleic and linolenic acids to their long-chain metabolites [21,22]. The restoration of normal plasma EFA levels following supplemental zinc administration seems to precede resolution of the skin lesions [21].

The diagnosis of acrodermatitis enteropathica is usually clinical. Laboratory evidence of plasma zinc deficiency supports the diagnosis; other useful indicators include deficiency of zinc-dependent enzymes such as alkaline phosphatase, and alterations in the plasma fatty acid profile [13]. An *in vitro* or *in vivo* zinc absorption test using radioisotopes (^{65}Zn or ^{69m}Zn) may be helpful, but the simplest test may be the clinical response to replacement with 3 to 30 μmol/kg of zinc per day over a 5-day period [13,16•].

Diagnosis of acrodermatitis enteropathica is of utmost importance, because death may occur in 1 to 3 years if the condition is left untreated. Therapy for inherited disease is lifelong. Oral zinc supplementation is the treatment of choice, with the dosage adjusted according to demand, secondary growth, and stressors [13].

Biotin deficiency and biotin-responsive inborn errors of metabolism

Biotin is part of the vitamin B complex and is required as a cofactor for the function of four carboxylase enzymes in humans. These include three mitochondrial enzymes, *ie*, β-methylcrotonyl coenzyme A carboxylase, propionylcoenzyme A carboxylase, and pyruvic acid carboxylase, and one cytosolic enzyme, acetylcoenzyme A carboxylase [23,24]. The mitochondrial enzymes are essential for the catabolism of leucine, isoleucine, threonine, valine, and methionine, and for gluconeogenesis and carbohydrate metabolism. Acetylcoenzyme A carboxylase catalyzes the first committed step in the biosynthesis of fatty acids [23].

Biotin deficiency may be induced by a diet deficient in biotin, by an avidin-rich diet with large quantities of raw egg whites, or by prolonged parenteral nutrition with inadequate biotin replacement [14,24–26]. Deficiencies of individual biotin-dependent enzymes in this pathway do not respond to biotin replacement [23]. There are, however, two autosomal recessive defects of human biotin utilization that are biotin-responsive. The first is known as holocarboxylase or early-onset (*ie*, neonatal) multiple carboxylase deficiency. It is a disorder of biotinylation resulting from deficient activities of the three mitochondrial carboxylases. Clinical symptoms of holocarboxylase deficiency include difficulties in feeding and breathing, hypotonia, seizures, lethargy or coma, and altered immune function [23,24,27–29]. Roughly half of the few reported patients developed skin rash and alopecia [23,27,28]. Affected children exhibit metabolic acidosis, hyperammonemia, and organic aciduria.

Biotinidase deficiency, also known as late-onset (*ie*, juvenile) multiple carboxylase deficiency, is a disorder of biotin recycling leading to biotin deficiency [14,23,24,28]. Biotinidase deficiency commonly presents with seizures, hypotonia, ataxia, breathing problems, keratoconjunctivitis, glossitis, hearing loss, optic atrophy, developmental delay, and recurrent fungal infections. Alopecia and dermatitis have been reported in 22 (53%) of 38 of such patients [23,30•]. Most symptomatic children exhibit metabolic ketolactic acidosis and organic aciduria.

Biotin deficiency and biotin-dependent carboxylase deficiencies can produce a periorificial, erythematous rash with mild scaling and crusted erosions resembling acrodermatitis enteropathica, sometimes involving the trunk and extremities [14,27,29,30•,31•].

It has been suggested that disturbances in the metabolism of polyunsaturated and odd-chain fatty acids have a role in the cutaneous manifestations of biotin deficiency and biotin-responsive inborn errors of metabolism. Dermatitis and alopecia in one patient with probable biotinidase deficiency improved with administration of oral and topical unsaturated fatty acids prior to biotin treatment [28,32]. Evidence from animal studies also suggests that the eruption of biotin deficiency may be mediated by acquired abnormalities in polyunsaturated EFA metabolism, with correction of the cutaneous findings by replacement of EFAs despite persistent biotin deficiency [30•,31•].

Biotin deficiency is treated by replacement; biotin-responsive syndromes are treated by biotin supplementation [14,23,28]. Biotin replacement can prevent but cannot reverse any neurologic deficits already manifest, and therefore benefits of therapy depend on timing of biotin replacement.

Inherited aminoacidurias and protein deficiency syndromes

In inherited aminoacidurias, the defect may be in an enzymatic step in the metabolic pathway of one or more amino acids. Cutaneous manifestations have been reported with several different syndromes [27]. However, only three syndromes produce NME-like eruptions: maple syrup urine disease (MSUD), neonatal citrullinemia, and Hartnup disease. In MSUD, the defect is in the branched chain keto acid decarboxylase responsible for the metabolism of leucine, isoleucine, and valine. This catabolic blockade results in the accumulation of these amino acids in tissues and blood, followed by aminoaciduria due to increased glomerular filtration [33].

Reports of cutaneous disease with MSUD are few, but such cases, when they do occur, are described as acrodermatitis-like manifestations (Fig. 2) [34••,35]. Histologic features have not been described. Importantly, the eruption in MSUD does not appear to result directly from the metabolic defects described. Instead, the development and resolution of the eruption parallel the development and resolution of plasma isoleucine deficiency during dietary therapy (Fig. 2) [34••,35].

Neonatal citrullinemia is sometimes although rarely associated with an eruption closely resembling NME or acrodermatitis enteropathica both clinically and histologically [36]. This heritable disorder of the urea cycle results from an argininosuccinic acid synthetase deficiency, which in turn leads to hyperammonemia and low plasma arginine levels. The eruption can be corrected with arginine replacement. Because arginine is a component of epidermal keratins, an abnormality of keratin structure has been postulated as a cause of the eruption.

A number of protein-dependent syndromes have been reported to produce NME-like eruptions, including kwashiorkor, protein-energy malnutrition in infants with cystic fibrosis, and nephrotic syndrome [14,37]. Because albumin is the major carrier for zinc in the

serum, hypoalbuminemia causes low serum zinc levels [14,38]. Obviously, diseases of protein-energy malnutrition are nutritionally quite complex. Zinc speeds the healing of kwashiorkor lesions in humans [39]. In infants with cystic fibrosis and severe malnutrition secondary in part to pancreatic enzyme deficiency with malabsorption, it is unclear whether their acrodermatitis enteropathica-like eruption occurs owing to zinc deficiency, EFA deficiency, protein and amino acid deficiency, or a combination of these and other factors [40••,41••].

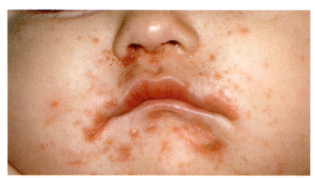

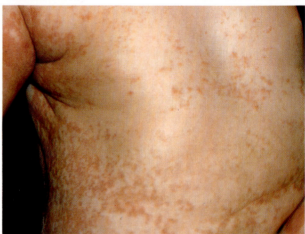

Fig. 2. An infant with maple syrup urine disease. **Top,** Rash of isoleucine deficiency during dietary therapy. **Bottom,** Axillary and inguinal accentuation of generalized eruption. (*Courtesy of* K. Madison, Iowa City, IA.)

Essential fatty acid deficiency

The major EFAs in human are the ω-6 fatty acid linoleic acid and its products linolenic and arachidonic acid [42]. EFA deficiency in humans, first described in 1963, manifests with scaling, erythema, thinning and loss of hair, poor wound healing, growth failure, and increased infections [43,44]. Eruptions closely mimicking NME have been associated with EFA deficiency in humans, which is often complicated by protein and zinc deficiency [4,40••,41••]. Descriptions of human histologic features are sparse but include epidermal hyperplasia, acanthosis, and hyperkeratosis [45]. Laboratory findings include decreased plasma levels of linoleic, linolenic, and arachidonic acids, and elevated levels of palmitoleic, oleic, and 5,8,11-(ω-6) eicosatrienoic acid [42,46].

Essential fatty aids are important as precursors to prostaglandins, because linoleic and γ-linolenic acids may increase tissue biosynthesis of prostaglandin E_1 with anti-inflammatory effects. EFAs also have a structural role in phospholipid membranes [47]. Skin changes in EFA deficiency have been attributed both to altered prostaglandin synthesis and to direct effects of linoleic acid [40••,42,44,45]. Treatment of EFA-deficient rats with prostaglandin E_1 or E_2 reverses the cutaneous scaliness but does not restore the epidermal barrier function [47]. When prostaglandin synthesis is blocked by indomethacin, however, administration of linoleic acid can correct this scaling [47,48]. Reversal of the cutaneous manifestations in patients with EFA deficiency follows intravenous, topical, or oral administration of linoleic acid [44,47].

Pellagra

Pellagra is the clinical syndrome of severe niacin deficiency. Niacin (also called vitamin B_3, nicotinamide, or nicotinic acid) deficiency can occur by several mechanisms: an inadequate dietary supply of niacin and tryptophan (which the body can convert to niacin), increased utilization in patients with malignant tumors of the intestinal tract (*ie*, carcinoid), intestinal parasites, Hartnup disease, and altered metabolism due to a variety of medications, such as isoniazid, 6-mercaptopurine, azathioprine, phenobarbital, and chloramphenicol [14,49•]. Although pellagra may not be due to a single vitamin or nutritional deficiency, most of the clinical signs of pellagra seem to disappear when niacin alone is administered, unless there are coexisting nutritional deficiencies that interfere with the response to niacin.

Clinical manifestations of pellagra include the classic triad of dermatitis, diarrhea, and dementia. The dermatitis may follow exposure to sunlight, heat, friction, or pressure. It is sharply marginated and symmetrical, with erythematous patches involving the face, extremities, inguinal region, and, in infants, the diaper area. There is superficial scaling with or without vesiculation and resolution with areas of hyperpigmentation. Lesions may progress to ulceration, exudation, and cracking with secondary infection. Cheilitis and glossitis are usually present. The histopathology of pellagra can be similar to that observed in glucagonoma and acrodermatitis enteropathica [49•].

Niacin is an essential precursor of NAD+ and NADP, which are involved in glycolysis and lipid, amino acid, and protein metabolism. Tryptophan, an essential amino acid, is converted to niacin. Normally, 1.5% of dietary tryptophan is converted to niacin [50]. Other alterations in dietary amino acid intake may be factors in the pathogenesis of pellagra, because diets high in leucine inhibit the conversion of tryptophan to niacin,

whereas isoleucine seems to facilitate this conversion [49•].

Diagnosis is clinical and supported by low levels of *N*-methylnicotinamide or 2-pyridone, which are urinary metabolites of niacin [49•]. Treatment consists of replacement; 15 mg/d of niacinamide is usually sufficient. Protection from sun exposure is important during the active phase of this disease.

Hartnup disease, an inborn error of metabolism, can produce a pellagra-like syndrome [49•]. An enzymatic defect in the intestinal and renal tubular transport is thought to cause inadequate reabsorption of tryptophan and several other amino acids. There is abnormal excretion of tryptophan, indole, leucine, isoleucine, valine, phenylalanine, tyrosine, alanine, threonine, histidine, glutamine, glycine, and serine [51].

Pyridoxine deficiency (presumably a result of a defect in niacin metabolism) and riboflavin deficiency may also at times mimic certain of the more distinctive aspects of NME or acrodermatitis enteropathica eruptions [49•,50]. Kynureninase, the enzyme that catalyzes the reaction leading to NAD+ synthesis, requires a vitamin B_6 (pyridoxine)–derived coenzyme. If this vitamin is deficient, niacin (and NAD) synthesis from tryptophan will be decreased, leading to pellagra.

Conclusions

Cutaneous eruptions mimicking NME can occur with a variety of metabolic disorders that initially appear to share little in common: glucagonoma syndrome or hyperglucagonemia, acrodermatitis enteropathica, biotin deficiency and biotin-responsive inborn errors of metabolism, EFA deficiency, some aminoacidurias and other conditions of altered protein metabolism, and even niacin, pyridoxine, or riboflavin deficiencies. However, anemia, weight loss, mental changes, alopecia, and increased susceptibility to infection are noted in many of these diseases. Diarrhea is common in glucagonoma, acrodermatitis, and pellagra. Eruptions in Hartnup disease and pellagra are photosensitive.

Many of these eruptions may present very similar histologic findings; epidermal necrosis or pallor, neutrophil infiltration of the epidermis, and vesicle formation are some of the more distinctive features. Given the clinical and histopathologic similarities of the cutaneous eruptions that develop in these syndromes, it is reasonable to suspect some shared pathways of cutaneous syndrome development. The most obvious links include altered amino acid metabolism or altered EFA metabolism.

Zinc deficiency and cutaneous improvement with zinc repletion have been noted in glucagonoma, inherited and acquired acrodermatitis enteropathica, hypoalbuminemia (occurring with cirrhosis or other liver disease, nephrotic syndrome, or starvation), and nutritional depletion or malabsorption (*eg*, cystic fibrosis). The cutaneous effects of tryptophan deficiency may be mediated in part through an alteration of zinc metabolism by loss of a tryptophan metabolite, picolinic acid, an apparent zinc ligand [5,40,41,52].

Altered amino acid metabolism links glucagonoma syndrome, acrodermatitis enteropathica, kwashiorkor (protein-energy malnutrition), nephrotic syndrome and other protein-wasting states, MSUD, Hartnup disease, and pellagra. Niacin and pyridoxine are important cofactors in glycolysis, fatty acid metabolism, and amino acid and protein metabolism. Moreover, the pellagra-like eruption of Hartnup disease seems to result from inadequate niacin resorption, perhaps complicated by urinary loss of several amino acids. Defects in MSUD do not produce the cutaneous eruption, however; this develops from dietary isoleucine deficiency during therapy. Given the role of isoleucine deficiency in the eruption in MSUD, it is interesting that isoleucine may facilitate the conversion of dietary tryptophan to niacin, which suggests an additional link between niacin and altered amino acid metabolism. High dietary intake of leucine can induce pellagra through this altered tryptophan metabolism, and the cutaneous manifestations of pellagra have resolved with isoleucine supplementation alone [53].

The most intriguing associations concern alterations in EFA metabolism, because of the role of EFA in epidermal integrity and inflammation. Zinc deficiency is associated with reduced absorption of unsaturated fatty acids and impaired desaturation of linoleic acid; cutaneous remission follows restoration of EFA [15]. Biotin-responsive inborn errors of metabolism decrease EFA synthesis, and the cutaneous manifestations respond to the administration of unsaturated fatty acids prior to biotin treatment [22,32]. In pellagra, NAD and NADP are decreased, and they are needed for fatty acid metabolism. Pyridoxine, or vitamin B_6, is utilized during conversion of tryptophan to niacin by the enzyme kynureninase. A deficiency blocks the tryptophan pathway, also resulting in abnormalities in fatty acids [50,52].

The clinical similarities between the syndromes surveyed in this paper dictate a broadening of the differential diagnosis of NME or acrodermatitis enteropathica beyond glucagonoma and zinc depletion, particularly in the younger or malnourished patient. While the metabolic links between these syndromes are far from clear, the recurring themes of altered metabolism suggest that the shared clinical and histologic cutaneous findings in these disorders may be more than coincidental.

References and recommended reading

Papers of particular interest, published within the annual period of review, have been highlighted as:
- Of special interest
- • Of outstanding interest

1. Becker SW, Kahn D, Rothman S: **Cutaneous Manifestations of Internal Malignant Tumors.** *Arch Dermatol Syphilol* 1942, **45**:1069–1080.
2. Hunt S, Vitold T, Abell E: **Necrolytic Migratory Erythema: Dyskeratotic Dermatitis, a Clue to Early Diagnosis.** *J Am Acad Dermatol* 1991, **24**:473–477.
3. Goodenberger D, Lawley T, Strober W, Wyatt L, Sangree MH Jr, Sherwen R, Rosenbaum H, Braverman I, Katz SI: **Necrolytic Migratory Erythema Without Glucagonoma.** *Arch Dermatol* 1979, **115**:1429–1431.
4. Blackford S, Wright S, Roberts D: **Necrolytic Migratory Erythema Without Glucagonoma: The Role of Dietary Essential Fatty Acids.** *Br J Dermatol* 1991, **125**:460–462.
5. Doyle J, Schroeter A, Rogers R III: **Hyperglucagonaemia and Necrolytic Migratory Erythema in Cirrhosis: Possible Pseudoglucagonoma Syndrome.** *Br J Dermatol* 1979, **101**:581–587.
6. Wynick D, Hammond P, Bloom S: **The Glucagonoma Syndrome.** *Clin*
•• *Dermatol* 1993, **11**:93–97.
Current and complete review of this syndrome.
7. Wells S, Austen W, Fonkalsvud E, Polk H, Scott H: **Functional En-**
•• **docrine Tumors of the Pancreas: Clinical Presentation, Diagnosis, and Treatment.** *Curr Probl Surg* 1990, **27**:303–385.
In-depth review of all endocrine pancreatic tumors, with a nice section on glucagonoma, plus color illustrations.
8. Almdal T, Heindorff H, Bardram L, Vilstrup H: **Increased Amino Acid Clearance and Urea Synthesis in a Patient With Glucagonoma.** *Gut* 1990, **31**:946–948.
9. Klein S, Jahoor F, Baba H, Townsend C Jr, Shepherd M, Wolfe R: **In vivo Assessment of the Metabolic Alterations in Glucagonoma Syndrome.** *Metabolism* 1992, **41**:1171–1175.
10. Norton J, Kahn C, Schiebinger R, Gorschboth C, Brennan M: **Amino Acid Deficiency and the Skin Rash Associated With Glucagonoma.** *Ann Intern Med* 1979, **91**:213–215.
11. Kheir S, Omura E, Grizzle W, Herrera G, Lee I: **Histologic Variation in the Skin Lesions of the Glucagonoma Syndrome.** *Am J Surg Pathol* 1986, **10**:445–453.
12. Shepherd M, Raimer S, Tyring S, Smith E: **Treatment of Necrolytic Migratory Erythema in Glucagonoma Syndrome.** *J Am Acad Dermatol* 1991, **25**:925–928.
13. Van Wouwe J: **Clinical and Laboratory Diagnosis of Acrodermatitis Enteropathica.** *Eur J Pediatr* 1989, **149**:2–8.
14. Weismann K: **Nutrition and the Skin.** In *Textbook of Dermatology,* vol 4, edn 5. Edited by Champion R, Burton J, Ebling F. Oxford: Blackwell Scientific Publications; 1992: 2358–2381.
15. Niemi K, Anttila P, Kanerva L, Johansson E: **Histopathological Study of Transient Acrodermatitis Enteropathica Due to Decreased Zinc in Breast Milk.** *J Cutan Pathol* 1989, **16**:382–387.
16. Kuramoto Y, Igarashi Y, Tagami H: **Acquired Zinc Deficiency in**
• **Breast-Fed Infants.** *Semin Dermatol* 1991, **10**:309–312.
Emphasizes that even breast-fed infants can develop zinc deficiency.
17. Gonzalez J, Botet M, Sanchez J: **The Histopathology of Acrodermatitis Enteropathica.** *Am J Dermatopathol* 1982, **4**:303–311.
18. Horn T: **Non-inflammatory Disorders of the Skin.** In *Pathology of the Skin,* edn 1. Edited by Farmer E, Hood A. Norwalk: Appleton & Lange; 1990: 402–403.
19. Lever W, Schaumburg-Lever G: *Histopathology of the Skin,* edn 7. Philadelphia: JB Lippincott Co.; 1990:211–212.
20. Ackerman A: **Intraepidermal Vesicular and Pustular Dermatitis.** In *Histologic Diagnosis of Inflammatory Skin Diseases: A Method by Pattern Analysis.* Philadelphia: Lea & Febiger; 1978: 497–581.
21. Mack D, Koletzko B, Cunnane S, Cutz E, Griffiths A: **Acrodermatitis Enteropathica With Normal Serum Zinc Levels: Diagnostic Value of Small Bowel Biopsy and Essential Fatty Acid Determination.** *Gut* 1989, **30**:1426–1429.
22. Cunnane S: **Role of Zinc in Lipid and Fatty Acid Metabolism and in Membranes.** *Prog Food Nutr Sci* 1988, **12**:151–158.
23. Wolf B, Heard G: **Disorders of Biotin Metabolism.** In *The Metabolic Basis of Inherited Disease,* edn 6. Edited by Scriver C, Beaudet A, Sly W, Valle D. New York: McGraw-Hill; 1989: 2083–2103.
24. Nyhan W: **Inborn Errors of Biotin Metabolism.** *Arch Dermatol* 1987, **123**:1696a–1698a.
25. Mock D, Baswell D, Baker H, Holman RT, Sweetman L: **Biotin Deficiency Complicating Parenteral Alimentation: Diagnosis, Metabolic Repercussions, and Treatment.** *J Pediatr* 1985, **106**:762–769.
26. Hebert A, Esterly N: **Mucous Membrane Disorders.** In *Pediatric Dermatology* vol 1, edn 1. Edited by Schnachner L, Hansen R. New York: Churchill Livingstone; 1988: 513–519.
27. Williams M, Packman S, Cowan M: **Alopecia and Periorificial Dermatitis in Biotin-Responsive Multiple Carboxylase Deficiency.** *J Am Acad Dermatol* 1983, **9**:97–103.

28. Mock D: **Skin Manifestations of Biotin Deficiency.** *Semin Dermatol* 1991, **10**:296–302.

29. Cowan M, Packman S, Wara D, Ammann A: **Multiple Biotin-Dependent Carboxylase Deficiencies Associated With Defects in T-Cell and B-Cell Immunity.** *Lancet* 1979, **ii**:115–118.

30. Mock N, Mock D: **Biotin Deficiency in Rats: Disturbances of Leucine**
• **Metabolism Are Detectable Early.** *J Nutr* 1992, **122**:1493–1499.
Explores links between amino acid biochemistry and EFA metabolism.

31. Mock D: **Evidence for a Pathogenic Role of ω-6 Polyunsaturated Fatty**
• **Acid in the Cutaneous Manifestations of Biotin Deficiency.** *J Pediatr Gastroenterol Nutr* 1990, **10**:222–229.
Essential fatty acid metabolism in humans seems to explain eruption of biotin disorders.

32. Munnich A, Saudubray J, Conde F, Charpentier C, Saurat JH, Frezal J: **Fatty Acid Responsive Alopecia in Multiple Carboxylase Deficiency [Letter].** *Lancet* 1980, **i**:1080–1081.

33. Efron M, Ampola M: **The Aminoacidurias.** *Pediatr Clin North Am* 1967, **14**:881–896.

34. Giacoia G, Berry G: **Acrodermatitis Enteropathica–Like Syndrome**
•• **Secondary to Isoleucine Deficiency During Treatment of Maple Syrup Urine Disease.** *Am J Dis Child* 1993, **147**:954–956.
Extremely interesting linkage of isoleucine deficiency to eruption reported in MSUD.

35. Thomas E: **Dietary Management of Inborn Errors of Amino Acid Metabolism With Protein Modified Diets.** *J Child Neurol* 1992, **7(suppl 1)**:S92–S111.

36. Goldblum O, Brusilow S, Maldonado Y, Farmer E: **Neonatal Citrullinemia Associated With Cutaneous Manifestations and Arginine Deficiency.** *J Am Acad Dermatol* 1986, **14**:321–326.

37. Latham M: **The Dermatosis of Kwashiorkor in Young Children.** *Semin Dermatol* 1991, **10**:270–272.

38. Jacobs R, Sandstead H, Solomons N, Rieger C, Rothberg R: **Zinc Status and Vitamin A Transport in Cystic Fibrosis.** *Am J Clin Nutr* 1978, **31**:638–644.

39. Golden M, Golden B, Jackson A: **Skin Breakdown in Kwashiorkor Responds to Zinc [Letter].** *Lancet* 1980, **i**:256.

40. Hansen R: **Dermatitis and Nutritional Deficiency: Diagnostic**
•• **and Therapeutic Considerations [Editorial].** *Arch Dermatol* 1992, **128**:1389–1390.
Very nice discussion of the complexity of nutritional deficiencies, as an editorial to the following paper.

41. Darmstadt G, Schmidt C, Wechsler D, Tunnessen W, Rosenstein B:
•• **Dermatitis as a Presenting Sign of Cystic Fibrosis.** *Arch Dermatol* 1992, **128**:1358–1364.
NME or acrodermatitis enteropathica-like eruptions in cystic fibrosis are linked to zinc and fatty acid derangements secondary to zinc malabsorption.

42. Hay R, Champion R, Greaves M: **Systemic Therapy.** In *Textbook of Dermatology*, vol 4, edn 5. Edited by Champion R, Burton J, Ebling F. Oxford: Blackwell Scientific Publications; 1992: 2927–2960.

43. Hansen A, Wiese H, Boelsche A, Haggard M, Adam DJD, Davis H: **Role of Linoleic Acid in Infant Nutrition.** *Pediatrics* 1963, **31**:171–191.

44. Horrobin D: **Essential Fatty Acids in Clinical Dermatology** *J Am Acad Dermatol* 1989, **20**:1045–1053.

45. Ziboh V, Chapkin R: **Biological Significance of Polyunsaturated Fatty Acids in the Skin.** *Arch Dermatol* 1987, **123**:1686a–1690a.

46. Riella M, Broviac J, Wells M, Scribner B: **Essential Fatty Acid Deficiency in Human Adults During Total Parenteral Nutrition.** *Ann Intern Med* 1975, **83**:786–789.

47. Wertz R, Swartzendruber D, Abraham W, Madison K, Downing D: **Essential Fatty Acids and Epidermal Integrity.** *Arch Dermatol* 1987, **123**:1381–1384.

48. Elias P, Brown B, Ziboh V: **The Permeability Barrier in Essential Fatty Acid Deficiency: Evidence for a Direct Role for Linoleic Acid in Barrier Function.** *J Invest Dermatol* 1980, **74**:230–233.

49. Hendricks W: **Pellagra and Pellagralike Dermatoses: Etiology, Differ-**
• **ential Diagnosis, Dermatopathology, and Treatment.** *Semin Dermatol* 1991, **10**:282–292.
Current and focused summary of clinical syndromes linked by altered niacin metabolism.

50. Rivlin R: **Disorders of Vitamin Metabolism: Deficiencies, Metabolic Abnormalities, and Excesses.** In *Cecil Textbook of Medicine*, edn 19. Edited by Wyngaarden J, Smith L, Bennett J. Philadelphia: WB Saunders Co.; 1992:1173–1175.

51. Halvorsen K, Halvorsen S: **Hartnup Disease.** *Pediatrics* 1963; 29–35.

52. Krieger I, Statter M: **Tryptophan Deficiency and Picolinic Acid: Effect on Zinc Metabolism and Clinical Manifestations of Pellagra.** *Am J Clin Nutr* 1987, **46**:511–517.

53. Krishnaswamy K, Gopalan C: **Effect of Isoleucine on Skin and Electroencephalogram in Pellagra.** *Lancet* 1971, **ii**:1167–1169.

Warren W. Piette, MD, Department of Dermatology, University of Iowa College of Medicine, Iowa City, IA 52242-0001, USA.

Pathogenesis and treatment of cutaneous calciphylaxis

Susan D. Laman, MD

Johns Hopkins Medical Institute and Francis Scott Key Hospital, Baltimore, Maryland, USA

In this update of developments in cutaneous calciphylaxis, the entity is defined and illustrated. Its epidemiologic, clinical, and histopathologic natures are discussed. Also reviewed are the old and new theories of pathogenesis and treatment, and the proposed method of diagnosis.

Current Opinion in Dermatology 1995:94–96

Description

Cutaneous calciphylaxis is a rare phenomenon clinically characterized by painful retiform purpura [1–3] most commonly located on the medial thighs or buttocks [4•]. Progression results in development of eschar, central necrosis, and ulceration (Fig. 1). In addition, peripheral gangrene of the toes and fingers can develop [3,5,6]. Calciphylaxis occurs most commonly in patients with end-stage renal disease (ESRD), those on hemodialysis or peritoneal dialysis, and those having undergone renal transplantation [1,2,5–8,9•,10–18]. Frequently, although not always, these patients have secondary or tertiary hyperparathyroidism associated with ESRD and an elevated calcium phosphate product [1,6–8,9•,16,18]. The renal failure appears to be of varying causes [1,2,5–8,9•,11–20], and there does not appear to be a preponderance of patients of a certain sex or age [8]. Aggravating factors include systemic corticosteroids and other immunosuppressive medications [3,21]. Systemic manifestations include skeletal muscle involvement, manifesting as muscle weakness, tenderness, or severe myositis [9•]; and pulmonary involvement [6]. Patients will often die, most commonly from sepsis, with the bacterial port of entry being the skin ulcerations.

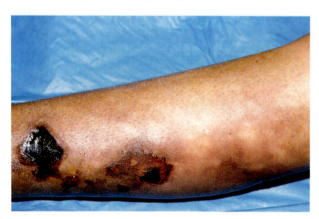

Fig. 1. Pattern of livido reticularis and dark red-brown mottling is associated with large areas of eschar and ulceration on the medial thigh.

Histopathologically, bland thrombi are noted in the superficial dermal vessels, and vascular calcification, ischemic epidermolysis, and rarely a perivascular lymphocytic infiltrate are seen in association with the subcutaneous vessels. In some cases, calcification of the deep vessels is not apparent, but there appears to be interstitial deposition of calcium in the subcutaneous adipose tissue, which affects mainly the subcutaneous septa and the elastin fibers (Fig. 2) [22]. Laboratory evaluation in these patients is remarkable for changes consistent with hyperparathyroidism, but occasionally, normal parathyroid hormone, calcium, and phosphate levels are noted [7]. Changes consistent with renal failure are also present.

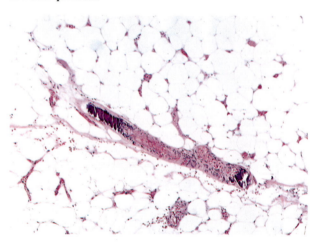

Fig. 2. Subcutaneous blood vessels demonstrate calcium in the vessel walls and clotting in the vessel lumen.

Theories of pathogenesis

Vascular calcification is common in patients with chronic renal failure and seldom resolves with renal transplantation or parathyroidectomy [6,10,23]. The calcium deposition can be located in the intima or media [10] and is rarely associated with histopathologic evi-

---

Abbreviations
DIC—disseminated intravascular coagulation; ESRD—end-stage renal disease.

dence of thrombosis or clinical tissue necrosis [6,10,11]. In calciphylaxis, by contrast, both vascular calcification and thrombosis are noted histopathologically. Clinically, moreover, patients can develop tissue necrosis overlying their lesions. Therefore, in the attempt to identify the causative factors in the development of calciphylaxis, the mechanisms of tissue calcification, thrombosis, and tissue necrosis must be addressed.,

In 1962, Selye *et al.* [24] first described calciphylaxis as a condition of induced systemic hypersensitivity in which the response to a sensitizing agent, a critical period, and a challenging agent was a precipitous albeit sometimes evanescent local calcification. Their proposed sensitizing agents included parathyroid hormone and vitamin D, and their proposed challenging agents included egg white, metallic salts, and trauma [25]. Other studies in animals, mostly rats, have supported this theory [26–30].

Although this theory would account for the occurrence of calciphylaxis in ESRD patients with hyperparathyroidism, it does not explain the histopathologic finding of thrombosis, the clinical finding of tissue necrosis, or the occasional progression to tissue necrosis following parathyroidectomy [10,31]. The thrombosis in calciphylaxis, which in turn might result in ischemia and tissue necrosis, might be explained by the theory proposed by Mehta *et al.* [32], who noted the similarity in the skin lesions of warfarin necrosis and calciphylaxis. Because warfarin necrosis is associated with a hypercoagulable state following a decrease in levels of functional protein C, they sought a similar mechanism in calciphylaxis. They measured antigenic and functional protein C levels in patients with ESRD and systemic calciphylaxis undergoing hemodialysis, patients without calciphylaxis undergoing dialysis, and normal volunteers. Antigenic levels of protein C were normal in all patients, while functional levels were significantly reduced in patients with calciphylaxis compared with those of the other groups.

Protein C is a strong, natural anticoagulant that inactivates factors Va and VIIIa and stimulates fibrinolysis by neutralizing plasminogen activator inhibitors. The synthesis of protein C in the liver is vitamin K–dependent. Deficiency of antigenic protein C might result in a hyperthrombotic state. Both congenital and acquired states of protein C deficiency exist. Conditions or factors that can be associated with skin lesions similar to those seen in calciphylaxis and a hyperthrombotic state include homozygous protein C deficiency (neonatal purpura fulminans), some forms of disseminated intravascular coagulation (DIC), hepatic dysfunction, institution of warfarin therapy, and vitamin K deficiency [33•].

Diagnosis and treatment

Diagnosis of cutaneous calciphylaxis should include history, physical examination, laboratory evaluation, and skin biopsy. Because the disease mimics vasculitis in some cases, antinuclear antibodies, cryoglobulins, cryofibrinogens, and rheumatoid factor may be helpful [6]. Skin biopsy should be an excisional biopsy extending to subcutaneous fat.

The differential diagnosis of retiform purpura includes any entity that occludes superficial and deep dermal vasculature, resulting in a livido-like pattern. Such entities can include those associated with occlusion due to microvascular platelet plugs, cold-related gelling or agglutination, organisms in the vessels, local or systemic alterations in control of coagulation, embolization, and crystal deposition. Vessel occlusion in combination with a decrease in functional protein C would narrow the differential diagnosis to entities associated with local or systemic alterations in control of coagulation such as DIC, homozygous protein C or protein S deficiency, acquired protein C deficiency, warfarin necrosis, and antiphospholipid antibody syndrome [4•].

Based on the theory of Selye *et al.* [24] and the fact that calciphylaxis has been found most commonly in ESRD patients with secondary or tertiary hyperparathyroidism and an elevated calcium phosphate product, parathyroidectomy and control of the calcium phosphate product have been the standard treatment. As already mentioned, however, the outcome of parathyroidectomy is unpredictable [10,31]; patients with calciphylaxis may or may not respond, and progression of the necrosis, lesion ulceration, and death have occurred following parathyroidectomy [5,10,11,31,34].

Therapy based on the histopathologic finding of thrombosis might include anticoagulation. The findings of Mehta *et al.* [32] suggest that treatment to increase the level of functional protein C and thus to decrease the proposed hypercoagulable state might be helpful. Such therapy might include discontinuation of warfarin therapy, treatment to help resolve DIC, and replacement of protein C [35].

In the past, replacement of protein C has been accomplished with factor IX concentrate and fresh frozen plasma [36], large volumes of which are required, because the concentration of actual protein C within these substances is low. In November 1991, Dreyfus *et al.* [37] described replacement and long-term maintenance therapy of protein C deficiency in neonatal purpura fulminans with a purified protein C concentrate. Protein C concentrate has been used in four other cases associated with protein C deficiency: in a patient with metastatic prostate cancer [38], in a pregnant woman with protein C deficiency and thrombosis [39••], in a boy with purpura fulminans, DIC, and severe protein C deficiency [40••], and most recently in an elderly woman with a deep venous thrombosis and warfarin necrosis [41••]. Thus, protein C concentrate appears to be of great benefit in treating the entities associated with protein C deficiency, and controlled studies of its use in the treatment of calciphylaxis need to be done.

Conclusions

Cutaneous calciphylaxis is an entity seen most commonly in patients with ESRD, and possibly in those with hyperparathyroidism or functional protein C deficiency. The skin lesions begin as retiform purpura and progress to ulcerated necrotic lesions. They occur most commonly on the inner, upper thighs and buttocks. Occasionally, an associated distal digital gangrene is seen. Death, associated with sepsis, is a common occurrence in these patients. Histopathologically, one notes vascular calcification (commonly seen in patients with ESRD) and vascular thrombotic occlusion (not commonly seen in ESRD). The theories of pathogenesis have attempted to explain the calcification, and more recently the thrombosis and tissue necrosis. Treatment to remedy the vascular calcification has been based on Selye's theory and includes parathyroidectomy, which does not always prevent progression to death. A more recent theory suggest treatment with heparin and substances containing protein C (*ie,* fresh-frozen plasma and factor IX concentrate). Although a protein C concentrate has been used to treat entities with similar pathophysiologic mechanisms and might be beneficial in treating calciphylaxis, more controlled studies need to be done in this regard.

References and recommended reading

Papers of particular interest, published within the annual period of review, have been highlighted as:
• Of special interest
•• Of outstanding interest

1. Asmundsson P, Eliasson G, Pordarson H: **A Case of Calciphylaxis.** *Scand J Urol Nephrol* 1988, 22:155–157.

2. Lugo-Somolinos A, Sanchez J, Mendez-Coll J, Joglar F: **Calcifying Panniculitis Associated With Polycystic Kidney Disease and Chronic Renal Failure.** *J Am Acad Dermatol* 1990, 22:743–747.

3. Lafeuillade A, Alessi M, Poizot-Martin I, Dhiver C, Quilichini R, Aubert L, Gastaut J, Juhan-Vague I: **Protein S Deficiency and HIV Infection.** *N Engl J Med* 1991, 324:1220.

4. Piette W: **The Differential Diagnosis of Purpura From a Morphologic**
• **Perspective.** *Adv Dermatol* 1994, 9:3–23.
A morphologic description of the differential diagnosis of purpura.

5. Sheinman Q, Helm K, Fairley J: **Acral Necrosis in a Patient With Chronic Renal Failure.** *Arch Dermatol* 1991, 127:247–252.

6. Androgue H, Frazier M, Zeluff B, Sucki W: **Systemic Calciphylaxis Revisited.** *Am J Nephrol* 1981, 1:177–183.

7. Ross C, Cassidy M, Thompson M, Jones R, Rees A: **Proximal Cutaneous Necrosis Associated With Small Vessel Calcification in Renal Failure.** *Q J Med* 1991, 79:443–450.

8. Gipstein R, Cobrun J, Adams D, Lee D, Parsa K, Sellers A, Suki W, Massry S: **Calciphylaxis in Man.** *Arch Intern Med* 1976, 136:1273–1280.

9. Edelstein C, Wickham M, Kirby P: **Systemic Calciphylaxis Presenting**
• **as a Painful Proximal Myopathy.** *Postgrad Med J* 1992, 68:209–211.
A case report on the myopathy associated with systemic calciphylaxis.

10. Chan Y, Mahony J, Turner J, Posen S: **The Vascular Lesions Associated With Skin Necrosis in Renal Disease.** *Br J Dermatol* 1983, 109:85–95.

11. Conn J, Krumlovsky F, Greco F, Simon N: **Calciphylacation: Etiology of Progressive Calciphylacation and Gangrene?** *Ann Surg* 1973, 177:206–210.

12. Rees J, Coles G: **Calciphylaxis in Man.** *BMJ* 1969, 2:670–672.

13. Ramakishna B, Pierides J, Disney A, Dymock R: **Calciphylaxis in a Renal Dialysis Patient With Secondary Hyperparathyroidism.** *Australas J Dermatol* 1987, 28:68–71.

14. Grob J, Legre R, Brotocchio P, Payan M, Andrac L, Bonerandi J: **Calcifying Panniculitis and Kidney Failure.** *Int J Dermatol* 1989, 28:129–131.

15. Rubinger D, Friedlaender M, Silver J, Kopoloric Y, Czacvkes W, Popovtzer M: **Progressive Vascular Calcification With Necrosis of the Extremities in Hemodialysis patients: A Possible Role of Iron Overload.** *Am J Kidney Dis* 1986, 7:125–129.

16. Duh Q, Lim R, Clark O: **Calciphylaxis in Secondary Hyperparathyroidism.** *Arch Surg* 1991, 126:1213–1219.

17. Mehregan D, Winkelmann R: **Cutaneous Gangrene, Vascular Calcification and Hyperparathyroidism.** *Mayo Clin Proc* 1989, 64:211–215.

18. Wenzel-Siefert K, Harwig S, Keller F: **Fulminant Calcinosis in Two Patients After Kidney Transplantation.** *Am J Nephrol* 1991, 11:497–500.

19. Lowry L, Tschen J, Wolf J, Yen A: **Calcifying Panniculitis and Systemic Calciphylaxis in a End Stage Renal Patient.** *Cutis* 1993, 51:245–247.

20. Cockerell C, Dolan E: **Widespread Cutaneous and Systemic Calcification(Calciphylaxis) in Patients With Acquired Immunodeficiency Syndrome and Renal Disease.** *J Am Acad Dermatol* 1992, 6:559–562.

21. Khafif R, DeLima C, Silverberg A, Frankel R: **Calciphylaxis and Systemic Calcinosis.** *Arch Intern Med* 1990, 150:956–959.

22. Johnson W, Alkek D: **Histopathology and Histochemistry of Cutaneous Calciphylaxis.** *Clin Orthop* 1970, 69:75–86.

23. Soloman A, Colmite S, Headington T: **Epidermal and Follicular Calciphylaxis.** *J Cutan Pathol* 1988, 15:282–285.

24. Selye H, Gobbiani G, Strebel R: **Sensitization to Calciphylaxis by Endogenous Parathyroid Hormones.** *Endocrinology* 1962, 71:554–558.

25. Selye H, Berczi I: **The Present Status of Calciphylaxis and Calcergy.** *Clin Orthop* 1970, 69:28–54.

26. Sukuma Y, Mori M: **Experimental Calcification in Rat Submandibular Gland.** *Cell Mol Biol* 1992, 38:413–427.

27. Raica M: **Experimental Skin Calciphylaxis Induced by Iron Citrate Sorbitol in Young Dogs.** *Rom J Morphol Embryol* 1991, 37:15–18.

28. Boivin G, Walzer C, Vand C: **Ultrastructure Study of the Long-Term Development of Two Experimental Cutaneous Calcinosis (Topical Calciphylaxis and Topical Calcergy) in the Rat.** *Cell Tissue Res* 1987, 247:525–532.

29. Rosenblum I, Black H, Ferrell J: **The Effects of Various Disphonates on a Rat Model of Cardiac Calciphylaxis.** *Calcif Tissue Res* 1977, 23:151–159.

30. Raica M: **Calciphylaxis Induced by Iron Citrate Sorbitol.** *Exp Pathol* 1990, 38:196–200.

31. Poch E, Almirall J, Alsina M, del Rio R, Cases A: **Calciphylaxis in a Hemodialysis Patient: Appearance After Parathyroidectomy During a Psoriatic Flare.** *Am J Kidney Dis* 1992, 19:285–288.

32. Mehta R, Scott G, Sloand J, Charles W: **Skin Necrosis Associated With Acquired Protein C Deficiency in Patients With Renal Failure and Calciphylaxis.** *Am J Med* 1990, 88:252–257.

33. Soundaravajan R, Leehey D, Yu A, Ing T, Miller J: **Skin Necrosis and**
• **Protein C Deficiency Associated With Vitamin K Depletion in a Patient With Renal Failure.** *Am J Med* 1992, 93:467–470.
A case report of a patient with necrotic skin lesions associated with protein C deficiency and vitamin K depletion.

34. Grob J, Legre R, Bertoccio P: **Calcifying Panniculitis and Kidney Failure: Considerations on Pathogenesis and Treatment of Calciphylaxis.** *Int J Dermatol* 1989, 28:129–131.

35. Vukovich T, Auberger K, Weil J, Engelmann H, Knobl P, Hadorn H: **Replacement Therapy for a Homozygous Protein C Deficient State Using a Concentrate of Human Protein C and S.** *Br J Dermatol* 1998, 70:435–440.

36. Marlar R: **Protein C in Thromboembolic Disease.** *Semin Thromb Hemost* 1985, 11:387–393.

37. Dreyfus M, Magny J, Bridey F, Schwarz, Planche C, Dehan M, Tchernia G: **Treatment of Homozygous Protein C Deficiency and Neonatal Purpura Fulminans With a Purified Protein C Concentrate.** *N Engl J Med* 1991, 325:1565–1568.

38. Okajimi K, Imamura H, Koga S, Inoue M, Takatsuki K, Aoki N: **Treatment of Patients With Disseminated Intravascular Coagulation by Protein C.** *Am J Hematol* 1990, 33:277–278.

39. Manco-Johnson M, Nuss R: **Protein C Concentrate Prevents Peripartum**
•• **Thrombosis.** *Am J Hematol* 1992, 40:69–70.
A case report on the use of protein C concentrate to treat protein C deficiency.

40. Gerson W, Dickerson J, Bovill E, Golden E: **Severe Acquired Protein**
•• **C Deficiency in Purpura Fulminans Associated With Disseminated Intravascular Coagulation: Treatment With Protein C Concentrate.** *Pediatrics* 1993, 91:418–422.
Case report of severe protein C deficiency associated with DIC and purpura fulminans and the use of purified protein C concentrate to treat this patient.

41. Shramm W, Spannagl M, Bauer K, Rosenberg R, Berkner B, Linnau
•• Y, Schwarz P: **Treatment of Coumarin Induced Skin Necrosis With Monoclonal Ab Purified Protein C Concentrate.** *Arch Dermatol* 1993, 129:753–756.
Case report on the use of protein C concentrate to treat warfarin-induced skin necrosis. No further skin lesions appeared during therapy, and the healing process of the necrotic lesions appeared to be enhanced.

Susan D. Laman, MD, Department of Dermatology, Johns Hopkins Outpatient Center, 601 North Caroline Street, Baltimore, MD 21287, USA.

Neurofibromatosis: correlating molecular genetic findings with the disease

Mary A. Curtis, MD

University of Iowa Hospitals and Clinics, Iowa City, Iowa, USA

Contrary to prior expectations, two genes (rather than many) account for the majority of neurofibromatosis seen in families studied to date. Some very interesting findings regarding the structure and function of these two genes have been reported. Linkage testing has become available for some families. Attempts to correlate a neurofibromatosis phenotype with the molecular genetic findings have been frustrating because of intrafamily heterogeneity and the limited number of gene mutations identified to date. Clinical findings, imaging studies, and potential treatment options continue to fascinate and baffle us. Careful evaluation and documentation of each patient is very important in sorting out subtypes and related conditions.

Current Opinion in Dermatology 1995:97–104

Clinical description

Counseling the parents of an infant exhibiting multiple café au lait spots (possible or probable neurofibromatosis) remains difficult. One reason is that we cannot confirm the diagnosis (or refute it) with certainty, unless other signs of neurofibromatosis are present or the family has other affected members. Linkage testing has become available for families in which two or more affected individuals are present. Within a few years, however, molecular genetics may be sufficiently advanced to allow such a diagnosis in an isolated case. Another reason is the marked intrafamily phenotypic heterogeneity (Fig. 1), which makes it difficult to be totally comforting to parents of an affected infant. I like to compartmentalize the information for families into categories such as physical manifestations, mental and social aspects, and tumor risks (Table 1).

The likelihood of neurofibromatosis type 1 (NF1) is often apparent when a physical examination is completed. The diagnostic criteria (Table 2) for neurofibromatosis should be adhered to. In addition to these criteria, however, there are many "soft signs" that may make it easier for the clinician to proceed with counseling. Height, weight, and blood pressure measurements should be routine. The average head circumference in children with NF1 is at the 87th percentile, while the average height is at the 34th percentile [1]. When children with NF1 also have the occasional benign hypotonia and coordination and learning problems, a major central nervous system (CNS) lesion might be suspected, although such symptoms are common and usually uneventful. A few infants and children have the benign cutaneous neurofibromas, although these typically begin to show up later. The larger plexiform neurofibromas often are inconspicuous soft prominences in infancy, which progress and may be life threatening if encompassing a tracheal, spinal or other vital area. Such tumors are highly vascular and bleed heavily upon trauma or during surgery. Regrowth after surgery is usual. Café au lait spots may become less noticeable with time, although freckling may become more apparent, sometimes becoming confluent in intertriginous areas, which may give a dirty appearance. In addition to café au lait spots and freckles, one may observe a number of other skin lesions including nevoxanthoendotheliomas and fuscoceruleus spots [2•], described as being blue-brown in color with coarse hairs and having a histopathologic appearance of dermal melanocytosis. Often a patient with neurofibromatosis will have a "tanned" appearance. While the skin appears more pigmented, there is often a subtle yellowish cast to it with dark circles under the eyes (Fig. 2). Scoliosis, often a tight thoracic curve with rapid progression, is most commonly noted around 6 years of age [3] (Fig. 3). For this reason, a spinal examination should be part of the routine toddler's or child's physical. Precocious puberty, visual disturbance, and alterations of growth pattern (slowed or accelerated) may be signs of a CNS glioma. A pheochromocytoma or renal vascular anomaly should be considered when hypertension is noted, although "benign essential" hypertension without a discernible cause is more common in NF1 than in the average population, as are severe headaches. Lisch nodules (Fig. 4) are age-dependent, as are cutaneous neurofibromas, and must be determined by an ophthalmologist or an individual skilled in use of a slit lamp.

Abbreviations

CNS—central nervous system; **NF1**—neurofibromatosis type 1; **NF2**—neurofibromatosis type 2.

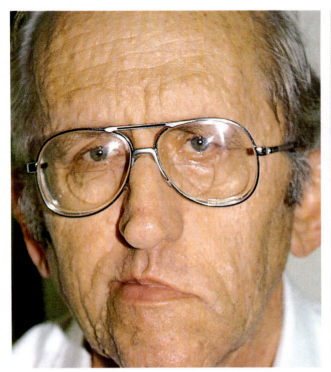

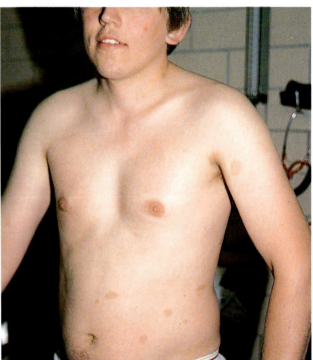

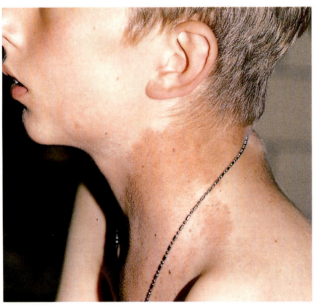

Fig. 1. Upper left, Father with neurofibromatosis type 1 manifested by multiple cutaneous neurofibromas, café au lait spots, and unilateral acoustic neuroma (after surgery). **Upper right**, Nineteen-year-old son with café au lait spots. **Bottom**, Eleven-year-old son with café au lait spots and a plexiform tumor extending into hypopharynx, cervical spinal cord, and thoracic cavity.

Close to 50% of children with NF1 have a learning disability or attention deficit disorder [4]. This is often the most distressing problem for parents of a child with a new mutation. Impulsiveness and social imperceptions combined with a learning disability and perhaps some physical manifestations of NF1 may give the bystander the impression that such a child is retarded. Most patients, however, do become self-supporting as adults and perform well as parents.

Some malignancies are associated with neurofibromatosis. In a review of 26,084 patients with cancer under 15 years of age, the incidence of NF1 was 6.45 times higher than expected [5]. The tumors in NF1 tended to be type- and site-specific. Of these tu-

mors, 31.4% were malignant schwannomas (Fig. 5), 1.36% were rhabdomyosarcomas (especially urogenital), 12.5% were optic gliomas, and 0.9% were other CNS gliomas.

In neurofibromatosis type 2 (NF2), it has recently been decided that "vestibular schwannoma" accurately describes the pathology and is the preferred term [6]. In the largest clinical study of NF2 to date, 150 patients were evaluated [7•], and the birth incidence was estimated to be one in 35,000 with 50% representing new mutations. In this study, 43% had café au lait patches. Of these, 24 patients had one patch, 11 had two, four had three, three had four, and one had six. No intertriginous freckling or plexiform tumors were noted, al-

Table 1. Characteristics of neurofibromatosis type 1

Physical manifestations
  Growth
    Height
    Head circumference
  Skin
    Café au lait
    Neurofibromas
    Freckles
    "Hairy" fuscoceruleus spots
    Nevoxanthoendotheliomas
  Orthopedic and neurologic
    Scoliosis
    Pseudarthrosis
    Hypotonia
Mental and social aspects
  Learning disability
  Attention deficit disorder
  Social imperceptions
  Speech alterations
Tumor and cancer risks
  Benign
    Cutaneous neurofibromas
    Plexiform neurofibromas
    Central nervous system and spine
      Glioma
      Meningioma
      Neurofibroma
      Schwannoma
      Neurilemmoma
  Malignant
    Malignant schwannoma
    Sarcomas (many types)
Other
  Phenochromocytoma
  Vascular anomalies
    Renal
    Brain
    Other
  "Benign essential" hypertension
  "Migraine" headaches

though 68% had skin tumors (average 5.8). The majority were simple schwannomas. Deafness and loss of balance are eventual outcomes and many patients are severely debilitated by CNS and spinal cord tumors (Fig. 6). The ophthalmologic findings in NF2 are juvenile cataracts, combined pigment epithelial and retinal hamartomas, and epiretinal membranes [8].

Molecular genetics

Neurofibromatosis type 1

Neurofibromatosis type 1 is caused by the alteration of a gene on chromosome 17 (17q11.2). The existence of more than one *NF1* locus is "highly unlikely judged by molecular genetic evaluation of mutations in over 170 families" [9•]. Attempts to correlate specific mutations (alleles) with particular clinical features have been hampered by the finding of a limited number of mutations to date and observed intrafamily phenotypic

heterogeneity [10]. The *NF1* gene spans 300 kb of DNA, encodes for a protein of 2818 amino acids [11••], and is organized into 50 exons. Of these, 48 are always found and two alternatively spliced are found in some only [11••]. In a large intron are three imbedded genes that are transcribed in the opposite direction from the *NF1* gene [11••]. *EV12A* and *EV12B* are human homologues of putative mouse protooncogenes involved in murine leukemias, while *OMGP* is expressed in myelin-producing cells of the central and peripheral nervous systems [11••]. The *NF1* gene protein product, neurofibromin, shows homology to the GTPase-activating protein (GAP) involved in regulation of ras activity [10]. The ras proteins are important in processes of cell proliferation, cell differentiation, cyclic adenosine monophosphate production, and the formation of tumors [11••]. Different isoforms of neurofibromin caused by alternative splicing of two exons are found in various body parts and are expressed at different times in development, suggesting distinct functions in proliferating versus differentiating cells [11••,12••]. Loss of control of proliferation or differentiation may lead to tumor development, café au lait spots, or cerebral hamartomatous lesions [13]. Strong support for the tumor suppressor gene hypothesis for NF1 comes from evidence of double inactivation of NF1 at the molecular level in malignant tumors in patients with NF1 [14,15]. Mutations in the *NF1* gene have also been identified in other types of malignant tumors including malignant melanoma cell lines [16,17] and neuroblastoma cell lines [17]. Easton *et al.* [18] suggested that genes unlinked to the *NF1* locus are important determinants of heterogeneic traits.

Fascinating bits of the human genetic puzzle are being teased out by comparing ongoing research results in the laboratory with unexpected findings in the human story. It has been noted that certain parts of the mammalian genome can be affected by "genomic imprinting" [19•], which is described as the modification of certain genes resulting in differential functional expression of those genes, depending on their parental origin (*ie*, from the mother or father) [20•]. "Although the specific genes and molecular processing involved in imprinting are as yet unknown, selective 'turning off' of genes through DNA methylation appears to play a role" [20•]. The methylation may be reversed during gametogenesis and the imprint erased depending on the sex of the parent [19•]. Methylation may be a secondary phenomena and is not the only alteration associated with imprinting. Others have been detected or suspected. Human conditions known to be associated with imprinting include Huntington disease, myotonic dystrophy, Wilms tumor, Prader-Willi syndrome, fragile X syndrome, and Beckwith-Wiedemann syndrome. Although neurofibromatosis has not been thoroughly studied for imprinting, very preliminary reports are beginning to suggest a possible association. In all 10 families examined by Stephens *et al.* [21], the apparent new *NF1* mutation occurred in the paternally derived chromosome, suggesting imprinting. In another recent study, DNA methylation has been found in exons 28 and 29 of the *NF1* gene and flanking genes [22].

Table 2. Criteria for clinical diagnosis of neurofibromatosis types 1 and 2*

Neurofibromatosis 1 may be diagnosed in white persons when two or more of the following are present:
Six or more café au lait macules whose greatest diameter is more than 5 mm in prepubescent patients and more than 15 mm in postpubescent patients
Two or more neurofibromas of any type or one plexiform neurofibroma
Freckling in the axillary or inguinal region
A distinctive osseous lesion such as sphenoid dysplasia or a thinning of long-bone cortex, with or without pseudarthrosis
Optic glioma
Two or more Lisch nodules (iris hemartomas)
A parent, sibling, or child with neurofibromatosis 1 on the basis of the previous criteria

Neurofibromatosis 2 may be diagnosed when one of the following is present:
Bilateral eighth cranial nerve masses seen by magnetic resonance imaging with gadolinium
A parent, sibling, or child with neurofibromatosis 2 and either unilateral eighth cranial nerve mass or any one of the following:
    Neurofibroma
    Meningioma
    Glioma
    Schwannoma
    Posterior capsular cataract or opacity at a young age

*From National Institutes of Health [53].

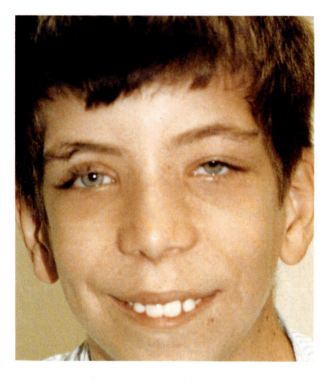

Fig. 2. An adolescent with neurofibromatosis type 1 after surgery for ptosis repair exhibits a characteristic increased pigment, yellowish cast, and dark circles under the eyes.

Neurofibromatosis type 2
Molecular genetic studies in NF2 were initially directed by the study of meningiomas, a common tumor in NF2, and led to the discovery of deletions in chromosome 22 [23,24]. Narod *et al.* [25] performed linkage analysis on 12 affected families. Their results "confirmed the assignment of the gene for NF2 to chromosome 22." A patient with NF2 was found to have a chromosomal translocation involving 22q12.2, which suggests this specific location for the gene [26]. A healthy 25-year-old man undergoing an infertility work up was found to have none of his father's chromosome 22. He did have an isochromosome derived from one of the maternal 22 chromosomes (*ie*, a balanced Robertsonian t(22q;22q) translocation), suggesting lack of maternally imprinted genes on chromosome 22 [27]. Rey *et al.* [28] made the second report of an intriguing chromosome 22 deletion in a neurofibrosarcoma in a patient with NF1.

Other subtypes
Some families have been described in which affected persons have only café au lait spots. Two recent reports exclude the *NF1* gene in several such families [29,30]. It appears that affected individuals in these families had fewer than 10 café au lait spots (often 4 to 6) and that other signs for neurofibromatosis were either not examined for or were likely not present. In a follow-up of 21 children who presented with café au lait spots as the single clinical finding, the majority had developed other signs of neurofibromatosis [31]. Niimura [2•] also noted that all of their patients who had six or more café au lait spots developed neurofibromas in their adolescence.

Watson syndrome and neurofibromatosis-Noonan syndrome are occasionally seen in members of otherwise typical NF1 families and are apparently part

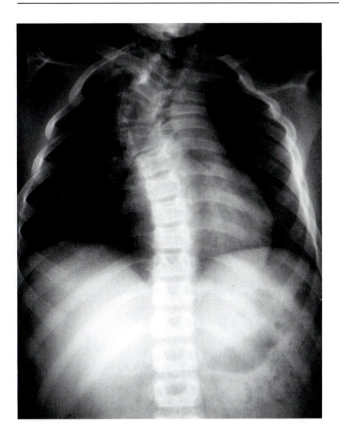

Fig. 3. Radiograph shows thoracic curve over a limited number of vertebral bodies in a child with neurofibromatosis.

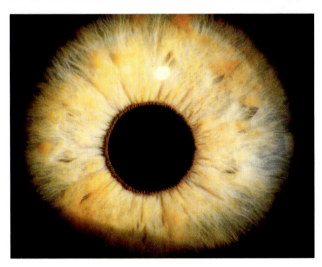

Fig. 4. Lisch nodules seen with a slit lamp.

of the heterogeneity of the *NF1* gene. Watson syndrome is said to be characterized by café au lait spots, pulmonary valve stenosis, and lowered intellect. In a recent review of the patients initially described with Watson syndrome, it was found that they had features more typical of NF1, including Lisch nodules and neurofibromas [32]. Linkage of neurofibromatosis-Noonan syndrome and Watson syndrome to the *NF1* gene has been accomplished in two three-generation families [32,33]. Sharland *et al.*

[34] recently evaluated 11 families who had Noonan syndrome without neurofibromatosis using probes at the *NF1* locus and found absence of linkage. None of these families were known to have multiple café au lait patches, neurofibromas, or Lisch nodules.

Pulst *et al.* [35] described a two-generation family in which three persons developed spinal meningiomas, one had multiple cranial meningiomas, and one had a spinal ependymoma, all as adolescents. None were noted to have vestibular schwannomas or other findings of neurofibromatosis. By genetic linkage analysis, the mutation in this family was excluded from the NF2 region. In the clinical study by Niimura [2•], 10 cases of "multiple neurilemmomatosis or schwannomatosis" were noted. Neurofibromas and bilateral vestibular tumors were not found.

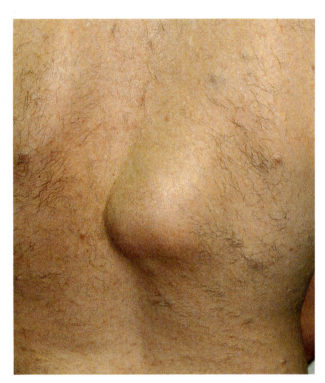

Fig. 5. A paraspinal malignant schwannoma in a young neurofibromatosis patient.

Information on "segmental" or "localized" neurofibromatosis is still very sketchy, with less than adequate documentation of clinical findings or outcome of the progeny of the affected person [36–38]. Café au lait spots have been reported in other unrelated conditions such as Soto syndrome, Proteus syndrome, Russell-Silver syndrome, and McCune Albright syndrome. Two recent additions to this list include Johnson-McMillin syndrome [39] and ring chromosome 7 syndrome [40]. Use of good clinical skills should allow easy differentiation in most cases.

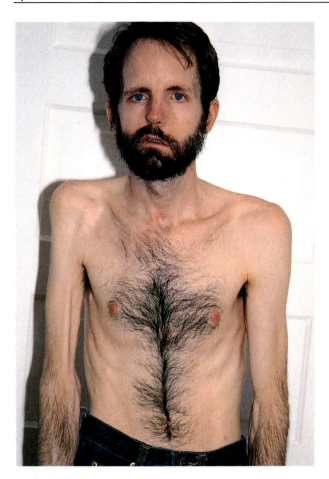

Fig. 6. A 27-year-old man with neurofibromatosis type 2 exhibited by bilateral vestibular schwannomas and spinal cord meningiomas with resulting deafness, weakness, and loss of balance.

Central nervous system imaging in neurofibromatosis type 1

Since the use of magnetic resonance imaging became widespread, 75% to 80% of patients with NF1 have been found to have an abnormality of the CNS [41]. Areas with increased signals on T2-weighted images called "unidentified bright objects" (Fig. 7) are frequently found in the basal ganglia, internal capsule, brain stem, and cerebellum. They do not demonstrate mass effect and are not associated with developmental disabilities [41]. In a series of 24 patients, an optic glioma was noted in six. In three of these patients, the gliomas were not noted on the first examination, and in one, the gliomas became symptomatic [42].

Treatment for neurofibromatosis type 1

Apparently, some patients in Japan routinely undergo general anesthesia for removal of up to 200 to 300 neurofibromas at a time [2•]. It was noted that injections of bleomycin were not as effective [2•]. Use of keto-

tifen in an attempt to decrease neurofibroma-associated itching, pain, tenderness, and tendency for bleeding has been debated, although one researcher seems convinced that it has been helpful [43]. A novel and potentially useful treatment for the future is the inhibition of angiogenesis and secondarily of tumors through treatment with AGM-1470, a potent fungus-derived inhibitor of angiogenesis [44]. Evaluation in the laboratory setting has been encouraging. Attempts at cosmetic improvement of café au lait spots include use of 510-nm wavelength nonpigmented dye laser [45], Q-switched ruby laser [46], copper vapor laser [47], carbon dioxide laser [48], argon laser [49], 300-ns pulse and 510-nm wavelength laser [50], Hexascan (Lihtan Technologies, San Rafael, CA) [51], and others. Some complications occur, such as recurrence, scarring, or deepening of the pigment color in some cases. Perhaps continued improvements will make these complications more predictable. A national multicenter drug treatment trial has started recently with participation of 10 institutions to evaluate chemotherapy for plexiform neurofibromas and optic gliomas [52].

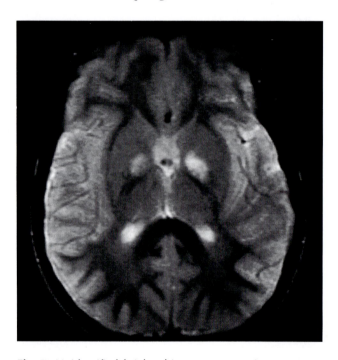

Fig. 7. Unidentified bright objects on magnetic resonance imaging of patient with neurofibromatosis.

Conclusions

Neurofibromatosis is one of the most common genetic disorders known. The varied manifestations of this condition bring such patients to all kinds of specialists, but the skin manifestations are by far the most common, the best known, and often the most feared. Marked variation in signs and symptoms makes diagnosis, prognosis, and treatment difficult. Although a great deal is now known about the two neurofibromatosis genes, we are not yet generally able to correlate gene alteration with manifestations and prognosis. It is hoped, however, that continued clinical and molecular genetic research will bring improved diagnosis and treatment possibilities to affected persons and families.

References and recommended reading

Papers of particular interest, published within the annual period of review, have been highlighted as:
*   Of special interest
** Of outstanding interest

1.   Riccardi V, Eichner J: *Neurofibromatosis Phenotype, Natural History and Pathogenesis*. Baltimore:Johns Hopkins University Press; 1986.

2.   Niimura M: **Aspects in Neurofibromatosis From the Viewpoint of**
•   **Dermatology**. *J Dermatol* 1992, 19:868–872.
An excellent clinical report of 1200 patients with neurofibromatosis followed up by one investigator over a 25-year period.

3.   Crawford A: **Pitfalls of Spinal Deformities Associated With Neurofibromatosis in Children**. *Clin Orthop* 1989, 245:29–42.

4.   Samango-Sprouse C, Rosenbaum K, Rodman L, Saal H, Stern H: **Incidence of Developmental Disabilities in Infants and Toddlers With von Recklinghausen Neurofibromatosis**. *Am J Hum Genet* 1988, 43:68A.

5.   Matsui I, Tanimura M, Kobayashi N, Sawada T, Nagahara N, Akatsuka J: **Neurofibromatosis Type 1 and Childhood Cancer**. *Cancer* 1993, 72:2746–2754.

6.   Eldridge R, Parry D: **Summary: Vestibular Schwannoma (Acoustic Neuroma)**. **Consensus Development Conference**. *Neurosurgery* 1992, 30:961–963.

7.   Evans D, Huson S, Donna D, Neary W, Blair V, Newton V, Harris
•   R: **A Clinical Study of Type 2 Neurofibromatosis**. *Q J Med* 1992, 84:603–618.
A population-based study of NF2 and the largest individual study of the condition. A comprehensive report of clinical features, age of onset, and survival.

8.   Landau K, Yasargil G: **Ocular Fundus in Neurofibromatosis Type 2**. *Br J Ophthalmol* 1993, 77:646–649.

9.   Kayes L, Burke W, Riccardi V, Bennett R, Ehrlich P, Rubenstein
•   A, Stephens K: **Deletions Spanning the Neurofibromatosis 1 Gene: Identification and Phenotype of Five Patients**. *Am J Hum Genet* 1994, 54:424–436.
A report on a study done to investigate the contribution to variability in NF1 by genes either contiguous to or contained within the *NF1* gene. Five patients carried a deletion greater than 700 kb in size. A variable number of physical anomalies were present that did not correlate with the extent of the deletion. Excellent references.

10.   Shen M, Harper P, Upadhyaya, M: **Neurofibromatosis Type 1 (NF1): the Search for Mutations by PCR-Heteroduplex Analysis on Hydrolink Gels**. *Hum Mol Genet* 1993, 2:1861–1864.

11.   Gutmann D, Collins F: **Neurofibromatosis Type 1: Beyond Positional**
••   **Cloning**. *Arch Neurol* 1993, 50:1185–1193.
In this review of current understanding of the molecular genetics of NF1 and its clinical implications, the authors clearly describe "identification of the protein product, determination of its relation to other known proteins, analysis of its distribution in tissues, within cells and over development with dissection of its role in producing the disease phenotype."

12.   Andersen L, Ballester R, Marchuk D, Chang E, Gutmann D, Saulino
••   A, Camonis J, Wigler M, Collins F: **A Conserved Alternative Splice in the von Recklinghausen Neurofibromatosis (NF1) Gene Produces Two Neurofibromin Isoforms, Both of Which Have GTPase-Activating Protein Activity**. *Mol Cell Biol* 1993, 13:487–495.
By using the RNA polymerase chain reaction with primers flanking the NF1 GTPase-activating protein–related domain, these investigators identified evidence for alternative splicing in this region of the *NF1* gene. Strong conservation of this alternative splicing was felt to suggest that both type 1 and 2 isoforms mediate important biological functions of neurofibromin. This article gives an in-depth description of the molecular genetics and potential implications.

13.   Nishi T, Saya H: **Neurofibromatosis Type 1 (NF1) Gene: Implication in Neuroectodermal Differentiation and Genesis of Brain Tumors**. *Cancer Metastasis Rev* 1991, 10:301–310.

14.   Legius E, Marchuk, D, Collins F, Glover T: **Somatic Deletion of the Neurofibromatosis Type 1 Gene in a Neurofibrosarcoma Supports a Tumour Suppressor Gene Hypothesis**. *Nat Genet* 1993, 3:122–126.

15.   Lothe R, Saeter G, Danielsen H, Stenwig A, Hoyheim B, O'Connell P, Borresen L: **Genetic Alterations in a Malignant Schwannoma From a Patient With Neurofibromatosis (NF1)**. *Pathol Res Pract* 1993, 189:465–471.

16.   Andersen L, Fountain J, Gutmann D, Tarle S, Glover T, Dracopoli C, Housman D, Collins F: **Mutations in the Neurofibromatosis 1 Gene in Sporadic Malignant Melanoma Cell Lines**. *Nature Genet* 1993, 3:118–121.

17.   Johnson M, Look T, DeClue J, Valentine M, Lowy D: **Inactivation of the NF1 Gene in Human Melanoma and Neuroblastoma Cell Lines Without Impaired Regulation of GTP Ras**. *Proc Natl Acad Sci U S A* 1993, 90:5539–5543.

18.   Easton D, Ponder M, Huson S, Ponder B: **An Analysis of Variation in Expression of Neurofibromatosis (NF) Type 1 (NF1): Evidence for Modifying Genes**. *Am J Hum Genet* 1993, 53:305–313.

19.   Driscoll D: **Genomic Imprinting and Human Disease**. *Int Pediatr*
•   1993, 8:6–13.
An easy-to-read summary article with 71 references.

20.   Engel E, Delozier-Blanchet C: **Uniparental Disomy, Isodisomy, and**
•   **Imprinting: Probable Effects in Man and Strategies for Their Detection**. *Am J Med Genet* 1991, 40:432–439.
This relatively short article is packed with information on the "new genetics."

21.   Stephens K, Kayes L, Riccardi V, Rising, M, Sybert V, Pagon, R: **Preferential Mutation of the Neurofibromatosis Type 1 Gene in Paternally Derived Chromosomes**. *Hum Genet* 1992, 88:279–282.

22.   Rodenhiser D, Coulter-Mackie M, Singh S: **Evidence of DNA Methylation in the Neurofibromatosis Type 1 (NF1) Gene Region of 17q11.2**. *Hum Mol Genet* 1993, 2:439–444.

23.   Schneider G, Lutz S, Henn W, Zang K, Blin N: **Search for Putative Suppressor Genes in Meningioma: Significance of Chromosome 22**. *Hum Genet* 1992, 88:579–582.

24.   Wolff R, Frazer K, Jackler R, Lanser M, Pitts L, Cox D: **Analysis of Chromosome 22 Deletions in Neurofibromatosis Type 2-Related Tumors**. *Am J Hum Genet* 1992, 51:478–485.

25.   Narod S, Parry D, Parboosingh J, Lenoir G, Ruttledge M, Fischer G, Eldridge R, Martuza R, Frontali M, Haines J, Gusella J, Rouleau G: **Neurofibromatosis Type 2 Appears to Be a Genetically Homogeneous Disease**. *Am J Hum Genet* 1992, 51:486–496.

26.   Arai E, Ikeuchi T, Karasawa S, Tamura A, Yamamoto K, Kida M, Ichimura K, Yuasa T, Tonomura A: **Constitutional Translocation t(4;22) (q12;q12.2) Associated With Neurofibromatosis Type 2**. *Am J Med Genet* 1992, 44:163–167.

27.   Schinzel A, Basaran S, Bernasconi F, Karaman B, Yuksel-Apak M, Robinson W: **Maternal Uniparental Disomy 22 Has No Impact on the Phenotype**. *Am J Hum Genet* 1994, 54:21–24.

28.   Rey J, Bello M, Kusak, M, de Campos J, Pestana A: **Involvement of 22q12 in a Neurofibrosarcoma in Neurofibromatosis Type 1**. *Cancer Genet Cytogenet* 1993, 66:28–32.

29.   Brunner H, Hulsebos T, Steijlen P, der Kinderen D, Steen A, Hamel B: **Exclusion of the Neurofibromatosis 1 Locus in a Family With Inherited Cafe-au-Lait Spots**. *Am J Med Genet* 1993, 46:472–474.

30.   Charrow J, Listernick R, Ward K: **Autosomal Dominant Multiple Cafe-au-Lait Spots and Neurofibromatosis-1: Evidence of Non-linkage**. *Am J Med Genet* 1993, 45:606–608.

31.   Fois A, Calistri L, Balestri P, Vivarelli R, Bartalini G, Mancini L, Berardi A, Vanni M: **Relationship Between Cafe-Au-Lait Spots as the Only Symptom and Peripheral Neurofibromatosis (NF1): A Follow-Up Study**. *Eur J Pediatr* 1993, 152:500–504.

32.   Tassabehji M, Strachan T, Sharland M, Colley A, Donnai D, Harris R, Thakker N: **Tandem Duplication Within a Neurofibromatosis Type 1 (NF1) Gene Exon in a Family With Features of Watson Syndrome and Noonan Syndrome**. *Am J Hum Genet* 1993, 53:90–95.

33.   Stern H, Saal H, Lee J, Fain P, Goldgar D, Rosenbaum K, Barker D: **Clinical Variability of Type 1 Neurofibromatosis: Is There a Neurofibromatosis-Noonan Syndrome?** *J Med Genet* 1992, 29:184–187.

34.   Sharland M, Taylor R, Patton M, Jeffrey S: **Absence of Linkage of Noonan Syndrome to the Neurofibromatosis Type 1 Locus**. *J Med Genet* 1992, 29:188–190.

35.   Pulst S, Rouleau G, Marineau C, Fain P, Sieb J: **Familial Meningioma Is Not Allelic to Neurofibromatosis 2**. *Neurology* 1993, 43:2096–2098.

36.   Micali G, Lembo D, Giustini S, Calvieri S: **Segmental Neurofibromatosis With Only Macular Lesions**. *Pediatr Dermatol* 1993, 10:43–45.

37.   Goldberg N: **What is Segmental Neurofibromatosis?** *J Am Acad Dermatol* 1992, 16:638–640.

38.   Mohri S, Atsusaka K, Sasaki, T: **Localized Multiple Neurofibromas**. *Clin Exp Dermatol* 1992, 17:195–196.

39. Hennekam R, Holtus F: **Johnson-McMillin Syndrome: Report of Another Family.** *Am J Med Genet* 1993, 47:714–716.

40. Vollenweider Roten S, Masouye I, Delozier-Blanchet C, Saurat, J: **Cutaneous Findings in Ring Chromosome 7 Syndrome.** *Dermatology* 1993, 186:84–87.

41. Balestri L, Calistri R, Vivarelli G, Bartalini L, Mancini A, Berardi A: **Central Nervous System Imaging in Reevaluation of Patients With Neurofibromatosis Type 1.** *Childs Nerv Syst* 1993, 9:448–451.

42. Listernick R, Charrow J, Greenwald M: **Emergence of Optic Pathway Gliomas in Children With Neurofibromatosis Type 1 After Normal Neuroimaging Results.** *J Pediatr* 1992, 121:584–587.

43. Riccardi V: **A Controlled Multiphase Trial of Ketotifen to Minimize Neurofibroma-Associated Pain and Itching.** *Arch Dermatol* 1993, 129:577-581.

44. Takamiya Y, Friedlander R, Brenl, H, Malick A, Martuza R: **Inhibition of Angiogenesis and Growth of Human Nerve-Sheath Tumors by AGM-1470.** *J Neurosurg* 1993, 78:470–476.

45. Grekin R, Shelton R, Geisse J, Frieden I: **510-nm Pigmented Lesion Dye Laser: Its Characteristics and Clinical Uses.** *J Dermatol Surg Oncol* 1993, 19:380–387.

46. Goldberg J: **Benign Pigmented Lesions of the Skin.** *J Dermatol Surg Oncol* 1993, 19:376-379.

47. Dinehart S, Waner M, Flock S: **The Copper Vapor Laser for Treatment of Cutaneous Vascular and Pigmented Lesions.** *J Dermatol Surg Oncol* 1993, 19:370–375.

48. Olbricht S: **Use of the Carbon Dioxide Laser in Dermatologic Surgery: A Clinically Relevant Update for 1993.** *J. Dermatol Surg Oncol* 1993, 19:364–369.

49. McBurney, E: **Clinical Usefulness of the Argon Laser for the 1990s.** *J Dermatol Surg Oncol* 1993, 19:358–362.

50. Fitzpatrick R, Goldman, M, Ruiz-Esparza J: **Laser Treatment of Benign Pigmented Epidermal Lesions Using a 300 Nsecond Pulse and 510 nm Wavelengths.** *J Dermatol Surg Oncol* 1993, 19:341–347.

51. McDaniel D: **Clinical Usefulness of the Hexascan: Treatment of Cutaneous Vascular and Melanocytic Disorders.** *J Dermatol Surg Oncol* 1993, 19:312–319.

52. Rubenstein A: **First Multi Center Drug Treatment Trials Have Begun.** *Newsletter Natl Neurofibromatosis Found* Winter 1994: 1,9.

53. Neurofibromatosis. *NIH Consensus Statement* July 13–15 1987, 6(12):1–7.

Mary A. Curtis, MD, Department of Pediatrics, Division of Medical Genetics, University of Iowa Hospitals and Clinics, 200 Hawkins Drive, Iowa City, IA 52242-1083, USA.

Pediatrics and genodermatoses

Edited by

Moise Levy
Texas Children's Hospital
Houston, Texas, USA

CURRENT SCIENCE

The cause and treatment of vitiligo

Joseph G. Morelli, MD

University of Colorado School of Medicine, Denver, Colorado, USA

Vitiligo is a common skin disorder characterized clinically by the progressive development of depigmented macules. Many theories regarding the cause of vitiligo have been postulated. It is likely that vitiligo is a heterogenous disease and that portions of all of the theories are correct in given subsets of patients. The initial section of this article will review recent evidence supporting the various hypotheses on the cause of vitiligo. Regardless of the cause, vitiligo remains a difficult disease to treat. The latter portion of this article will discuss recent treatment advances as well as some of the basic science of melanocyte movement as it pertains to the repigmentation of vitiligo.

Current Opinion in Dermatology 1995:105–108

Vitiligo occurs in 1% to 2% of the population worldwide, and there is an equal racial distribution [1••]. It is characterized by the development of usually asymptomatic white spots that may be a few millimeters to several centimeters in size. Occasionally, vitiligo macules will be surrounded by a raised erythematous border (inflammatory vitiligo). In some patients there will be a transition zone from depigmented skin to various stages of hypopigmentation to normal-appearing skin (trichrome vitiligo [Fig. 1]). Over one half of the cases of vitiligo begin prior to 20 years of age. There are two classically described types of vitiligo: segmental and generalized. Generalized vitiligo often begins symmetrically and acrally (Fig. 2) and may occur anywhere on the body. The clinical course is usually one of slow, intermittent spread over years. Occasionally there will be depigmentation of the total cutaneous surface. On the other hand, spontaneous repigmentation also occurs. Despite years of study, the cause of vitiligo remains a mystery, and treatment of the condition is difficult. This article reviews recent evidence supporting various theories of the pathogenesis of vitiligo, discusses recent trends in treatment, and reports on some of the research into the basic science of melanocyte movement as it pertains to repigmentation in vitiligo.

Pathogenesis

One of the most basic questions in the pathogenesis of vitiligo is whether the melanocytes are destroyed or are just damaged and not functioning. This question has once again been recently addressed. When discussing the presence or absence of melanocytes in vitiligo, one must be careful to differentiate stable depigmented vitiligo from actively depigmenting vitiligo. By either electron microscopy or immunohistochemical staining, three separate groups concluded

that there were no identifiable melanocytes present in long-standing, stable vitiligo lesions [2•–4•]. Immunohistochemical staining of an expanding lesion revealed abnormal melanocyte morphology consistent with ongoing melanocyte destruction [4•]. By electron microscopy, melanocytes within areas of early active vitiligo demonstrated multiple degenerative changes including vacuolization, fatty degeneration, autophagic vesicles, pyknosis, and homogenous cytoplasmic degeneration [2•]. In addition to the changes seen in melanocytes, normal-appearing skin adjacent to early lesions of vitiligo reveal vacuolar changes in basal keratinocytes, epidermal infiltration of lymphocytes, and melanophages in the upper dermis [3•]. Thus, it appears that vitiligo is a disease of melanocyte damage leading to total melanocyte destruction in areas of long-standing depigmentation.

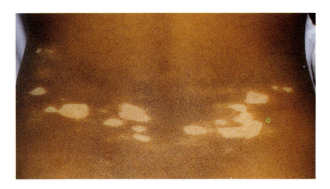

Fig. 1. Trichrome vitiligo.

There is no doubt that the immune system is involved in the melanocyte destruction in certain patients with vitiligo. Vitiligo is seen in association with a number of autoimmune diseases [1••], as in the case of a pa-

---

Abbreviation
PUVA—psoralens and ultraviolet A.

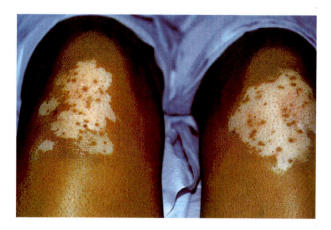

Fig. 2. Symmetrical, acral vitiligo.

tient with autoimmune thyroiditis and circulating anti-NuMA (nuclear mitotic apparatus) antibodies [5], and antibodies to pigment cells are present in the sera of patients with vitiligo [6,7•]. Recently, these antibodies were shown to be present in 78% of patients with vitiligo compared with only 14% of control patients [6]. There were several different antibodies present, but the most common were directed to 40- to 45-kD, 75-kD, and 90-kD antigens. These antigens were present in 74%, 57%, and 35% of patients respectively and were thought to be cell surface antigens. Sera from patients with vitiligo was demonstrated to cause complement-mediated cell lysis in 85% of those patients with active disease, 44% of those patients with inactive disease, and in only 6% of control patients [7•]. Antikeratinocyte antibodies have also been demonstrated in sera of patients with vitiligo, but these antibodies are not cytotoxic to keratinocytes *in vitro* [8]. Therefore, it appears that a large number of patients with vitiligo have circulating antimelanocyte antibodies, which are capable of aiding in melanocyte destruction.

Other findings support an autoimmune hypothesis in the pathogenesis of vitiligo. There is a sixfold increase in the number of melanocytes expressing the intercellular adhesion molecule-1 in perilesional skin of patients with vitiligo compared with unaffected skin of patients with vitiligo and with skin from control subjects [9]. Intercellular adhesion molecule-1 is important in lymphocyte interaction with target cells, and the increase expression of this molecule by melanocytes in patients with vitiligo may be part of the immune-mediated destruction of melanocytes in these patients. Natural killer cell activity has also been shown to be higher in patients with vitiligo than in control subjects, but interestingly, higher activity was seen in those patients with stable vitiligo compared with those with active disease [10]. There is also a marked decrease in the migration of epidermal Langerhans cells out of vitiligo skin stimulated with interferon γ [11]. This reaction is likely related to the abnormal response of vitiliginous skin to contact allergens and is another sign of an altered immune response in patients with vitiligo.

Vitiligo-like depigmentation in certain animal models appears to be transmitted as an autosomal recessive

trait. The depigmenting mouse is also known as the *vit/vit* mouse. The *vit* gene has now been shown to be an allele of the microphthalmia (*mi*) gene on mouse chromosome 6 [12•].

Although vitiligo-like depigmentation is an autosomal recessive trait in animals, no such data exist for human vitiligo. It has been believed by some that human vitiligo is an autosomal dominant disorder with incomplete penetrance [13••]. Although familial aggregation exists in patients with vitiligo, it is unlikely that a single gene locus is responsible for human vitiligo [13••]. The relative risk of first-degree relatives for developing vitiligo is 7 for parents, 12 for siblings, and 36 for children [13••]. This extent of familial aggregation of vitiligo is statistically significant. Also supporting the genetic theory for human vitiligo is the increase in HLA-A30, -Cw6, and -DQw3 and a decrease in C4A*QO in northern Italian patients with vitiligo [14]. It is likely that human vitiligo is a polygenic disease.

Because melanocytes are neural crest–derived cells, abnormal neural control has been suggested as playing a role not only in the pathogenesis of segmental vitiligo, but also in generalized vitiligo. Catecholamines are neurotransmitters that bind to β-adrenoreceptors. Patients with active vitiligo have a significant increase in urinary metabolites of catecholamines [15]. Differentiated cultured keratinocytes from lesional skin of patients with vitiligo show a significant increase in β_2-adrenoreceptors [16]. Patients with vitiligo also have increased plasma levels of the neuropeptides β-endorphin and met-enkephalin [10]. How these alterations in catecholamine metabolism, catecholamine binding, and altered neuropeptides contribute to the pathogenesis of vitiligo remains to be elucidated.

Treatment

Because the pathogenesis of vitiligo is unknown, there are no therapies directed at the primary cause of the disease. Therefore, all medical treatments are empiric, and their mechanisms of action are also unknown. There are four recent excellent reviews covering the spectrum of vitiligo treatment [17••–20••].

Psoralen photochemotherapy (psoralens and ultraviolet A [PUVA]) is regarded as the most efficacious treatment for vitiligo available in the United States. Historically, approximately 50% of patients respond to PUVA therapy. In a recent report, 61% of patients achieved greater than 25% repigmentation [17••]. In another study, 44% of patients repigmented with treatment, and half of those patients achieved greater than 50% repigmentation [21]. There was no difference in the response rates between topical and oral psoralen with topical therapy used for those patients with less than 20% involvement [17••,21].

Khellin has been used in Europe for photochemotherapy as an alternative to psoralens. Khellin has been advocated for photochemotherapy of vitiligo, because unlike psoralens, it does not require a phototoxic response to achieve repigmentation. As with psoralens, khellin may be used topically or orally and with ultraviolet A radiation or natural sunlight. Topical khellin used with natural sunlight has recently been shown to be no different than natural sunlight alone in the treatment of vitiligo [22]. At this time, because of questions of liver toxicity, khellin is not available in the United States.

There has been much debate about the efficacy of Melagenina in the treatment of vitiligo. There are many anecdotal reports about its efficacy in the treatment of vitiligo [23], but no controlled studies verifying these reports have been published [24]. Like khellin, Melagenina is not available in the United States.

An interesting approach to the treatment of vitiligo is the nutritional one, which consists of oral folic acid (2 mg twice a day) and vitamin C (500 mg twice a day) along with vitamin B_{12} (100 mg intramuscularly every 2 weeks). This regimen was reported to achieve steady and significant repigmentation in eight of 15 patients followed up over a 3-year period [25].

Several surgical approaches have been used to repigment small, stable, cosmetically important areas that have not responded to medical therapy [17••]. These approaches include autologous suction blister grafting, autologous minigrafting, autologous melanocyte transplants, and mixed epidermal transplants [17••]. The vitiliginous epidermis can be removed either by suction [26,27], liquid nitrogen [28–30], or dermabrasion [31,32]. Donor areas are harvested by dermatome [29,31,32], suction [26,27,30], or liquid nitrogen [28], and autologous epidermal grafts [26,27,30,31], epidermal suspensions [28], or cultured melanocytes [26,29,32] are transferred to the donor site. Debate continues over which technique gives the best result.

Basic science of melanocyte migration

Repigmentation in vitiligo takes place predominantly in a perifollicular fashion (Fig. 3). Although interfollicular epidermal melanocytes are destroyed in vitiligo, there remains a reservoir of inactive melanocytes in the outer root sheath of the hair follicle. During repigmentation these cells are activated, proliferate, and migrate into the depigmented epidermis. An understanding of the factors involved in these processes may lead to improved methods of treatment. First, there must be some signal to begin migration. Leukotriene C_4 and transforming growth factor-α have been demonstrated to enhance melanocyte random movement in vitro [33•]. Once cells are stimulated to migrate, they must move through a complex environment, and this movement requires the interaction of melanocytes with keratinocytes and basement membrane matrix proteins. The interaction of cells with matrix proteins is in part regulated by cell surface receptors called integrins. Melanocytes preferentially migrate over a matrix of type IV collagen, and this migration is blocked by antibodies to α_2- and α_3-integrins, but not by antibodies to α_5-integrins [34•]. Thus, we know now some

factors that enhance migration, and we understand which matrix proteins of the basement membrane allow for melanocyte movement. There is still much to be learned about all of the factors necessary to activate a hair follicle outer root sheath melanocyte, the stimuli for migration of these cells, and the changes required in the melanocyte itself and the environment to allow for this migration.

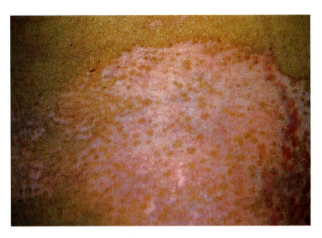

Fig. 3. Perifollicular repigmentation during psoralens and ultraviolet A treatment of vitiligo.

References and recommended reading

Papers of particular interest, published within the annual period of review, have been highlighted as:
- •   Of special interest
- ••   Of outstanding interest

1. Mosher DB, Fitzpatrick TB, Hori Y, Ortonne J-P: **Disorders of**
•• **Melanocytes.** In *Dermatology in General Medicine*, edn 4. Edited by Fitzpatrick TB, Eisen AZ, Wolff K, Freedberg IM, Austen KF. New York: McGraw-Hill; 1993:723–733.
Excellent textbook description covering all aspects of vitiligo.

2. Galadari E, Mehregan AH, Hashimoto K: **Ultrastructural Study of**
• **Vitiligo.** *Int J Dermatol* 1993, 32:269–271.
This article, along with those of Hann *et al.* (*J Dermatol* 1992, 19:217–222) and Le Poole *et al.* (*J Invest Dermatol* 1993, 100:816–822), presents convincing evidence that melanocytes are absent in long-standing, stable vitiligo lesions.

3. Hann SK, Park Y-K, Lee K-G, Choi EO, Im S: **Epidermal Changes**
• **in Active Vitiligo.** *J Dermatol* 1992, 19:217–222.
This article, along with those of Galadari *et al.* (*Int J Dermatol* 1993, 32:269–271) and Le Poole *et al.* (*J Invest Dermatol* 1993, 100:816–822), presents convincing evidence that melanocytes are absent in long-standing, stable vitiligo lesions.

4. Le Poole IC, van den Wijngaard RMJGJ, Westerhop W, Dutrieux
• RP, Das PK: **Presence of Absence of Melanocytes in Vitiligo Lesions: An Immunohistochemical Investigation.** *J Invest Dermatol* 1993, 100:816–822.
This article, along with those of Galadari *et al.* (*Int J Dermatol* 1993, 32:269–271) and Hann *et al.* (*J Dermatol* 1992, 19:217–222), presents convincing evidence that melanocytes are absent in long-standing, stable vitiligo lesions.

5. Auer-Grumbach P, Stangl M: **Autoantibodies to Nuclear Mitotic Apparatus in a Patient With Vitiligo and Autoimmune Thyroiditis.** *Dermatology* 1993, 186:229–231.

6. Cui J, Harning R, Henn M, Bystryn J-C: **Identification of Pigment Cell Antigens Defined by Vitiligo Antibodies.** *J Invest Dermatol* 1992, 98:162–165.

7. Cui J, Arita Y, Bystryn J-C: **Cytolytic Antibodies to Melanocytes in**
• **Vitiligo.** *J Invest Dermatol* 1993, 100:812–815.
Presents further evidence that antibodies in vitiligo are melanocytotoxic.

8.   Yu H-S, Kao C-H, Yu C-L: **Coexistence and Relationship of Antik-eratinocyte and Antimelanocyte Antibodies in Patients With Non-segmental-type Vitiligo.** *J Invest Dermatol* 1993, 100:823–828.

9.   Al Badri AMT, Foulis AK, Todd PM, Garioch JJ, Gudgeon JE, Stewart DG, Gracie JA, Goudie RB: **Abnormal Expression of MHC Class II and ICAM-1 by Melanocytes in Vitiligo.** *J Pathol* 1993, 169:203–206.

10.   Mozzanica N, Villa ML, Foppa S, Vignati G, Cattaneo A, Diotti R, Finzi AF: **Plasma α-Melanocyte Stimulating Hormone, β-Endorphin, Met-Enkephalin, and Natural Killer Cell Activity in Vitiligo.** *J Am Acad Dermatol* 1992, 26:693–700.

11.   Gilhar A, Aizen E, Ohana N, Etzioni A: **Vitiliginous Vs Pigmented Skin Response to Intradermal Administration of Interferon Gamma.** *Arch Dermatol* 1993, 129:600–604.

12. • Lamoreaux ML, Boissy RE, Womack JE, Nordlund JJ: **The *vit* Gene Maps to the *mi* (Microphthalmia) Locus of the Laboratory Mouse.** *J Hered* 1992, 83:435–439.
Identifies the gene responsible for vitiligo in the mouse.

13. •• Majumder PP, Nordlung JJ, Nath SK: **Pattern of Familial Aggregation of Vitiligo.** *Arch Dermatol* 1993, 129:994–998.
Excellent discussion on the familial patterns seen in vitiligo.

14.   Orecchia G, Perfetti L, Malagoli P, Borghini F, Kipervag Y: **Vitiligo is Associated With a Significant Increase in HLA-A30, Cw6 and DQ3w and a Decrease on C4AQO in Northern Italian Patients.** *Dermatology* 1992, 185:123–127.

15.   Morrone A, Picardo M, de Luca C, Terminali O, Passi S, Ippolito F: **Catecholamines and Vitiligo.** *Pigment Cell Res* 1992, 5:65–69.

16.   Schallreuter KU, Wood JM, Pittlekow MR, Swanson NN, Steinkraus V: **Increased In Vitro Expression of β₂-Adrenoreceptors in Differentiating Lesional Keratinocytes of Vitiligo Patients.** *Arch Dermatol Res* 1993, 285:216–220.

17. •• Grimes PE: **Vitiligo: An Overview of Therapeutic Approaches.** *Dermatol Clin* 1993, 11:325–338.
This article, together with those of Nordlund et al. (*Dermatol Clin* 1993, 11:27–33) and Goldstein et al. (*Int J Dermatol* 1992, 31:229–236;314–319), covers all aspects of current vitiligo therapy.

18. •• Nordlund JJ, Halder RM, Grimes PE: **Management of Vitiligo.** *Dermatol Clin* 1993, 11:27–33.
This article, together with those of Grimes et al. (*Dermatol Clin* 1993, 11:325–338) and Goldstein et al. (*Int J Dermatol* 1992, 31:229–236;314–319), covers all aspects of current vitiligo therapy.

19. •• Goldstein E, Haberman HF, Menon IA, Pawlowski D: **Non-psoralen Treatment of Vitiligo: Part I. Cosmetics, Systemic Coloring Agents and Corticosteroids.** *Int J Dermatol* 1992, 31:229–236.
This article, together with those of Grimes et al. (*Dermatol Clin* 1993, 11:325–338), Nordlund et al. (*Dermatol Clin* 1993, 11:27–33), and Goldstein et al. (*Int J Dermatol* 1992, 31:314–319), covers all aspects of current vitiligo therapy.

20. •• Goldstein E, Haberman HF, Menon IA, Pawlowski D: **Non-psoralen Treatment of Vitiligo: Part II. Less Commonly Used and Experimental Therapies.** *Int J Dermatol* 1992, 31:314–319.
This article, together with those of Grimes et al. (*Dermatol Clin* 1993, 11:325–338), Nordlund et al. (*Dermatol Clin* 1993, 11:27–33), and Goldstein et al. (*Int J Dermatol* 1992, 31:229–236), covers all aspects of current vitiligo therapy.

21.   Wildfang IL, Jacobsen FK, Thestrup-Pedersen K: **PUVA Treatment of Vitiligo: A Retrospective Study of 59 Patients.** *Acta Derm Venereol (Stockh)* 1992, 72:305–306.

22.   Orrecchia G, Perfetti L: **Photochemotherapy With Topical Khellin and Sunlight in Vitiligo.** *Dermatology* 1992, 184:120–123.

23.   Azambuja RD: **Melagenina and Vitiligo [Letter].** *Dermatology* 1992, 184:153.

24.   Nordlund JJ: **Melagenina and Vitiligo [Reply].** *Dermatology* 1992, 184:154–155.

25.   Montes LF, Diaz ML, Lajous J, Garcia NJ: **Folic Acid and Vitamin B₁₂ in Vitiligo: A Nutritional Approach.** *Cutis* 1992, 50:39–42.

26.   Zachariae H, Zachariae C, Deleuran B, Kristensen P: **Autotransplantation in Vitiligo: Treatment With Epidermal Grafts and Cultured Melanocytes.** *Acta Derm Venereol (Stockh)* 1993, 73:46–48.

27.   Mutalki S: **Transplantation of Melanocytes by Epidermal Grafting: An Indian Experience.** *J Dermatol Surg Oncol* 1993, 19:231–234.

28.   Gauthier Y, Surleve-Bazeille J-E: **Autologous Grafting With Noncultured Melanocytes: A Simplified Method for Treatment of Depigmented Lesions.** *J Am Acad Dermatol* 1992, 26:191–194.

29.   Falabella R, Escobar C, Borrero I: **Treatment of Refractory and Stable Vitiligo by Transplantation of In Vitro Cultured Epidermal Autografts Bearing Melanocytes.** *J Am Acad Dermatol* 1992, 26:230–236.

30.   Skouge JW, Morison WL, Diwan RV, Rotter S: **Autografting and PUVA: A Combination Therapy for Vitiligo.** *J Dermatol Surg Oncol* 1992, 18:357–360.

31.   Kahn AM, Cohen MJ, Kaplan L, Highton A: **Vitiligo: Treatment by Dermabrasion and Epithelial Sheet Grafting: A Preliminary Report.** *J Am Acad Dermatol* 1993, 28:773–774.

32.   Olsson MJ, Juhlin L: **Repigmentation of Vitiligo by Transplantation of Cultured Autologous Melanocytes.** *Acta Derm Venereol (Stockh)* 1993, 73:49–51.

33. • Morelli JG, Kincannon J, Yohn JJ, Zekman T, Weston WL, Norris DA: **Leukotriene C₄ and TGF-α Are Stimulators of Human Melanocyte Migration In Vivo.** *J Invest Dermatol* 1992, 98:290–295.
This article is an early attempt to understand the biology of pigment cell migration in vitiligo repigmentation.

34. • Morelli JG, Yohn JJ, Zekman T, Norris DA: **Melanocyte Movement In Vitro: Role of Matrix Proteins and Integrin Receptors.** *J Invest Dermatol* 1993, 101:605–608.
This article is an early attempt to understand the biology of pigment cell migration in vitiligo repigmentation.

Joseph G. Morelli, MD, Department of Dermatology B-153, University of Colorado Health Sciences Center, 4200 East Ninth Avenue, Denver, CO 80262, USA.

Pharmacologic therapy for endangering hemangiomas

John B. Mulliken, MD, Laurence M. Boon, MD,
Kazue Takahashi, PhD, Laurie A. Ohlms, MD, Judah
Folkman, MD, and R. Alan B. Ezekowitz, MD, DPhil

Children's Hospital, Harvard Medical School, Boston, Massachusetts, USA

The common cutaneous hemangioma of infancy rarely requires therapeutic intervention. These tumors proliferate rapidly and invariably involute slowly. Approximately 10% of hemangiomas cause tissue destruction, obstruct a vital structure, or threaten life. Pharmacologic intervention may be indicated for these problematic tumors. The first-line drug therapy remains high-dose corticosteriods. Accelerated regression is seen in 30% of infants within 2 weeks. If the response is equivocal or growth continues, there is no advantage to continuing corticosteroid therapy. Interferon alfa-2a is the second-line drug for endangering hemangiomas. The response rate is greater than 80%, but acceleration of involution with this recombinant protein is slow. Interferon therapy must be given for 6 to 8 months as a daily subcutaneous injection. Side effects for both agents must be considered.

Current Opinion in Dermatology 1995:109–113

The diagnosis and natural history of hemangioma, the most common tumor of infancy, are well known [1]. Fortunately, most hemangiomas are small, harmless vascular birthmarks. Nevertheless, there is often parental pressure to do something about them, usually coupled with a physician's natural desire to intervene. The majority of cutaneous hemangiomas, however, should be left alone to proliferate and involute naturally, for they will leave normal or only slightly blemished skin.

Because of their location, size, or behavior, approximately 10% to 20% of hemangiomas require treatment. Ulceration, particularly in the ears, lips, and anogenital areas, occurs in 5% of hemangiomas [2]. Ulcerations are usually minor and heal with cleansing and topical antibiotics. Sometimes a wet-to-dry dressing regimen is necessary. Major ulcerations are often associated with other endangering problems that necessitate therapy. Obstruction and distortion are hemangiomatous complications unique to the cervicofacial region. Even a small hemangioma in the upper eyelid can distort the cornea and produce astigmatism and possible amblyopia [3]. Subglottic hemangioma is a potentially life-threatening lesion that presents insidiously as biphasic stridor at 6 to 8 weeks of age. Large facial hemangiomas grow to expand the skin and distort normal anatomic structures.

Infants with multiple cutaneous hemangiomas are at high risk for visceral lesions, particularly intrahepatic hemangiomas. These infants typically present several weeks after birth with congestive heart failure, hepatomegaly, and anemia. Hepatic hemangiomas have a mortality rate of 30% to 80% [4,5]. High-output cardiac decompensation can also occur with a large cutaneous hemangioma in the absence of visceral lesions.

Platelet-trapping coagulopathy (ie, Kasabach-Merritt syndrome) is another life-threatening complication.

The infant is at risk for gastrointestinal, pleuropulmonic, peritoneal, or intracranial hemorrhage. The mortality rate for this thrombocytopenic complication is 30% to 40%, despite corticosteroid therapy [6].

Basic mechanisms

Terminologic and clinical confusion between hemangioma and vascular malformation has been responsible for improper diagnosis, illogical treatment, and misdirected research efforts. Over one decade ago, it was shown that hemangiomas and malformations are entirely different biologically, as demonstrated by clinical-cellular [7,8], in vitro [9], and radiologic [10–12] studies.

Immunohistochemical cellular markers also differentiate hemangioma from vascular malformation and further elucidate the clinical phases of hemangioma [13••]. Hemangiomas in the rapid-growth phase are defined by high expression of proliferating cell nuclear antigen, type IV collagenase and vascular endothelial growth factor. Elevated expression of the tissue inhibitor of metalloproteinase, TIMP-1 (an inhibitor of new blood vessel formation), is observed only in involuting lesions. Basic fibroblast growth factor (bFGF), endothelial markers, CD31, and von Willebrand factor are coexpressed in the proliferating and involuting phases. Vascular malformations, in contrast, do not manifest any of these histologic signs, other than the phenotypic endothelial markers, CD31, von Willebrand factor, and a pericyte marker called α–smooth muscle actin.

Preliminary studies indicate that the angiogenic peptide bFGF is elevated in the urine and serum of cancer patients [14] and also in infants with even small proliferating hemangiomas. In contrast, urinary bFGF is normal

---

Abbreviations
bFGF—basic fibroblast growth factor; IFN-α2a—interferon alfa-2a.

in patients with large vascular malformations, of either the slow-flow or the fast-flow type (Folkman *et al.*, unpublished data). Thus, bFGF levels are potentially useful in distinguishing hemangiomas from other vascular anomalies.

Corticosteroid therapy

The optimum corticosteroid regimen is prednisone (or prednisolone) given orally, 2 to 3 mg/kg per day, either as a single morning dose or divided into two doses. Intravenous therapy may be used, if necessary, but there is no evidence that it is more effective. A sensitive hemangioma exhibits signs of regression within several days to 1 week. As a general rule, 30% of the lesions respond dramatically, 40% respond equivocally, and 30% do not respond at all [15••]. If there is no effect, *ie*, no lightening of color, softening, or diminished growth, then corticosteroid therapy should be discontinued, in a rapid taper, after a 2-week trial. Anecdotal evidence suggests that in some instances, corticosteroids may accelerate hemangiomatous growth. If there is a therapeutic response, the drug should be continued and gradually tapered over the subsequent weeks and months. Alternate-day therapy diminishes the side effects, viz, anorexia, weight loss, growth retardation, Cushingoid facies, and immunosuppression [16]. Rebound growth may occur during the first (proliferative) phase if the drug level is lowered too rapidly. Corticosteroid treatment must be continued until involution is well under way, usually for 8 to 10 months.

Intralesional corticosteroids are preferred for well-localized cutaneous hemangiomas. Triamcinolone is injected slowly at low-pressure, and no more than 3 to 5 mg/kg are given. The response rate is similar to that for systemic corticosteroids; usually two or three injections given everyday for 6 to 8 weeks are needed [17,18]. Caution is necessary when injecting intralesional corticosteroids. The drug is a colloidal suspension. Cases of obstruction of the retinal artery, causing blindness (even in the contralateral eye), have been reported with periorbital injection [19,20]. Other complications of intralesional therapy include cutaneous atrophy (usually temporary), skin necrosis, cholesterol plaque deposition, and Cushingoid facies.

Interferon therapy

There is accumulating evidence that recombinant interferon alfa-2a (IFN-α2a) effective treatment for site-threatening or life-threatening hemangiomas, even after failure of corticosteroid therapy (Figs. 1 and 2) [21–23,24••,25–28]. At this writing, IFN-α2a is considered a second-line drug, used most often for endangering lesions that do not respond to corticosteroids. The dosage is not yet well established. The empiric range is 3 MU/m² daily, given subcutaneously. There is a reported failure of IFN-α2a therapy when given only three times a week [29]. Interferon alfa-2b also has been used successfully [30,31••], although there is a report of failure [32].

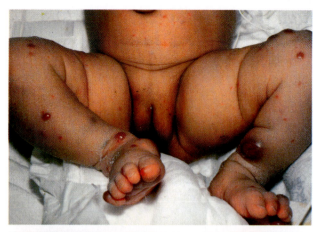

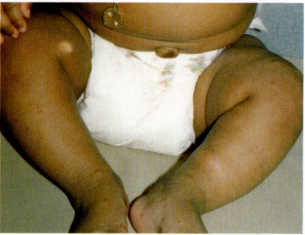

Fig. 1. Top, One-month-old girl with multiple cutaneous hemangiomas and lesion of the right atrium causing congestive heart failure. **Bottom,** At age 6 months, rapid regression of cutaneous lesions is seen after 6 months of interferon alfa-2a therapy.

We documented accelerated regression in 18 of 20 treated infants and children with site-threatening and life-threatening hemangiomas in various cutaneous and visceral locations [24••]. Our ongoing experience in another 28 patients confirms this response. IFN-α2a therapy must be continued, on average, for 6 to 10 months. Accelerated regression is less dramatic in tumors treated with IFN-α2a than in tumors highly responsive to corticosteroids. For hemangiomas of the upper eyelid, however, pressure on the cornea must be relieved rapidly to prevent astigmatism. This need, coupled with the relative contraindication (*ie*, retinal embolization) to local corticosteroids, has stimulated revival of surgical excision for periorbital lesions [33]. Other novel pharmacologic approaches include a gonadotropin hormone release antagonist (Lupron R; TAP Pharmaceuticals, Chicago, IL) which is under investigation in our ophthalmology department for the treatment of periorbital hemangiomas (L. Smith, Personal communication).

Interferon alfa-2a appears to be particularly effective in the treatment of large cutaneous hemangiomas with associated Kasabach-Merritt syndrome. Platelets and

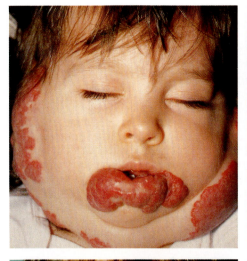
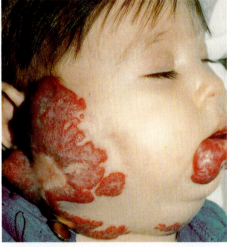
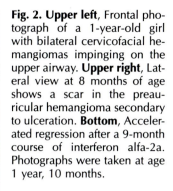

Fig. 2. Upper left, Frontal photograph of a 1-year-old girl with bilateral cervicofacial hemangiomas impinging on the upper airway. **Upper right,** Lateral view at 8 months of age shows a scar in the preauricular hemangioma secondary to ulceration. **Bottom,** Accelerated regression after a 9-month course of interferon alfa-2a. Photographs were taken at age 1 year, 10 months.

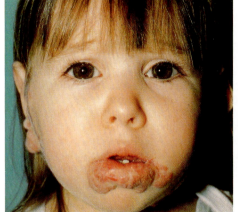
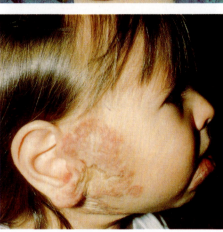

blood products should be avoided in infants with this type of thrombocytopenic coagulopathy, particularly in the absence of clinical bleeding. Infused blood components and platelets are trapped within the lesion, and transfusion often accelerates capillary growth with rapid enlargement of the hemangioma. Packed erythrocytes may be required if the hematocrit falls to the low 20% range.

Kasabach-Merritt thrombocytopenia should not be confused with disseminated intravascular coagulopathy, a hematologic disorder that sometimes occurs with venous malformations. Heparin therapy, a mainstay for treatment of this condition, is specifically contraindicated in infants with Kasabach-Merritt coagulopathy. There is experimental evidence that heparin potentiates the effect of growth factors on cultured endothelium [34,35] and accelerates tumor angiogenesis in mice [36]. Furthermore, heparin also mobilizes bFGF, a potent angiogenic protein, from its storage site in the extracellular matrix [37]. In our early clinical experience, we noted apparent accelerated growth of hemangiomas when heparin was used as conventional therapy for Kasabach-Merritt coagulopathy. We therefore stopped using heparin in infants with hemangioma-causing thrombocytopenia. We have also seen immediate improvement of a platelet-trapping hemangioma coincident with discontinuation of heparin and platelet transfusions in an infant referred to us.

In a rare tumor known as Kaposi-like infantile hemangioendothelioma, all therapies, including corticosteroids, embolization, and irradiation, have been unsuccessful [38–40]. This tumor appears later in infancy than a typical hemangioma. In most cases, Kasabach-Merritt syndrome is evident. The "unfavorable" microscopic features are infiltrative sheets and nodules of slender endothelial cells, and areas of spindle cells, surrounded by dilated lymphatic-like spaces. We have tried IFN-α2a in four children with these highly lethal tumors. Two died from extensively invasive retroperitoneal tumor. Another child is alive at 3 years with a cervicomediastinal tumor, thrombocytopenia, and a tracheostomy. She failed to respond to corticosteroids, IFN-α2a, and embolization. Another child 5 years of age is doing well after surgical excision of a thoracic Kaposi-like hemangioendothelioma.

Toxicities

Most of the children given IFN-α2a have fever for the first 1 to 2 weeks of therapy, with temperatures of up to 39°C. Pretreatment with acetaminophen 1 to 2 hours prior to injection seems to ameliorate the febrile response.

Interferon alfa-2a causes reversible toxicoses. These include an up to fivefold induction in liver transaminases, transient neutropenia, and anemia. Neutropenia is ascribed to "margination" not to suppression of bone marrow, and usually it resolves on treatment. None of these effects have required termination of therapy. Most infants on IFN-α2a seem to gain weight and to grow normally, in contrast to infants on prolonged high-dose corticosteroids. In two infants who had accelerated regression of their lesions, loss of appetite required withdrawal of therapy.

In one patient, a treatment failure, a higher dose of 6 MU/m² resulted in hyperactivity for 1 day. This effect resolved the day following the withdrawal of therapy. A more worrisome possible adverse reaction is spastic diplegia [41]. We have observed mild long tract signs in one child. Two other patients developed signs of spastic diplegia but had confounding factors, *eg*, prematurity in one child and spinal venous malformations in the other. We are also aware of two children with similar neurologic symptoms treated at other centers. The signs improved after termination of therapy. We therefore strongly advise careful neurologic and developmental assessment prior to initiation of IFN-α2a therapy. Assessments should be done at least every 3 months during therapy, followed by yearly evaluations.

The "cotton wool" retinal spots have been noted in adults on IFN-α2a therapy [42]. To our knowledge, these retinal signs have not been reported in children on IFN-α2a, nor have they been seen in the children examined in our study.

Current protocol

Infants with destructive, distorting, endangering, or life-threatening hemangiomas are eligible for the IFN-α2a protocol. We first try a 2-week course of corticosteroids at a dosage of 2 to 3 mg/kg a day. If the tumor displays an obvious response, then corticosteroids are continued and gradually tapered off.

There are four indications for interferon treatment of an endangering hemangioma: 1) failure of or equivocal response to corticosteroids, 2) contraindication to several months of corticosteroid therapy, 3) complication of corticosteroid administration, and 4) parental refusal of a corticosteroid trial.

A 2-week tapering off of corticosteroids is begun at or prior to initiation of IFN-α2a therapy. The initial dosage of IFN-α2a is 1 to 2 MU/m². The dosage is gradually increased to 3 MU/m² per day. IFN-α2a can be given during the corticosteroid taper, but we do not recommend coadministration of therapeutic doses of interferon and corticosteroids.

Our current preprotocol evaluation includes complete blood count, liver transaminases, thyroid function tests, urinary bFGF measurements, photography, and radiography, if indicated. All infants have a baseline developmental and neurologic assessment.

The infants are seen every 3 months, if possible; all the tests and examinations are repeated at these intervals. Children are maintained on interferon therapy until the lesion is no longer endangering or life-threatening. If IFN-α2a is discontinued prematurely, there may be rebound growth necessitating reinstitution of the drug. Effective therapy involves several months of subcutaneous injections. We have never seen regrowth of hemangioma after successful completion of IFN-α2a therapy. After the conclusion of IFN-α2a therapy, the children are examined again at 3 months and at yearly intervals.

Conclusions

Interferon alfa, the first cytokine to be produced by recombinant DNA technology, is an important regulator of growth and differentiation [43•]. IFN-α2a treatment of endangering hemangiomas is a paradigm of the antiangiogenesis concept. The precise cellular and molecular mechanisms by which interferon alfa affects angiogenesis are unknown. There are at least nine homologous type 1 interferon genes clustered on the long arm of chromosome 9, which suggests that interference with viral replication is only one of many biologic properties of the "interferon cluster." There is evidence that interferon downregulates production of bFGF [44].

The future holds the possibility for more specific antiangiogenic molecules and other chemotypes for the treatment of hemangiomas. The exponential increase in our knowledge of regulation of angiogenesis points the way to safe, effective pharmacologic agents for control of hemangioma. It must be emphasized that hemangiomas invariably regress, and drugs have potential side effects. Treatment must be reserved for distorting, endangering, or obstructing hemangiomas. The relative advantages and disadvantages of corticosteroids, interferon, and other treatment modalities require large prospective, randomized, interinstitutional clinical trials.

Acknowledgments

The authors thank the following for their valued participation in the IFN-α2a protocol: Dr. Charles Barlow, Dr. Connie Keefer, Dr. Lois Smith, Dr. Patricia Burrows, Dr. Harriet Paltiel, Dotty MacDonald, RN, Terry Law, Susan Connors, and Jennifer Fortin and her colleagues in the General Clinical Research Center. We gratefully acknowledge the support and advice of Dr. Judy Prestofillipo. This work is supported by grants from the National Institutes of Health including a grant in support of the General Clinical Research Center. Dr. Takahashi is a Hoffmann-LaRoche postdoctoral fellow.

References and recommended reading

Papers of particular interest, published within the annual period of review, have been highlighted as:
•   Of special interest
••   Of outstanding interest

1.   Mulliken JB, Young AE: *Vascular Birthmarks: Hemangiomas and Malformations.* Philadelphia: WB Saunders Co.; 1988.

2.   Margileth AM, Museles M: **Cutaneous Hemangiomas in Children: Diagnosis and Conservative Management.** *JAMA* 1965, **194**:523–526.

3.   Robb RM: **Refractive Errors Associated With Hemangiomas of the Eyelids and Orbit in Infancy.** *Am J Ophthalmol* 1977, **83**:52–58.

4.   Berman B, Lim HW-P: **Concurrent Cutaneous and Hepatic Hemangiomata in Infancy: Report of a Case and Review of the Literature.** *J Dermatol Surg Oncol* 1978, **4**:869–873.

5.   Cohen RC, Myers NA: **Diagnosis and Management of Massive Hepatic Hemangiomas in Childhood.** *J Pediatr Surg* 1986, **21**:6–9.

6.   El-Dessouky M, Azmy AF, Raine PAM, Young DG: **Kasabach-Merritt Syndrome.** *J Pediatr Surg* 1980, **23**:109–111.

7. Mulliken JB, Glowacki J: **Hemangiomas and Vascular Malformations of Infants and Children: A Classification Based on Endothelial Characteristics.** *Plast Reconstr Surg* 1982, 69:411–420.

8. Glowacki J, Mulliken JB: **Mast Cells in Hemangiomas and Vascular Malformations.** *Pediatrics* 1982, 70:48–51.

9. Mulliken JB, Zetter BR, Folkman J: **In Vitro Characteristics of Endothelium From Hemangiomas and Vascular Malformations.** *Surgery* 1982, 92:348–353.

10. Burrows PE, Mulliken JB, Fellows KE, Strand RE: **Childhood Hemangiomas and Vascular Malformations: Angiographic Differentiation.** *AJR Am J Roentgenol* 1983, 141:483–488.

11. Huston J III, Forbes GS, Ruefenacht DA, *et al.*: **Magnetic Resonance Imaging of Facial Vascular Anomalies.** *Mayo Clin Proc* 1992, 67:739–747.

12. Meyer JS, Hoffer FA, Barnes PD, Mulliken JB: **MR Correlation of the Biological Classification of Soft Tissue Vascular Anomalies.** *Am J Radiol* 1991, 157:559–564.

13. Takahashi K, Mulliken JB, Kozakewich HPW, Rogers RA, Folkman J,
•• Ezekowitz RAB: **Cellular Markers That Distinguish the Phases of Hemangioma During Infancy and Childhood.** *J Clin Invest* 1994, in press.
Examines immunohistochemical differentiation of vascular malformations from hemangiomas with characterization of the growth phases of hemangiomas.

14. Nguyen M, Watanabe H, Budson AE, Richie JP, Hayes DF, Folkman J: **Elevated Levels of An Angiogenic Peptide, Basic Fibroblast Growth Factor, in the Urine of Patients With a Wide Spectrum of Cancers.** *J Natl Cancer Inst* 1994, 85:356–361.

15. Enjolras, O, Riché MC, Merland JJ, Escanda JP: **Management of Alarming Hemangiomas in Infancy: A Review of 25 Cases.** *Pediatrics* 1990,
•• 85:491–498.
Defines the corticosteroid responsiveness.

16. Hyams, JS, Carey DE: **Corticosteroids and Growth.** *J Pediatr* 1980, 113:249–253.

17. Kushner BJ: **The Treatment of Periorbital Infantile Hemangioma With Intralesional Corticosteroids.** *Plast Reconstr Surg* 1985, 76:517–526.

18. Sloan GM, Reinisch JF, Nichter LS, Saber WL, Lew K, Marwood DT: **Intralesional Corticosteroid Therapy for Infantile Hemangiomas.** *Plast Reconstr Surg* 1989, 83:459–467.

19. Shorr N, Seiff SR: **Central Retinal Artery Occlusion Associated With Periocular Corticosteroid Injection for Juvenile Hemangioma.** *Ophthalmic Surg* 1986, 17:229–231.

20. Ruttum MS, Abrams GW, Harris GJ, Ellis MR: **Bilateral Retinal Embolization Association With Intralesional Corticosteroid Injection for Capillary Hemangioma of Infancy.** *J Pediatr Ophthalmol Strabismus* 1993, 30:4–7.

21. White CW, Sondheimer HM, Crouch EC, Wilson H, Fan LL: **Treatment of Pulmonary Hemangiomatosis With Recombinant Interferon α-2a.** *N Engl J Med* 1989, 320:1197–2000.

22. Orchard, PJ, Smith CM III, Woods WG, Day DL, Dehner LP, Shapiro, R: **Treatment of Hemangioendotheliomas With Alfa Interferon.** *Lancet* 1989, 2:565–567.

23. White CW, Wolf SJ, Korones DN, Sondheimer HM, Tosi MF, Yu A: **Treatment of Childhood Angiomatous Diseases With Recombinant Interferon Alfa-2a.** *J Pediatr* 1991, 118:59–66.

24. Ezekowitz RAB, Mulliken JB, Folkman J: **Interferon Alfa-2a Therapy
•• for Life-Threatening Hemangiomas of Infancy.** *N Engl J Med* 1992, 326:1456–1463. [Published erratum appears in *N Engl J Med* 1994, 330:300.]
A series of 20 infants and children with endangering hemangiomas treated with IFN-α2a.

25. Spiller JC, Sharma V, Woods GM, Hall JC, Seidel FG: **Diffuse Neonatal Hemangiomatosis Treated Successfully With Interferon Alfa-2a.** *J Am Acad Dermatol* 1992, 27:102–104.

26. Blei F, Orlow SJ, Geronemus RG: **Supraumbilical Midabdominal Raphe, Sternal Atresia, and Hemangioma in an Infant: Response of He-**
mangioma to Laser and Interferon Alfa-2a. *Pediatr Dermatol* 1993, 10:71–76.

27. Blei F, Orlow SJ, Geronemus RG: **Interferon Alfa-2a Therapy for Extensive Perianal and Lower Extremity Hemangioma.** *J Am Acad Dermatol* 1993, 23:98–99.

28. Ohlms LA, Jones DT, McGill TJI, Healy GB: **Interferon Alfa-2a Therapy for Airway Hemangiomas.** *Ann Otol Rhinol Laryngol* 1994, 103:1–8.

29. de Castelbajac D, Teillac D, Bodemer C, Brunelle F, Marcombes F, de Prost Y: **Hemangiomé céphalique tubéreux d'Evolution fatale: Inefficacité du Traitment par Interféron alpha.** *Ann Dermatol Venereol* 1990, 117:821–822.

30. Loughnan MS, Elder J, Kemp A: **Treatment of a Massive Orbital Capillary Hemangioma With Interferon Alfa-2b: Short-Term Results.** *Arch Ophthalmol* 1992, 110:1366–1367.

31. Dubois J, Leclerc JBM, Garel L, Filiatrault D, Hershon K, Hamel P:
•• **Radiologic Modifications Induced by Interferon Alfa-2b in Progressive Hemangioma: Clinical and CT Correlation [Abstract].** In *Thirty-sixth Annual Meetng of the American Society for Pediatric Radiology, May 12–15, 1993.* Seattle: American Society for Pediatric Radiology; 1993: abstract 35.
Examines a series of 19 problematic hemangiomas treated with interferon alfa-2b.

32. Teillac-Hamel D, De Prost Y, Bodemer C, Andry P, Enjolras O, Sebag G, Brunelle F, Hubert P, Nihoul-Fekete C: **Serious Childhood Angiomas: Unsuccessful Alpha-2b Interferon Treatment. A report of 4 cases.** *Br J Dermatol* 1993, 129:473–476.

33. Deans RM, Harris GJ, Kivlin JD: **Surgical Dissection of Capillary Hemangiomas: An Alternative to Intralesional Corticosteroids.** *Arch Ophthalmol* 1992, 110:1743–1749.

34. Taylor S, Folkman J: **Protamine Is an Inhibitor of Angiogenesis.** *Nature* 1982, 297:307–312.

35. Sudhalter J, Folkman J, Svahn CM, Bergendal K, D'Amore P: **Importance of Size, Sulfation and Anticoagulant Activity in the Potentiation of Acidic Fibroblast Growth Factor by Heparin.** *J Biol Chem* 1989, 264:6892–6897.

36. Folkman J, Langer R, Linhardt R, Haudenschild C, Taylor S: **Angiogenesis Inhibition and Tumor Regression Caused by Heparin or a Heparin Fragment in the Presence of Cortisone.** *Science* 1983, 221:719–725.

37. Folkman J, Klagsbrun M, Sasse J, Wadzinski M, Ingber DE, Vlodavsky I: **A Heparin-Binding Angiogenic Protein: Basic Fibroblast Growth Factor Is Stored Within Basement Membrane.** *Am J Pathol* 1988, 130:393–400.

38. Niedt GW, Greco MA, Wieczorek R, Blanc WA, Knowles DM II: **Hemangioma With Kaposi's Sarcoma-like Features: Report of Two Cases.** *Pediatr Pathol* 1989, 9:567–575.

39. Tsang, WYW, Chan JKC: **Kaposi-like Infantile Hemangioendothelioma.** *Am J Surg Pathol* 1991, 15:982–989.

40. Zukerberg LR, Nicoloff BJ, Weiss SW: **Kaposiform Hemangioendothelioma of Infancy and Childhood.** *Am J Surg Pathol* 1983, 17:321–328.

41. Vesikari T, Nuutila A, Cantell K: **Neurologic Sequelae Following Interferon Therapy of Juvenile Laryngeal Papilloma.** *Acta Paediatr Scand* 1988, 77:619–22.

42. Guyer DR, Tiedeman J, Yannuzzi LA, Slakter JS, Parke D, Kellay J, Tang RA, Marmor M, Abrams G, Miller JW: **Interferon-Associated Retinopathy.** *Arch Ophthalmol* 1993, 111:350–356.

43. Gutterman JU: **Cytosine Therapeutics: Lessons From Interferon Alfa.**
• *Proc Natl Acad Sci U S A* 1994, 91:1198–1205.
A general review on the therapeutic potential of interferon.

44. Fidler IJ: **Role of the Organ Environment in the Pathogenesis of Cancer Metastasis [Abstract].** *Proc Annu Meet Am Assoc Cancer Res* 1993, 34:570.

R. Alan B. Ezekowitz, MD, DPhil, Division of Hematology and Infectious Diseases, Children's Hospital, Enders Building, 300 Longwood Avenue, Boston, MA 02115, USA.

Kawasaki syndrome

Laurie O. Beitz, MD, and Karyl S. Barron, MD

Children's National Medical Center, Washington, DC, USA

Kawasaki syndrome is an acute systemic vasculitis of childhood. Children are predominantly affected at less than 5 years of age, and coronary artery involvement is responsible for most of the morbidity and mortality of the disease. Since the institution of intravenous γ-globulin in the treatment of the disease, outcome has significantly improved. Although multiple infectious agents and toxins have been implicated in the etiology of the disease, none has been identified. Activation of the immune system is known to occur in the acute stage of the disease, and plays an important role in the pathogenesis of the disease.

Current Opinion in Dermatology 1995:114–122

Kawasaki syndrome is an acute febrile illness of childhood and is the primary cause of acquired heart disease in children in the United States and Japan. Initially described by Dr. Tomisaku Kawasaki in 1967 [1], the syndrome was thought to be a benign, self-limited febrile illness. It is now known to be a systemic vasculitis occurring predominantly in small and medium-sized muscular arteries, especially the coronary vasculature. Specific epidemiologic evidence suggests an infectious etiology, but a causative organism or toxin has not been identified. Morbidity and mortality of the disease are most often due to cardiac sequelae, and treatment is based on prevention of aneurysm formation. Recent investigation is focused on identifying the etiologic agent through examination of immune system aberrations.

Epidemiology

Eighty percent of cases of Kawasaki syndrome occur in children less than 5 years of age. The peak incidence is in children 2 years of age and younger, with boys affected 1.5 times as often as girls. Recurrences occur in 2% to 4% of cases [2,3], and familial incidence is approximately 2% [4]. The population most affected is Asian, with the incidence in the Japanese being highest at approximately 50 to 200 per 100,000 children less than 5 years of age (nonepidemic vs epidemic years) [5]. The incidence in the United States is 5 to 10 cases per 100,000 children [6–8] with Asian Americans being proportionately overrepresented and white Americans underrepresented. Compared with Asians, whites are affected at an older age and have an older distribution of disease [9]. Of note, cases in the United States seem to cluster in the winter and spring [10•], and epi-demics have been reported in the United States, Japan, and other countries.

Mortality rates have been shown to be higher in boys with most deaths occurring in the first 2 months of illness. Nakamura *et al.* [11••] have recently shown that if deaths in the first few months of illness are excluded, the death rate for both boys and girls was not statistically different than the control population. With the institution of therapy with intravenous γ-globulin (IVGG), case fatality has improved from 2% to 0.3% or less [10•].

Clinical features

The clinical features of Kawasaki syndrome mimic many childhood illnesses, and the differential diagnosis includes infections, toxicosis, drug reactions, and connective tissue diseases, as summarized in Table 1 [12]. The principle diagnostic criteria are shown in Table 2 [13] along with other associated manifestations. Five of the six criteria, with fever being an absolute, must be present for diagnosis. "Atypical" cases may be diagnosed with fewer criteria when coronary artery aneurysms are noted by echocardiography or angiography. Figure 1 reveals the typical nonpurulent bulbar conjunctivitis, and oral pharyngeal changes are demonstrated in Figure 2.

Kawasaki syndrome is a systemic illness, and abnormalities have been described in all organ systems. Cardiac abnormalities are numerous and are described in full later in the text. Other vascular abnormalities include aneurysmal dilation of the abdominal aorta, and the superior mesenteric [14•], axillary, subclavian, brachial (Fig. 3, *top*), iliac, renal, and other arteries. Pe-

---

Abbreviations

ICAM-1—intracellular adhesion molecule-1; **IL**—interleukin; **IVGG**—intravenous γ-globulin; **MHC**—major histocompatibility complex; **TNF-α**—tumor necrosis factor-α.

Table 1. Differential diagnosis of Kawasaki syndrome

Infection
  Bacterial
    Streptococcus sp
    Staphylococcus sp
    Proprionibacterium acnes
  Spirochetal
    Leptospira sp
  Rickettsial
    Rocky Mountain spotted fever
  Viral
    Measles
    Adenovirus
    Parainfluenza
    Epstein-Barr virus
    Cytomegalovirus
    Retroviruses
  Fungal
    Candida sp
Toxicosis
  Mercury
Drug reactions
  Antibiotics
  Antifungals
    Griseofulvin
  Anticonvulsants
Connective tissue disease
  Systemic onset juvenile rheumatoid arthritis
  Other vasculitides
Malignancies
  Leukemia
  Lymphomas

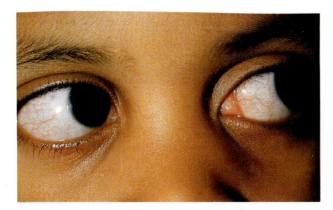

Fig. 1. Bilateral, nonpurulent conjunctival injection is one of the clinical criteria in the diagnosis of Kawasaki syndrome.

ripheral extremity ischemia rarely occurs, but it may result in gangrene of the affected area (Fig. 3, *bottom*). Vasculitis with resultant vessel spasm is thought to be responsible [15••]. Skin involvement is frequently seen early in the disease course and is polymorphous. The typical rash is macular or morbilliform and involves the trunk and extremities (Fig. 4) [13]. Rarely, the rash may be pustular (Fig. 5), but it is neither vesicular nor bullous in nature. A large portion of children will initially develop erythema of the perineum which evolves

into desquamation within 48 hours (Fig. 6). In the first days of disease, there may be brawny induration of the hands and feet, and in the convalescent stage of the disease, characteristic periungual desquamation occurs and may involve the entire hand or foot (Fig. 7). Beau's lines (transverse grooves) of the nails occur several months later as a testament to the acute illness. Central nervous system disease includes aseptic meningitis, facial palsy, subdural effusion, and symptomatic and asymptomatic cerebral infarction [16•]. Pulmonary infiltrates and pleural effusions may be present. Gastrointestinal manifestations include hepatomegaly (which is sometimes associated with jaundice [17]), hydrops of the gallbladder [18], diarrhea, and pancreatitis [19]. Renal manifestations range from sterile pyuria (most likely secondary to urethral inflammation), with or without proteinuria, to acute renal insufficiency with interstitial nephritis proven by biopsy [20]. Ocular findings range from inflammatory, nonpurulent conjunctival injection to anterior uveitis [21]. Sensorineural hearing loss has been reported, albeit in conjunction with aspirin therapy [22]. Uvulitis and supraglottitis have also been described [23].

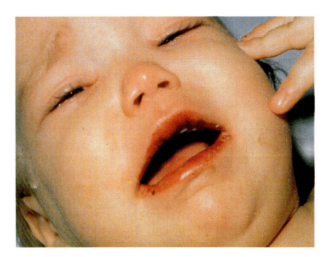

Fig. 2. Classic erythema of the oral mucosa and fissuring of the lips in an infant with Kawasaki syndrome.

Laboratory findings

Early in the course of disease, laboratory evaluation reveals a leukocytosis with a left shift, normochromic normocytic anemia, increased sedimentation rate, increased α_1-antitrypsin (as an acute phase reactant), and depressed albumin. In the subacute stage of the disease, the platelet count increases and frequently reaches the one million range or greater by the 3rd week of illness. Lipid metabolism has been found to be abnormal in the acute stage, with a decrease in high-density lipoprotein cholesterol and total cholesterol. Months later, total cholesterol levels return to normal, but high-density lipoprotein levels may remain depressed for several years [24]. A mild hepatitis is evident by elevated transaminases, and direct bilirubin

Table 2. Characteristics of Kawasaki syndrome*

Principal diagnostic criteria
  Fever lasting more than 5 days
  Conjunctival injection
  Oropharyngeal changes
    Erythema, swelling, and fissuring of the lips
    Diffuse erythema of the oropharynx
    Strawberry tongue
  Peripheral extremity changes
    Erythema of the palms and soles
    Induration of the hands and feet
    Desquamation of the skin of the hands and feet
    Beau's lines
  Polymorphous rash
  Cervical lymphadenopathy, usually a single
    node >1.5 cm
Associated manifestations
  Irritability, mood swings
  Pyuria
  Arthralgia, arthritis
  Abdominal pain, diarrhea
  Aseptic meningitis
  Hepatitis
  Obstructive jaundice
  Hydrops of the gallbladder
  Uveitis
  Cardiovascular changes

*From Barron and Murphy [13]; with permission.

and urobilinogen may be elevated secondary to hydrops of the gallbladder with functional biliary tract obstruction. Urinalysis may show mild proteinuria and sterile pyuria, but creatinine is rarely elevated. Cerebrospinal fluid shows a mononuclear pleocytosis with normal protein and glucose, and joint fluid shows predominantly polymorphonuclear neutrophil leukocytes with 50,000 to 300,000 cells/mm³ [10•]. Other findings associated with aberrant immune regulation include increased levels of serum interleukin (IL)–1 [25], soluble IL-2 receptors [26], IL-6 [27], tumor necrosis factor-α (TNF-α) [28], and interferon gamma [29]. CD4+ T cells are increased, as is the percentage of monocytes/macrophages (compared with the total number of monocytes) and B cells [28,30–32]. A nonspecific hypergammaglobulinemia also occurs. Antineutrophil cytoplasmic antibodies may be present, but they are distinct from those associated with adult vasculitides [33•]. Angiotensin-converting enzyme activity is decreased along with increased levels of von Willebrand factor, indicating endothelial cell damage [34•]. Finally, recent studies show elevation of urine neopterin, which is thought to be a marker of activation of the cellular immune response [35•].

Cardiac disease

Cardiac abnormalities are numerous and varied. Acute stage manifestations include pericardial effusions in approximately 30% of cases. Myocarditis is also common in the acute phase and manifests by frequent tachy-

cardia and gallop rhythm. Congestive heart failure and atrial and ventricular arrhythmias can occur. Electrocardiogram findings include decreased R wave voltage, ST segment depression, and T wave flattening or inversion. Slowed conduction can also occur with PR or QT prolongation [36••]. When valvular involvement occurs it is usually mitral, although aortic valve involvement has been described [37]. Recent evidence suggests mitral regurgitation may be present in approximately 30% of patients, although it is usually mild [38].

Coronary artery lesions are responsible for most of the morbidity and mortality of the disease. They developed in approximately 15% to 25% of patients prior to the widespread use of IVGG, but now occur in less than 10%. Aneurysms usually appear from 1 to 4 weeks after the onset of fever, and it is rare to detect new lesions after 6 weeks (Fig. 8). Aneurysms are most easily detected by transthoracic two-dimensional echocardiography, but other imaging techniques are being evaluated [39,40•,41–43].

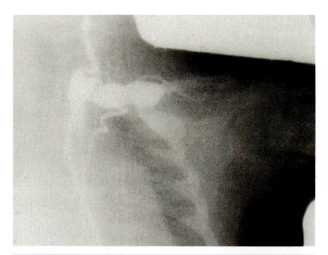

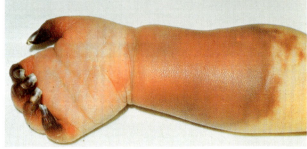

Fig. 3. Top, Aneurysms can occur in arteries other than the coronaries in Kawasaki syndrome. This radiograph shows aneurysms in the subclavian artery. **Bottom**, Vasculitis with probable vasospasm of peripheral arteries in Kawasaki syndrome may lead to compromised perfusion distal to the lesion with consequent ischemic changes, as illustrated in this infant's arm.

Aneurysms are described as small (<4 mm), medium (4 to 8mm), or giant (>8 mm), and are more commonly proximal than distal. Ectasia of the vessels (vessel size larger than age-matched controls) is also a

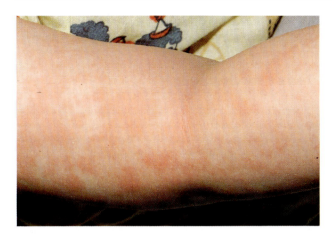

Fig. 4. A polymorphous rash occurs early in patients with Kawasaki syndrome, here consisting of nonpruritic, erythematous plaques.

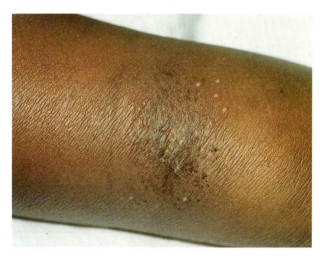

Fig. 5. The skin lesions in Kawasaki syndrome may rarely be pustular.

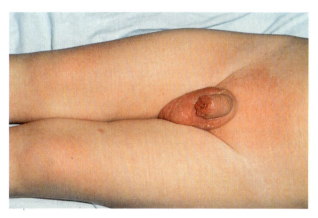

Fig. 6. Perineal erythema is a common finding in Kawasaki syndrome.

common finding. Small and medium-sized aneurysms generally regress radiographically within 5 years of follow-up [44•]; however, these vessels most likely remain abnormal, because response to pharmacologic dilation may remain impaired [45•]. Pathologically regressed aneurysms may reveal abnormal intimal proliferation [46]. Although they are more at risk of developing aneurysms, children with onset at less than 1 year of age and those with saccular or distal lesions generally have the best rate of aneurysm regression [10•]. Therapy with IVGG has decreased the incidence of giant aneurysms [44•], which rarely regress and frequently develop complicating thromboses, stenosis, or total occlusion. Myocardial infarction may result; when it occurs, it is most likely to be in the 1st year, with 40% occurring in the first 3 months of illness [47]. There are, however, case reports of young adults suffering myocardial infarctions over a decade after their initial dis-

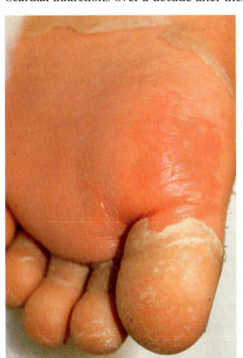

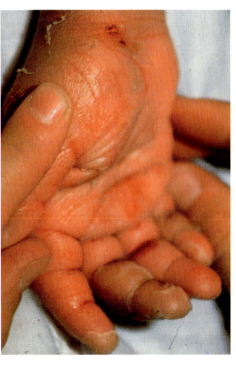

Fig. 7. Periungual desquamation frequently occurs in the convalescent stage of Kawasaki syndrome, and may involve the palm of the hand or the sole of the foot.

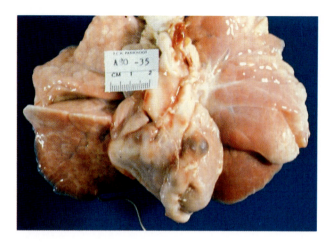

Fig. 8. Coronary artery aneurysms in a pathologic specimen from a child with Kawasaki syndrome.

ease [48,49], and others with coronary artery aneurysms who were not known to have had Kawasaki syndrome as children [50•,51].

Treatment and long-term follow-up

Treatment in the acute phase of the disease is aimed at limiting inflammation. Treatment with IVGG in various regimens has been shown to significantly reduce the incidence of coronary artery aneurysm formation, as well abate the fever and reduce myocardial inflammation [52•,53,54]. In the United States, the standard of care is 2 g/kg IVGG as a single infusion [55]. This regimen decreases the cost of hospitalization as compared with the regimen of 400 mg/kg per day for 4 days. Aspirin is given concurrently at a dosage of 80 to 100 mg/kg/d orally until the fever has subsided; the dosage is then changed to 3 to 5 mg/kg/d, which is sufficient for the antiplatelet effect. If the fever persists, a second dose of IVGG at 1 g/kg may result in defervescence, although it is unknown whether retreatment prevents the development of coronary artery lesions [56••].

The duration, frequency, and best imaging methods for long-term follow-up are still a matter of debate. Of greatest concern are those children with initial coronary artery aneurysms, because thrombosis or segmental stenosis may occur in the chronic phase of disease. The American Heart Association has recently recommended guidelines for long-term follow-up, as summarized in Table 3 [57••]. Children with multiple aneurysms, giant aneurysms, or known coronary artery obstruction require close follow-up and possible long-term anticoagulation therapy. Stress testing in the adolescent years is important, especially in those patients with a history of coronary artery involvement, because abnormalities may require limitations in physical activity and may indicate the need for angiography to assess the degree of coronary artery stenosis or obstruction.

Finally, children with Kawasaki syndrome should not receive live virus vaccines (eg, measles-mumps-rubella) for 11 months after treatment with IVGG, be-

cause the preparation may contain neutralizing antibodies, thus preventing the proper immune response.

Disease mechanisms

Although the etiologic agent of the disease remains a mystery, epidemiologic data indicate that there may be an infectious cause. Many organisms and toxins have been reported as possible agents in the disease and include *Staphylococcus* species, *Streptococcus* species, *Candida* species, *Rickettsia* species, retroviruses, Epstein-Barr virus, and others [58]. Enterotoxins and exotoxins of staphylococci and streptococci have recently been identified from cultures, predominantly of the rectum and oral pharynx, in a small cohort of children with Kawasaki syndrome. It is speculated that the toxins may be acting as superantigens in the disease process, but these findings remain to be confirmed [59••]. Infection with Epstein-Barr virus has also been implicated as the etiologic agent in Kawasaki syndrome, and the viral genome has been identified in renal cells of a child with interstitial nephritis [60] and in the aorta and cardiac tissues of three children [61] all with Kawasaki-like coronary aneurysms. Viruslike particles with reverse transcriptase activity [62], extracellular products of oral *Streptococcus viridans* strains [63], and antibodies to heat shock protein 65 [64] have all been described in children with Kawasaki syndrome. Finally, the role of *Streptococcus pyogenes* has again been questioned [65]. Unfortunately, none of these hypotheses has been proven as yet.

Kawasaki syndrome has a high incidence in the Japanese as well as a disproportionately high attack rate among Japanese Americans. For this reason, a number of investigators have searched for evidence of genetic susceptibility. Whereas some reports suggest a major histocompatibility class association with susceptibility to Kawasaki syndrome [66,67], others have failed to find a significant association [68,69•,70].

Although we have yet to determine the initiating factor, immune activation may play a major role in Kawasaki syndrome pathogenesis. Acute phase leukocytosis is accompanied by increased numbers of circulating helper T cells, increased monocytes and macrophages, and polyclonal activation of B cells [28,30–32]. Serum levels of soluble IL-2 receptors are increased (most significantly in those who develop aneurysms), indicating lymphocyte activation [26], and HLA-DR–positive T cells have been found in skin biopsy specimens, suggesting possible sequestration of activated T cells [71]. As a consequence of activation of the cellular immune system, the levels of various cytokines are increased in the acute phase serum, including IL-1 [25], TNF-α [28], interferon gamma [29], IL-6 [27], and IL-8 [72]. Increased levels of IL-6 and IL-8 in the first week of illness have been shown to be associated with increased risk of coronary artery aneurysms [72]. Cytokines have also been detected in skin lesions of patients in the acute phase of disease, again suggesting that they play a role in the inflammatory process in the skin of Kawasaki syndrome patients [73•].

Table 3. Guidelines of the American Heart Association for the long-term follow-up of patients with Kawasaki syndrome*

Risk level	Pharmacologic therapy	Physical activity	Follow-up and diagnostic testing	Invasive testing
I (No coronary artery changes at any stage of illness)	None beyond initial 6 to 8 weeks	No restrictions beyond 6 to 8 weeks	None beyond 1st year unless cardiac disease suspected	None recommended
II (Transient coronary artery ectasia that disappears during acute illness)	None beyond initial 6 to 8 weeks	No restrictions beyond initial 6 to 8 weeks	None beyond 1st year unless cardiac disease suspected Physician may choose to see patient at 3- to 5-year intervals	None recommended
III (Small to medium solitary coronary artery aneurysm)	3 to 5 mg/kg/d aspirin at least until abnormalities resolve	For patients in 1st decade of life, no restriction beyond initial 6 to 8 weeks	Annual follow-up with echocardiogram ± electro-cardiogram in 1st decade of life	Angiography, if stress testing or echocardio-graphy suggests stenosis
IV (One or more giant coronary artery aneurysms, or multiple small to medium aneurysms, without obstruction)	Long-term aspirin (3 to 5 mg/kg/d) ± warfarin	For patients in 2nd decade, physical activity guided by stress testing every other year Competitive contact athletics with endurance training discouraged For patients in 1st decade of life, no restriction beyond initial 6 to 8 weeks For patients in 2nd decade, annual stress testing guides recommendations Strenuous athletics are strongly discouraged If stress test rules out ischemia, noncontact recreational sports allowed	Annual follow-up with echocardiogram ± electrocardiogram ± chest radiogram ± additional electrocardiogram at 6-month intervals For patients in 1st decade of life, pharmacologic stress testing should be considered	Angiography, if stress testing or echocardiography suggests stenosis Effective catheterization may be done in certain circumstances
V (Coronary artery obstruction)	Long-term aspirin (3 to 5 mg/kg/day) ± warfarin Use of calcium channel blockers should be considered to reduce myocardial oxygen consumption	Contact sports, isometrics, and weight training should be avoided Other physical activity recommendations guided by outcome of stress testing or myocardial perfusion scan	Echocardiogram and electrocardiogram at 6-month intervals and annual Holter and stress testing	Angiography recommended for some patients to aid in selecting therapeutic options Repeat angiography with new-onset or worsening ischemia

*From Dajani *et al.* [57••]; with permission.

The pathologic consequences of immune system activation in Kawasaki syndrome are well described, consisting primarily of findings one would expect from a vasculitis that affects small and medium-sized blood vessels. Skin biopsies from children in the acute stage of Kawasaki syndrome are characterized by extensive edema in the papillary dermis with marked dilation of the capillaries. Neutrophil emigration is slight, and the predominant cellular infiltrate is mononuclear [74]. Immunohistochemical findings show that the infiltrating mononuclear cells are predominantly monocytes/macrophages and CD4+ T cells. HLA-DR is expressed on the epidermal keratinocyte surface and on the walls of small blood vessels and the infiltrating cells around them [73•]. Major histocompatibility complex (MHC) class II antigens have also been described on coronary artery endothelium in Kawasaki syndrome patients but not in control subjects [75]. Furthermore, circulating antibodies cytotoxic toward both resting and cytokine-pretreated vascular endothelial cells are seen in the acute phase of the disease [76–78]. Interferon gamma induces MHC class II antigen expression on endothelial cells, increases IL-1 and IL-6 production by endothelial cells, and increases intracellular adhe-

sion molecule-1 (ICAM-1) on endothelial cells. ICAM-1 is involved in the adhesion of polymorphonuclear neutrophil leukocytes, monocytes and lymphocytes to endothelial cells by interaction with leukocyte cell surface molecules [75]. Finally, in the acute stage of Kawasaki syndrome, increased serum levels of soluble ICAM-1 have been described, with the highest levels found in patients who subsequently develop coronary artery lesions [79••].

In summary, it is hypothesized that Kawasaki syndrome is due to immune system activation, probably initiated by a toxin or infectious agent. In response to the offending agent, activated T cells, monocytes, and macrophages secrete a variety of cytokines, which are thought to mediate the clinical features of the disease (*eg*, fever, rash, and inflammatory changes). In the acute phase of the disease, cytokine stimulation results in B-cell proliferation and induces vascular endothelial cells to express class II MHC antigens. The induction of ICAM-1 by IL-1, TNF-α, and interferon gamma leads to the influx of more inflammatory cells, potentiating the vascular damage seen in the acute phase of the disease. This inflammatory process may then result in eventual aneurysm formation. Therapy with IVGG may act in a number of ways to abate the inflammatory response, including neutralizing an infectious agent or toxin, providing negative feedback to B cells secreting immune globulin, preventing platelet adhesion to vascular wall endothelium, and inducing an anticytokine effect [80].

Conclusions

In conclusion, Kawasaki syndrome is an immunologically mediated diffuse vasculitis of childhood with generally self-limited clinical features. Morbidity and mortality are primarily due to cardiovascular complications, and current therapy with aspirin and IVGG has significantly improved the long-term morbidity of affected children. Although immune system activation occurs in the acute stage of the disease, the initiating factor is yet to be identified.

References and recommended reading

Papers of particular interest, published within the annual period of review, have been highlighted as:
- Of special interest
- • Of outstanding interest

1. Kawasaki T: **Acute Febrile Mucocutaneous Lymph Node Syndrome, With Accompanying Specific Peeling of the Fingers and the Toes [in Japanese].** *Allergy* 1967, 16:178–222.

2. Mason W, Takahashi M, Schneider T: **Recurrence of Kawasaki Disease in a Large Urban Cohort in the United States.** In *Proceedings of the Fourth International Symposium on Kawasaki Disease.* Edited by Takahashi M, Taubert K. Dallas: American Heart Association; 1993:21–26.

3. Yanagawa H, Nakamura Y, Yashiro M, Fujita Y, Nagai M, Kawasaki T, Aso S, Imada Y, Shigematsu I: **A Nationwide Incidence Survey of Kawasaki Disease in 1985-1986 in Japan.** *J Infect Dis* 1988, 158:1296–1301.

4. Fujita Y, Nakamura Y, Sakata J, Hara N, Kobayashi M, Nagai M, Yanagawa H, Kawasaki T: **Kawasaki Disease in Families.** *Pediatrics* 1989, 84:666–669.

5. Yanagawa H: **Epidemiological Picture of Kawasaki Disease in Japan.** In *Proceedings of the Fourth International Symposium on Kawasaki Disease.* Edited by Takahashi M, Taubert K. Dallas: American Heart Association; 1993:1–5.

6. Shulman S, McAuley J, Pachman L, Miller M, Ruschhaupt D: **Risk of Coronary Abnormalities Due to Kawasaki Disease in Urban Area With Small Asian Population.** *Am J Dis Child* 1987, 141:420–425.

7. Rauch A, Kaplan S, Nihill M, Pappas P, Hurwitz E, Schonberger L: **Kawasaki Syndrome Clusters in Harris County, Texas, and Eastern North Carolina: A High Endemic Rate and a New Environmental Risk Factor.** *Am J Dis Child* 1988, 142:441–444.

8. Taubert K, Rowley A, Shulman S: **Nationwide Survey of Kawasaki Disease and Acute Rheumatic Fever.** *J Pediatr* 1991, 119:279–282.

9. Lu C, Lee W, Hwang K, Salo E: **Kawasaki Disease in Finland in 1982-1992.** *Scand J Infect Dis* 1993, 25:497–502.

10. Sundel R, Newburger J: **Kawasaki Disease and Its Cardiac Sequelae.**
- *Hosp Pract (Off Ed)* 1993, 28:51–66.
This is a good review of the clinical disease, laboratory findings, therapy, and outcome of Kawasaki disease. The authors touch on possible pathophysiology and etiology of the disease.

11. Nakamura Y, Yanagawa H, Kawasaki T: **Mortality Among Children**
- • **With Kawasaki Disease in Japan.** *N Engl J Med* 1992, 326:1246–1249.
The investigators asked whether patients with Kawasaki disease had a higher death rate than age-matched healthy control subjects. This was a multicenter trial with 4608 Kawasaki patients enrolled. The authors found mortality among boys with Kawasaki syndrome was twice that of control subjects, with most of the deaths occurring in the first 2 months of the illness. If the first 2 months were excluded from analysis, there was no statistically significant difference found in mortality.

12. Amita D, Danon Y, Garty B: **Kawasaki-like Syndrome Associated With Griseofulvin Treatment.** *Clin Exp Dermatol* 1993, 18:389–392.

13. Barron K, Murphy D: **Kawasaki Syndrome: Still a Fascinating Enigma.** *Hosp Pract (Off Ed)* 1989, 13:51–60.

14. Nemoto S, Toyoda S, Katayama A, Sakuma S, Hamada R: **Ultrasono-**
- **graphic Evaluation of Abdominal Vessels in Kawasaki Disease.** *Acta Paediatr Jpn* 1993, 35:68–71.
The authors describe 21 patients on whom serial coronary and abdominal ultrasonography was performed. They report two patients with abdominal vessel abnormalities—one with aortic and superior mesenteric aneurysms and one with superior mesenteric artery disease. Presence of these lesions did not correlate with severity of coronary disease.

15. Tomita S, Chung K, Mas M, Gidding S, Shulman S: **Peripheral**
- • • **Gangrene Associated With Kawasaki Disease.** *Clin Infect Dis* 1992, 14:121–126.
Eleven cases of peripheral gangrene are discussed in this paper. This is a very rare finding in Kawasaki syndrome, but is responsible for a significant morbidity due to amputation. Only one Japanese child had been described with this complication. Treatment strategies are described.

16. Fujiwara S, Yamano T, Hattori M, Fujiseki Y, Shimada M: **Asymp-**
- **tomatic Cerebral Infarction in Kawasaki Disease.** *Pediatr Neurol* 1992, 8:235–236.
The authors discuss the case of a child with Kawasaki syndrome and asymptomatic cerebral infarction. They recommend the use of routine radiologic screening for any child with vascular abnormalities and also discuss other neurologic complications described in Kawasaki syndrome.

17. Bader-Meunier B, Hadchouel M, Fabre M, Arnoud MD, Dommergues JP: **Intra-hepatic Bile Duct Damage in Children With Kawasaki Disease.** *J Pediatr* 1992, 120:750–752.

18. Falcini F, Trapani S, Pampaloni A, Ienuso R, Pollini I, Bartolozzi G: **Hydrops of Gallbladder Requiring Cholecystomy in Kawasaki Syndrome.** *Clin Exp Rheumatol* 1993, 11:99–100.

19. Lanting W, Mulnos W, Kamani N: **Pancreatitis Heralding Kawasaki Disease.** *J Pediatr* 1992, 121:743–744.

20. Veiga P, Pieroni D, Maier W, Field L: **Association of Kawasaki Disease and Interstitial Nephritis.** *Pediatr Nephrol* 1992, 6:421–423.

21. Germaine B, Moroney J, Guggino G, Cimino L, Rodriquez C, Bocanegra T: **Anterior Uveitis in Kawasaki Disease.** *J Pediatr* 1980, 97:780–781.

22. Sundel R, Cleveland S, Beiser A, Newburger J, McGill T, Baker A, Koren G, Novak R, Harris J, Burns J: **Audiologic Profiles of Children With Kawasaki Disease.** *Am J Otol* 1992, 13:512–515.

23. Kazi A, Gauthier M, Lebel M, Farrell C, Lacroix J: **Uvulitis and Supraglottitis: Early Manifestations of Kawasaki Disease.** *J Pediatr* 1992, 120:564–567.

24. Newburger J, Burns J, Beriser A, Loscalzo J: **Altered Lipid Profile After Kawasaki Syndrome.** *Circulation* 1991, 84:625–631.

25. Maury C, Salo E, Pelkonen P: **Circulating Interleukin-1 Beta in Patients With Kawasaki Disease [Letter].** *N Engl J Med* 1988, 319:1670–1671.

26. Barron K, Montalvo J, Joseph A, Hilario M, Saadeh C, Giannini E, Orson F: **Soluble Interleukin-2 Receptors in Children With Kawasaki Disease.** *Arthritis Rheum* 1990, 33:1371–1377.

27. Ueno Y, Takano N, Kanehane H, Yokoi T, Yachie A, Miyawaki T, Taniguchi N: **The Acute Phase Nature of Interleukin-6: Studies in Kawasaki Disease and Other Febrile Illness.** *Clin Exp Immunol* 1989, 76:337–342.

28. Furukawa S, Matsubara T, Jujoh K, Yone K, Sagomara T, Sasai K, Kato H, Yabuta K: **Peripheral Blood Monocyte/Macrophage and Serum Necrosis Factor in Kawasaki Disease.** *Clin Immunol Immunopathol* 1988, 48:247–251.

29. Rowley A, Shulman S, Preble O, Poiesz B, Ehrlich G, Sullivan J: **Serum Interferon Concentrations and Retroviral Serology in Kawasaki Syndrome.** *Pediatr Infect Dis J* 1988, 7:663–665.

30. Leung D, Siegel R, Grady S, Krensky R, Meade R, Reinherz E, Geha R: **Immunoregulatory Abnormalities in Mucocutaneous Lymph Node Syndrome.** *Clin Immunol Immunopathol* 1982, 23:100–112.

31. Leung D, Chu E, Wood N, Grady S, Krensky A, Meade R, Geha R: **Immunoregulatory T Cell Abnormalities in Mucocutaneous Lymph Node Syndrome.** *J Immunol* 1983, 130:2002–2004.

32. Barron K: **Immune Abnormalities in Kawasaki Disease: Prognostic Implications and Insight Into Pathogenesis.** *Cardiol Young* 1991, 1:206–211.

33. Kaneko K, Shah G, Gaskin G, Pusey C, Dillon M: **Kawasaki Disease**
- **Has Distinct Antineutrophil Cytoplasmic Antibodies.** In *Proceedings of the Fourth International Symposium on Kawasaki Disease.* Edited

by Takahashi M, Taubert K. Dallas: American Heart Association; 1993:192–197.

This is the first report of antineutrophil cytoplasmic antibody in Kawasaki syndrome. Fifteen samples from 14 patients with Kawasaki syndrome were studied. All had a positive weak diffuse staining by acid extraction, and six had positive cytoplasmic antineutrophil cytoplasmic antobodies as well. The specificity of these antibodies has not yet been defined.

34. Matucci-Cernic M, Jaffa A, Kahaleh B: **Angiotensin Converting Enzyme: An In Vivo and In Vitro Marker of Endothelial Injury.** *J Lab Clin Med* 1992, 120:428–433.

Plasma from seven children in the acute stage of Kawasaki syndrome was studied. Von Willebrand factor and angiotensin-converting enzyme levels were measured; the former increased and the latter decreased. Endothelial cells produce both proteins, and the authors propose from *in vitro* studies with human umbilical vein endothelial cells that activation of endothelial cells leads to increases in angiotensin-converting enzyme levels, whereas injury leads to a decrease. Von Willebrand factor is not differentially produced; increased values are seen with activation as well as injury.

35. Iizuka T, Minatogawa Y, Suzuki H, Itoh M, Nakamine S, Hatanake Y, Uemura S, Koike M: **Urinary Neopterin as a Predictive Marker of Coronary Artery Abnormalities in Kawasaki Syndrome.** *Clin Chem* 1993, 39:600–604.

These authors studied urinary neopterin in 29 Kawasaki syndrome patients and 174 control subjects. They found that in the acute stage of disease, children with Kawasaki had urine neopterin levels 2 SD greater than that of control subjects. Sixty-three percent of patients with levels greater than 5000 μM per mole creatinine developed coronary artery dilation, compared with 23% with levels less than 5000 μM. The authors hypothesize that increased neopterin concentrations may be secondary to activation of monocytes/macrophages, and that the correlation with fever may be indicative of high concentrations of circulating cytokines.

36. Dajani A, Taubert K, Gerber M, Shulman S, Ferrieri P, Freed M, Takahashi M, Bierman F, Karchmer A, Wilson W, *et al.*: **Diagnosis and Therapy of Kawasaki Disease in Children.** *Circulation* 1993, 87:1776–1780.

This is an excellent overview of the diagnostic features and clinical and laboratory findings of Kawasaki disease. Particular attention is paid to the principal cardiac findings and sequelae of the disease, as well as on acute management.

37. Nakano H, Nojima K, Saito A, Ueda K: **High Incidence of Aortic Regurgitation Following Kawasaki Disease.** *J Pediatr* 1985, 107:59–63.

38. Usami H, Ryo S, Harada K, Okuni M: **Mitral Regurgitation in the Acute Phase of Kawasaki Disease.** In *Proceedings of the Fourth International Symposium on Kawasaki Disease.* Edited by Takahashi M, Taubert K. Dallas: American Heart Association; 1993:370–373.

39. Schwartz S, Gillam L, Weintraub A, Sanzobrino B, Hirst J, Hsu T, Fisher J, Marx G, Fulton D, McKay R, Pandian W: **Intracardiac Echocardiography in Humans Using a Small-Sized (6F), Low Frequency (12.5MHz) Ultrasound Catheter.** *J Am Coll Cardiol* 1993, 21:189–198.

40. Sugimura T, Kato H, Inoue O, Fukuda T, Sato N, Ishii M, Takagi J, Akagi T, Moeno Y, Kawano T, *et al.*: **Intravascular Ultrasound of Coronary Arteries in Children: Assessment of the Wall Morphology and the Lumen After Kawasaki Disease.** *Circulation* 1994, 89:258–265.

Angiography is used extensively in evaluation of coronary artery aneurysms. This study tried to determine the degree of intimal proliferation in regressed aneurysms appearing normal by angiography, those regressed but still with slight angiographic abnormalities, and those continuing. Regressed aneurysms with visible abnormalities had intimal proliferation, whereas those no longer visible showed mild thickening at most. Walls of current unhealed aneurysms showed no thickening.

41. Ishikawa S, Takamoto S, Nozaki Y, Iwasaki A, Kim YW, Okuyama K, Kawauchi A: **Evaluation of Coronary Artery Aneurysm in Children With Kawasaki Disease: Transesophageal Doppler Color Flow Mapping.** In *Proceedings of the Fourth International Symposium on Kawasaki Disease.* Edited by Takahashi M, Taubert K. Dallas: American Heart Association; 1993:402–403.

42. Kuroe K, Kohata T, Ono Y, Echigo S, Kamiya T, Naitoh H, Takamiya M: **Myocardial and Coronary Arterial Imagings on Ultrafast Computed Tomography in Patients With a History of Kawasaki Disease.** In *Proceedings of the Fourth International Symposium on Kawasaki Disease.* Edited by Takahashi M, Taubert K. Dallas: American Heart Association; 1993:270–277.

43. Uemura S, Yoshida S, Suzuki H, Negoro H, Minami Y, Koike M: **Evaluation of the Coronary Arterial Lesions With Kawasaki Disease by Magnetic Resonance Imaging.** In *Proceedings of the Fourth International Symposium on Kawasaki Disease.* Edited by Takahashi M, Taubert K. Dallas: American Heart Association; 1993:284–289.

44. Akagi T, Rose V, Benson L, Newman A, Freedom R: **Outcome of Coronary Artery Aneurysms After Kawasaki Disease.** *J Pediatr* 1992, 121:689–694.

The authors describe 583 children who had Kawasaki disease from 1974 to 1991. This group found that greater than 80% of small or moderate-sized aneurysms regressed in 5 years, but giant aneurysms did not. The regression of an aneurysm was related to the initial patient treatment, the size of the aneurysm, and the gender of the patient.

45. Sugimura T, Kato H, Inoue O, Takagi J, Fukuda T, Sato N: **Vasodilatory Response of the Coronary Arteries After Kawasaki Disease: Evaluation by Intracoronary Injection of Isosorbide Dinitrate.** *J Pediatr* 1992, 121:684–688.

These authors found that despite regression of coronary artery aneurysms, those patients who had been followed up for more than 5 years showed statistically poorer distensibility with isosorbide injection than those patients who had Kawasaki syndrome and never experienced coronary artery lesions. These findings functionally confirm pathohistologic data showing abnormal vessels after regression of aneurysms (*see* Sasaguri and Kato: *J Pediatr* 1982, 100:225–231.)

46. Sasaguri Y, Kato H: **Regression of Aneurysms in Kawasaki Disease: A Pathologic Study.** *J Pediatr* 1982, 100:225–231.

47. Kato H, Ichinose E, Kawasaki T: **Myocardial Infarction in Kawasaki Disease: Clinical Analyses in 195 Cases.** *J Pediatr* 1986, 108:923–927.

48. Kodama K, Okayama H, Tamura A, Suetsugu M, Honda T, Doiuchi J, Hamada N, Nomoto R, Akamatsu A, Jo T: **Kawasaki Disease Complicated by Acute Myocardial Infarction Due to Thrombotic Occlusion of Coronary Aneurysms 19 Years After Onset.** *Intern Med* 1992, 31:774–777.

49. Kato H, Inoue O, Kawasaki T, Fujiwara H, Watanabe T, Toshima H: **Adult Coronary Artery Disease Probably due to Childhood Kawasaki Disease.** *Lancet* 1992, 340:1127–1129.

50. Shaukat N, Syed A, Mebewu A, Freemont A, Keenan D: **Myocardial Infarction in a Young Adult due to Kawasaki Disease: A Case Report and Review of the Late Cardiological Sequelae of Kawasaki Disease.** *Int J Cardiol* 1993, 39:222–226.

The case of a 24-year-old man with fatal myocardial infarction due to thrombotic occlusion of multiple aneurysms is described. There was no previous history of Kawasaki syndrome. Also described are methods used to assess myocardial ischemia, management issues of obstructive or stenotic lesions, and coronary artery bypass outcomes.

51. Smith B, Grider D: **Sudden Death in a Young Adult: Sequelae of Childhood Kawasaki Disease.** *Am J Emerg Med* 1993, 11:381–383.

52. Kao C, Hsieh K, Wang Y, Chen C, Liao S, Wan S, Yeh S: **Tc-99m HMPAO Imaging to Detect Carditis and to Evaluate the Results of High Dose Gamma Globulin Treatment in Kawasaki Disease.** *Clin Nucl Med* 1992, 17:623–626.

The authors study cardiac uptake of traced white blood cells. In the early stages of disease, uptake is increased, consistent with active carditis. After IVGG treatment, this uptake is significantly reduced in approximately 40%, giving credence to the role of IVGG in abating the acute inflammatory response.

53. Barron K, Murphy D, Silverman E, Rattenberg H, Wright G, Franklin W, Goldberg S, Higashino S, Cox D, Lee M: **Treatment of Kawasaki Syndrome: A Comparison of Two Dosage Regimes of Intravenous Immune Globulin.** *J Pediatr* 1990, 117:638–644.

54. Newburger J, Takahashi M, Burns J, Beiser A, Chung K, Duffy E, Glode M, Mason W, Reddy V, Sonders S, *et al.*: **The Treatment of Kawasaki Syndrome With Intravenous Gamma Globulin.** *N Engl J Med* 1986, 315:341–347.

55. Newburger J, Takahashi M, Beiser A, Burns J, Bastian J, Chung K, Colan S, Duffy E, Fulton O, Glode M, *et al.*: **A Single Infusion of Gamma Globulin as Compared With Four Infusions in the Treatment of Kawasaki Syndrome.** *N Engl J Med* 1991, 324:1633–1639.

56. Sundel R, Burns J, Baler A, Beiser A, Newburger J: **Gamma Globulin Retreatment in Kawasaki Disease.** *J Pediatr* 1993, 123:657–659.

This is a retrospective analysis of the use of a second and in some instances third dose of IVGG in children with continued fever and signs of inflammation in Kawasaki syndrome. This was a limited study of 13 patients, with 10 initially defervescing after the second dose; the fever recurred in one patient after 5 days. Third-dose treatment resulted in prompt response. A third dose was given to the three patients who did not respond to the second; one child responded. Larger prospective trials with long-term follow-up are needed.

57. Dajani A Tauber K, Takahashi M, Bierman F, Freed M, Ferrieri P, Gerber M, Shulman S, Karchmer A, Wilson W, *et al.*: **Guidelines for Long-Term Management of Patients With Kawasaki Disease.** *Circulation* 1994, 89:916–922.

This document outlines current recommendations for long-term follow-up of patients with Kawasaki syndrome from the Committee on Rheumatic Fever, Endocarditis, and Kawasaki Disease, Council on Cardiovascular Disease in the Young, American Heart Association. Specifically addressed are the need for long term anticoagulation, frequency of cardiac catheterization, and recommendations on physical activity.

58. Barron K: **Kawasaki Disease: Epidemiology, Late Prognosis, and Therapy.** *Rheum Dis Clin North Am* 1991, 17:907–919.

59. Leung D, Meissner H, Fulton D, Murray D, Kotzin B, Schlievert
•• P: **Toxic Shock Syndrome Toxin-Secreting Staphylococcus aureus in Kawasaki Syndrome.** *Lancet* 1993, 342:1385–1388.
This paper describes the isolation of toxic shock syndrome toxin secreting *Staphylococcus aureus* in 11 of 16 children, and pyrogenic exotoxin secreting *Streptococcus* (streptococcal pyrogenic exotoxin B and C) from two of 16 patients with acute Kawasaki syndrome. Staphylococcal isolates were unusual in that they were white, and could easily be mistaken for coagulase-negative staphylococcus. The authors speculate that these toxins may be acting as superantigens in the pathogenesis of the disease, especially in light of the recent evidence for selective expansion of T cells expressing Vβ2 and Vβ8 T-cell receptors in patients with Kawasaki syndrome.

60. Muso E, Fujiwara H, Yoshida R, Hosokawa R, Yashiro M, Hongo Y, Matumiya T, Yamabe H, Kikuta H, Hironaka T, Hirai K, Kawai C: **Epstein-Barr Virus Genome-Positive Tubulointerstitial Nephritis Associated With Kawasaki Disease-like Coronary Aneurysms.** *Clin Nephrol* 1993, 40:7–15.

61. Kikuta H, Sakiyama Y, Matsumoto S, Hamada I, Yazaki M, Iwaki T, Nakano M: **Detection of Epstein-Barr Virus DNA in Cardiac and Aortic Tissues From Chronic, Active Epstein-Barr Virus Infection Associated With Kawasaki Disease-like Coronary Aneurysms Artery.** *J Pediatr* 1993, 123:90–92.

62. Lin CY, Chen IC, Cheng TI, Liu WT, Hwang B, Chiang B: **Virus-Like Particles With Reverse Transcriptase Activity Associated With Kawasaki Disease.** *J Med Virol* 1992, 38:175–182.

63. Takada H, Kawabata Y, Tamura M, Matsushita K, Igarashi H, Ohkuni H, Todome Y, Uchiyama T, Kotani S: **Cytokine Induction by Extracellular Products of Oral Viridans Group Streptococci.** *Infect Immun* 1993, 61:5252–5260.

64. Yokota S, Tsubaki K, Kuriyama T, Shimizu H, Ibe M, Mitsuda Y, Aihara Y, Kosug K, Nomaguchi H: **Presence in Kawasaki Disease of Antibodies of Mycobacterial Heat-Shock Protein HSP65 and Autoantibodies to Epitopes of Human HSP65 Cognate Antigen.** *Clin Immunol Immunopathol* 1993, 67:163–170.

65. Akiyama T, Yashiro K: **Probable Role of Streptococcus Pyogenes in Kawasaki Disease.** *Eur J Pediatr* 1993, 152:82–92.

66. Barron K, Silverman E, Gonzales J, St. Clair M, Anderson K, Reveille J: **Major Histocompatibility Complex Class II Alleles in Kawasaki Syndrome: Lack of Consistent Correlation With Disease or Cardiac Involvement.** *J Rheumatol* 1992, 19:1790–1793.

67. Kato S, Kumira M, Tsuji K, Kusakawa S, Asai T, Juji T, Kawasaki T: **HLA Antigens in Kawasaki Disease.** *Pediatrics* 1978, 61:252–255.

68. Fildes N, Burns J, Newburger J, Klitz W, Begovich B: **The HLA Class II Region and Susceptibility to Kawasaki Disease.** *Tissue Antigens* 1992, 39:99–101.

69. Chang C, Hawkins B, Kao H, Chow C, Lau Y: **Human Leukocyte**
• **Antigens in Southern Chinese With Kawasaki Disease.** *Eur J Pediatr* 1992, 151:866–868.
The authors of this paper briefly discuss their findings that no HLA associations exist in Southern Chinese patients. They also discuss previous HLA findings and include a very good reference list.

70. Iwasa M, Sahashi N, Kamura H, Ando T: **Association of Kawasaki Disease With Human Lymphocyte Antigen.** In *Proceedings of the Fourth International Symposium on Kawasaki Disease.* Edited by Takahashi M, Taubert K. Dallas: American Heart Association; 1993:217–218.

71. Furukawa S, Matsubara T, Obara T, Okumura K, Yabuta K: **Soluble CD2 Levels in Serum During Acute Kawasaki Disease and Infectious Mononucleosis.** *J Infect Dis* 1993, 67:778–779.

72. Lin CY, Lin CC, Hwang B, Chiang B: **Cytokines Predict Coronary Artery Aneurysm Formation in Kawasaki Disease Patients.** *Eur J Pediatr* 1993, 152:309–312.

73. Sato N, Sagawa K, Sasaguri Y, Inoue O, Kato H: **Immunopathol-**
• **ogy and Cytokine Detection in the Skin Lesions of Patients With Kawasaki Disease.** *J Pediatr* 1993, 122:198–203.
Skin specimens of 10 patients with Kawasaki disease were studied. Most of the cellular infiltrate was CD4+ T lymphocytes and CD13+ macrophages. IL-1 and TNF-α were strongly positive in skin lesions in the acute phase, whereas IL-2 and interferon gamma were weakly detected. No cytokines were detected in the convalescent stage of the disease. The authors suggest cell activation with cytokine secretion may be involved in the pathogenesis of the disease.

74. Hirose S, Hamashima Y: **Morphologic Observations on the Vasculitis in the Mucocutaneous Lymph Node Syndrome: A Skin Biopsy Study of 27 Patients.** *Eur J Pediatr* 1978, 129:17–27.

75. Leung D: **Immunologic Aspects of Kawasaki Syndrome.** *J Rheumatol* 1990, 17[Suppl 24]:15–18.

76. Leung D, Collins T, Lapierre L, Geha R, Pober J: **Immunoglobulin M Antibodies Present in the Acute Phase of Kawasaki Syndrome Lyse Cultured Vascular Endothelial Cells Stimulated by Gamma Interferon.** *J Clin Invest* 1986, 77:1428–1435.

77. Leung D, Geha R, Newburger J, Burns J, Fiers W, LaPierre L, Pober J: **Two Monokines, Interleukin 1 and Tumor Necrosis Factor, Render Cultured Vascular Endothelial Cells Susceptible to Lysis by Antibodies Circulating During Kawasaki Syndrome.** *J Exp Med* 1986, 164:1958–1972.

78. Kaneko K, Savage C, Pottinger B, Shah V, Pearson J, Dillon M: **Cytotoxic Antiendothelial Cell Antibodies in Kawasaki Disease can be Detected by Two Different Methods: A Cellular Based ELISA and Cytotoxicity Studies.** In *Proceedings of the Fourth International Symposium on Kawasaki Disease.* Edited by Takahashi M, Taubert K. Dallas: American Heart Association; 1993:185–191.

79. Furukawa S, Matsubara T, Yabuta K: **Immunological Parameters in**
•• **Determining the Severity of Vascular Damage During Acute Kawasaki Disease.** In *Proceedings of the Fourth International Symposium on Kawasaki Disease.* Edited by Takahashi M, Taubert K. Dallas: American Heart Association; 1993:149–154.
This is a good overview of immune dysregulation in Kawasaki syndrome. Discussion focuses on changes in peripheral blood cells, soluble antigens, cytokines, and adhesion molecules.

80. Barron K, Sher M, Silverman E: **Intravenous Immunoglobulin Therapy: Magic or Black Magic.** *J Rheumatol* 1992, 19(suppl 33):94–97.

Karyl S. Barron, MD, Children's National Medical Center, Department of Rheumatology, 111 Michigan Avenue NW, Washington, DC 20010, USA.

Disorders of the skin in HIV-infected children

Margarita Silio, MD, and Russell B. Van Dyke, MD

Tulane University School of Medicine, New Orleans, Louisiana, USA

The prevalence of HIV infection in children is rising at an alarming rate. Dermatologic manifestations seen in HIV-infected children are usually the same as those seen in immunocompetent children, but they tend to be severe and difficult to treat. This review discusses diagnosis and current treatment guidelines for these infections as well as for less common skin conditions seen only in immunocompromised patients.

Current Opinion in Dermatology 1995:123–128

As of September 1993, nearly 5000 cases of AIDS had been reported in children less than 13 years old in the United States. The actual number of HIV-infected children is estimated to be three to five times higher and increasing rapidly as the number of HIV-infected women also increases. Perinatal transmission now accounts for nearly all new infections in children [1]. Mucocutaneous and cutaneous infections are very common in HIV-infected children, and these infections are frequently of increased severity and recalcitrant to therapy. Dermatologic manifestations may lead to the initial consideration of HIV infection, and familiarity with these manifestations will facilitate the early diagnosis and treatment of these children.

Fungal infections of the skin

Candida

Oral candidiasis is the most common mucocutaneous disease in HIV-infected children. Oral thrush is common in healthy newborns and usually responds rapidly to oral therapy with nystatin. In HIV-infected children, however, thrush is often recurrent and resistant to topical antifungal treatment (Fig. 1). If oral thrush is seen in infants older than 6 months, particularly in those not receiving antibiotic therapy, immunodeficiency states including HIV infection should be considered. Typical lesions are white plaques covering the oropharyngeal mucosa, with friable underlying mucosa. Punctuate mucosal erythema, diffuse mucosal erythema, and angular cheilitis may be present. If dysphagia or substernal pain is present, esophageal candidiasis should be considered.

Candidiasis lesions can also be seen in the neck folds (Fig. 2), diaper area, and nails. Candidal diaper dermatitis presents as an erythematous plaque with satellite lesions (Fig. 3). If diaper dermatitis is resistant to therapy, a biopsy should be considered to establish the presence of herpes simplex virus or cytomegalovirus [2].

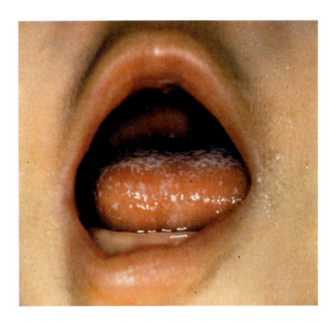

Fig. 1. Recurrent oral candidiasis in a 3-month-old child with HIV infection. (*Courtesy of* J. Junprasert, New Orleans, LA.)

Initial therapy of oral thrush consists of oral nystatin or clotrimazole troches. As the child's immune status worsens, the lesions tend to be recurrent and resistant to conventional therapy. Ketoconazole (5 to 10 mg/kg per day orally) and fluconazole (10 mg/kg oral loading dose, then 5 mg/kg per day) have been shown to be effective. There is a propensity for relapse unless suppressive therapy with topical antifungal agents is used. If there is no response to initial therapy, a scraping or biopsy should be performed to rule out coinfections with cytomegalovirus or herpes simplex virus.

For esophageal candidiasis, ketoconazole or fluconazole is administered until there is a resolution of symptoms. Chronic maintenance therapy with either nystatin or clotrimazole may be considered. As with oral lesions, a biopsy for cytomegalovirus and herpes simplex should be performed if there is no response to initial

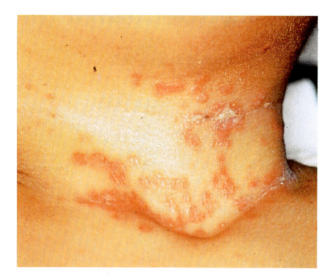

Fig. 2. Candidiasis in the neck folds of a 1-year-old HIV-infected child. (*Courtesy of* J. Junprasert, New Orleans, LA.)

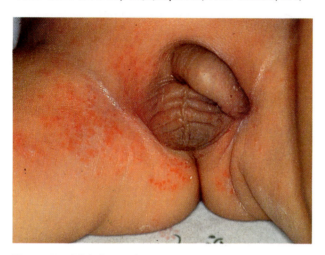

Fig. 3. Candidal diaper dermatitis in a 1-year-old child with AIDS. (*Courtesy of* J. Junprasert, New Orleans, LA.)

antifungal therapy [3]. Some isolates of *Candida krusei* and *Torulopsis glabrata* are resistant to fluconazole and require amphotericin B therapy. Diaper dermatitis requires frequent diaper changes to prevent maceration as well as treatment with a topical antifungal cream, such as nystatin, clotrimazole, or miconazole.

Dermatophytes

Cell-mediated immunity plays an important role in resistance to dermatophytes. HIV-infected patients and others with depressed cell-mediated immunity have an increased susceptibility to dermatophyte infections that are often of increased severity [4]. Children commonly present with tinea capitis (Fig. 4), tinea corporis, or onychomycosis.

Tinea capitis is treated with griseofulvin (15 to 20 mg/kg per day) for 4 to 6 weeks. Tinea corporis, often caused by *Trichophyton rubrum*, may not respond to topical imidazole creams when infection is widespread, and systemic therapy may be required. Infections of the

nail (Fig. 5) and paronychia are treated with systemic griseofulvin or ketoconazole, but recurrences are common [5].

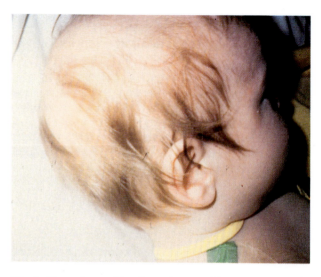

Fig. 4. Alopecia resulting from tinea capitis in an 18-month-old child with AIDS. (*Courtesy of* W. K. Galen, New Orleans, LA.)

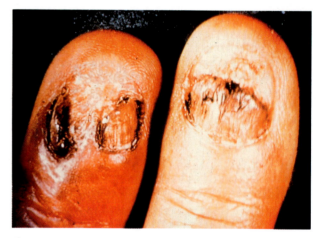

Fig. 5. Tinea unguium in an HIV-infected patient. (*Courtesy of* D. Greer, New Orleans, LA.)

Penicillium marneffei

Penicillium marneffei is a dimorphic saprophyte endemic to Southeast Asia that causes systemic infections. Over half of the reported cases are in HIV-infected adults and children [6,7]. The clinical manifestations are nonspecific: fever, weight loss, anemia, hepatomegaly, adenopathy, pulmonary infiltrates, and skin lesions. The skin lesions can present as pustules, papules, or nodules (Fig. 6). Mucosal ulcers and papules are seen as well. Diagnosis is made by examination of biopsy specimens or culture. The fungus is found intercellularly in histiocytes and appears as yeastlike oval and rectangular forms but reproduces by transverse septation (Fig. 7). They measure 1 to 3 μm in diameter and can easily be confused with *Histoplasmosis capsulatum* in tissue. This disease should be suspected in patients who have either migrated from Southeast Asia or traveled there in the recent past. Therapy has been successful with 2 to 8 weeks of amphotericin B, or 2 months of itraconazole or ketoconazole. Maintenance therapy may be required.

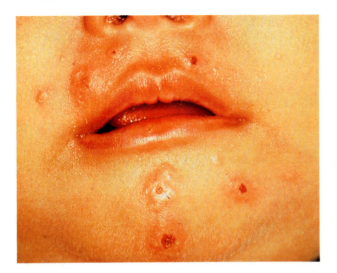

Fig. 6. Skin lesions in a 10-month-old child with AIDS diagnosed as *Penicillium marneffei* infection. The infant had disseminated fungal infection involving liver, spleen, and bone. (*From* Sirisanthana and Sirisanthana [7]; with permission.)

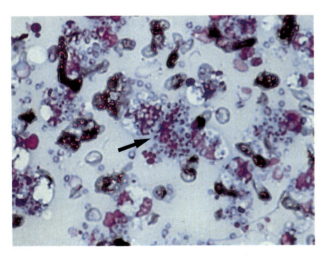

Fig. 7. Wright stain of a skin lesion positive for *Penicillium marneffei* (arrow). (*From* Sirisanthana and Sirisanthana [7]; with permission.)

Herpesvirus infections

Varicella-zoster virus

Varicella in HIV-infected children may have a prolonged course with persistent fever and continued eruption of new lesions for more than 2 weeks (Fig. 8). Patients with low CD4 counts may have an extremely large number of skin lesions ($>400/m^2$). Visceral dissemination to the lungs, liver, and central ner-

vous system can occur. In mild cases, oral acyclovir will shorten the course of the infection (20 mg/kg four times a day); severe disease requires intravenous acyclovir (500 mg/m^2 every 8 hours). HIV-infected children who are susceptible to varicella should receive varicella-zoster immune globulin within 72 hours of exposure to an infected child.

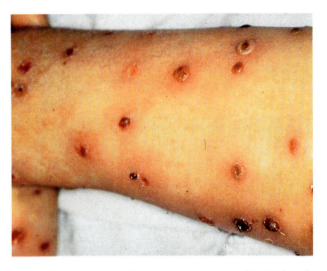

Fig. 8. Extensive varicella-zoster in a 1-year-old child with end-stage AIDS. (*Courtesy of* J. Junprasert, New Orleans, LA.)

The appearance of herpes zoster in a child less than 1 year of age with no history of varicella should raise the clinical suspicion of HIV infection (Fig. 9). HIV-infected children may have persistent lesion formation intermittently for months despite antiviral therapy. Chronic zoster lesions are initially varicelliform but eventually develop into deep, non-healing ulcers that become necrotic and crusted [8]. Chronic hyperkeratosis has also been described [9•]. These lesions may be difficult to recognize, and they need to be examined in biopsy to rule out other causes. Testing of varicella-zoster virus isolate for resistance to acyclovir should be performed if lesions recur or fail to heal with appropriate therapy.

Zoster is usually treated with oral acyclovir (20 mg/kg every 4 hours). Severe or disseminated disease should be treated with high-dose intravenous acyclovir (500 mg/m^2 every 8 hours) for 7 to 10 days. Long-term suppressive oral therapy may occasionally be required for recurrent disease. The management of chronic varicella ulcers can be complicated by poor bioavailability or oral acyclovir or emergence of varicella-zoster strains resistant to acyclovir. Foscarnet has been used successfully to treat infections with acyclovir-resistant strains of the virus [10•].

Herpes simplex virus

As in immunocompetent children, the primary lesion in HIV-infected children is usually gingivostomatitis, but the infection may be more severe. Other mani-

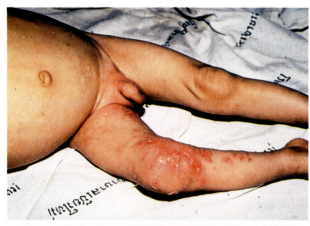

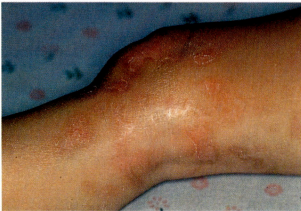

Fig. 9. Top, Herpes zoster in a 1-year-old child with end-stage AIDS. **Bottom,** Scarred healed lesions in the same child. (*Courtesy of* J. Junprasert, New Orleans, LA.)

festations consist of perineal ulcerations and herpetic whitlow. Treatment with intravenous acyclovir (250 mg/m² every 8 hours) or oral acyclovir (250 mg/m² every 6 hours) results in prompt healing. Strains of herpes simplex virus that fail to respond to acyclovir are increasingly being recognized in HIV-infected individuals. Infections with acyclovir-resistant virus will respond to intravenous foscarnet (40 mg/kg every 8 hours). Other drugs are currently under investigation for the treatment of acyclovir-resistant herpes simplex virus [10•].

Human papillomavirus

Human papillomavirus infections have four common clinical presentations: verruca vulgaris (common wart), verruca plana juvenilis (flat wart [Fig. 10]), verruca plantaris (plantar wart), and condyloma acuminatum (anogenital wart). In HIV-infected individuals, the lesions are often widespread. Human papillomavirus elicits both a cellular and humoral immune response [11]. The defective immune response in HIV-infected individuals may predispose them to frequent human papillomavirus infections that are difficult to treat [12]. In these difficult cases, multiple intralesional injections of interferon alfa may be effective, but recurrences are frequent [13]. Condyloma acuminatum in a child should raise the possibility of sexual abuse.

Molluscum contagiosum

Molluscum is a common cutaneous viral infection caused by a DNA poxvirus. The lesions are pearly, dome-shaped papules with central umbilication. In the normal host, the papules vary in size from 1 to 5 mm. The usual sites of involvement in children are the trunk, face, and extremities. In the HIV-infected child, the lesions tend to be numerous and unusually large. If the number of lesions is small, treatment consists of removal of each lesion with a sharp curette. In widespread disease, the application of tretinoin cream, 10% benzoyl peroxide, salicylic acid, or liquid nitrogen has been suggested [14].

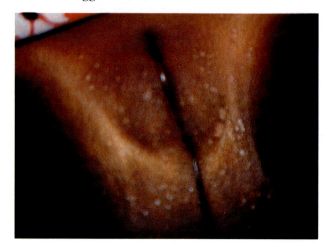

Fig. 10. Verruca plana (flat warts) in the perineum of a 2-year-old child infected with HIV. (*Courtesy of* L. Harrington, New Orleans, LA.)

Bacterial infections

HIV-infected children have an increased frequency of common bacterial infections, presumably resulting in part from defective antibody production. *Staphylococcus aureus* is the organism that most commonly causes skin infections, which present as impetigo, ecthyma, cellulitis, or persistent folliculitis [15]. *Pseudomonas aeruginosa* is an uncommon cause of bacteremia, but HIV-infected children are at increased risk for disseminated disease [16]. In a review of five HIV-infected children with life-threatening pseudomonal infections, four of the five presented with cutaneous manifestations [17].

The etiologic agents implicated in bacillary angiomatosis are *Rochalaca henselae* and *Rochalimaea quintana* [18]. The infection is most common in adults with advanced AIDS and CD4 counts of less than 200 cells/mm³. The skin lesions are purplish-red papules that increase in size and number over time, becoming nodular in consistency. Lesions may resemble pyogenic granulomas. The differential diagnosis is extensive and includes Kaposi sarcoma; definitive diagnosis requires a biopsy [19]. Treatment consists of oral erythromycin for a minimum of 4 weeks. Bacillary angiomatosis has not yet been reported in an HIV-infected child, but it has been described in an adolescent undergoing chemotherapy [20].

Hypersensitivity reactions

Trimethoprim-sulfamethoxazole is commonly administered to HIV-infected individuals for the prevention of *Pneumocystis carinii* pneumonia. Eruptions in reaction to trimethoprim-sulfamethoxazole are extremely common in this population, occurring in 40% to 80% of HIV-infected adults and at least 15% of infected children. The most common reaction is a simple morbilliform rash, but fatal Stevens-Johnson syndrome has been reported [21•]. Toxic epidermal necrolysis is a rare disease with an increased incidence in HIV-infected individuals [22]. A recent review of this disease in France reported an increasing number of patients who were HIV-infected. The most common offending drug was a sulfonamide.

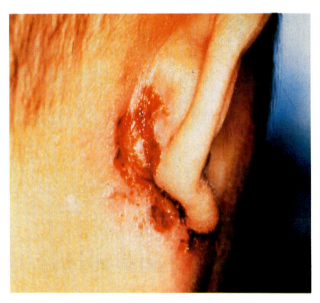

Fig. 11. Postauricular seborrheic dermatitis in a 2-year-old child with AIDS. She also presented with thrombocytopenia. (*Courtesy of* J. Junprasert, New Orleans, LA.)

Amithiozone, an inexpensive antituberculosis medication in use outside of the United States, has been implicated in causing adverse skin reactions in African children [23]. The majority of the affected children were HIV-infected. The cutaneous lesions are extensive and maculopapular in nature. Half of the children with skin manifestations developed Stevens-Johnson syndrome and died.

Inflammatory and infectious skin conditions

Seborrheic dermatitis is a common inflammatory skin disorder in the pediatric age group. In normal infants, it presents as a diffuse or local scaling and crusting of the scalp ("cradle cap"). The adult form of seborrheic

dermatitis is distinctly unusual in children, but it may present in those with HIV infection. It appears as dry, scaly erythematous dermatitis of the nasolabial folds, glabella, and postauricular areas (Fig. 11) [15].

Scabies is a common disease in children; although in HIV infection, infestation of the *Sarcoptes scabiei* mite usually results in a severe, generalized papular eruption. Norwegian scabies has been described in children with AIDS [24]. The lesions are hyperkeratotic crusted plaques primarily on the face, scalp and trunk. This form of scabies is highly contagious, because the child harbors thousands of mites. Treatment consists of a single overnight application of permethrin cream. Recurrences are common.

Acne rosacea has been described in HIV-positive adult patients with low CD4 counts [25]. The cutaneous manifestations developed after HIV-seroconversion.

Granulomatous rosacea has been described in an HIV-infected child [26]. The child presented with an erythematous papular and papulopustular eruption on her cheeks. A biopsy revealed tuberculoid granulomas and *Demodex* mites. Therapy with isoniazid and rifampin resulted in no improvement. When a second biopsy again revealed the mites, which are usually considered part of the normal flora of the face, a course of oral erythromycin resulted in clinical improvement. Two studies by Dominey *et al.* [27,28] confirmed the role of this ectoparasite as an etiologic agent.

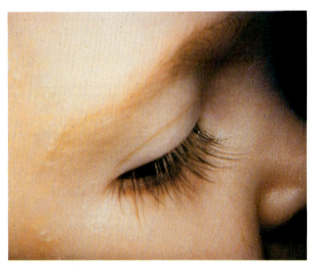

Fig. 12. Elongated eyelashes in an 18-month-old child with AIDS. (*Courtesy of* W. K. Galen, New Orleans, LA.)

Kaposi sarcoma

Kaposi sarcoma is common in adults with AIDS, but rare in children; only 33 cases have been reported in children. Orlow *et al.* [29•] observed that children with predominant lymph node involvement of Kaposi sarcoma had been infected perinatally. In contrast, children who were infected postnatally presented with the typical skin manifestations seen in adults.

Acquired trichomegaly

Elongation of eyelashes has been reported in both adults and children with AIDS (Fig. 12). Sadick [30] found that six of 500 HIV-infected individuals had acquired trichomegaly. These patients had advanced disease, with severe depletion of CD4 counts, high levels of p24 antigenemia, and intolerance to zidovudine (AZT). Regression of trichomegaly occurred when alternate antiretroviral agents were administered.

Conclusions

The cutaneous diseases seen in HIV-infected children are similar to those of immunocompetent children, but they often have more dramatic presentations and may be more resistant to treatment. Many, including oral candidiasis in children over 6 months of age, recurrent oral candidiasis, and herpes zoster, should prompt an investigation for HIV. Because of aggressive treatment of HIV-related diseases, HIV-infected children are surviving longer. It can be expected that many of the skin manifestations seen in adults will become more common in HIV-infected children.

References and recommended reading

Papers of particular interest, published within the annual period of review, have been highlighted as:
•   Of special interest
••   Of outstanding interest

1. Centers for Disease Control and Prevention: *HIV/AIDS Surveillance Report* Oct. 1993, **5**(3).

2. Thiboutot DM, Beckford A, Mart CR, Sexton M, Maloney ME: **Cytomegalovirus Diaper Dermatitis.** *Arch Dermatol* 1991, **127**:396–398.

3. Indacochea F, Scott G: **Recent Advances in the Management of the HIV-Infected Infant.** *AIDS* 1990, **4**:S227–S234.

4. Jones HE, Reinhardt JH, Rinaldi MG: **Immunologic Susceptibility to Chronic Dermatophytosis.** *Arch Dermatol* 1974, **110**:213–220.

5. Zalla MJ, Daniel Su WP, Fransway AF: **Subject Review: Dermatologic Manifestations of Human Immunodeficiency Virus Infection.** *Mayo Clin Proc* 1992, **67**:1089–2208.

6. Hilmarsdottir I, Meynard JL, Rogeaux O, Guermonprez G, Datry A, Katlama C, Brucker G, Coutellier A, Danis M, Gentilini M: **Disseminated Penicillium Marneffei Infection Associated With Human Immunodeficiency Virus: A Report of Two Cases and a Review of 35 Published Cases.** *J Acquir Immune Defic Syndr* 1993, **6**:466–471.

7. Sirisanthana V, Sirisanthana T: **Penicillium Marneffei Infection in Children Infected With Human Immunodeficiency Virus.** *Pediatr Infect Dis J* 1993, **12**:1021–1025.

8. Leibovitz E, Kaul A, Rigaud M, Bebenroth D, Krasinski K, Borkowsky W: **Chronic Varicella Zoster in a Child Infected With Human Immunodeficiency Virus: Case Report and Review of the Literature.** *Cutis* 1992, **49**:27–31.

9. Grossman MC, Grossman ME: **Chronic Hyperkeratotic Herpes Zoster**
•   **and Human Immunodeficiency Virus Infection.** *J Am Acad Dermatol* 1993, **28**:306–308.
Case report and discussion of unusual presentations of herpes zoster commonly seen in HIV-infected children.

10. Balfour HH, Benson C, Braun J, Cassens B, Erice A, Friedman-Kien
•   A, Klein T, Polsky B, Safrin S: **Management of Acyclovir-Resistant Herpes Simplex and Varicella-Zoster Virus Infections.** *J Acquir Immune Defic Syndr* 1994, **7**:254–260.

A round-table symposium concerning management of acyclovir-resistant herpes simplex virus and varicella-zoster virus infection. Algorithms were developed concerning the management of these lesions.

11. Bender ME, Ostrow RS, Watts S, Zachow K, Faras A, Pass F: **Immunology of Human Papillomavirus: Warts.** *Pediatr Dermatol* 1983, **2**:121–126.

12. Morison WL: **Viral Warts, Herpes Simplex, and Herpes Zoster in Patients With Secondary Immune Deficiencies and Neoplasms.** *Br J Dermatol* 1975, **92**:625–630.

13. Vance JC, Bart BJ, Hansen RC, Reichman RC, McEwen C, Hatch KD, Berman B, Tanner DJ: **Intralesional Recombinant Alpha-2 Interferon for the Treatment of Patients With Condyloma Acuminatum or Verruca Plantaris.** *Arch Dermatol* 1986, **122**:272–277.

14. Prose NS: **Skin Diseases in Infancy and Childhood.** In *Color Atlas of Pediatric Dermatology*, edn 2. Edited by Weinberg S, Prose NS. New York: McGraw-Hill; 1990:535–546.

15. Prose NS: **HIV Infections in Children.** *J Am Acad Dermatol* 1990, **22**:1223–1231.

16. Roilides E, Butler KM, Husson RN, Mueller BU, Lewis LL, Pizzo PA: **Pseudomonas Infections in Children With Human Immunodeficiency Virus Infection.** *Pediatr Infect Dis J* 1992, **11**:547–553.

17. Flores G, Stavola JJ, Noel GJ: **Bacteremia Due to Pseudomonas Aeruginosa in Children With Aids.** *Clin Infect Dis* 1993, **16**:706–708.

18. Birtles RJ, Harrison TG, Taylor AG: **Cat Scratch Disease and Bacillary Angiomatosis: Aetiological Agents and the Link With AIDS.** *Commun Dis Rep CDR Rev* 1993, **3**:R107–R110.

19. Spach DH: **Review: Bacillary Angiomatosis.** *Int J Dermatol* 1992, **31**:19–24.

20. Myers SA, Prose NS, Garcia JA, Wilson KH, Dunsmore KP, Kamino H: **Bacillary Angiomatosis in a Child Undergoing Chemotherapy.** *J Pediatr* 1992, **121**:574–578.

21. Chanock SJ, Luginbuhl LM, McIntosh K, Lipshultz SE: **Life-Threaten-**
•   **ing Reaction to Trimethoprim/Sulfamethoxazole in Pediatric Human Immunodeficiency Virus Infection.** *Pediatrics* 1994, **93**:519–520.
This article reports on the rare occurrence of life-threatening reactions to trimethoprim-sulfamethoxazole in two HIV-infected children. Rechallenge of trimethoprim-sulfamethoxazole after a skin rash should be avoided if at all possible.

22. Correia O, Chosidow O, Saiag PH, Bastuji-Garin S, Revuz J, Roujeau JC: **Evolving Pattern of Drug-Induced Toxic Epidermal Necrolysis.** *Dermatology* 1993, **186**:32–37.

23. Chinto C, Luo C, Bhat G, Raviglione M, DuPont H, Zumla A: **Cutaneous Hypersensitivity Reactions Due to Thiacetazone in the Treatment of Tuberculosis in Zambian Children Infected With HIV-I.** *Arch Dis Child* 1993, **68**:665–668.

24. Jucowics P, Ramon ME, Don PC, Stone RK, Bamji M: **Norwegian Scabies in an Infant With Acquired Immunodeficiency Syndrome.** *Arch Dermatol* 1989, **125**:1670–1671.

25. Vin-Christian K, Maurer TA, Berger TG: **Acne Rosacea as a Cutaneous Manifestation of HIV Infection.** *J Am Acad Dermatol* 1994, **30**:139–140.

26. Sanchez-Viera M, Hernanz JM, Sampelayo T, Gurbindo MD, Lecona M, Soto-Melo J: **Granulomatous Rosacea in a Child Infected With the Human Immunodeficiency Virus.** *J Am Acad Dermatol* 1992, **27**:1010–1011.

27. Dominey A, Tschen J, Rosen T, Batres E, Stern JK: **Pityriasis Folliculorum Revisited.** *J Am Acad Dermatol* 1989, **21**:81–84.

28. Dominey A, Rosen T, Tschen J: **Papulonodular Demodicidosis Associated With Acquired Immunodeficiency Syndrome.** *J Am Acad Dermatol* 1989, **20**:197–201.

29. Orlow SJ, Cooper D, Petrea S, Kamino H, Popescu V, Lawrence R,
•   Leibovitz E: **AIDS-Associated Kaposi's Sarcoma in Romanian Children.** *J Am Acad Dermatol* 1993, **28**:449–453.
This article reviews all the reported cases of AIDS-associated Kaposi sarcoma in children and discusses the different clinical manifestations of each. The authors contend that Kaposi sarcoma is caused by a secondary infectious agent in HIV-infected patients.

30. Sadick N: **Clinical and Laboratory Evaluation of AIDS Trichopathy.** *Int J Dermatol* 1993, **32**:33–38.

Margarita Silio, MD, and Russell B. Van Dyke, MD, Section of Pediatric Infectious Diseases, Department of Pediatrics, Tulane University School of Medicine, 1430 Tulane Avenue, New Orleans, LA 70131, USA.

Surgery

Edited by

Duane C. Whitaker
University of Iowa College of Medicine
Iowa City, Iowa, USA

CURRENT SCIENCE

Developments and techniques in general dermatologic surgery

Eckart Haneke, MD

Kliniken der Universität Witten-Herdecke and Lehrkrankenhaus
der Universität Düsseldorf, Wuppertal, Germany

Dermatologic surgery has become a major portion of dermatologists' daily workload. Attention must therefore be paid to postoperative wound care and to new dressing materials that have been made available to dermatologists. New suture and knotting techniques further enhance the functional and aesthetic results in dermatologic surgery. Some experimental techniques offer possibilities for enhancing flap viability. A new technique called dermatography can be used to color-match distant flaps and grafts in exposed areas.

Current Opinion in Dermatology 1995:129–136

Surgical treatment modalities once performed by only a few dermatologists in the United States have become more and more popular. A recent analysis of the most frequently cited clinical dermatology articles revealed that dermatologic surgery is now an integral and respected part of dermatology. The *Journal of Dermatologic Surgery and Oncology* ranks as the seventh most cited clinical dermatology journal, with an immediacy index in 1990 of 0.167 (rank 5), an impact factor of 1.61 (rank 5), and a scope-adjusted impact factor of 5.978 (rank 2). A 1991 commercial survey noted that 88% of all dermatologists read an average issue of the *Journal of Dermatologic Surgery and Oncology* (whereas 90% read the *Archives of Dermatology*; 92%, the *Journal of the American Academy of Dermatology*; and 24%, *Journal of Investigative Dermatology* [1•].

The importance of surgical treatment in dermatology in other countries has been documented by a survey comparing the number of surgical operations performed in Germany, Austria, and the German-speaking part of Switzerland in 1984 and 1991. Dermatologic surgery, which is defined as surgical treatment of the epidermis, dermis, and subcutaneous tissue, with all of their structures included, as well as of the mucous membranes adjacent to the skin, is aimed at treating benign and malignant neoplasms, congenital and acquired cutaneous malformations, and cicatricial and inflammatory sequelae of skin diseases. It also includes surgical phlebology and proctology and aesthetic skin surgery. Dermatologic departments performed 58% more surgical operations in 1991 than in 1984, with more dramatic increases in medium-sized and large operations: 60.6% and 173%, respectively. Dermatologists in private practice performed more skin excisions with primary reconstruction than surgeons (per capita, 76% more) [2].

Wound care after office procedures

Whereas preoperative planning and surgical performance receive much attention, postoperative wound care, wound dressing, and advice on how to behave after surgery are often treated as being of lesser importance. However, postoperative care may be as important as the surgical procedure itself and should therefore not be neglected. An explosion of research in this field is not necessarily made known to dermatologic surgeons, who are frequently confronted with new materials and techniques by representatives of manufacturing companies [3••].

It is essential to differentiate between wound types, both between partial-thickness, full-thickness, subdermal, and sutured wounds and between sterile, contaminated, and infected wounds. Partial-thickness wounds are produced by excoriations, curettage, shave excisions, dermabrasion, chemical peel, and laser abrasion. They heal rapidly because reepithelialization takes place from the wound edges and the remaining deep portions of the adnexal structures.

The more superficial a wound, the more rapidly it heals. In cosmetic procedures such as dermabrasions and chemical peels, scarring is usually absent. The same results should be sought for after shave excisions; I have found, however, that hemostatic solutions such as Monsel's, which are in fact caustic, significantly prolong wound healing and increase scarring. Although they are very convenient for hemostasis of shave ex-

Abbreviations
CGRP—calcitonin gene–related peptide; **PDS**—polydioxanone suture.

© 1995 Current Science ISBN 1-85922-686-8 ISSN 1068–381X

cision wounds, these solutions are no longer used after shave excisions of seborrheic keratoses, actinic keratoses, and so on. Instead, nonadherent gauze impregnated with antibiotic ointment and a thick pad of gauze to absorb the blood are used for a pressure dressing, which is replaced after 24 hours with just a small piece of tape. Hemostasis is improved by the patient's exerting a gentle, even pressure for approximately 10 minutes. To maintain a moist wound environment, an ointment is put on the wound at least twice a day. There is usually no need to apply antimicrobial antiseptic agents to the wound: their use often delays healing by preventing or slowing reepithelialization, increasing inflammation and tissue necrosis, and inducing endothelial damage and thrombosis [4•]. The amount of devitalized tissue, which is also influenced by the use of toxic topical agents, is critical, permitting bacteria of the local microbial flora to grow and eventually to cause an infection. Patients may take their daily shower before replacing an antibiotic ointment and a sterile adhesive bandage, for instance a Band-Aid (Johnson & Johnson, New Brunswick, NJ). Large partial-thickness wounds, such as split-thickness skin graft donor sites, should be covered with one of the various proprietary semipermeable dressings, preferably a translucent one that allows wound inspection. Any collection of serous exudate may be drawn by sterile puncture, as one would puncture a large, tense bulla. A mesh version of siliconized synthetic dressing that sticks gently to the surrounding skin but not to the wound allows blood and serum to ooze through, and an absorbent layer of gauze can be changed as often as necessary.

Large wound areas profit considerably from the use of semiocclusive dressings, by a 50% reduction in healing time [5]. However, a recent study of 50 shave biopsy sites did not show a significant difference between conventional therapy (bacitracin ointment plus a sterile adhesive bandage) and the use of a hydroactive semipermeable or semiocclusive dressing (Cutinova Hydro; Beiersdorf, Norwalk, CT); it must be taken into account that the authors used Monsel's solution or aluminum chloride hexahydrate solution (Drysol; Person & Covey, Glendale, CA) for hemostasis and that they are caustic because of the oxidative potency of ferric chloride. The hydroactive dressing did not cause discomfort on removal, a feature often observed with conventional ointment and an adhesive dressing. Semiocclusive dressings were more convenient and saved time in dressing changes. The number of dressing changes per week was 2.1 for semiocclusive dressings and 10.3 for conventional dressings [6•].

In recent years, many different new synthetic dressing materials have been developed [7]. It is usually not possible for the individual dermatologist to achieve enough experience with all products; therefore, each dermatologist should limit him- or herself to the use of one or two of the different classes of synthetic dressings [8•].

Full-thickness wounds reach down to the subcutis. If left to heal naturally, the defect starts to be filled with granulation tissue and contracts because of the effect of myofibroblasts. Contraction can account for approximately half of the wound area, and the rest is covered by reepithelialization. Although wound contraction aids considerably in the reduction of full-thickness skin defects, it may result in the crucial distortion of critical structures; cicatricial ectropion or eclabium is very difficult to repair. The new dressings also facilitate reepithelialization of full-thickness wounds and thus reduce contraction [3••].

Another issue to be discussed in postoperative wound care is the patient's behavior after surgery. Excessive alcohol intake must be avoided. Wound healing is much worse in smokers: scars are three to seven times wider in smokers than in nonsmokers. Smoking must be prohibited after flap and graft surgery. It is particularly deleterious in trained flaps and after surgery of acral structures such as digits and nails. Scar dehiscence is common on the back and deltoid regions; in addition to sutures, which are stable for several weeks, and suture strips, stretching perpendicular to the scar line must be reduced to a minimum because at 14 days a scar has only 5% to 10% of the stability of the normal skin, and it achieves its 80% maximal stability only after many months. Sports activities must therefore be reduced to those that do not interfere with healing.

Tumescent anesthesia

Liposuction has become the most frequently performed cosmetic operation. Its greatest risks were general anesthesia and excessive bleeding. The tumescent technique developed by dermatologic surgeons has been shown to virtually eliminate these risks and to allow greater amounts of fat to be removed. In two prospective studies carried out on patients who underwent high-volume liposuction (>1500 mL), Klein [9••] showed that the direct infiltration into subcutaneous fat of copious amounts of very dilute anesthetic solutions permitted the injection of 400 to 1000 mg of lidocaine and 0.5 to 1 mg of epinephrine without systemic toxicity. The mean total amount of lidocaine injected was 33.3 mg/kg (range, 11 to 52.1) dissolved in a mean volume of 4609 mL (range, 2050 to 7275). The mean volume of aspirate was 2657 mL (range, 1840 to 4575), giving 1945 mL (range, 1500 to 3400) of fat. The mean volume of calculated blood loss was only 18.5 mL, and the hematocrit did not indicate a loss of body fluids. Neither infections nor seromas or hematomas were observed. In contrast, the "dry technique" causes great blood loss, with 20% to 45% of the aspirate being blood. The advantages of the tumescent technique can be summarized as follows:

1. Profound local anesthesia without the risk of general anesthesia

2. Reduced surgical blood loss

3. Lower intravenous fluid requirements

4. Considerably less postoperative pain because anesthesia usually wanes only after 12 hours

5. Enhanced aesthetic results due to an increase in the suctioned fat volume

This article was discussed by one of the leading plastic surgeons, who despite some criticisms had to admit that this innovative study of lidocaine pharmacokinetics is "particularly praiseworthy" and added that plastic surgeons have been using variations of this technique [10].

Wound closure

Sutureless tissue repair has been used in many areas during the last 10 years. Concentrated human fibrinogen has been used to glue grafts and flaps to their recipient site. In addition to fixing wound edges together, this technique also seals blood vessels and provides perfect hemostasis. Sutureless tissue repair has also been tried with lasers. A new approach is dye-enhanced laser welding using indocyanine green (a nontoxic, US Food and Drug Administration–approved dye with an absorption peak of 780 to 805 nm) and a tunable alexandrite laser operated at 780 nm with 250-μs pulses and a 4-mm spot size. Full-thickness skin incisions were made in albino guinea pigs; the wound edges were stained with indocyanine green, abutted with forceps, and treated with a laser. The optimal tensile strength of 30 to 60 g was achieved at dye concentrations of 0.1 to 1 mg and a laser irradiance of 8 to 12 W/cm^2. This resulted in slight thermal damage. More damage inhibited welding, whereas less laser irradiance resulted in only very weak tensile strength. The inverse relationship of dye concentration and laser irradiance is consistent with a concept of selective photothermolysis. Although the mechanism of welding is still poorly understood, the thermal behavior of collagen may be an explanation: the melting of collagen fibers occurs just below tissue shrinkage temperatures and provides large quantities of denatured proteins in the region of the incision, which may cause adhesion on cooling and coagulation. With further optimization, indocyanine green dye–enhanced laser welding may become clinically practicable [11•].

Sutures

Monofilament suture material has several advantages over braided materials, but because of general concern about knot security, multiple throws are often added, or the cut suture ends are left long, resulting in excessive amounts of foreign material in the wound. A study was performed to identify the holding capacity of different knots made with a variety of suture materials. The nonabsorbable materials used were polypropylene (Prolene; Ethicon, Norderstedt, Germany) and nylon (Dermalon: Cyanamid of Great Britain, Gosport, UK; and Ethilon: Ethicon, Norderstedt, Germany), the monofilament absorbable materials were polydioxanone suture (PDS) and polyglyconate (Maxon; Cyanamid of Great Britain, Gosport, UK), and the braided materials were coated polyglycolic acid (Dexon; Cyanamid of Great Britain, Gosport, UK) and polyglactin (Vicryl; Ethicon, Norderstedt, Germany). All materials examined were metric 4 (no. 1 size). It was found that the knot-holding capacity increased rapidly with the number of throws until it equaled the breaking force.

The breaking point was reached without additional throws for Dexon with all knots tested, and it was reached with double knots with all materials except for Ethilon and PDS. The surgeon's knot required one additional throw with all materials except for Ethilon, which required two throws. Thus, the double knot has the greatest knot-holding capacity when its parallel configuration is not distorted by overtightening. With respect to knot-holding capacity, Dexon was superior to Vicryl, Maxon was superior to PDS, and Prolene was the best nonabsorbable material. Knot slippage was followed by immediate total knot disruption with Ethilon, Dermalon, Prolene, and PDS but by knot recomposition with Maxon and Vicryl. For the latter group, long cut ends may be better, but they are not superior in the former group [12•].

The study showed that a maximum of two additional throws yields a knot-holding capacity that equals the breaking force, and more throws are unnecessary. Long uncut ends of suture are also unnecessary. With respect to these results, the operation time may be shortened and less foreign material will be left in the wounds. Both buried interrupted dermal and buried running sutures are increasingly being used in dermatologic surgery. However, knot tying may be difficult, resulting in incomplete coaptation of wound edges.

The buried parallel pulley suture has already been demonstrated [7]. A modification was recently proposed by Motley and Holt [13•] (Fig. 1). Multiple bites of tissue from each side of the wound are taken, creating a pulley configuration (Fig. 1B). The suture, preferably a 3-0 PDS, is passed into the undersurface of the dermis 1 to 2 cm away from the wound edge. When the suture is pulled taut, the edges of the wound are powerfully apposed and gently everted, with an even tension across several strands of suture and through several points in the skin. This prevents breakage of the suture material or cutting out of the tissue. An elongated pulley or bootlace suture can be used for the largest wounds (Fig. 1C). This technique is particularly useful for wounds on the back, scalp, and proximal limbs.

The running meander-like subcuticular suture placed parallel to the skin surface cannot take up wound tension without wavelike deformation of the wound margins. The stitches are usually not locked and tend to loosen. Additional transepidermal sutures may be necessary for exact wound apposition. In contrast, simple buried interrupted sutures leave a great deal of suture material in the wound. Cosmetically and functionally optimal sutures ensure exact coaptation of wound margins, atraumatic tissue handling, less foreign material in the wound, and uptake of tissue tension. A running intradermal suture with "overthrow" to overcome the disadvantage of the running subcuticular suture was pro-

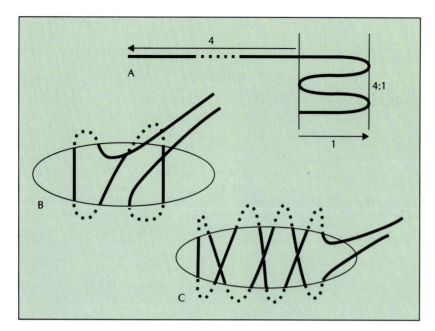

Fig. 1. A, Illustration of the pulley effect. The greater the number of loops of suture, the higher the ratio of suture "pull" to wound closure, and the more powerful the pulley effect. **B,** A double loop forms the simplest pulley suture. **C,** An elongated subcutaneous pulley or "bootlace" suture. (*From* Motley and Holt [13•]; with permission.)

posed by Groth *et al.* [14]. This suture begins on the wound end away from the surgeon and is carried out in his or her direction. The needle is inserted into the dermis from the subcutis, as if a simple buried suture were being used, and a surgeon's knot is tied. The nonneedle end is cut short, and the long end is held at an angle of 20° to 30° with the skin along the axis of the wound. The suture is advanced as if another such stitch is to be placed. When the needle is inserted into the dermis from its undersurface, it is crossed over the holding thread, a new vertical buried suture is performed, and the needle is pulled out under the central axial thread, thus automatically yielding the first throw of a knot. The assistant leaves the central thread and the suture is pulled tight and the suture is held again. The procedure is repeated, giving a tight wound closure with excellent coaptation. No subcutaneous stitches are necessary. The suture is completed with a second double square knot, which is formed by using a loop as a counterpart to the suture's needle end. This knot is slightly more bulky than the first one. To avoid a superficial knot position and possible spitting, the loop is cut close to the knot, and the needle may be inserted vertically into the wound between the margins right behind the knot (into the subcutaneous fat and through the dermis and epidermis) and pulled out away from the wound but in the axis of the wound. When the suture material is pulled tight, the bulky knot is buried deep in the subdermal tissue. The suture is cut directly over the epidermis and slips back into or under the skin (Fig. 2).

Because the axial suture thread is held tight, the simple throws are fixed and keep their position, so that the distance between two bites remains constant and waviness is avoided. To prevent breaking of the suture material during tightening of the axial thread, the surgeon may approximate the wound margins with the left thumb and index finger.

This suture is performed with monofilament absorbable material, which is superior with respect to stability, durability, and slippage. If the suture ruptures when it has been incidentally cut with the needle, the suture ends are tied together and the procedure continues.

The suture material used is metric 6-0 PDS or polyglyconate for the face, 5-0 for the extremities and the ventral aspect of the trunk, and 4-0 for the back. This technique is applicable for closure of excisions as well as for skin flaps.

A running locked intradermal suture was proposed by Wong [15•]. This suture provides dermal support to reduce tension, allows good wound edge apposition, avoids superficial stitches, and reduces postoperative wound care. This suture, again, begins like a buried intradermal suture. A surgeon's knot is tied, and the nonneedle end of the suture is cut short. At an adequate distance, the needle is inserted again, as if another buried intradermal suture were being placed. A good-sized bite of dermis is taken, the suture is pulled through the upper dermis, the needle is crossed to the opposite edge in the upper dermis, the needle is inserted at the same level, an equal bite of dermis is taken, and the suture is pulled through in the dermis-hypodermis plane. A short length of connecting thread between the first and second sutures is left exposed above the skin, and the needle is passed backward and under this thread. The needle is continued around and hooked under the connecting thread to catch it. The loop is then pulled tight until the connecting thread retracts into the wound and the wound edges are apposed. The needle is then passed through the new loop, and by pulling at the free end of the suture, a complete knot is tied. To continue the suture, the needle is hooked under the new suture and the procedure is repeated until the wound is completely closed (Fig. 3). The thread is then cut close to the knot. To facilitate this suture, the needle must be curved

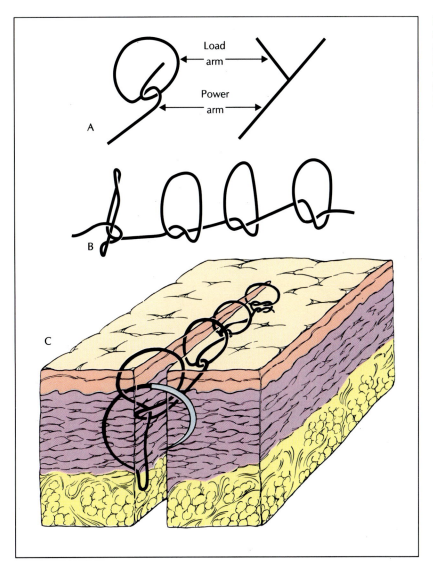

enough; it should preferentially be semicircular. Coated braided absorbable suture material such as polyglactin or polyglycolic acid was used and gave good support for 7 to 15 days, with minimal inflammation and fibrous reaction. For the face and neck 4-0 to 5-0 suture material was used, and for the scalp 3-0 to 4-0 material was employed.

Adequate undermining, minimal tension of the surrounding tissue, and excellent hemostasis are crucial. Antibiotic ointment and a clear adhesive dressing are applied to the wound. The latter is left in place for more than 5 days or until it is loose; the wound is then cleaned, and antibiotic ointment and a new dressing are applied.

Advantages of this suture are that 1) precise epidermal wound edge apposition is achieved; 2) closure of dermal dead space is obtained because the suture has a vertical and a horizontal component; 3) suture marks are avoided; 4) minimal postoperative wound care is needed because a clear occlusive dressing and antibiotic ointment reduce the risk of bacteria entry and allow inspection of wound healing; 5) if a needle or

thread breaks, the wound does not need to be sutured from the beginning; and 6) no sutures have to be removed. Disadvantages of this suture are that 1) more material is buried in the wound; 2) the suture is more time consuming and more difficult to learn; and 3) the suture must be aligned correctly.

Table 1 compares different buried suture techniques. Running subcuticular sutures are being increasingly used because they provide excellent cosmetic results. When the suture slips, however, the wound becomes dehiscent. Several devices are commercially available to secure the loose end of a running suture, but a simple knot appears to be the cheapest and most practical method. To avoid a bulky knot that may cause an unsightly scar at the end of the suture line, a new adjustable knot was proposed by Di Saverio *et al.* [16•]. After the subcuticular suture has been completed, it is pulled through the epidermis and its end is cut at 10 to 15 cm from the point of exit. The redundant free suture is then tied around the end of the suture exiting the skin with a sliding knot made of two simple half-hitches. This knot is slid along the suture until it is against the skin. When the correct tension on the suture

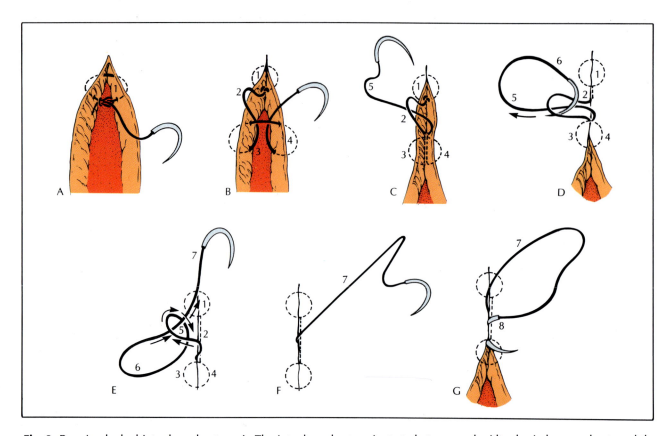

Fig. 3. Running locked intradermal suture. **A,** The intradermal suture is started at one end with a buried square knot, and the nonneedle end is cut short (1). **B,** Another intradermal suture is placed (3, 4), leaving a short length of connecting thread exposed over the skin (2). **C,** The needle is passed back (5) and under the connecting thread (2). **D,** The needle is hooked around the connecting thread once again (6), and the suture is pulled taut from the first loop (5). **E,** The needle is passed behind and through the new loop (5,6). **F,** The suture is pulled tight (7). **G,** To continue, the needle is hooked under the new suture, and steps *B* to *F* are repeated; at the end of the suture (8), cut close to the knot. (*From* Wong [15•]; with permission.)

Table 1. Comparison of various buried intradermal suture techniques*

	Simple interrupted	Parallel pulley	Boot lace	Running subcuticular	Running overthrow	Running locked
Epidermal apposition	Usually	Yes	Usually	Yes	Yes	Yes
Dermal apposition	Yes	Excellent	Excellent	No	Yes	Yes
Avoids external sutures	Yes	Yes	Yes	Often†	Yes	Yes
Avoids puncture of epidermis	Yes	Yes	Yes	Often†	Yes	Yes
Minimizes wound care	No	Yes	Yes	Yes†	Yes	Yes
Avoids suture removal	Yes	Yes	Yes	Often†	Yes	Yes
Takes up wound tension	Little	Excellent	Excellent	No	Good	Good
Foreign material in wound	Much	Little	Little	No‡	Moderate	Moderate to much
Remains stable†	Weeks	Months	Months	Days‡	Weeks to months	Weeks to months

*Data from Haneke [7], Groth *et al.* [14], and Wong [15•].
†Depends on whether absorbable or nonabsorbable suture material is used.
‡If nonabsorbable suture material is removed.

has been achieved, the sliding knot is secured in position by two hitches between the exiting skin suture and the redundant suture. This simple and effective knotting technique leaves little or no scar at the end of the subcuticular suture line. It can also be employed when a running suture breaks or is cut accidentally. In these circumstances, the broken ends of the running suture can be joined in a similar fashion to continue the running suture.

Scar stretch depends not only on suture technique but also on the amount of skin available on both sides of the wound. Most skin excisions leave a defect that requires some tension for closure. A skin-stretching device for harnessing the viscoelastic properties of skin was designed by Hirshowitz et al. [17•]. The device consists of two pins that are threaded through the dermis of the wound edges on either side of the defect. Two U-shaped arms on the undersurface are inward-facing sharp cutting hooks that engage the pins through the skin surface overlying the pins. A threaded screw that passes through the center of the arms pulls the loose distal arm riding over the screw closer when the screw is turned by a tension knot at its free end. The device can be left in place during suturing by placing sutures both between and at the sides of the U-arms. Because both skin undermining and traction may be detrimental to the vitality of the wound margins, the risk is reduced by this nonundermining approach. This device has been successfully used for the closure of skin defects after the removal of skin carcinomas; over exposed bone, joints, plates, and screws; and after dehiscence of a surgical wound that was sutured under tension. This device appears to be more complicated than the suture tension adjustment reel described by Cohen and Cosmetto [18]. (The suture tension adjustment reel was extensively described in my first review for *Current Opinion in Dermatology* [7].)

Attempts to improve flap viability

Flap survival depends on a minimum of blood circulation, and wound edge necrosis observed after suture under too high a tension is probably also due to compromised circulation. Topical prostaglandin E_1 has been shown to improve flap survival [19•]. Another study was performed to evaluate the effect of the continuous topical application of heparin on flap survival. Rectangular flaps were raised on the backs of rats and sutured back into place. Either the proximal third or the middle third was covered with a silicon gel drug delivery system containing 25,000 U of heparin in a sheet of approximately 12×15 cm. The length of the surviving flap portion was increased only when the heparin was delivered to the critical midportion of the flap. This effect was probably due to platelet disaggregation maintaining vascular patency. Heparin accelerates antithrombin action, influences endogenous endothelial prostanoid synthesis, reduces platelet adhesiveness, inhibits the conversion of fibrin from fibrinogen, stimulates the release of tissue-type plasminogen activator, decreases leukocyte-mediated free radical injury, and promotes the migration and proliferation of the capillary endothelium as well as neovascularization on topical application, but it has no vasodilatory effect like prostaglandin E_1. Thus, blood clotting appears to be the major risk factor for the critical flap area.

A clinical study used calcitonin gene–related peptide (CGRP), which is the most potent sensory vasodilatory peptide, to increase the viability of flaps with compromised circulation in humans [20•]. CGRP infusion significantly increased blood flow as measured by laser Doppler flowmetry and was beneficial in terms of blood flow, reflow, and survival of flaps. Particularly compromised regions responded to CGRP, which was already known from patients with Raynaud's disease. In the study on flaps at risk, CGRP was significantly more efficacious than transcutaneous electrical nerve stimulation. It was observed that when blood flow was not improved by the first treatment, the flap at risk did not survive. CGRP infusion was thus also a predictor of flap viability.

Table 2. Factors affecting scarring*

Uncontrollable
  Race
  Age
  Body region
  Skin type
  Skin disorder
  Infection
  Impaired blood supply
  Idiosyncratic (hereditary?)
Controllable
  Atraumatic technique
  Evenness
  Direction according to relaxed skin tension lines
  Sutures and their handling
  Postoperative immobilization and splinting
  Smoking

*From Callan and Morrison [21•]; with permission.

Treatment of scars and other sequelae of surgery

Because the surgeon cannot operate through the skin without leaving a scar, it must be decided, particularly in treating benign lesions, whether the cure is worse than the disease [21•]. People with dark skin often scar unpredictably, leaving a hyperpigmented or even a keloidal scar. Scars on the back and shoulders stretch considerably; those over the sternum frequently become hypertrophic or even keloids (Table 2). The clinical observation that prolonged wound support by deep sutures and adhesive tapes helps to prevent scar stretching has been proven. Absence of inflammation is another important factor in optimal wound healing. Whenever scar revision is considered, it must be kept in mind that the results are often unrewarding because the conditions that made the scar wide or hypertrophic usually still pertain. The nature of scars is predictable to a large degree; they are usually fine in the face, wide on the back, and hypertrophic on the sternum and deltoid regions. Therefore, lesions in these locations should not be removed for cosmetic reasons alone. Scars in children that become hypertrophic may eventually fade, flatten, and soften but then frequently become wide.

The treatment of keloids is still extremely delicate. Simple excision is almost always followed by a recurrence that is larger than before. Injection with corticosteroid crystal suspension right into (not under) the keloid, the application of long-term pressure, cryosurgery, and recently the use of silicone gel sheets have been proposed, and often a combination of these methods is necessary. The mechanism of action of the silicone gel sheet is poorly understood. Because it is usually applied without pressure, probably the occlusion and hydration explain the therapeutic effect. This was recently shown experimentally because no difference was found between the occlusive treatment of keloid with silicone oil–containing cream and oil-in-water cream [22•].

Free flaps and grafts transposed to the face, as well as wide scars, usually have another color than the surrounding skin and thus appear like a strange patch. A refined tattoo method called dermatography was described by Van der Velden *et al.* [23•]. They designed an electromotor-driven dermoinjector with seven needles in two rows that allows fine staining of skin and scars. Flaps and grafts that are paler need only low-intensity coloration, thus permitting the seasonal fluctuation of natural skin pigmentation to shine through. Even freckles can be tattooed to match the normal appearance [23•].

References and recommended reading

Papers of particular interest, published within the annual period of review, have been highlighted as:
- Of special interest
- • Of outstanding interest

1. Dubin D, Hafner AW, Arndt KA: **Citation Classics in Clinical Dermatologic Journals: Citation Analysis, Biomedical Journals, and Landmark Articles, 1945-1990.** *Arch Dermatol* 1993, 129:1121–1129.
This evaluation of the most cited articles and journals in clinical dermatology shows the importance of dermatologic surgery.

2. Petres J, Rompel R: **Relative Importance of Dermatosurgery in Hospital and Private Practice of Dermatology [in German With English Summary].** *Hautarzt* 1994, 45:113–139.

3. •• Telfer NR, Moy RL: **Wound Care After Office Procedures.** *J Dermatol Surg Oncol* 1993, 19:722–731.
The importance of postoperative wound care to maintain a good surgical result is emphasized.

4. • Brown CD, Zitelli JA: **A Review of Topical Agents for Wounds and Methods of Wounding.** *J Dermatol Surg Oncol* 1993, 19:732–737.
Many topical agents for treatment of wounds may delay wound healing; thus, detailed knowledge is mandatory.

5. Roenigk RK: **Dermabrasion: State of the Art.** *J Dermatol Surg Oncol* 1985, 11:306–314.

6. • Phillips TJ, Kapoor V, Provan A, Ellerin T: **A Randomized Prospective Study of a Hydroactive Dressing Vs Conventional Treatment After Shave Biopsy Excision.** *Arch Dermatol* 1993, 129:859–860.
Hydroactive dressings did not accelerate wound healing but were considerably more comfortable and required fewer dressing changes.

7. Haneke E: **Developments and Techniques in General Dermatologic Surgery.** *Curr Opin Dermatol* 1994, 1:145–151.

8. • Eaglstein WH: **Occlusive Dressings.** *J Dermatol Surg Oncol* 1993, 19:716–720.
Review of new dressing materials and their specific indications and advantages.

9. •• Klein JA: **Tumescent Technique for Local Anesthesia Improves Safety in Large-Volume Liposuction.** *Plast Reconstr Surg* 1993, 92:1085–1098.
Excellent study on the pharmacokinetics and toxicity of large amounts of lidocaine, as needed for large-volume liposuction.

10. Pitman GH: **Tumescent Technique for Local Anesthesia Improves Safety in Large-Volume Liposuction [Discussion].** *Plast Reconstr Surg* 1993, 92:1099–1100.

11. • Decorte SD, Farinelli W, Flotte T, Anderson R: **Dye-Enhanced Laser Welding for Skin Closure.** *Lasers Surg Med* 1993, 12:25–32.
Interesting study in experimental animals on the use of dye-enhanced laser to weld wound edges.

12. • Brown RP: **Knotting Technique and Suture Material.** *Br J Surg* 1992, 79:399–400.
Systematic study of the holding capacity of different knots with various suture materials.

13. • Motley RJ, Holt PJA: **Subcutaneous Pulley and "Bootlace" Sutures.** In *Abstracts of the XIV Congress of the International Society of Dermatologic Surgery.* Edited by Camacho F. Sevilla: International Society of Dermatologic Surgery; 1993:117.
Variation of a horizontal pulley suture to appose skin defects under tension.

14. Groth W, Hecker CH, Henn M, Quinkler C: **Wundnaht-Intradermal-Naht.** *Z Hautkr* 1991, 66(suppl 3):65–68.

15. • Wong NJ: **The Running Locked Intradermal Suture.** *J Dermatol Surg Oncol* 1993, 19:30–36.
Running intradermal suture with vertical and horizontal components is knotted after each stitch.

16. • Di Saverio G, De Soras X, Guidicelli H: **New Adjustable Knot for Securing Subcuticular Running Sutures.** *Br J Surg* 1993, 80:873.
Simple technique to secure the exited thread of running subcuticular sutures.

17. • Hirshowitz B, Lindenbaum E, Har-Shai Y: **A Skin-Stretching Device for the Harnessing of the Viscoelastic Properties of Skin.** *Plast Reconstr Surg* 1993, 92:260–270.
Device for immediate preoperative and intraoperative skin expansion.

18. Cohen BH, Cosmetto AJ: **The Suture Tension Adjustment Reel: A New Device for the Management of Skin Closure.** *J Dermatol Surg Oncol* 1992, 18:112–132.

19. • Sawada Y, Hatayama I, Sone K: **The Effect of Continuous Topical Application of Heparin on Flap Survival.** *Br J Plast Surg* 1993, 45:515–518.
Topical heparin can increase the length of flaps at risk when it is applied to the risk zone.

20. • Jernbeck J, Dalsgaard CJ: **Calcitonin Gene-Related Peptide Treatment of Flaps With Compromised Circulation in Humans.** *Plast Reconstr Surg* 1993, 91:236–244.
Infusion of CGRP increases flap viability in humans.

21. • Callan PP, Morrison WA: **Recent Advances in Plastic Surgery.** *Aust Fam Physician* 1992, 21:950–961.
Review of certain aspects of dermatologic surgery from the plastic surgeon's point of view.

22. • Sawada Y, Sone K: **Hydration and Occlusion Treatment for Hypertrophic Scars and Keloids.** *Br J Plast Surg* 1992, 45:599–603.
This study indicates that occlusion and hydration may be responsible for the effect of silicone cream on keloids.

23. • Van der Velden EM, Wittkampf ARM, de Jong BD, van der Putte SCJ, van der Dussen FN: **Dermatography, a Treatment for Sequelae After Head and Neck Surgery: A Case Report.** *J Craniomaxillofac Surg* 1992, 20:273–278.
Artful tattooing may improve the cosmetic appearance of grafts and free flaps in the face.

Eckart Haneke, MD, Department of Dermatology, Ferdinand-Sauerbruch-Klinik, Kliniken der Universität Witten-Herdecke, Lehrkrankenhaus der Universität Düsseldorf, 42117 Wuppertal, Germany.

Diagnosis and therapeutics
in nonmelanoma skin cancer

Ira C. Davis, MD, and Barry Leshin, MD

Wake Forest University Medical Center, Winston-Salem, North Carolina, USA

Nonmelanoma skin cancer is the most common malignancy in the world. True incidence rates can be determined only by large population-based studies in which registry of the tumor type is mandated. Studies of subgroups of patients with nonmelanoma skin cancer, such as the young and renal transplant patients, can allow the clinician to adapt care to the specific patient population. Sunscreens and protective clothing provide the foundation for effective prevention of nonmelanoma skin cancer. Improvements in the clinician's understanding of the effectiveness of these products results in better advice to the patient. Laser Doppler velocimetry and B-scan ultrasonography improve preoperative assessment of tumors. Fine-needle aspiration biopsy is being increasingly used for examining skin nodules.

Current Opinion in Dermatology 1995:137–141

Nonmelanoma skin cancer (NMSC) is the most common cancer in the United States. A better understanding of patient populations, the use of prevention strategies, and new technology aid in the advancement of care for this common tumor.

Epidemiology

Studies of defined populations can aid the dermatologist in adapting his or her clinical practice beyond anecdotal experience and reports. This information can result in improved counseling of patients who may be part of more defined subpopulations.

Incidence of basal cell carcinoma
Although the recorded incidence of skin cancer is increasing, an accurate accounting of the true incidence is lacking because these cancers are variably reported in cancer registries [1].

In a study of the population of Malmö, Sweden (population 250,000) conducted by Dahl et al. [2•], the age-standardized basal cell carcinoma (BCC) incidence rate per 100,000 persons doubled between 1970 and 1986 for both males (from 78 to 163) and females (from 63 to 121). Four 2-year periods (1970 to 1971, 1975 to 1976, 1980 to 1981, and 1985 to 1986) were studied. An accurate account of the skin cancer incidence was possible because all histopathologic specimens in Malmö were sent to one of two laboratories, enabling identification of all histologically confirmed BCCs. A population-based study in Rochester, Minnesota, reported similar incidence rates for the white population of the United States [1]. The Malmö study noted that only 66% of the

reported tumors were located on the head and neck, in contrast to the commonly reported 80% (Fig. 1). This distribution difference may reflect the broader patient base of this study, which included patients treated by physicians other than dermatologists. Forty-one percent of the patients developed more than one tumor, reaffirming the need for continued surveillance of patients who develop BCC.

Basal cell carcinoma and the young
Young patients with BCC compose a small percentage of the total patient population with BCC. Two studies examined this subpopulation of patients who developed BCC and excluded patients with genodermatoses, such as xeroderma pigmentosum and basal cell nevus syndrome [3,4••].

A study of the United Kingdom Northern Regional Cancer Registry for the incidence of BCC over an 11-year period noted that young patients (aged 15 to 34 years) composed 1.2% of the total patient population with BCC [3]. The registry recorded cancers of patients treated by a variety of physicians, including dermatologists, plastic and general surgeons, and radiotherapists. A slight majority of females were noted in the group under 35-years of age. Detailed 5-year follow-up was available for 39 patients. Of these patients, 9% had a morpheaform BCC, and 28% required further treatment for potential or actual recurrences, for metastasis, or for a second primary BCC. The author emphasizes the importance of continued follow-up of this patient population.

Dinehart et al. [4••] studied patients younger than 30 years of age with BCC who were referred for Mohs micrographic surgery and compared this group with

---

Abbreviations
BCC—basal cell carcinoma; **NMSC**—nonmelanoma skin cancer; **SPF**—sun protection factor.

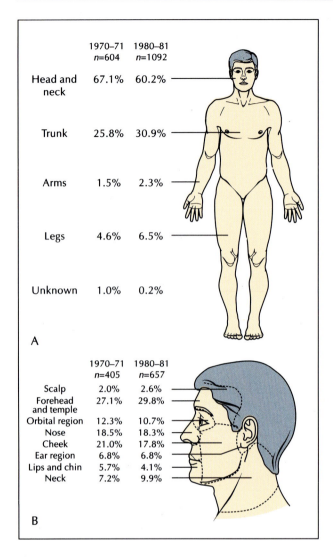

	1970–71 n=604	1980–81 n=1092
Head and neck	67.1%	60.2%
Trunk	25.8%	30.9%
Arms	1.5%	2.3%
Legs	4.6%	6.5%
Unknown	1.0%	0.2%

A

	1970–71 n=405	1980–81 n=657
Scalp	2.0%	2.6%
Forehead and temple	27.1%	29.8%
Orbital region	12.3%	10.7%
Nose	18.5%	18.3%
Cheek	21.0%	17.8%
Ear region	6.8%	6.8%
Lips and chin	5.7%	4.1%
Neck	7.2%	9.9%

B

Fig. 1. A, Total body distribution of 1696 basal cell carcinomas. **B**, Head and neck distribution of basal cell carcinomas. (*From* Dahl *et al.* [2•]; with permission.)

an older control group (56 to 70 years of age). The younger group (15 to 30 years of age) was predominantly female (63%), in contrast to the older control group, in which a majority of patients were male (56%). The increased use of tanning booths and hair dyes was noted in the younger group. The tumors and their consequent defects were smaller in the younger group than in the older comparison group. No difference in time to diagnosis or recurrence rate was noted between the two groups.

Giant basal cell carcinoma

Giant BCC is defined as tumors of greater than 5 cm in diameter (T3 tumors). Randle *et al.* [5] retrospectively analyzed a patient population prone to giant BCC. Fifty consecutive patients with giant BCC were compared with three other groups: those with small BCC (average size, 1 cm) who were treated with excision or electrodesiccation and curettage; those with T1 tumors (< 2

cm in diameter) who were treated with Mohs micrographic surgery; and those with T2 tumors (2 to 5 cm in diameter) who were treated with Mohs micrographic surgery. Aggressive histologic subtype, recurrence after previous treatment, history of exposure to ionizing radiation, and neglect of the tumor were risk factors associated with giant BCC. No patient with a giant BCC was younger than 45 years of age.

Nonmelanoma skin cancer and renal transplant patients

Renal transplant patients with NMSC require close surveillance and aggressive treatment of their malignancies. A study of 167 randomly selected patients with renal allografts in a regional transplantation clinic revealed a lag time of 3.5 years after transplantation before the development of solar keratoses [6•]. Up to 40% of renal transplant patients will develop NMSC 10 years after transplantation [7]. Knowledge of the factors that predispose renal transplant patients to the development of NMSC would allow some stratification within this population.

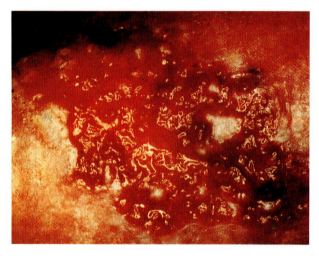

Fig. 2. Basal cell carcinoma developing in a venous leg ulcer: translucent and exuberant granulation tissue extend beyond the clinical margin of the ulcer. (*From* Harris *et al.* [9]; with permission.)

Bouwes Bavinck *et al.* [8••] studied 36 renal transplant patients with NMSC and 101 patients without skin cancer. A high level of exposure to sunlight before 30 years of age was more significant than sunlight exposure after 30 years of age for the development of NMSC. The relative risk for the development of NMSC increased in patients with 50 to 99 keratotic lesions (warts and actinic keratoses). The relative risk for the development of NMSC was highest in patients with 100 or more keratotic lesions. Gender, number of treatments for rejection, and daily doses of azathioprine or prednisone did not affect the development of NMSC. Patients with skin type I or II are at increased risk for developing squamous cell carcinoma [7,8••]. Finally, patients likely to develop NMSC are older at the time of transplantation (35 to 37 vs 31 years of age) [8••].

Basal cell carcinoma and venous stasis ulcers

Basal cell carcinomas may arise in venous stasis ulcers. Harris *et al.* [9] reported a series of five cases with such an occurrence. The presence of translucent and exuberant granulation-like tissue with extension beyond the clinical margin of the ulcer suggests the diagnosis of BCC (Fig. 2).

Skin cancer prevention

Sunscreens

Sunscreens and protective clothing are the mainstays of skin cancer prevention for NMSC. Schlesinger *et al.* [10] reviewed basic information about the use of sunscreens. Sunscreens should be applied to children as young as 6 months of age. Oral vitamin D supplementation in elderly patients is suggested. The use of sun protection factors (SPFs) of greater than 15 should be considered for people who live in tropical climates. In addition, an individual's method of applying sunscreens can result in a lower effective SPF because laboratory measurements may not be replicated. Furthermore, SPF 30 sunscreens more efficiently prevent sunburn cell production than of SPF 15 sunscreens.

Wolf *et al.* [11,12••] examined the protection against immunosuppression delivered by the sunscreens para-aminobenzoic acid, cinnamate, and benzophenone in mice. These agents offer limited protection against the immunosuppressive properties of ultraviolet radiation when compared with their sunburn-protective properties. Hence, if patients gauge their sun exposure solely on preventing sunburn, they will probably not obtain adequate protection against the immunosuppressive properties of ultraviolet radiation. The investigators noted that liposomes containing T4 endonuclease V, a DNA excision repair enzyme, afforded better protection than sunscreens against ultraviolet-induced immunosuppression but inferior protection against ultraviolet-induced erythema. A combination of conventional sunscreens and newer agents such as the T4-containing liposomes may be necessary to protect the patient from the carcinogenic effects of ultraviolet irradiation.

The development of increasingly effective sunscreens without due attention to adverse reactions will decrease their use. Sixteen percent (90 of 603) of participants developed an adverse reaction in a randomized, double-blinded, longitudinal, population-based study comparing the daily use of a sunscreen containing 8% 2-ethylhexyl-*p*-methoxycinnamate and 2% 4-*t*-butylmethoxydibenzoylmethane with the use of its placebo base in the prevention of actinic keratoses [13]. Reactions were equally divided between the sunscreen and the vehicle groups. Of those affected, 50% had a personal history consistent with atopy. Only four patients had positive patch tests results, although none were to the sunscreens active ingredients. The high frequency of adverse reactions may result in failure to comply with the recommended daily use of sunscreens.

Ultraviolet indicators

Ultraviolet indicators that change color when exposed to sunlight have been introduced for use by the public in order to determine the exposure to sunlight. Moseley *et al.* [14] studied the reliability of Suncheck patches (Sherwood Skin Care, Nottingham, UK) and Tanscan cards (B & H Group, London, UK). Although these indicators provide useful information on ultraviolet in-

Table 1. Predicted sun protection factors of various garments*					
Garment type	Color	Fabric	Test condition	SPF (predicted)[†]	UVA PF (predicted)[†]
Famous-maker T-shirt sold at Hawaiian resort	White	Cotton knit	Side of shirt; dry	7.4	7.3
			Side of shirt; wet	5.5	4.3
California long-sleeved lifeguard T-shirt	Blue	Cotton knit	Side of shirt; dry	7.0	5.2
			Side of shirt; wet	5.2	3.9
Polo shirt	White	Cotton piqué	Side of shirt; dry	31.0	33.3
			Side of shirt; wet	17.9	26.3
			Shoulder of shirt; dry	8.7	8.5
			Shoulder of shirt; wet	6.8	6.6
Gardening shirt	White	Woven cotton	Dry	5.1	6.0
			Wet	2.6	2.6
Shirt	White	Woven polyester	Dry	3.7	3.4
Solumbria fabric[‡]	White	Woven nylon	Dry	74.6	85.2
			Wet	66.6	77.9
SPF 15 sunscreen, standard				11.6	4.1

*From Sayre and Hughes [15•]; with permission.
†Risk is calculated using sunlight.
‡Sun Precautions, Seattle, WA.
SPF—sun protection factor; UVA PF—ultraviolet A protective factor.

Table 2. Sun protection factors at various sites on the head and neck provided by different types of hats*

Style of hat	Typical sun protection factor				
	Forehead	Nose	Cheek	Chin	Back of neck
Small-brimmed hat (<2.5 cm)	15	1.5	1	1	1
Medium-brimmed hat (2.5–7.5 cm)	>20	3	2	1	2
Large-brimmed hat (>7.5 cm)	>20	7	3	1.2	5
Peaked cap	>20	5	1.5	1	1

*From Diffey and Cheeseman [16••]; with permission.

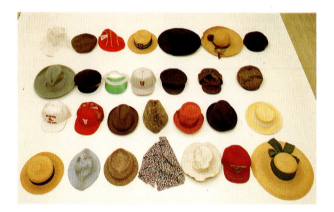

Fig. 3. The 28 hats tested in a study of their sun-protective potential. (*From* Diffey and Cheeseman *et al.* [16••]; with permission.)

tensity, the authors noted that these devices can give the patient a false sense of security. The amount of sunscreen applied to the device may not be the same as that applied to the individual. Additional applications of sunscreen on the indicator result in additional layers of sunscreen and do not mirror the additional applications to the skin.

Sun-protective clothing

Sayre and Hughes [15•] performed *in vitro* measurements of ultraviolet transmission through various fabrics (Table 1). Predicted SPFs were less than the standard SPF 15 of sunscreen. The SPF decreased when the clothing was moistened with tap water. Clothing manufactured by Sun Precautions (Seattle, WA) afforded an SPF of 74.6 when dry and 66.6 when wet.

Wearing a hat with a brim is highly recommended. A recent study evaluated the sun protection provided by 28 different hats (Fig. 3) [16••]. Headgear was divided into four categories: small-brimmed hats (<2.5 cm), medium-brimmed hats (2.5 to 7.5 cm), large-brimmed hats (<7.5 cm), and peaked caps. All headgear tested afforded adequate protection to the forehead. Only large-brimmed hats provided some protection to the nose and cheek (Table 2). The use of a hat cannot be recommended as the sole means of sun protection for the face and neck.

Diagnostic techniques

Assessment of tumor margin

The objective of ablative and surgical treatments is the complete destruction or removal of tumor, with the removal of minimal tumor-free tissue. Newer technologies such as laser Doppler velocimetry and high-frequency digital B-scan ultrasonography aid in tumor margin assessment.

Tumor growth is accompanied by increased vascularization and concomitant increased blood flow. Laser Doppler velocimetry can delineate areas of increased blood flow that represent tumor neovascularization. Clinically predicted size, laser Doppler velocimetry–predicted size, and actual postoperative defect size were measured in 10 patients with 14 biopsy-proven BCCs who were referred to a university center for Mohs micrographic surgery [17]. Only the laser Doppler velocimetry–predicted size correlated with the Mohs surgery postoperative defect size. The postoperative defect size may lead one to overestimate the actual tumor dimensions because the surgery removes a margin of normal tissue and tissue removal usually results in wound relaxation.

High-frequency B-scan ultrasonography provides a two-dimensional cross-sectional image that correlates well with tumor thickness and width [18]. Hoffman *et al.* [19] used B-scan ultrasonography to assess tumor thickness and width before cryosurgery in 80 patients with BCC. This information aided in their selection of the number of cryocycles, probe size, and freezing temperatures. Scanning was performed several times during the course of wound healing over a 3-week period. Ultrasonography detected reepithelialization better than clinical observation. In addition, ultrasonography monitored continued wound healing in the dermis even after complete clinical reepithelialization, providing a means of objectively monitoring wound healing.

Fine-needle aspiration biopsy

Fine-needle aspiration biopsy is commonly used to confirm the metastatic nature of skin nodules [20]. Samples of primary skin tumors may inadvertently or purposely be examined in this manner [20,21]. Powers *et al.* [21] described the use of fine-needle aspiration biopsy in six cases of dermatofibrosarcoma protuberans. Four of the six cases were initially diagnosed with fine-needle aspiration biopsy. Layfield and Glasgow [20] retrospectively reviewed 558 aspirates of subcutaneous and cutaneous nodules suspected of being metastatic tumors. Ninety-four lesions (17%) proved to be primary cutaneous tumors. The benign or malignant nature of the primary skin neoplasm was identified in 89% of cases; 81% of neoplasms were specifically diagnosed. Primary skin tumors included epidermal inclusion cysts, pilomatrixoma, BCC, squamous cell carcinoma, sebaceous carcinoma, Merkel cell tumor, melanoma, lymphoma, hemangioma, pyogenic granuloma, Kaposi's sarcoma, angiosarcoma, dermatofibrosarcoma protuberans, granular cell tumor, and chalazion.

Clinical history and immunohistochemical data are likely to be necessary to differentiate primary and metastatic squamous cell carcinoma, lymphomas, mesenchymal and fibrohistiocytic tumors, and some neuroendocrine tumors. Additional factors that can contribute to increased diagnostic accuracy include accurately assessing the tissue plane sampled and allowing the pathologist to perform the procedure to allow better clinicopathologic correlation [22].

Conclusions

Population-based studies accurately assess the magnitude of the rising incidence of BCC. A better understanding of the behavior of NMSC in patient subgroups when compared with the general population can help tailor care to these patients, resulting in appropriate therapy. An improved understanding of the mechanism of action and use of sunscreens will allow the physician to advise patients better in regard to skin cancer prevention. Newer technologies and techniques can result in more optimal patient care.

References and recommended reading

Papers of particular interest, published within the annual period review, have been highlighted as:
•   Of special interest
•• Of outstanding interest

1.   Chuang TS, Popescu A, Su WPD, Chute CG: **A Population-Based Incidence Study in Rochester, Minnesota**. *J Am Acad Dermatol* 1990, 22:413–417.

2.   Dahl E, Aberg M, Rausing A, Rausing E-L: **Basal Cell Carcinoma: An Epi-**
•   **demiologic Study in a Defined Population**. *Cancer* 1992, 70:104–108.
Determines the age-standardized incidence rates for BCC in Malmö, Sweden, because the population could be easily defined and all histopathologic specimens could be traced.

3.   Cox HN: **Basal Cell Carcinoma in Young Adults**. *Br J Dermatol* 1992, 127:26–29.

4.   Dinehart S, Dodge R, Stanley W, Franks HH, Pollack SV: **Basal Cell**
••   **Carcinoma Treated With Mohs Surgery: A Comparison of 54 Younger Patients With 1050 Older Patients**. *J Dermatol Surg Oncol* 1992, 18:560–566.

Compares BCCs in a group of patients younger than 30 years of age with those in an older group (56 to 70 years of age). The lesions are not more aggressive in the younger patient population.

5.   Randle HW, Roenigk RK, Brodland DG: **Giant Basal Cell Carcinoma (T3): Who Is at Risk?** *Cancer* 1992, 72:1624–1630.

6.   Taylor AM, Shuster S: **Skin Cancer After Renal Transplantation: The**
•   **Causal Role of Azathioprine**. *Acta Derm Venereol (Stockh)* 1992, 72:115–119.
Solar keratoses do not develop in 167 randomly selected patients with renal allografts until 3.5 years after transplantation. The prevalence of patients with dyskeratotic lesions increases linearly by 6.8% per year.

7.   Glover MT, Deeks J, Kwan J, Proby C, Leigh IM: **Identification and Management of Renal Transplant Recipients With a High Risk of Skin Cancer [Abstract]**. *Br J Dermatol* 1993, 129(suppl 42):29.

8.   Bouwes Bavinck JN, Boer ADE, Vermeer BJ, Hartevelt MM, Van Der
••   Woude FJ, Claas FHJ, Wolerbeek R, Vandenbroucke JP: **Sunlight, Keratotic Skin Lesions and Skin Cancer in Renal Transplant Recipients**. *Br J Dermatol* 1993, 129:242–249.
Retrospective study of 136 renal transplantation patients: 36 with NMSC and 101 without skin cancer. An increased relative risk for NMSC was noted in patients with exposure to sunlight before 30 years of age and in patients with more than 50 keratotic lesions (warts and actinic keratoses).

9.   Harris B, Eaglstein WH, Falanga V: **Basal Cell Carcinoma Arising in Venous Ulcers and Mimicking Granulation Tissue**. *J Dermatol Surg Oncol* 1993, 19:150–152.

10.   Schlesinger IH, Wagner RF Jr, Tyring SK: **Potential and Limitations of Topical Sunscreens**. *Skin Cancer* 1993, 8:19–32.

11.   Wolf P, Kripke ML: **Sunscreens and Immunity**. *Skin Cancer* 1993, 8:33–40.

12.   Wolf P, Yarosh DB, Kripke ML: **Effects of Sunscreens and a DNA Ex-**
••   **cision Repair Enzyme on Ultraviolet Radiation-Induced Inflammation, Immune Suppression, and Cyclobutane Pyrimidine Dimer Formation in Mice**. *J Invest Dermatol* 1993, 101:523–527.
This animal study demonstrates that sunscreens are not as effective in protecting against ultraviolet-induced immunosuppression as in protecting against ultraviolet-induced erythema.

13.   Foley P, Nixon R, Marks R, Frowen K, Thompson S: **The Frequency of Reactions to Sunscreens: Results of a Longitudinal Population-Based Study on the Regular Use of Sunscreens in Australia**. *Br J Dermatol* 1993, 128:512–518.

14.   Moseley H, Mackie RM, Ferguson J: **The Suitability of Suncheck Patches and Tanscan Cards for Monitoring the Sunburning Effectiveness of Sunlight**. *Br J Dermatol* 1993, 128:75–78.

15.   Sayre RM, Hughes S: **Sun Protective Apparel: Advancements in Sun**
•   **Protection**. *Skin Cancer* 1993, 8:41–47.
Tests the ultraviolet protection of various types of clothing.

16.   Diffey BL, Cheeseman J: **Sun Protection With Hats**. *Br J Dermatol* 1992,
••   127:10–12.
Studies the sun-protective potential of various types of headgear.

17.   Haiken M, Garland LD: **Margin Assessment of Selected Basal Cell Carcinomas Utilizing Laser Doppler Velocimetry**. *Int J Dermatol* 1993, 32:290–292.

18.   Harland CC, Bamber JC, Gusterson BA, Mortimer PS: **High Frequency High Resolution B-Scan Ultrasound in the Assessment of Skin Tumors**. *Br J Dermatol* 1993, 128:525–532.

19.   Hoffman K, Winkler K, El-Gammal S, Altmeyer P: **A Wound Healing Model With Sonographic Monitoring**. *Clin Exp Dermatol* 1993, 18:217–225.

20.   Layfield LJ, Glasgow BJ: **Aspiration Biopsy Cytology of Primary Cutaneous Tumors**. *Acta Cytol* 1993, 37:679–688.

21.   Powers CN, Hurt MA, Frable WJ: **Fine-Needle Aspiration Biopsy: Dermatofibrosarcoma Protuberans**. *Diagn Cytopathol* 1993, 9:145–150.

22.   Kinsey W, Coghill SB: **A Case of Pilomatrixoma Misdiagnosed as Squamous Cell Carcinoma**. *Cytopathology* 1993, 4:167–171.

Ira C. Davis, MD, 1365 York Avenue, Apartment 8M, New York, NY 10021, USA.

Barry Leshin, MD, Dermatology Department, Wake Forest University Medical Center, Department of Dermatology, Medical Center Boulevard, Winston-Salem, NC 27157, USA.

Diagnostic and therapeutic surgical interventions in pediatric dermatology

Elaine C. Siegfried, MD

St. Louis University Health Sciences Center, St. Louis, Missouri, USA

Although surgical intervention is required less often in pediatric than adult dermatology patients, several aspects of dermatologic surgery in children deserve special consideration. This article defines absolute and relative indications for cold-steel and laser surgery in pediatric patients. Technical issues are also discussed, including aspects of wound healing and wound care unique to infants and children, practical considerations for performing potentially painful or frightening procedures in different age groups, and important details about pharmacologic sedation in children.

Current Opinion in Dermatology 1995:142–154

Pediatricians are well aware that children are not merely "small adults." Their presentation and variety of diseases, range of treatment options, and responses to medical management are unique [1]. The decision to intervene surgically is usually more difficult for children than adults, because fear, pain, and lifelong scarring are of relatively greater concern. Often, anxiety centered on a surgical approach will overshadow the clinical indication for an invasive procedure. Children are almost always opposed to the procedure, while parents may be biased for or against it. Unrecognized, this emotional overlay can influence a physician's perception of the medical problem, prompting a more or less aggressive course of action. The following guidelines were designed to separate surgical from emotional issues and provide practical suggestions for successful pediatric dermatologic surgery.

Indications for surgery

The most common dermatologic surgical procedures in children are cold steel and laser. Each modality has unique indications and offers unique advantages. Cold steel is used diagnostically, most commonly for skin biopsy, and therapeutically for excision. Laser ablation offers the advantage of selective therapeutic tissue destruction with minimal risk of scarring, but it cannot provide the diagnostic information essential for certain types of lesions. There are widely accepted, absolute indications for each modality, as well as relative indications.

Diagnostic skin biopsy

In many cases, the clinical appearance of a skin lesion may be ambiguous or misleading. A recent prospective study assessed 134 adults with facial cutaneous lesions who underwent surgical excision with margins and complex repairs planned on the basis of clinical judgment alone. Twenty-one percent of the preoperative diagnoses were incorrect, resulting in poor surgical planning [2]. In infants and children, clinical diagnosis may be more difficult. Several common problems prompt diagnostic skin biopsies prior to definitive therapy. For example, it may be impossible to clinically distinguish a plexiform neurofibroma from a smooth muscle hamartoma, a lightly pigmented congenital nevus, or a café au lait macule in a neonate (Fig. 1). Appropriate management for each lesion is very different. Although a biopsy of the anogenital area is emotionally and physically uncomfortable in children, skin and mucosal changes in the area often warrant it. Anogenital vitiligo, steroid atrophy, and lichen sclerosis may also be clinically indistinguishable (Fig. 2). If vulvar lesions are purpuric, eroded, or hypopigmented, then contact dermatitis, bullous pemphigoid, and sexual abuse must also be added to the differential diagnosis [3]. Other clinically confusing anogenital lesions are those associated with condyloma acuminatum and agminated molluscum (Fig. 3). Both of these infections may be acquired innocently or through sexual abuse, and accurate diagnosis is essential for appropriate referral and treatment [4–6]. Careful inspection for isolated primary lesions may help the physician to avoid biopsy, and it is especially important for children who may be victims of abuse. Occasionally, it may be impossible to distinguish a Spitz nevus from a pilomatricoma, juvenile xanthogranuloma, or pyogenic granuloma. If the lesion is too large to remove by punch biopsy, a diagnostic biopsy is indicated to plan appropriate therapy.

Ichthyoses may not be clinically distinguishable during the first few years of life or at initial presentation. Often, ascertaining the family history will help to verify the diagnosis, but a biopsy can be definitive for several types of ichthyoses. Light microscopy alone can distinguish among ichthyosis vulgaris, lamellar ichthyosis, and epidermolytic hyperkeratosis. Tissue must be appropriately processed to differentiate other types, based on biochemical defects [7]. Light microscopy is not valuable in differentiating among the abnormalities that cause the collodion baby phenotype. If the family history does not help, biopsy should be postponed for at least 6 months in these infants, so that a more directed laboratory assessment may be performed.

Diffuse alopecias are another diagnostically challenging group of disorders that present in childhood. The differential diagnosis includes telogen effluvium, tinea capitis, traction alopecia trichotillomania, and alopecia areata [8]. A deep punch biopsy through the subcutaneous layer is often essential for accurate diagnosis. In addition to routine vertical sections, horizontal sections of these specimens provide valuable diagnostic information when interpreted by a dermatopathologist experienced in the technique [9,10].

Blistering disorders can also be clinically confusing, especially in neonates. The timely recognition of acute, potentially life-threatening, treatable conditions such as herpes simplex, staphylococcal scalded skin syndrome, and toxic epidermal necrolysis is imperative [11]. Superficial skin samples may be obtained for immediate microscopic analysis by scraping, but if history, physical examination, and initial laboratory evaluation are not diagnostic, skin biopsy is essential. Appropriate tests include light microscopy and bacterial, fungal, and viral cultures. Immunofluorescent mapping or electron microscopy is indicated if epidermolysis bullosa is suspected.

Congenital midline masses are a distinct group of diagnostically and therapeutically challenging conditions. These abnormalities are located deep in the dermis and occur at the cranial or caudal midline. Some of the lesions mark an underlying central nervous system anomaly or even an intracranial connection [12•]. The differential diagnosis includes lesions that occasionally occur in the midline by serendipity; hemangioma is the most common. Vascular malformations, hair tufts, dimples and lipomas may also occur at the cranial or caudal midline and can mark underlying central nervous system anomalies [12•,13–15]. A midline mass in the nasal area may represent a dermoid, encephalocele, or glioma [16]. Occipital lesions include aplasia cutis congenita, encephalocele, or heterotopic brain tissue [17]. A biopsy of an occipital midline mass should not be performed unless an imaging study has been obtained to clarify the nature of the lesion. If the possibility of an intracranial connection exists, the patient should be referred to a neurosurgeon.

Therapeutic excision

For several dermatologic conditions in children, a surgical approach is first line therapy. Although each of these conditions is uncommon, vigilance and a high degree of suspicion are important when monitoring these children.

Most primary cutaneous malignancies are treated by therapeutic excision. Skin cancers are rare prior to adulthood, occurring only in 0.14% of pediatric dermatology patients [18•]. Primary cutaneous tumors are seen more often than cutaneous metastases. The most frequently reported cutaneous malignant tumors in children are unlike those seen in the adult population. In the largest series reported, 53 tumors were diagnosed during a 22-year period at a large pediatric tertiary care center. Primary rhabdomyosarcoma was the most frequent tumor (25%), followed by primary and metastatic lymphomas (19%), basal cell carcinomas (13%), and leukemia (13%), and metastatic neuroblastoma (10%). Melanoma in childhood is rare, but *de novo* tumors probably occur more often than those associated with congenital nevi [19]. Mortality associated with malignant skin tumors in children is high and is often related to late recognition [18•]. The need for caution and prudent use of excisional surgery is therefore evident.

Multiple primary skin cancers are expected in children with such cancer-prone genodermatoses as basal cell nevus syndrome, xeroderma pigmentosum, Bazex syndrome, Rombo's syndrome, Rothmund-Thomson syndrome, oculocutaneous albinism, and epidermolysis bullosa dystrophica [20,21]. Children who have received therapeutic irradiation for systemic malignancies are another group at risk for developing skin cancers after an interval as short as 8 years [22,23]. In contrast, children who have received chemotherapy have a higher number of nevocellular nevi than their healthy siblings, but a higher incidence of skin cancers has not been reported for them [24]. Surgical excision of individual tumors is used routinely to control rapidly enlarging or symptomatic lesions on children with cancer-prone conditions. Aggressive surgery can be severely disfiguring, however, and must be considered carefully for slowly growing, asymptomatic tumors, especially those on the face. Nonsurgical approaches are also important, including prophylactic avoidance of sunlight and radiation. Oral retinoids have been used to control tumor growth in patients with xeroderma pigmentation and basal cell nevus system [25–27].

Other skin lesions predisposed to tumorigenesis are nevus sebaceus of Jadassohn and congenital nevocellular nevi. Routine prophylactic surgical excision for these conditions is a matter of controversy. Tumor nodules arising within either type of birthmark may be benign or malignant but they should always be sampled for histologic examination. Subclinical basal cell carcinoma has been reported in nevus sebaceus as early as age 8 years [28]. Other malignant neoplasms have also been reported in association with nevus sebaceus, including squamous cell carcinoma, apocrine carcinoma, and adnexal carcinoma. Benign neoplasms more commonly arise within these birthmarks, eg, syringocystadenoma papilliferum, keratoacanthoma, hidradenomas, apocrine cystadenoma, syringoma, sebaceous epithelioma, trichilemmoma, and hidrocystoma [21].

Giant congenital nevi are rare, occurring in one of 20,000 neonates. The lifetime incidence of malignant melanoma arising within giant congenital nevi is 5% with a bimodal distribution; peaks occur prior to age 3

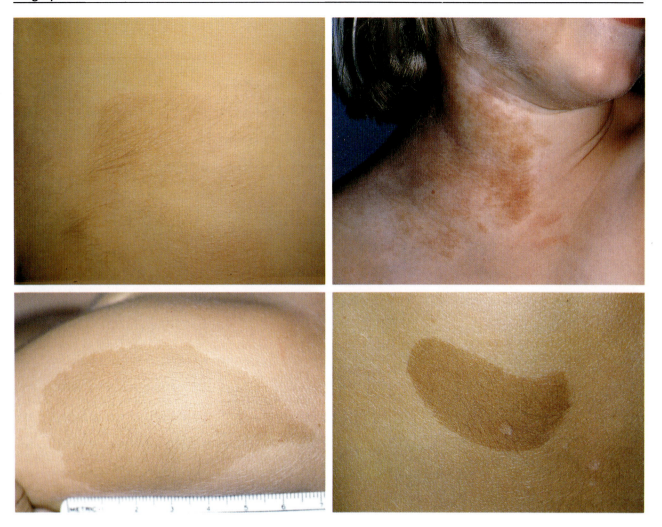

Fig. 1. It may be difficult to distinguish clinically between a smooth muscle hamartoma (*top left panel*), plexiform neurofibroma (*top right panel*), congenital nevus (*bottom left panel*), and café au lait macule (*bottom right panel*), especially in a neonate. The management of each of these lesions is different.

years and again after puberty [1]. Small congenital nevi are, by definition, nevocellular tumors measuring less than 1.5 cm in diameter present at birth or arising before age 2 years. These lesions are common, occurring in 1% of white and 2% of black children. The incidence of malignant transformation in small congenital nevi is unknown. Asymptomatic, stable congenital nevi and nevus sebaceus may be excised electively or monitored for change. Other surgical modalities, including dermabrasion, curettage, and selective laser ablation have been used [29,30]. These modalities do not allow histologic examination of the tissue and should be reserved for locations where excisional surgery would result in severe disfigurement or functional impairment. Elective excision of these lesions is easiest, safest, and most cost-effective when the patient is old enough to tolerate the procedure under local anesthesia. However, hypertrophic scars and widened "scar spread" are common in children [31]. The reasons for this are unclear; intrinsic factors (*see* "Wound healing") as well as difficulty with wound care probably contribute to the problem in active, growing children and adolescents. Early infancy may be an optimal time to remove birthmarks,

especially those located on the scalp. During the first 2 months of life, hair is sparse, and the scalp is relatively slack, minimizing closing tension and the need for undermining. The patient has no anxiety or fear, local anesthesia is well tolerated, and excision can often be performed when the patient is asleep. Wound care is relatively uncomplicated, because young infants have limited mobility, and healing is surprisingly rapid.

Surgical excision is also indicated for several benign cutaneous lesions that do not resolve spontaneously and are prone to bleeding, drainage, or ulceration. Often, the clinical appearance is diagnostic. In these cases, excisional surgery with appropriate margins can be performed without prior biopsy. Examples include typical pilomatrixoma, keratoacanthoma, Spitz nevus, and pyogenic granuloma. A patient's age and level of maturity, as well as the size and location of the lesion, dictate the need for anesthesia and sedation. Office-based excision under local anesthesia can be reliably performed for non-facial lesions less than one centimeter in small infants and most children over five years of age (*see* "Sedation in an office setting").

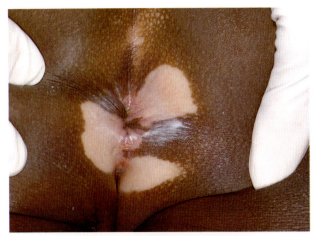

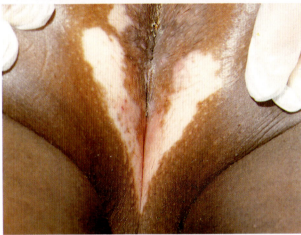

Fig. 2. Anogenital vitiligo (*top panel*) and lichen sclerosis (*bottom panel*) may be clinically indistinguishable, and a biopsy is required to confirm the diagnosis.

Lasers

The rapid evolution of laser surgery has been both miraculous and risky for children. Early, overly enthusiastic use of the continuous-wave argon laser to treat port wine stains caused a high incidence of scarring and permanent pigment change in children [32•]. The design and development of more selective laser systems has greatly improved the clinical outcomes and decreased the cutaneous risk [33]. However, many new lasers are being marketed and used to treat a variety of skin lesions in children, despite the paucity of clinical experience and published data. Uncertainty remains about the short-term and long-term benefits of these treatments. The availability and cost of laser treatment are controversial issues [34••], as is the need for sedation or anesthesia, with their additional risks [35].

In 1986, the yellow-light pulsed dye laser was approved by the US Food and Drug Administration for the treatment of nevus flammeus, as early as the neonatal period. The copper vapor laser and the argon pumped tunable dye laser are also yellow-light lasers. Most of the published data on laser treatment of port wine stains in children are from studies of the pulsed-

dye laser. Children require an average of four or five pulsed-dye laser treatments for maximum lightening. The best results have been seen in children under 4 years old. In this age group, 20% can expect 95% clearing [36]. Pulsed-dye laser therapy is less effective for facial port wine stains that are close to midline or those on the extremities [37,38]. Although remarkable improvement of laser-treated port wine stains has been reported, none of the currently available lasers is capable of erasing port wine stains in the majority of patients. Important unanswered questions remain: How long should treatment continue when complete resolution is not achieved? Does early laser therapy prevent subsequent soft-tissue hypertrophy? What constitutes the "ideal" laser system?

Yellow lasers deliver a beam with wavelengths that range from 570 to 590 nm, which corresponds to the second peak of the oxyhemoglobin absorption spectrum. Longer wavelengths allow maximum penetration to aberrant blood vessels in the dermis with relatively less interference from melanin. The systems also vary in emission patterns; irradiance, spot size, and pulse duration further influence the efficacy and adverse effects of laser therapy [39•]. The shorter, 360 to 450 μs (10^{-6} second) pulses delivered by the pulsed-dye laser are believed to cause selective microvaporization of smaller vessels, such as normal capillaries, and of the majority of proliferative vessels in the uniformly pink, macular juvenile port wine stains. The immediate clinical effect is purpura. The other yellow lasers, when coupled with automatic scanners, emit chopped pulses of 20 to 200 ms (10^{-3} second), 60 to 100 times longer than those of the pulsed-dye system. Longer pulses with higher fluences are believed to cause a less selective microcoagulation of larger, ectatic blood vessels and surrounding tissue. The immediate clinical effect is blanching [39•]. These lasers are more effective for telangiectasias and mature port wine stains [40]. The optimal exposure time for treating ectatic vessels is 1 to 10 ms [41]. None of the currently available lasers can deliver a pulse of this duration with adequate power to selectively destroy the majority of these vessels in one treatment.

The range of skin conditions that may benefit from yellow-light laser therapy is expanding rapidly to include a variety of skin lesions with vascular components, including nevus araneus, lymphangioma circumscriptum, pyogenic granuloma, scars, lichen sclerosis, papillomatous epidermal nevi, and verruca vulgaris [1,42–45]. Infantile hemangiomas have been treated with yellow lasers in a variety of ways. Early treatment will prevent growth of the superficial, but not of the deep, component of proliferating hemangiomas [46–48]. Later treatment of persistent hemangiomas may hasten or ensure resolution (M. Waner, Personal communication). The pain associated with ulceration is immediately relieved following laser treatment, and healing may be hastened [32•,47]. Laser treatment of hemangiomas remains a controversial subject; this form of therapy should be reserved for patients for whom more conservative therapy has failed (Fig. 4). The magnitude of growth of these lesions, the timing

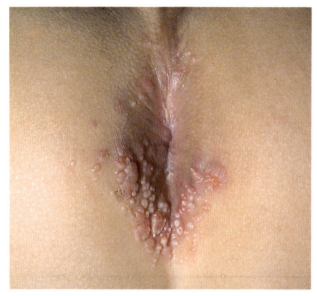

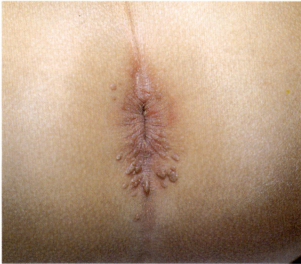

Fig. 3. Agminated perianal molluscum (*top panel*) may mimic perianal condyloma (*bottom panel*).

of involution, and the severity of sequelae are variable and unpredictable. Large, prospective, controlled studies are necessary to determine the true efficacy of laser treatment of hemangiomas.

Green-light lasers, such as the argon (514 nm) and the frequency-doubled (532 nm), emit beams in the range of the first peak oxyhemoglobin absorption spectrum, with relatively greater competitive absorption by melanin. These lasers have been used to treat vascular as well as pigmented lesions [39•]. Several other lasers have been used to treat a variety of benign pigmented lesions, including the 511-nm copper vapor, the 694-nm ruby, the 1064-nm neodymium:yttrium-aluminum-garnet, and the 510-nm pulsed dye systems. Published data on the use and the short-term outcomes of these treatments have been limited, especially in children. Much controversy surrounds laser therapy of the two most important pigmented lesions of childhood: café au lait macules and congenital nevi. Laser

treatment will cause café au lait macules to fade [49], but anecdotal reports suggest that there is a high incidence of recurrence. A small percentage of patients with congenital nevocellular nevi are at risk of developing malignant melanoma. It is not known how laser therapy will alter this risk; small numbers of patients have been treated, often with disappointing results [30]. Many more data are needed before laser treatment of these lesions can be recommended.

The CO_2 laser, with a wavelength of 10,600 nm (far infrared), causes nonspecific thermal damage to its target tissues. It is useful for vaporizing several superficial skin lesions in children, including recalcitrant, symptomatic condylomata acuminata, hyperkeratotic epidermal nevi, [50] and extensive, immature nevus sebaceus [51]. However, severe scarring can result from CO_2 laser surgery. The proper output parameters will minimize damage to surrounding tissue. Postsurgical wound care is equally important. Glabrous skin is most easily cared for with bioocclusive dressings (see "Postoperative wound care"). Children treated for anogenital condyloma deserve special postoperative consideration. Care is aimed at pain relief to maintain normal patterns of defecation and to prevent withholding of stool and development of anal stricture. Analgesics (*eg*, acetaminophen or ibuprofen) should be given liberally. Codeine may be used initially, but its usefulness should be weighed against its constipating effects. Frequent sitz baths are comforting and promote wound healing. A topical anesthetic, 1% pramoxine in zinc oxide ointment (*eg*, Anusol; Parke Davis, Morris Plains, NJ) can be applied as often as necessary. Plain zinc oxide ointment or white petrolatum should be applied following cleansing. Soft, formed bowel movements should be promoted at least daily. Often, dietary management with high-fiber foods will be sufficient. Some children will require additional bulk-forming agents such as psyllium, which is available in a palatable "cookie" form for children that should be taken only with adequate fluid. Stimulant laxatives and stool softeners are not recommended. They do not promote anal dilatation, and they can be habit-forming.

Technical and practical considerations

Wound healing

Mechanisms of wound healing evolve with age. Wounded skin in neonatal animals heals earlier and has a more complex collagen structure than mature skin [52]. Wounds can cause scars in some human infants [53], but prospective examination of sternotomy scars [54], and bacille Calmette-Guérin vaccinations [55] in children found a direct correlation between increasing age and more prominent scarring. Human fetal-skin wounds heal without scarring. This clinical observation, first made by surgeons pioneering antenatal diagnosis and treatment, has been followed by an explosion of experimental data elucidating the unique aspects of fetal wound healing [56–59]. Wound healing in the fetus differs from that of the adult by tissue environment, inflammatory response, and components of

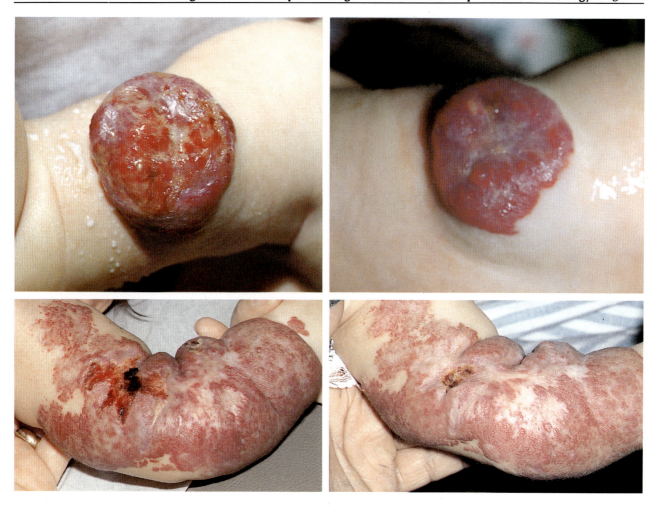

Fig. 4. Top left, Painful ulcerated hemangioma on the arm of a 1-month-old infant prior to treatment. **Top right**, Complete epithelialization after 6 weeks of wound care with hydrocolloid bioocclusive dressing. **Bottom left**, Painful ulcerated hemangioma on the arm of a 6-month-old infant. This lesion failed to improve after 1 month of wound care with hydrocolloid dressing. Immediately after pulsed dye laser therapy, an eschar formed, and the infant's agitation was dramatically reduced. **Bottom right**, Three weeks after laser therapy, the ulcer was healed.

the dermal extracellular matrix (Table 1). There are also defined differences between fetal and adult epidermal keratinization (Table 2) [60••], and although the fetus and newborn are growing rapidly, they have limited mobility and loose skin. These factors decrease wound tension simplify postoperative wound care, and probably contribute to the observed decrease in scarring [61]. In addition, infants do not require preoperative sedation (*see* "Sedation in an office setting"). For all these reasons, the early neonatal period is an optimal time to remove small congenital skin lesions and perform other uncomplicated surgical procedures.

The preoperative consultation

Ideally, the preoperative consultation is performed during a separate, initial visit, which allows time for parents to consider the details, risks, and benefits of the procedure and alternative forms of therapy before giving consent. Because anxious parents will hear and retain only a fraction of the information given in the clinic, a hand-written summary or preprinted handouts can be very helpful.

Plans for parental presence in the procedure room, conscious sedation, or anesthesia should be discussed at the preoperative visit. A delay before the scheduled procedure gives parents an opportunity to better evaluate their own and their child's emotional responses to help prepare for the experience. Based on this evaluation, plans can be modified as needed.

Approach to the pediatric patient

Unnecessary fear and discomfort should be avoided, but if an uncomfortable examination or procedure is necessary, it should not be omitted. In the past, the subject of pain control in infants and children was largely ignored. Recently, much more attention has been given to developing safe and effective strategies to minimize and control the apprehension, fear, and pain that destroy a child's cooperation. With the right combination of techniques, a wide range of procedures may be safely and comfortably performed on infants and children without the additional risks and expense of general anesthesia. Some of these techniques involve behavioral tactics suitable for children in spe-

Table 1. Comparison of fetal and adult wound repair

	Fetus (< 24 wk)	Adult
Tissue environment	Sterile Amniotic fluid rich in growth factors and hyaluronic acid Relative hypoxemia	Air
Inflammatory infiltrate	Limited Neutrophils and lymphocytes predominate	Macrophages predominate
Extracellular matrix	Hyaluronic acid Nonexcessive deposition of types III and V collagen organized into a reticular pattern	Abundant type I collagen deposited into disorganized bundles

cific age groups [62–64]. For children of all ages, a few guidelines are essential (Table 3). Verbal and nonverbal communication with the patient should be age-appropriate. In all cases, the goal is to gain trust. A physician should never lie to or threaten a child. "This won't hurt" is never germane before a painful maneuver. Demonstration is a valuable way to alleviate fear. For example, a puppet or doll can help a child know what to expect and what is expected of him or her [64,65]. Some children prefer to see a syringe and needle before an injection; others avoid looking. Asking a child his or her preference will enhance rapport. Consider using gentler techniques when they are just as effective as painful ones, eg, applying cantharidin to molluscum instead of freezing or curettage [66].

Table 2. Comparison of fetal and adult patterns of keratinization

Dermal area	Fetus (< 24 wk)	Adult
Basal layer	K5/K14	K5/K14
Intermediate cells	K1/K10 K4/K13	—
Periderm	K4/K13 K8/K18, K19	—
Stratum corneum	—	K1/K10

Parental attitudes and behavior can have a profound positive or negative effect on the ambience. Most dermatologic procedures can be done with parents present. Some parents and children prefer to be separated, however, and they should always be offered the option. For fast but uncomfortable procedures or anxious parents, returning the child to his or her care giver for solace after the fact may minimize a child's distress

Table 3. Age-appropriate interactions with children

Age	Age-appropriate behaviors	Interview and examination techniques	Procedure techniques
< 6 mo	Watches faces Dislikes sudden movements Poor short-term memory	Approach slowly Speak softly	Infants should be settled prior to the procedure Allow parents to hold and encourage them to talk or sing
6–16 mo	Stranger anxiety	Offer toys	Distract Encourage parents to maintain physical or eye contact
1.5–4 y	Seeks care givers and favorite objects for comfort Tantrums Magical thinking	Give directed attention Use simple language Provide a safe environment	Allow child to see and touch instruments Demonstrate Be truthful Look to parents for help with tantrums Give unconditional rewards
5–12 y	Fears physical harm and loss of control Coping strategies reflect past experiences Ability to reason Conscious of peer pressure	Speak to child Answer questions	Explain first Play preparation with dolls or models Allow choices Give positive reinforcement
Adolescent	Attempts self-control Seeks independence	Provide privacy Use open-ended questions	Expect temporary regression Encourage suggestions about how to manage pain and fear

[67]. A stable, supportive parent who prefers to remain with his or her child can often be a calming influence.

Unlike older children, infants have no and procedure-related anxiety or fear and are amnestic; therefore, uncomplicated procedures can usually be performed with local anesthesia alone. An infant or toddler may be held in the lap of his or her parent on the surgical table. Table, parent, patient, and physician must be comfortably and securely positioned to avoid a "moving target." Older children can be distracted with a favorite story, book, or song.

Physical strategies are also helpful, including application of heat, cold (*eg*, an ice pack, a chilled soft drink can, or fluoroethyl or ethyl chloride spray) [68,69], or vibration. Flexible, 0.5- to 1-inch 30-gauge siliconized needles should be used to administer local anesthesia. Pain from injection may be minimized by inserting the needle into a follicular orifice and delivering the volume in a slow, sustained fashion [70]. The hand used to hold the syringe must be supported on the patient, so that a sudden jerk will not disrupt the process.

There are also several improved pharmacologic approaches to local anesthesia. Commercially available lidocaine hydrochloride has a pH of 3.3 to 5.5. The acidic pH is responsible for the pain associated with infiltration [71]. This can be reduced by buffering 9 mL of 1% lidocaine with 1 mL of sodium bicarbonate (75 mg/mL) [72]. Warming the anesthetic solution to body temperature may also reduce the pain associated with local injection [73]. Eutectic mixture of local anesthetics (EMLA Cream; Astra Pharmaceutical Products, Westboro, MA) received the approval of the US Food and Drug Administration in 1993. A eutectic mixture is a unique combination of ingredients whose melting point is lower than the melting point of either chemical, alone which allows oil formation at room temperature. EMLA cream is an oil-in-water emulsion of lidocaine and prilocaine hydrochloride bases mixed in a ratio of one to one. Unlike other topical combinations, such as tetracaine, adrenaline, and cocaine [74], or either single anesthetic agent, the combination is effective on intact skin, especially after application under an occlusive dressing for 1 to 2 hours. It can reduce or eliminate the pain of curetting mollusca, visible-light laser treatments, or percutaneous injections [62,75].

Anesthetic agents have narrow margin of safety; the appropriate dosage for a child must always be calculated on a milligram-per-kilogram basis. The maximum recommended dosage of topical viscous or subcutaneously injected plain lidocaine is 3 mg/kg given every 2 to 3 hours. A 2% solution contains 20 mg/mL. For an infant weighing 5 kg, the maximum dose is only 0.75 mL. When epinephrine is added, local vasoconstriction will limit systemic absorption, and the dosage can be safely increased to 7 mg/kg. EMLA contains 25 mg/g prilocaine and an equal amount of lidocaine. The maximum recommended dose for an infant under 1 year of age is 2 g (less than half a tube). Methemoglobinemia is a rare adverse effect of prilocaine. EMLA is not recommended in pediatric patients at increased risk for this problem, *ie*, infants under 3 months of age or children receiving sulfonamides [76].

Despite all these tactics, fear of pain, especially from "shots," remains overwhelming in some children. Young children can safely be restrained and will calm down easily after they realize that the injection was not extremely uncomfortable. When older children become irrational, however, physical restraint will only exacerbate the problem. Sometimes a procedure must be rescheduled. Sedation or general anesthesia may be necessary.

Sedation in an office setting

A discussion of safe, effective alternatives for office sedation in children is a very important, evolving subject. Comparative data on the safety and efficacy of sedatives in children are limited. Pediatric responses to and risks of analgesics, anxiolytics, and anesthetics vary from those of adults. Children have increased oxygen requirements, with a resting oxygen consumption that is twice that of adults, coupled with decreased functional residual capacity and oxygen reserves. They also have a central respiratory drive that is less responsive to hypoxemia. When children are given sedative and anesthetic agents, these factors lead to a more rapid onset of hypoxia and a greater degree of respiratory depression. Children also have comparatively hyperreactive airway reflexes, with increased risk for laryngospasm. This tendency can be exacerbated by inadequate pain control in sedated patients.

The degree of cooperation required and the expected level of pain will define the necessary level of pharmacologic support. Conscious sedation causes drowsiness without loss of airway control. Deep sedation is needed for more invasive procedures. At this level, loss of respiratory drive and airway reflexes may occur unpredictably [77••]. Sedating antihistamines, such as hydroxyzine, can be used safely and sometimes successfully to achieve conscious sedation. Chloral hydrate is one of the most widely utilized sedatives, because it has a relatively wider margin of safety. Given orally, this drug is rapidly metabolized to trichloroethanol, which has pharmacologic effects similar to those of ethanol [78]. An appropriate starting dose is 75 mg/kg given 30 to 60 minutes before the procedure. If the child is not drowsy after 30 minutes, an additional 25 to 30 mg/kg may be given, with an absolute maximum total dose of 1 g. Responses to chloral hydrate are extremely variable. An idiosyncratic reaction to this and other sedatives is not uncommon in children who may experience agitation rather than drowsiness. In addition, the half-life of trichloroethanol can be as long as 40 hours. Prolonged drowsiness, requiring extended postoperative monitoring, can occur. Chronically administered chloral hydrate is carcinogenic in mice, raising concern about its use in humans [78]. However, epidemiologic data have not confirmed this risk.

Midazolam is a short-acting sedating benzodiazepine that has the added advantage of inducing amnesia [79]. It can be given orally or intranasally, 0.5 to 0.75 mg/kg, and the onset of action is rapid [80]. Sublingual or oral administration of the concentrated injectable solution (5 mg/mL) mixed in fruit juice concentrate or melted Popsicle juice is much more easily accomplished than intranasal administration. Respiratory depression can sometimes occur with the use of midazolam as a single agent.

Low-level (<50%) inhaled nitrous oxide is anxiolytic, sedating, and mildly analgesic. Given with at least 20% oxygen, it is extremely safe and has a rapid onset and recovery time; as a sole agent, it does not cause respiratory depression. In an uncooperative child, however, face-mask administration of nitrous oxide can be as challenging as anesthetic injection. For these difficult patients and up to 15% of the general population, a concentration of less than 50% nitrous oxide as a sole agent is less likely to be effective. Higher doses of nitrous oxide increase the risks of agitation, laryngospasm, and diffusion hypoxia [81]. Nitrous oxide has been widely used in children undergoing dental procedures, with an excellent safety profile, but when it is used in combination with narcotics, for deep sedation, there is a significant risk of cardiorespiratory depression. Portable nitrous oxide units cost $1000 to $2000, not including monitoring equipment. Specialized training is also important for physicians who plan to use this agent. Information on training courses can be obtained from the American Dental Association, (800) 621-8099, extension 2869.

Another cocktail that has been widely used for conscious and deep sedation consists of variable mixtures of meperidine hydrochloride, promethazine hydrochloride, and chlorpromazine given orally or intramuscularly. This combination is not optimal, with slow onset and long recovery time and life-threatening adverse reactions. These include respiratory depression, significant hypotension, lowered seizure threshold, and neuroleptic malignant syndrome [31]. Other regimens that have not been well studied or widely used in children include mild sedative-analgesic combinations such as hydroxyzine or codeine with acetaminophen, aspirin, ibuprofen, or ketorolac [82], and more deeply sedating anesthetic agents such as fentanyl, ketamine, and methohexital [83].

Specific guidelines for monitoring and management of pediatric patients under conscious and deep sedation have been defined [77••,84]. Normally healthy children or those with only mild systemic diseases are candidates for office sedation. Sedative medication should not be administered before the patient arrives at the health care facility. Presedation dietary precautions should be followed. The patient must be accompanied by a responsible care giver. The office must be furnished with equipment adequate to the management of emergency situations, such as a positive-pressure oxygen delivery system, suction apparatus, sphygmomanometer with pediatric cuffs, a pulse oximeter,

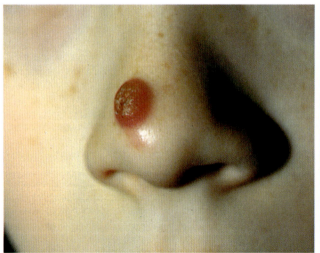
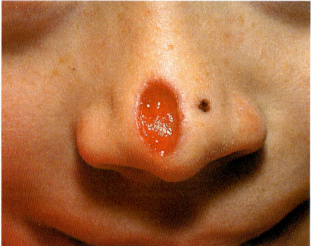
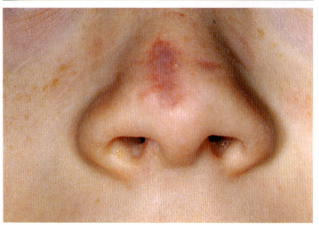

Fig. 5. Large, rapidly growing lesions on the nose of a 5-year-old child. **Top left,** The histopathology of a preliminary biopsy revealed a probable Spitz nevus with unusual features. The lesion was excised with 1-mm margins. **Top right,** The operative wound was allowed to heal by secondary intention, to simplify long-term monitoring. **Bottom,** Epithelialization was complete in 6 weeks.

and a crash cart. After the procedure, the patient must be observed in a suitably equipped facility.

General anesthesia, as supervised by trained personnel, is necessary when a procedure mandates deep sedation with loss of reflexes. There is a one-in-10,000 risk of mortality from general anesthesia in healthy children; the risk is somewhat increased in infants younger than 1 year old. This level of sedation is rarely needed for pediatric dermatologic procedures.

Wound closure

The usefulness of simple or rapid techniques of wound closure for pediatric excisions should be emphasized. Children are often more frightened of "stitches" than scalpels. Removal of nonabsorbable sutures can sometimes be more difficult than placement, especially for an anxious child who required preoperative sedation. For small wounds that are easily opposed, adhesive skin tapes (eg, Steristrips; 3M Health Care, St. Paul, MN) are acceptable. Their position can be secured and protected by a clear polyurethane dressing. In some cases, it may be beneficial to use absorbable suture for epidermal closure. Mild chronic gut, 5-0 or 6-0, will be absorbed within 2 weeks.

Increased tension on wound edges certainly contributes to poor scar quality. This problem is compounded in rapidly growing, active adolescent patients. Subcuticular sutures can reduce the problem. Selection of an absorbable suture with prolonged tensile strength, such as polydioxanone, may be an important factor in limiting scar spread. Whereas most absorbable suture has a 50% tensile strength after one week, polydioxanone retains a 50% tensile strength at 28 days. It must therefore be placed deep in the dermis. In a controlled study of surgical wounds closed under tension, the half closed with polyglycolic acid (Dexon; American Cyanamid Co., Wayne, NJ) healed with significantly wider scars than the half closed with polydioxanone [85].

Healing by secondary intention should be considered for surgical wounds in pediatric patients. The use of bioocclusive dressings greatly simplifies the care of these wounds, and the cosmetic results are often excellent (Fig. 5). Wounds located on concave surfaces heal especially well [86]. Lesions with ambiguous histology, or those at high risk for recurrence, such as unusual Spitz, congenital, or "dysplastic" nevi, may be more easily monitored after secondary intention healing; primary closure, flaps, or grafts might obscure regrowth.

Table 4. Properties of occlusive and semiocclusive wound dressings*

Dressing	Composition	Adhesiveness	Absorbency	Transparency
Polyurethane membranes Bioclusive (Johnson & Johnson, New Brunswick, NJ) Opsite (Smith & Nephew United, Largo, FL) Tegaderm (3M Health Care, St. Paul, MN) Acu-Derm (Acme United Corp., Fairfield, CT) Blister Film (Sherwood Medical Co., St. Louis, MO)	0.2-mm polyurethane with an adhesive backing	++	–	++
Hydrocolloids Duoderm (Convatec, Princeton, NJ) Comfeel (Coloplast, Tampa, FL) Cutinova Hydro (Beiersdorf, Norwalk, CT) Restore (Hollister, Libertyville, IL) J & J (Johnson & Johnson)	Carboxymethyl cellulose with an adhesive backing	+	+	–
Hydrogels Vigilon (Bard Home Health, Murray Hill, NJ) Second Skin (Spenco Medical Corp., Waco, TX) Nu-Gel (Johnson & Johnson) Clearsite (NDM Corp., Dayton, OH) Intrasite Gel (Smith & Nephew United)	Polyethylene oxide and saline gel sandwiched between polyethylene sheets	–	++	+
Alginates Sorbsan (Dow B. Hickham, Sugar Land, TX) Kaltostat (Calgon Vestal Laboratories, St. Louis, MO) Algosteril (Johnson & Johnson)	Alginic acid and mixed calcium and sodium salts	–	++++	–
Foams Lyofoam (Acme United Corp.) Cutinova Plus Foam Gel (Beiersdorf) Mitraflex (Calgon Vestal Laboratories) Epi-Lock (Calgon Vestal Laboratories)	Synthetic polymers and copolymers	–	++++++	–

*Adapted from Helfman *et al.* [91] and Falanga and Eaglstein [92]; with permission.
The *plus* and *minus* signs indicate the relative strength of each product with regard to each property.

Postoperative wound care

Traditional wound care consists of soaks, gentle debridement, topical antibiotic ointment, and dry gauze dressing changed three times a day. This method is inexpensive and utilizes readily available materials, but it is poorly tolerated by young children, disruptive to the wound bed, and very time-consuming. Bioocclusive dressing materials greatly simplify the process. They are impermeable to fluids, protect wounds from outside contamination, and allow accumulation of transudate, thus permitting autodebridement and enhancing reepithelialization [87,88]. They can be left in place for several days, which minimizes the pain and labor involved with traditional dressing changes. Bioocclusive dressings are appropriate for postsurgical, laser, or dermabrasion wounds. They can also be very helpful in the management of ulcerated hemangiomas (Fig. 4).

Each category of dressing material has unique properties with respect to adhesiveness, absorbency, and transparency (Table 4). These different properties are suitable for different kinds of wounds. Adhesive dressings (ie, polyurethanes and hydrocolloids) are easy to apply and remain secure for long periods of time. They are an excellent choice for punch biopsies and closed surgical wounds. Dressings with a capacity to absorb excess wound fluid (eg, foams, hydrocolloids, and especially calcium alginate) are appropriate for very transudative wounds such as open wounds allowed to heal by secondary intention. The absorptive capacity of hydrocolloid dressings can be augmented by supplementary use of absorbent granules or paste. Transparent dressings (ie, polyurethane and hydrogel) allow some visualization of the wound, although this is often obscured by exudate. Transparent, adhesive dressings are most cosmetically acceptable for use on the face.

Bioocclusive dressing materials have a few disadvantages. They may be expensive and difficult to obtain. Correct use requires special instructions. Care givers must be informed that accumulation of wound fluid is a normal, beneficial part of wound healing. The material accumulated under a bioocclusive dressing can be malodorous and appear purulent. This does not indicate infection without accompanying increases in redness, swelling, warmth, or tenderness.

Approach to scarring

Repeated local injection of corticosteroids is standard therapy for hypertrophic scars or keloids. This technique is inconvenient and poorly tolerated by children. A unique dressing containing silicone gel has recently been developed to prevent and treat hypertrophic scars [89]. Although its mechanism of action is unclear, it may work by generating and maintaining a field of static electricity from surface friction [92]. The dressing is applied and left in place for 12 to 24 hours a day, for a period of 2 to 7 months. It may be removed daily for cleansing. Compared with repeated injection of steroids, this treatment option is safe, painless, relatively cost-effective, and especially appropriate for children. Several variants of this prod-

uct are commercially available under the trade names Silastic (Dow Corning Corp., Midland, MI) and Morelle SOS (Pitt Enterprises, Queensbury, NY). Convenient, competitively priced products are Topigel (CUI Corp., Carpenteria, CA) and Epi-Derm (Biodermis, Las Vegas, NV). They are self-adherent, durable, and flexible.

References and recommended reading

Papers of particular interest, published within the annual period of review, have been highlighted as:
- •   Of special interest
- ••   Of outstanding interest

1.   Siegfried E: **Principles of Treatment.** In *Pediatric Dermatology*, edn 2. Edited by Schachner L, Hansen R. New York: Churchill Livingstone; 1994, in press.

2.   Smyth A: **A Prospective Study of 134 Consecutive Patients Requiring Diagnosis, Excision and Repair of a Facial Cutaneous Lesion.** *Br J Oral Maxillofac Surg* 1992, 30:157–160.

3.   Levine V, Sanchez M, Nestor M: **Localized Vulvar Pemphigoid in a Child Misdiagnosed as Sexual Abuse.** *Arch Dermatol* 1992, 128:804–806.

4.   Committee on Child Abuse and Neglect: **Guidelines for the Evaluation of Sexual Abuse of Children.** *Pediatrics* 1991, 87:254–260.

5.   Schachner L, Hankin D: **Correspondence.** *J Am Acad Dermatol* 1986, 14:848–849.

6.   Raimer S, Raimer B: **Family Violence, Child Abuse, and Anogenital Warts.** *Arch Dermatol* 1992, 128:842–844.

7.   Shwayder T, Ott F: **All About Ichthyosis.** *Pediatr Clin North Am* 1991, 38:835–857.

8.   Levy M: **Disorders of the Hair and Scalp in Children.** *Pediatr Clin North Am* 1991, 38:905–919.

9.   Headington J: **Transverse Microscopic Anatomy of the Human Scalp.** *Arch Dermatol* 1984, 120:449–456.

10.   Headington J: **Telogen Effluvium: New Concepts and Review.** *Arch Dermatol* 1993, 129:4;356–363.

11.   Frieden I: **Blisters and Pustules in the Newborn.** *Curr Probl Pediatr* 1989, 555–615.

12.   Martinez-Lage J, Capel A, Costa T, Perez-Espejo M, Poza M: **The Child With a Mass on Its Head: Diagnostic and Surgical Strategies.** *Childs Nerv Syst* 1992, 8:247–252.
• This article reviews the neurosurgical literature on 65 patients with scalp masses, including 30 midline lesions. The importance of both clinical and radiologic evaluation is stressed.

13.   Tavafoghi V, Ghandchi A, Hambrick G, Udverhelyi G: **Cutaneous Signs of Spinal Dysraphism.** *Arch Dermatol* 1978, 114:573–577.

14.   Hall D, Udvarhelyi G, Altman J: **Lumbosacral Skin Lesions as Markers of Occult Spinal Dysraphism.** *JAMA* 1981, 246:2606–2608.

15.   Hayashi T, Shyojima K, Honda E, Hashimoto T: **Lipoma of Corpus Callosum Associated With Frontoethmoidal Lipomeningocele: CT Findings.** *J Comput Assist Tomogr* 1984, 8:795–796.

16.   Paller A, Pensler J, Tomita T: **Nasal Midline Masses in Infants and Children.** *Arch Dermatol* 1991, 127:362–366.

17.   Commens C, Rogers M, Kan A: **Heterotrophic Brain Tissue Presenting as Bald Cysts With a Collar of Hypertrophic Hair.** *Arch Dermatol* 1989, 125:1253–1256.

18.   Orozco-Covarrubias M, Tamayo-Sanchez L, Duran-McKinster C, Ridaura C, Ruiz-Maldonado R: **Malignant Cutaneous Tumors in Children.** *J Am Acad Dermatol* 1994, 30:243–249.
• This is an analysis of all malignant cutaneous tumors seen at a major pediatric tertiary care center during a 20-year period.

19.   Mehregan A, Mehregan D: **Malignant Melanoma in Childhood.** *Cancer* 1993, 71:4096–4103.

20.   Goeteyn M, Geerts M, Kint A, Weert J: **The Bazex-Dupre-Christol Syndrome.** *Arch Dermatol* 1994, 130:337–342.

21.   Comstock J, Hansen R, Korc A: **Basal Cell Carcinoma in a 12-Year-Old Boy.** *Pediatrics* 1990, 86:460–463.

22.   Dinehart S, Anthony J, Pollack S: **Basal Cell Carcinoma in Young Patients After Irradiation for Childhood Malignancy.** *Med Pediatr Oncol* 1991, 19:508–510.

23. Whitmore S, Greer K: **Multiple Neck Papules in a Child With Acute Lymphocytic Leukemia: Multiple Basal Cell Carcinomas (BCCs).** *Arch Dermatol* 1990, 126:104–105.

24. DeWit P, DeVaan G, DeBoo T, Lemmens W, Rampen F: **Prevalence of Naevocytic Naevi After Chemotherapy for Childhood Cancer.** *Med Pediatr Oncol* 1990, 18:336–338.

25. Goldberg G, Hsu S, Alcalay J: **Effectiveness of Isotretinoin in Preventing the Appearance of Basal Cell Nevus Syndrome.** *J Am Acad Dermatol* 1989, 21:144–145.

26. Hodak E, Ginzburg A, David M, Sandbank M: **Etretinate Treatment of the Nevoid Basal Cell Carcinoma Syndrome: Therapeutic and Chemopreventive Effect.** *Int J Dermatol* 1987, 26:606–609.

27. Kraemer K, DiGiovanna J, Moshell A, Tarone R, Peck G: **Prevention of Skin Cancer in Xeroderma Pigmentosum With the Use of Oral Isotretinoin.** *N Engl J Med* 1988, 318:1633–1637.

28. Goldstein G, Whitaker D, Argenyi Z, Bardach J: **Basal Cell Carcinoma Arising in a Sebaceous Nevus During Childhood.** *J Am Acad Dermatol* 1989, 18:429–430.

29. DeMey A, Dupuis C, Lejeune F, Lejour M: **Neonatal Treatment of Giant Naevi.** *Dermatology* 1992, 185:300–301.

30. Scheeper J, Quaba A: **Clinical Experience With the PLDL-1 (Pigmented Lesion Dye Laser) in the Treatment of Pigmented Birthmarks: A Preliminary Report.** *Br J Plast Surg* 1993, 46:247–251.

31. Wheeland R: **Surgical Techniques.** In *Pediatric Dermatology,* edn 1. Edited by Schachner L, Hansen R. New York: Churchill Livingstone; 1988:209–264.

32. Geronemus R: **Pulsed Dye Laser Treatment of Vascular Lesions in**
• **Children.** *J Dermatol Surg Oncol* 1993, 19:303–310.
This paper reviews the indications for and details of pulsed dye laser treatment of vascular lesions in children. Port wine stains, telangiectases, and hemangiomas are discussed.

33. Nelson J: **Lasers: State of the Art in Dermatology.** *Dermatol Clin* 1993, 11:15–26.

34. Strauss R, Resnick S: **Pulsed Dye Laser Therapy for Port-Wine**
•• **Stains in Children: Psychosocial and Ethical Issues.** *J Pediatr* 1993, 122:505–510.
This is an editorial analysis providing historical perspectives and commentaries on pain control and anesthesia, rationale for treatment, expectations of care, equity, cost, and medical ethics.

35. Robinwitz L, Esterly N: **Anesthesia and/or Sedation for Pulsed Dye Laser Therapy.** *Pediatr Dermatol* 1992, 9:132–153.

36. Goldman M, Fitzpatrick R, Ruiz-Esparza J: **Treatment of Port-Wine Stains (Capillary Malformation) With the Flashlamp-Pumped Pulsed Dye Laser.** *J Pediatr* 1993, 122:71–77.

37. Renfro L, Geronemus R: **Anatomical Differences of Port-Wine Stains in Response to Treatment With the Pulsed Dye Laser.** *Arch Dermatol* 1993, 129:182–188.

38. Garden J, Bakus A: **Clinical Efficacy of the Pulsed Dye Laser in the Treatment of Vascular Lesions.** *J Dermatol Surg Oncol* 1993, 19:321–326.

39. Mordon S, Rotteleur G, Brunetaud J, Apfelberg D: **Rationale for Au-**
• **tomatic Scanners in Laser Treatment of Port Wine Stains.** *Lasers Surg Med* 1993, 13:113–123.
This overview of laser therapy includes an excellent discussion of basic skin optics, anatomic variations in port wine stains, and details of the microvaporization and coagulation laser treatment modalities.

40. Sheehan-Dare R: **Laser Treatment for Port Wine Stains.** *BMJ* 1993, 306:4–5.

41. Neumann R, Leonhartsberger H, Bohler-Sommeregger K, Knobler R, Kokoschka E, Hönigsmann H: **Results and Tissue Healing After Copper-Vapour Laser (at 578 nm) Treatment of Port Wine Stains and Facial Telangiectasias.** *Br J Dermatol* 1993, 128:306–312.

42. Glass A, Milgraum S: **Flashlamp-Pumped Pulsed Dye Laser Treatment for Pyogenic Granuloma.** *Cutis* 1992, 49:351–353.

43. Alster T, Kurban A, Grove G, Grove M, Tan O: **Alterations of Argon Laser-Induced Scars by the Pulsed Dye Laser.** *Lasers Surg Med* 1993, 13:368–373.

44. Tan O, Hurwitz R, Stafford T: **Pulsed Dye Laser Treatment of Recalcitrant Verrucae: A Preliminary Report.** *Lasers Surg Med* 1993, 13:127–137.

45. Rabinowitz L: **Lichen Sclerosus et Atrophicus Treatment With the 585-nm Flashlamp-Pumped Pulsed Dye Laser: Prospective Analysis.** *Arch Dermatol* 1993, 129:381–382.

46. Waner M: **Laser Photocoagulation of Superficial Proliferating Hemangiomas.** *J Derm Surg Oncol* 1994, 20:43–46.

47. Garden J, Bakus A, Paller A: **Treatment of Cutaneous Hemangiomas by the Flashlamp-Pumped Pulsed Dye Laser: Prospective Analysis.** *J Pediatr* 1992, 120:555–560.

48. Ashinoff R, Geronemus R: **Failure of the Flashlamp-Pumped Pulsed Dye Laser to Prevent Progression to Deep Hemangioma.** *Pediatr Dermatol* 1993, 10:77–80.

49. Fitzpatrick R, Goldman M, Ruiz-Esparza J: **Laser Treatment of Benign Pigmented Epidermal Lesions Using a 300 Nsecond Pulse and 510 nm Wavelength.** *J Dermatol Surg Oncol* 1993, 19:341–347.

50. Hohenleutner U, Landthaler M: **Laser Therapy of Verrucous Epidermal Naevi.** *Clin Exp Dermatol* 1993, 18:124–127.

51. Ashinoff R: **Linear Nevus Sebaceus of Jadassohn Treated With the Carbon Dioxide Laser.** *Pediatr Dermatol* 1993, 10:189–191.

52. Adzick N, Harrison M, Beckstead J, Villa R, Scheuenstuhl H, Goodson W: **Comparison of Fetal, Newborn, and Adult Wound Healing by Histologic, Enzyme-Histochemical, and Hydroxyproline Determinations.** *J Pediatr Surg* 1985, 20:315–319.

53. Den Ouden AL, Berger HM, Ruys JH: **Scarring of the Hands Resulting From Venipunctures in Babies.** *Eur J Pediatr* 1986, 145:58–59.

54. Lista FR, Thomson HG: **The Fate of Sternotomy Scars in Children.** *Plast Reconstr Surg* 1988, 81:35–39.

55. Sivarajah N, Jegatheesan J, Gnananathan V: **BCG Vaccinations and Development of a Scar.** *Ceylon Med J* 1990, 36:75–77.

56. Dostal G, Gamelli R: **Fetal Wound Healing.** *Surg Gynecol Obstet* 1993, 176:299–306.

57. Mast B, Diegelmann R, Krummel T, Cohen I: **Scarless Wound Healing in the Mammalian Fetus.** *Surg Gynecol Obstet* 1992, 174:441–451.

58. Longaker M, Adzick N: **The Biology of Fetal Wound Healing: A Review.** *Plast Reconstr Surg* 1991, 87:788–798.

59. Bleacher J, Adolph V, Dillon P, Krummel T: **Fetal Tissue Repair and Wound Healing.** *Dermatol Clin* 1993, 11:677–683.

60. Smack D, Korge B, James W: **Keratin and Keratinization.** *J Am Acad*
•• *Dermatol* 1994, 30:85–100.
An excellent review of recent information with a focus on the epithelial keratin polypeptides, keratin intermediate filaments, keratohyaline granule proteins, cell envelope proteins, "soft" keratinization, and disorders of keratinization.

61. Grinnell F: **Fibroblasts, Myofibroblasts, and Wound Contraction.** *J Cell Biol* 1994, 124:401–404.

62. Piedalue RJ, Millnes A: **An Overview of Non-pharmacological Pedodontic Behaviour Management Techniques for the General Practitioner.** *J Can Dent Assoc* 1990, 56:137–144.

63. Agency for Health Care Policy and Research: **Acute Pain Management in Infants, Children and Adolescents: Operative and Medical Procedures.** *Am Fam Physician* 1992, 46:469–479.

64. Zelter L, Altman A, Cohen D, Lebaron S, Munuksela L, Schechter N: **Report of the Subcommittee on the Management of Pain Associated With Procedures in Children With Cancer.** *Pediatrics* 1990, 86:826–831.

65. Rothman K, Nutile A, Appel C: **The Use of Dolls as a Teaching Aid for Children Undergoing Treatment With the Flashlamp-Pulsed Tunable Dye Laser.** *J Am Acad Dermatol* 1990, 22:854–855.

66. Epstein E: **Cantharidin Treatment of Molluscum Contagiosum.** *Acta Dermatol Venereol (Stockh)* 1989, 69:91–92.

67. Gonzalez JC, Routh DK, Saab PG, Armstrong FD, Shifman L, Guerra E, Fawcett N: **Effects of Parent Presence on Children's Reactions to Injections: Behavioral, Physiological, and Subjective Aspects.** *J Pediatr Psychol* 1989, 14:449–462.

68. Gedaly-Duff V, Burns C: **Reducing Children's Pain-Distress Associated With Injections Using Cold: A Pilot Study.** *J Am Acad Nurse Pract* 1992, 4:95–100.

69. Maikler V: **Effects of a Skin Refrigerant/Anesthetic and Age on the Pain Responses of an Infant Receiving Immunizations.** *Res Nurs Health* 1991, 14: 397–403.

70. Randle H: **Reducing the Pain of Local Anesthesia.** *Cutis* 1994, 53:167–170.

71. Bartfield J, Ford D, Homer P: **Buffered Versus Plain Lidocaine for Digital Nerve Blocks.** *Ann Emerg Med* 1993, 22:216–219.

72. Stewart JH, Cole G, Klein J: **Neutralized Lidocaine With Epinephrine for Local Anesthesia.** *J Dermatol Surg Oncol* 1989, 15:1081–1083.

73. Alonso PE, Perula LA, Rioja LF: **Pain-Temperature Relation in the Application of Local Anesthesia.** *Br J Plastic Surg* 1993, 46:76–78.

74. Bonadio W, Wagner V: **Adrenaline-Cocaine Gel Topical Anesthetic for Dermal Laceration Repair in Children.** *Ann Emerg Med* 1992, 21:1435–1438.

75. Tan O, Stafford T: **EMLA for Laser Treatment of Portwine Stains in Children.** *Lasers Surg Med* 1992, **12**:543–548.

76. Frayling IM, Addison GM, Chattergee K, Meaklin G: **Methaemoglobinaemia in Children Treated With Prilocainelignocaine Cream.** *BMJ* 1990, **301**:153–154.

77. Committee on Drugs: **Guidelines for Monitoring and Management of Pediatric Patients During and After Sedation for Diagnostic and Therapeutic Procedures.** *Pediatrics* 1992, **89**:1110–1115.
•• This paper details the updated recommendations from the American Academy of Pediatrics.

78. American Academy of Pediatrics Committee on Drugs and Committee on Environmental Health: **Use of Chloral Hydrate for Sedation in Children.** *Pediatrics* 1993, **92**:471–473.

79. Sievers TD, Yee JD, Foley ME, Blanding PJ, Berde CB: **Midazolam for Conscious Sedation During Pediatric Oncology Procedures: Safety and Recovery Parameters.** *Pediatrics* 1991, **88**:1172–1179.

80. Wilton NT, Leigh J, Rosen D, Pandit U: **Preanesthetic Sedation of Preschool Children Using Intranasal Midazolam.** *Anesthesiology* 1988, **69**:972–975.

81. Weber P, Weber M, Dzubow L: **Sedation for Dermatologic Surgery.** *J Am Acad Dermatol* 1989, **20**:815–826.

82. Cummings D, Amadio JR: **A Review of Selected Newer Nonsteroidal Anti-inflammatory Drugs.** *Am Fam Physician* 1994, 1197–1202.

83. Schwanda A, Freyer D, Sanfilippo D, Axtell R, Fahner J, Hackbarth R, Hassan N, Kopec J, Waskerwitz M: **Brief Unconscious Sedation for Painful Pediatric Oncology Procedures.** *Am J Pediatr Hematol Oncol* 1993, **15**:370–377.

84. Committee on Drugs: **Guidelines for the Elective Use of Conscious Sedation, Deep Sedation, and General Anesthesia in Pediatric Patients.** *Pediatrics* 1985, **76**:317–321.

85. Chantarasak N, Milner R: **A Comparison of Scar Quality in Wounds Closed Under Tension With PGA (Dexon) and Polydioxanone (PDS).** *Br J Plast Surg* 1989, **42**:687–691.

86. Zitelli J: **Wound Healing by Secondary Intention.** *J Am Acad Dermatol* 1983, **9**:407–415.

87. Reed B, Clark RF: **Cutaneous Tissue Repair: Practical Implications of Current Knowledge. II.** *J Am Acad Dermatol* 1985, **13**:919–941.

88. Misiani R, Bellayita T, Fenili D, Vicario O, Marchesi D, Sironi PL, Zilio P: **Interferon in Alpha 2a Therapy in Cryoglobulinemia Associated With Hepatitis C Virus.** *N Engl J Med* **330**:751–756.

89. Ahn S, Monafo W, Mustoe T: **Topical Silicone Gel for the Prevention and Treatment of Hypertrophic Scar.** *Arch Surg* 1991, **126**:499–504.

90. Hirschowitz B, Alimna Y, Har-Shai YE: **Silicone Occlusive Sheeting Is Recommended for the Treatment of Hypertrophic and Keloid Scars.** *Eur J Plast Surg* 1993, **16**:5–9.

91. Helfman T, Ovington L, Falanga V: **Occlusive Dressings and Wound Healing.** *Clin Dermatol* 1994, **12**:121–127.

92. Falanga V, Eaglstein WH: **Wound Healing: Practical Aspects.** *Progr Dermatol* 1988, **22**:1–10.

Elaine C. Siegfried, MD, St. Louis University Health Sciences Center, Division of Dermatology, 1402 South Grand Boulevard, St. Louis, MO 63104, USA.

Lasers in the treatment of vascular and pigmented cutaneous lesions

Suzanne Linsmeier Kilmer, MD

University of California, Davis Medical School, Sacramento, California, and Harvard Medical School, Boston, Massachusetts, USA

The use of lasers for cutaneous lesions has expanded rapidly since its inception in the early 1960s. The current focus is on refining the treatment of vascular and pigmented lesions with pulsed lasers and expanding the list of laser-responsive lesions. A review of the advances in cutaneous laser surgery during 1993 is presented.

Current Opinion in Dermatology 1995:155–161

Laser treatment of cutaneous lesions, initiated by Maiman [1] and Goldman et al. [2–4] in the 1960s, has expanded greatly in the past 30 years. The most remarkable growth has occurred in the past decade with the application of the principle of selective photothermolysis, described by Anderson and Parrish [5,6], which dramatically improved the efficacy and safety of dermatologic laser systems. Selective photothermolysis is accomplished by choosing an appropriate wavelength [7,8] and pulse duration [9,10] for a given target. Ideally, the wavelength should be preferentially absorbed by the intended target, and the pulse duration should be shorter than or equal to the target's thermal relaxation time, eg, the amount of time the target can absorb heat without dissipation to adjacent structures. Using this principle, it is possible to selectively target endogenous chromophores (ie, hemoglobin and melanin [Fig. 1]) [7,8,11–14], as well as exogenous chromophores (eg, tattoo inks) [15,16], with minimal potential for scarring.

Although pulsed lasers, with their inherent selectively and lower risk of scarring, are the preferred treatment modality in many cases, continuous-wave lasers remain an effective and inexpensive alternative. This article presents a review of the literature on cutaneous laser surgery published since January 1993, taking last year's section in Current Opinion in Dermatology [17] one year further. Several excellent review articles on laser treatment of cutaneous lesions were published in 1993 [18•,19••,20,21••].

Vascular lesions

The argon (wavelength 488 and 514 nm), copper vapor (511 and 578 nm), argon-pumped tunable dye, pulsed dye (577 to 585 nm), potassium titanylphosphate (532 nm), and frequency-doubled Q-switched neodymium:yttrium-aluminum-garnet (QS Nd:YAG) (532 nm) lasers all have wavelengths that are well absorbed by hemoglobin, but their pulse durations vary. To minimize thermal damage to the surrounding collagen, the optimal pulse duration for vessels ranges from 1 to 10 ms, depending on vessel size [5,6]. The flash-lamp pumped pulsed dye laser (PDL), continues to be the treatment of choice for pediatric and most adult port wine stains (PWSs) as its wavelength and pulse duration currently provide the best available combination for enhanced selectivity of vessels with minimal nonspecific thermal damage [5,8,9,18•,19••,20,21••,22–24,25•–29•,30,31••]. Melanin is a competing chromophore that may inhibit successful laser treatment of PWSs, if it is present in large quantities [32].

A recent study by Goldman et al. [27•] noted that PWSs in younger children (< 4 years old) were more likely to clear than those in older children (4 to 12 years old), and that lesions on the face, neck, and torso responded better than lesions on the arms or hands. Renfro and Geronemus [31••] also looked at the effect of anatomic location on treatment response with the PDL and found that midline lesions responded best to treatment and that centrofacial lesions and lesions in a V2 distribution responded less favorably. In a recent article, Strauss and Resnick [33] addressed psychosocial, ethical, and health policy issues with respect to PDL treatment of PWSs in children. Their interdisciplinary approach is helpful, and the need for pain management in these young patients is emphasized. Sherwood [34•] reported that use of a eutectic mixture of lidocaine and prilocaine (EMLA; Astra Pharmaceuticals, Westboro, MA) in children reduced mean pain scores 66% when compared with control subjects and noted pain-free treatments in 52% of the children.

Abbreviations

PDL—pulsed dye laser; **PLDL**—pigmented lesion dye laser; **PWS**—port wine stain;
QS Nd:YAG—Q-switched neodymium:yttrium-aluminum-garnet; **QSRL**—Q-switched ruby laser.

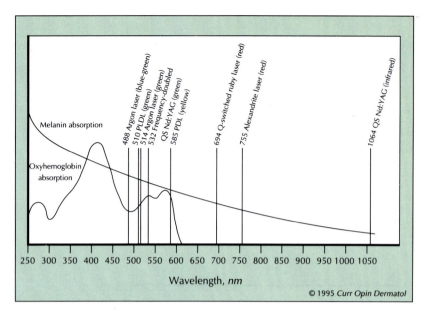

Fig. 1. Absorption spectrum for hemoglobin and melanin with respect to wavelength. Also shown are wavelengths of the lasers used in dermatology. PDL—pulsed dye laser; PLDL—pigmented lesion dye laser; QS Nd:YAG—Q-switched neodymium:yttrium-aluminum-garnet.

Several recent articles reviewed the use of continuous-wave lasers for the treatment of PWSs and other vascular lesions. McBurney [35•] elaborated on ways to enhance utility of the argon laser, and several others [36•,37,38•] commented on the varied uses of the copper vapor laser. Mordon et al. [39•] used argon (all lines), 532-nm, and 585-nm continuous wave lasers to treat PWSs. Immediate whitening, which is required for effective permanent blanching of the targeted vessel, correlated with a surface treatment temperature of 53°C, but the fluence threshold needed to achieve this temperature was lower at 532- and 585-nm wavelengths, for which hemoglobin absorption is stronger. Chilling the skin increased tolerance to thermal damage [39•]. Calcitonin gene–related peptide induced a long-lasting increase in blood flow in PWSs, according to Jernbeck and Malm [40•]; these areas often responded better to treatment, and results were achievable with lower energy levels.

The use of scanning devices with continuous-wave lasers can minimize laser-induced thermal damage [41•]. The Hexascan device (Lihtan Technologies, San Rafael, CA) in combination with a continuous-wave laser can treat PWS, with excellent results and no significant scarring, as noted by McDaniel [42•], Sheehan-Dare and Cotterill [37], and Apfelberg and Smoller [43•]. A comparison between the PDL and the argon-pumped tunable dye laser coupled to a robotized handpiece for treatment of facial telangiectasia demonstrated better clearing with the former but less bruising and fewer postinflammatory changes with the latter [44•].

The early treatment of proliferating hemangiomas remains controversial. Garden et al. [45••] performed a prospective analysis of the treatment of capillary and mixed hemangiomas with the PDL (wavelength 385 nm, pulse duration 360 to 400 μs) at 3- to 4-week intervals in infants ranging in age from 2 weeks to 7 months and concluded that this treatment may prevent enlargement and promote involution of these lesions. How-

ever, successful treatment of the capillary portion of the hemangioma does not preclude growth of the deeper component [46•].

It is of great interest that the reappearance of normal skin markings was noted by Alster et al. [47••] in argon laser–induced scars when patients were then treated with the PDL, suggesting that remodeling of scar tissue is possible with this laser. Also of great potential benefit is a preliminary report by Tan et al. [48•], who stated that 72% of recalcitrant verrucae cleared with PDL treatment, without generation of a potentially hazardous smoke plume. Other vascular entities that responded to various lasers include lichen sclerosis et atrophicus [49], blue rubber bleb nevus syndrome [50], angiokeratomas [51], and angiofibromas [52]. In contrast, a controlled, prospective study found that PDL offered only a short-term, cosmetic benefit for the treatment of Kaposi's sarcoma. Limited depth of penetration of the PDL's wavelength allowed recurrence of the lesion, and costly, long-term therapy would be necessary to maintain cosmetic improvement [53].

Pigmented lesions

Epidermal pigmented lesions are easy to treat with a variety of modalities including cryosurgery, curettage, topical agents, and now, with increasing frequency, laser surgery. The Q-switched ruby laser (QSRL), potassium titanylphosphate laser, pigmented lesion dye laser (PLDL), and frequency-doubled QS Nd:YAG laser all recently received the approval of the US Food and Drug Administration for the treatment of pigmented lesions. Many studies, including several recent ones [54,55,56•–58•,59,60•,61•,62,63,64•] have confirmed the efficacy of these lasers for the treatment of epidermal pigmented lesions, such as lentigines, ephelides, seborrheic keratosis, café au lait macules (Fig. 2), Becker's nevi, and postinflammatory hyperpigmentation. Similar findings are noted with the QSRL (694 nm) [54,61•], copper vapor laser (511,578 nm) [36•,42•,64•], argon laser (514 nm) [56•], and PLDL (510 nm, now frequently sold in combination with the Q-switched alexandrite [755 nm] laser) [57•,58•,59] for the treatment of benign epidermal pigmented lesions. The frequency-doubled QS Nd:YAG (532 nm) [60•] was recently proven to be similarly effective to the above lasers. Addition of a frequency-doubling crystal into the QS Nd:YAG laser reduces the wavelength by one half from 1064 to 532 nm, creating a visible green light that is well absorbed by melanin.

Dermal pigmented lesions are more difficult to treat successfully; the ability to insult the epidermis without residual scarring does not extend to the dermis. Melanin must be selectively targeted, yet the longer wavelengths required for increased depth of penetration are less well absorbed by melanin [7,8]. At 1064 nm, for instance, depth of penetration is good, but melanin absorption is lower, and much higher fluences are required for effective treatment. Nevus of Ota, a periorbital, deep, dermal nevocellular nevus occurring predominantly in Asians, was difficult to treat until the advent of Q-switched lasers. The QSRL has now been shown to remove these lesions effectively [62]. Postsclerotherapy hyperpigmentation has lightened with both the PLDL (50% of cases) [63] and the copper vapor laser (90% of cases) [64•]; serum ferritin levels may help predict the potential for postinflammatory hyperpigmentary changes [64•].

Tattoos

Tattoos, an exogenous source of dermal pigmentation, were previously considered to be permanent body markings because of the difficulty in removing them without significant scarring. In the past decade, we have progressed from gross tissue destruction to a more selective removal of tattoo inks by pulsed

lasers without scarring (Fig. 3). The QSRL (694 nm, 25 to 40 ns) [15,16,65•,66] was the only laser able to accomplish this until the recent introduction of the frequency-doubled QS Nd:YAG (532 and 1064 nm, 10 ns) [65•,67•,68•,69] and the Q-switched alexandrite (510 and 755 nm, 300 ns) lasers [70•]. The ink's absorption of the light from these three nanosecond-domain lasers leads to a large, rapid change in temperature, fracturing the ink particles. Because tattoos frequently have more than one color of ink, lasers that offer more than one wavelength enhance the ability of a particular system to remove different tattoo inks and may also offer the additional benefit of targeting melanin and hemoglobin.

The QSRL continues to treat professional and amateur tattoos successfully, especially when green, blue, and black inks are targeted [15,16,65•]. Medical and traumatic tattoos also clear quickly [66]. In a controlled, prospective study, Kilmer *et al.* [67•] demonstrated excellent removal of black ink with the 1064-nm QS Nd:YAG laser with minimal side effects. QSRL-resistant tattoos also responded, and pigmentary changes that had occurred during treatment with the QSRL improved during treatment with the QS Nd:YAG laser. To clear 95% of black tattoo ink, an average of four treatment sessions were needed. The frequency-doubled QS Nd:YAG laser (532 nm) produces a visible green light that is well absorbed by red pigments and has been shown to treat red-containing inks effectively [68•], sometimes with a single treatment.

The Q-switched alexandrite laser (510 and 755 nm, 300 ns) is similar to the QS Nd:YAG in that two wavelengths are available to target tattoo inks as well as melanin. Fitzpatrick *et al.* [70•] showed 755 nm to be effective for green, blue, and blue-black colors, whereas 510 nm will target melanin. Absorption spectra of these inks show the 510-nm wavelength to be promising for red ink [70•], as confirmed by Grekin [58•], and possibly for yellow ink. Again, side effects, including scarring, were rare.

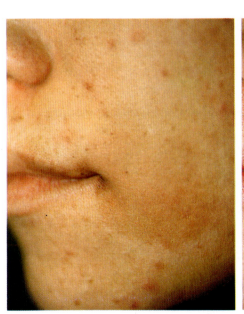 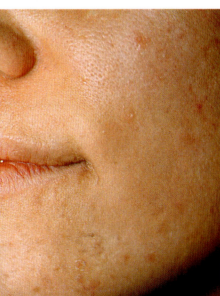

Fig. 2. Café au lait macule on the face of a 30-year-old woman shown before (*left panel*) and after (*right panel*) two treatments with the frequency-doubled Q-switched neodymium: yttrium- aluminum- garnet laser, which has a wavelength of 532 nm.

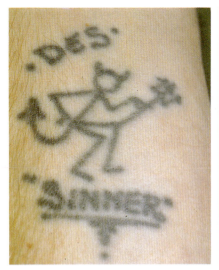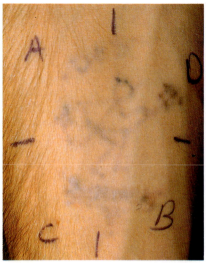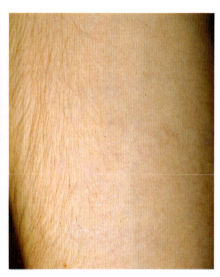

Fig. 3. Professional tattoo placed 15 years ago on the lower arm of a 36-year-old man. The tattoo is shown before treatment (*left panel*), after five treatments (*center panel*) with the Q-switched ruby laser (wavelength 694 nm), and after two treatments (*right panel*) with the Q-switched neodymium:yttrium-aluminum-garnet laser (1064 nm).

It is a matter of concern that pulsed and Q-switched lasers, with their high-intensity pulses, have been noted paradoxically to darken red, flesh, white, and brown inks to a slate-gray or black color. Repeated treatment usually removes the darkened ink, but test sites are recommended, because some inks can be quite recalcitrant to subsequent therapy [71•]. Another potential hazard of Q-switched lasers is their ability to produce fresh cutaneous debris, which may be potentially infective. For this reason, some type of "splatter shield" is needed [72•].

Carbon dioxide laser

An excellent review by Olbricht [73•] reintroduced us to the many uses for the CO_2 laser. Green *et al.* [74] demonstrated equivalent reepithelialization of pulsed CO_2 laser–ablated and dermatome-created wounds 1 week postoperatively; however, early phases of wound healing were delayed [75•]. In a separate study, Green *et al.* [76•] also showed that ablative lasers producing less than 160 ± 60 µm of thermal damage (pulsed CO_2 and excimer) allowed optimal skin graft take and healing. It is also of interest that the ultrashort, high-intensity, titanium-sapphire laser ablated *in vitro* rat skin to a depth of 0.1 µm per pulse, with damage contained within 0 to 30 µm of the adjacent tissue [77•]. This finding may prove helpful for epidermal ablation, perhaps for enhanced transepidermal drug delivery or surface recontouring, but the minimal thermal damage (less than 30 µm) is unlikely to seal blood vessels, and thus a bloodless environment would not be obtained.

Uses for the CO_2 laser continue to proliferate. Recalcitrant warts [78,79] continue to be one of the more frequently treated entities. In the past year, successful treatment of epidermal nevus [80•], linear nevus sebaceus of Jadassohn [81], porokeratosis of Mibelli [82],

and hemangioma-associated rhinophyma [83•] were reported. Malignant cutaneous tumors can be treated [84], and a European group reported effective treatment of nonnodal regional recurrence of cutaneous metastatic melanoma [85•] with the CO_2 laser.

Conclusions

The use of lasers for cutaneous lesions is on the rise. Vascular lesions can be treated with many lasers, but the PDL remains the laser of choice for PWSs. Use of scanning devices increases safety and versatility of several continuous-wave lasers. Greater availability of Q-switched lasers has enhanced our ability to treat pigmented lesions, especially tattoos. The CO_2 laser and other continuous-wave lasers continue to prove useful, and when they are coupled with a scanning device or used in a rapidly pulsed mode, safety and versatility are maximized. It is to be hoped that we shall continue to use good judgment to assess what is valid and useful and explore innovative techniques for laser treatment of cutaneous disorders.

References and recommended reading

Papers of particular interest, published within the annual period of review, have been highlighted as:
•   Of special interest
••   Of outstanding interest

1.   Maiman TH: **Stimulated Optical Radiation in Ruby.** *Nature* 1960, 187:493–494.

2.   Goldman L, Igelman JM, Richfield DF: **Impact of the Laser on Nevi and Melanomas.** *Arch Dermatol* 1964, 90:71–75.

3.   Goldman L, Hornby P, Meyer R: **Radiation From a Q-Switched Ruby Laser With a Total Output of 10 Megawatts on a Tattoo of a Man.** *Invest Dermatol* 1965, 44:69–71.

4.   Goldman L, Rockwell RJ, Meyer R, Otten R, Wilson RG, Kitzmiller KW: **Laser Treatment of Tattoos: A Preliminary Survey of Three Years' Clinical Experience.** *JAMA* 1967, 201:163–166.

5. Anderson RR, Parrish JA: **Microvasculature Can Be Selectively Damaged Using Dye Lasers: A Basic Theory and Experimental Evidence in Human Skin.** *Lasers Surg Med* 1981, 1:263–267.

6. Anderson RR, Parrish JA: **Selective Photothermolysis: Precise Microsurgery by Selective Absorption of Pulsed Irradiation.** *Science* 1983, 220:524–527.

7. Anderson RR, Margolis RJ, Watanabe S, Flotte TJ, Hruza GJ, Dover JS: **Selective Photothermolysis of Cutaneous Pigmentation by Q-switched Nd:YAG Laser Pulses at 1064, 532 and 355 nm.** *J Invest Dermatol* 1989, 93:28–32.

8. Sherwood KA, Murray S, Kurban AK, Tan OT: **Effect of Wavelength on Cutaneous Pigment Using Pulsed Irradiation.** *J Invest Dermatol* 1989, 92:717–720.

9. Garden JM, Tan OT, Kerschman R, Boll J, Furumoto H, Anderson RR, Parrish JA: **Effect of Dye Laser Pulse Duration on Selective Cutaneous Vascular Injury.** *J Invest Dermatol* 1986, 87:653–657.

10. Watanabe S, Flotte TJ, Margolis R, *et al.*: **The Effect of Pulse Duration on Selective Pigment Cell Injury by Dye Lasers [Abstract].** *J Invest Dermatol* 1987, 88:523.

11. Dover JS, Margolis RJ, Polla LL, Watanabe S, Hruza GJ, Parrish JA, Anderson RR: **Pigmented Guinea Pig Skin Irradiated With Q-switched Ruby Laser Pulses.** *Arch Dermatol* 1989, 125:43–49.

12. Hruza GJ, Dover JS, Flotte TJ, Goetschkes M, Watanabe S, Anderson RR: **Q-switched Ruby Laser Irradiation of Normal Skin: Histologic and Ultrastructural Findings.** *Arch Dermatol* 1991, 127:1799–1805.

13. Polla LL, Margolis RJ, Dover JS, Whitaker D, Murphy GF, Jacques SL, Anderson RR: **Melanosomes Are a Primary Target of Q-switched Ruby Laser Irradiation in Guinea Pig Skin.** *J Invest Dermatol* 1987, 89:281–286.

14. Murphy GF, Shepard RS, Paul BS, *et al.*: **Organelle-Specific Injury to Melanin-Containing Cells in Human Skin by Pulsed Laser Irradiation.** *Lab Invest* 1987, 49:680–685.

15. Reid WH, McLeod PJ, Ritchie A, Ferguson-Pell M: **Q-switched Ruby Laser Treatment of Black Tattoos.** *Br J Plast Surg* 1983, 36:455–459.

16. Taylor CR, Gange RW, Dover JS, Flotte TJ, Gonzalez E, Michaud N, Anderson RR: **Treatment of Tattoos by Q-switched Ruby Laser.** *Arch Dermatol* 1990, 126:893–899.

17. Kilmer SL: **Lasers in the Treatment of Vascular and Pigmented Cutaneous Lesions.** *Curr Opin Dermatol* 1994, 1:165–170.

18. Nelson JS: **Lasers: State of the Art in Dermatology.** *Dermatol Clin*
   • 1993, 11:15–26.
   Excellent discussion regarding the present use of cutaneous laser systems.

19. Dover JS, Kilmer SL, Anderson RR: **What's New in Cutaneous Laser**
   •• **Surgery.** *J Dermatol Surg Oncol* 1993, 19:295–298.
   Reviews the latest advances in dermatologic surgery and comments on future possibilities of diode lasers, photodynamic therapy, and laser diagnostics.

20. Sheehan-Dare RA, Cotterill JA: **Lasers in Dermatology.** *Br J Dermatol* 1993, 129:1–8.

21. Hruza GJ, Geronemus RG, Dover JS, Arndt KA: **Lasers in Dermatol-**
   •• **ogy: 1993.** *Arch Dermatol* 1993, 129:1026–1035.
   Excellent overview of the use of lasers in dermatology from its inception to current and possible future applications.

22. Ries WM: **Current Concepts in Cutaneous Laser Surgery.** *Facial Plast Surg* 1993, 9:58–67.

23. Tan OT, Sherwood K, Gilchrest BA: **Treatment of Children With Port-Wine Stains Using the Flash-Lamp Pulsed Tunable Dye Laser.** *N Engl J Med* 1989, 320:416–420.

24. Tan OT: **Lasers for Vascular Lesions in Pediatric Dermatology.** *Pediatr Dermatol* 1992, 9:358–360.

25. Garden JM, Bakus AD: **Clinical Efficacy of the Pulsed Dye Laser**
   • **in the Treatment of Vascular Lesions.** *J Dermatol Surg Oncol* 1993, 4:321–326.
   The PDL remains the laser of choice for treatment of PWSs and hemangiomas, especially in children.

26. Geronemus RG: **Pulsed Dye Laser Treatment of Vascular Lesions in**
   • **Children.** *J Dermatol Surg Oncol* 1993, 4:303–310.
   The PDL is the safest and most effective laser for treatment of PWSs. Multiple treatment sessions are usually required.

27. Goldman MP, Fitzpatrick RE, Ruiz-Esparza J: **Treatment of Port-Wine**
   • **Stains (Capillary Malformations) With the Flashlamp-Pumped Pulsed Dye Laser.** *J Pediatr* 1993, 122:71–77.
   Port wine stains in children under 4 years old respond better to treatment with the PDL than do those in children 4 to 12 years of age.

28. Wheeland RG: **Treatment of Port-Wine Stains for the 1990s.** *J Der-*
   • *matol Surg Oncol* 1993, 4:348–356.

29. Achauer BM, Vander-Kam VM: **Vascular Lesions.** *Clin Plast Surg*
   • 1993, 20:43–51.
   In children, early treatment of PWSs with the PDL is recommended.

30. Van Gemert MJC, Carruth JAS, Shakespeare PG: **Laser Treatment of Port Wine Stains: Newer Lasers Bring Better Treatments.** *BMJ* 1993, 306:4–5.

31. Renfro L, Geronemus RG: **Anatomical Differences of Port-Wine Stains**
   •• **in Response to Treatment With the Pulsed Dye Laser.** *Arch Dermatol* 1993, 129:182–188.
   The authors studied the effect of anatomic locations on treatment response with the PDL and found that the midline lesions responded best to treatment, and that centrofacial lesions and lesions in a V2 distribution respond less favorably.

32. Ashinoff R, Geronemus RG: **Treatment of a Port Wine Stain in a Black Patient With the Pulsed Dye Laser.** *J Dermatol Surg Oncol* 1992, 18:147–148.

33. Strauss RP, Resnick SD: **Pulsed Dye Laser Therapy for Port-Wine Stains in Children: Psychosocial and Ethical Issues.** *J Pediatr* 1993, 122:505–510.

34. Sherwood KA: **The Use of Topical Anesthesia in Removal of Port**
   • **Wine Stains in Children.** *J Pediatr* 1993, 122:S36–S40.
   EMLA (eutectic mixture of lidocaine and prilocaine) significantly reduced mean pain scores 66% when compared with control subjects. Pain-free treatments were noted in 52% of the cases.

35. McBurney EI: **Clinical Usefulness of the Argon Laser for the 1990s.**
   • *J Dermatol Surg Oncol* 1993, 4:358–362.
   The argon laser is an excellent choice for treatment of mature nodular PWSs, telangiectasia, small vascular lesions, and superficial pigmented lesions, when appropriate techniques are used.

36. Dinehart SM, Waner M, Flock S: **The Copper Vapor Laser for Treat-**
   • **ment of Cutaneous Vascular and Pigmented Lesions.** *J Dermatol Surg Oncol* 1993, 4:370–375.
   The copper vapor laser effectively treats vascular lesions (with a 578-nm wavelength) and pigmented lesions (with a 511-nm wavelength) and can be used in conjunction with a scanning device.

37. Sheehan-Dare RA, Cotterill JA: **Copper Vapor Laser Treatment of Port Wine Stains: Clinical Evaluation and Comparison With Conventional Argon Laser Therapy.** *Br J Dermatol* 1993, 128:546–549.

38. Neumann RA, Leonhartsberger H, Bohler-Sommeregger K, Knobler
   • R: **Results and Tissue Healing After Copper Vapor Laser (at 578 nm) Treatment of Port Wine Stains and Facial Telangiectasias.** *Br J Dermatol* 1993, 128:306–312.
   Fluences up to 12 J/cm² were vessel-selective, whereas fluences greater than or equal to 15 J/cm² resulted in nonselective coagulation necrosis, even though the theoretically correct wavelength (585 nm) was used.

39. Mordon S, Beacco C, Rotteleur G, Brunetaud JM: **Relation Between**
   • **Skin Surface Temperature and Minimal Blanching During Argon, Nd:YAG 532, and CW Dye 585 Laser Therapy of Port-Wine Stains.** *Lasers Surg Med* 1993, 13:124–126.
   Immediate whitening, required for effective treatment, correlated with a surface treatment temperature of 53°C. The fluence threshold to achieve this temperature was lower for 532- and 585-nm wavelengths, at which hemoglobin absorption is stronger.

40. Jernbeck J, Malm M: **Calcitonin Gene-Related Peptide Increases the**
   • **Blood Flow of Port-Wine Stains and Improves Continuous-Wave Dye Laser Treatment.** *Plast Reconstr Surg* 1993, 91:245–251.
   Calcitonin gene–related peptide induces a long-lasting increase in blood flow in PWS, these areas often had a better response to treatment, and the response was achievable with lower energy levels.

41. Mordon S, Rotteleur G, Brunetaud JM, Apfelberg DB: **Rationale for**
   • **Automatic Scanners in Laser Treatment of Port-Wine Stains.** *Lasers Surg Med* 1993, 13:113–123.
   Scanning devices can minimize laser-induced thermal damage, facilitate use, and optimize treatment of difficult areas.

42. McDaniel DH: **Clinical Usefulness of the Hexascan: Treatment of Cu-**
   • **taneous Vascular and Melanocytic Disorders.** *J Dermatol Surg Oncol* 1993, 4:312–319.
   The Hexascan increases the safety and potential uses of several continuous-wave lasers.

43. Apfelberg DB, Smoller B: **Preliminary Analysis of Histological Results**
   • **of Hexascan Device With Continuous Tunable Dye Laser at 514 (Argon) and 577 nm (Yellow).** *Lasers Surg Med* 1993, 13:106–112.
   Use of the Hexascan device with the tunable dye laser at 514 and 577 nm produced histologically similar results, ie, nearly normal-appearing skin with few residual vessels.

Although the PDL is the treatment of choice for PWSs, others including the argon, argon-pumped tunable dye, copper vapor, and potassium titanylphosphate lasers may be helpful, particularly if a scanner is used in conjunction with the continuous wave lasers.

44. Ross M, Watcher MA, Goodman MM: **Comparison of the Flashlamp-**
• **Pumped Pulsed Dye Laser With the Argon Tunable Dye Laser With Robotized Handpiece for Facial Telangiectasia.** *Lasers Surg Med* 1993, 13:374–378.
A comparison between the PDL and the argon-pumped tunable dye laser coupled to a robotized handpiece for treatment of facial telangiectasia demonstrated better clearing with the former (100% vs 47% had an excellent response) but less bruising and fewer postinflammatory changes with the latter.

45. Garden JM, Bakus AD, Pallor AS: **Treatment of Cutaneous Heman-**
•• **giomas by the Flashlamp-Pumped Pulsed Dye Laser: Prospective Analysis.** *J Pediatr* 1992, 120:555–560.
A prospective analysis of 33 capillary and mixed hemangiomas treated at 3- to 4-week intervals with the PDL in infants ranging in age from 2 weeks to 7 months concluded that treatment may prevent enlargement and promote involution.

46. Ashinoff R, Geronemus RG: **Failure of the Flashlamp-Pumped Pulsed**
• **Dye Laser to Prevent Progression to Deep Hemangioma.** *Pediatr Dermatol* 1993, 10:77–80.
The deeper component may enlarge in spite of clearing of the more superficial component when the PDL is used.

47. Alster TS, Kurban AK, Grove GL, Grove MJ, Tan OT: **Alteration of**
•• **Argon-Induced Scars by the Pulsed Dye Laser.** *Lasers Surg Med* 1993, 13:368–373.
Of great interest, reappearance of normal skin markings were noted in argon laser–induced scars when patients were subsequently treated with the PDL.

48. Tan OT, Hurwitz RM, Stafford TJ: **Pulsed Dye Laser Treatment of**
• **Recalcitrant Verrucae.** *Lasers Surg Med* 1993, 13:127–137.
Seventy-two percent of recalcitrant warts responded to PDL treatments, with the added advantage that no smoke plume was generated.

49. Rabinowitz LG: **Lichen Sclerosis et Atophicus: Treatment With the 585-nm Flashlamp-Pumped Pulsed Dye Laser.** *Arch Dermatol* 1993, 129:381–382.

50. Busund B, Stray-Pederson S, Iverson OH, Austad J: **Blue Rubber Bleb Nevus Syndrome With Manifestations in the Vulva.** *Acta Obstet Gynecol Scand* 1993, 4:310–313.

51. Lapins J, Emstestam L, Marcusson JA: **Angiokeratomas in Fabry's Disease and Fordyce's Disease: Successful Treatment With Copper Vapour Laser.** *Acta Derm Venereol (Stockh)* 1993, 73:133–135.

52. Kopera D: **Angiofibroma in Tuberous Sclerosis–Argon Laser.** *Int J Dermatol* 1993, 32:541–542.

53. Tappero JW, Grekin RC, Zanelli GA, Berger TG: **Pulsed-Dye Laser Therapy for Cutaneous Kaposi's Sarcoma Associated With Aquired Immunodeficiency Syndrome.** *J Am Acad Dermatol* 1992, 27:526–530.

54. Nelson JS, Applebaum: **Treatment of Superficial Cutaneous Lesions by Melanin-Specific Selective Photothermolysis Using the Q-switched Ruby Laser.** *Ann Plast Surg* 1992, 29:231–237.

55. Tan OT, Morelli JG, Kurban AK: **Pulsed Dye Laser Treatment of Benign Cutaneous Pigmented Lesions.** *Lasers Surg Med* 1992, 12:538–542.

56. Trelles MA, Verkruysse W, Pickering JW, Velez M, Sanchez J, Sala
• P: **Monoline Argon Laser (514 nm) Treatment of Benign Pigmented Lesions With Long Pulse Lengths.** *J Photochem Photobiol B* 1992, 16:357–365.
Using 1.5 W, 0.5-mm spot size, and pulse widths of 200 or 300 ms, researchers treated 620 cutaneous pigmented lesions successfully with little damage of adjacent structures histologically, normal pigmentation, and excellent cosmetic results.

57. Fitzpatrick RE, Goldman MP, Ruiz-Esparza J: **Treatment of Benign**
• **Pigmented Epidermal Lesions Using a 300 Nsecond Pulse and 510 nm Wavelength.** *J Dermatol Surg Oncol* 1993, 19:341–347.
Sixty-five patients with 492 pigmented lesions were treated with 50% complete clearing noted after a single treatment; the rest of the lesions cleared with subsequent treatments.

58. Grekin RC, Shelton RM, Geisse JK, Frieden I: **510 nm Pigmented**
• **Lesion Dye Laser: Its Characteristics and Clinical Uses.** *J Dermatol Surg Oncol* 1993, 19:380–387.
Facial and hand lentigines responded better than truncal or upper- and lower-extremity lesions. Café au lait macules responded inconsistently, those on the face responded best. Finally, red link cleared in three tattoos.

59. Day TW, Pardue CC: **Preliminary Experience With a Flashlamp-Pumped Tunable Dye Laser for Treatment of Benign Pigmented Lesions.** *Cutis* 1993, 51:188–190.

60. Kilmer SL, Wheeland RG, Goldberg DJ, Anderson RR: **Treatment**
• **of Epidermal Pigmented Lesions With the Frequency-Doubled Q-switched Nd:YAG Laser (532 nm): A Controlled, Dose-Response, Multi-center Trial.** *Arch Dermatol* 1993, in press.

A single treatment with the frequency-doubled QS Nd:YAG laser effectively treats most lentigines, as well as other benign epidermal pigmented lesions.

61. Goldberg DJ: **Benign Pigmented Lesions of the Skin: Treatment With**
• **the Q-switched Ruby Laser.** *J Dermatol Surg Oncol* 1993, 19:376–379.
The QSRL treats epidermal and dermal pigmented lesions.

62. Goldberg DJ, Nychay SG: **Q-switched Ruby Laser Treatment of Nevus of Ota.** *J Dermatol Surg Oncol* 1992, 18:817–821.

63. Goldman MP: **Postsclerotherapy Hyperpigmentation.** *J Dermatol Surg Oncol* 1992, 18:417–422.

64. Thibault P, Wlodarczyk J: **Postsclerotherapy Hyperpigmentation: The**
• **Role of Serum Ferritin Levels and the Effectiveness of Treatment With the Copper Vapor Laser.** *J Dermatol Surg Oncol* 1992, 18:47–52.
Postsclerotherapy hyperpigmentation lightened with the copper vapor laser in 90% of cases. Elevated serum ferritin levels correlated with increased chance for postinflammatory hyperpigmentary changes.

65. Kilmer SL, Anderson RR: **Clinical Use of the Q-switched Ruby (694**
• **nm) and the Q-switched Nd:YAG (532 and 1064 nm) Lasers for the Treatment of Tattoos.** *J Dermatol Surg Oncol* 1993, 19:330–338.
This overview of the treatment of tattoos with the QSRL and the QS Nd:YAG laser covers pretreatment expectations, anesthesia, treatment parameters, and intraoperative and postoperative courses.

66. Ashinoff R, Geronemus RG: **Rapid Response of Traumatic and Medical Tattoos to Treatment With the Q-switched Ruby Laser.** *Plast Reconstr Surg* 1993, 91:841–845.

67. Kilmer SL, Lee MS, Grevelink JM, Flotte TJ, Anderson RR: **Treat-**
• **ment of Tattoos With the Q-switched Nd:YAG (1064 nm) Laser: A Controlled, Dose-Response Study.** *Arch Dermatol* 1993, 129:971–978.
Controlled, dose-response study found that increasing fluences were more effective without an increase in side effects. QSRL-resistant tattoos responded to the 1064-nm wavelength, and the pigmentary changes initiated with QSRL treatment resolved during treatment with the QS Nd:YAG laser.

68. Kilmer SL, Lee MS, Anderson RR: **The Q-switched Nd:YAG Laser**
• **Effectively Treats Tattoos: A Controlled, Dose-Response Study.** *Lasers Surg Med* 1993, 5(suppl):54.
The frequency-doubled QS Nd:YAG laser (532 nm) most effectively treats red tattoo ink: the QSRL (694 nm) more effectively treats green ink. Yellow ink did not respond well to either wavelength. These results correlated with the individual ink's absorption spectrum.

69. Watts MT, Downes RN, Collin JR, Walker NP: **The Use of Q-switched Nd:YAG Laser for the Treatment of Permanent Eyeliner Tattoo.** *Ophthal Plast Reconstr Surg* 1992, 8:292–294.

70. Fitzpatrick RE, Goldman MP, Ruiz-Esparza: **Use of the Alexandrite**
• **Laser for Tattoo Pigment Removal in an Animal Model.** *J Am Acad Dermatol* 1993, 28:745–750.
The alexandrite laser was shown to be effective for the treatment of black, green, and blue tattoo pigments but minimally effective for red tattoo pigment.

71. Anderson RR, Geronemus RG, Kilmer SL, Farinelli W, Fitzpatrick RE:
• **Cosmetic Tattoo Ink Darkening: A Complication of Q-switched and Pulsed Laser Treatment.** *Arch Dermatol* 1993, 129:1010–1014.
Irreversible darkening of red, white, flesh-colored, and pink tattoo ink occurred with Q-switched and pulsed laser treatment. In most cases, subsequent laser treatment will remove the darkened ink. Test sites were recommended.

72. Kilmer SL, Casparian JC, Wimberly J, Anderson RR: **Hazards of Q-**
• **switched Lasers.** *Lasers Surg Med* 1993, 5(suppl):56.
This study examined the tissue splatter noted with Q-switched laser treatment and found that esterases in splattered cells maintain the ability to cleave fluorescein diacetate to fluorescein 15 minutes after treatment, demonstrating at least temporary cell viability and potential for infectivity.

73. Olbricht SM: **Use of the Carbon Dioxide Laser in Dermatologic**
• **Surgery: A Clinically Relevant Update for 1993.** *J Dermatol Surg Oncol* 1993, 19:364–369.
Reviews the many effective uses of the CO_2 laser for cutaneous lesions.

74. Green HA, Burd E, Nishioka NS, Bruggemann U, Compton CC: **Mid-**
• **dermal Wound Healing: A Comparison Between Dermatomal Excision and Pulsed Carbon Dioxide Laser Ablation.** *Arch Dermatol* 1992, 128:639–645.

75. Middleton WG, Tees DA, Ostrowski M: **Comparative Gross and Histo-**
• **logical Effects of the CO_2 Laser, NdYAG Laser, Scalpel, Shaw Scalpel and Cutting Cautery on Skin in Rats.** *J Otolaryngol* 1993, 22:167–170.
Instruments that provided hemostasis also delayed early phases of wound healing.

76. Green HA, Burd EE, Nishioka NS, Compton CC: **Skin Graft Take and**
• **Healing Following 193-nm Excimer, Continuous-Wave Carbon Dioxide (CO_2) and Pulsed CO_2, or Pulsed Holmium:YAG Laser Ablation of the Graft Bed.** *Arch Dermatol* 1993, 129:979–988.
Ablative lasers that produced less than 160 ± 60 μm of thermal damage (pulsed CO_2 and excimer) allow optimal skin graft take and healing.

77. Frederickson KS, White WE, Wheeland RG, Slaughter DR: **Pre-**
•   **cise Ablation of Skin With Reduced Collateral Damage Using the
      Femtosecond-Pulsed, Terawatt Titanium-Sapphire Laser.** *Arch Derma-
      tol* 1993, **129**:989–993.
This ultrashort, high-intensity laser ablated *in vitro* rat skin to a depth of 0.1
µm per pulse at threshold intensity, with damage contained within 0 to 30 µm
of the adjacent tissue.

78. Frega A, Di-Renzi F, Palazzeti PL, Pace S, Figliolini M, Stentella P:
      Vulvar and Penile HPV Lesions: Laser Surgery and Topical Anesthesia.
      Clin Exp Obstet Gynecol 1993, **20**:76–81.

79. Townsend DE, Smith LH, Kinney WK: **Condyloma Acuminata: Roles
      of Different Techniques of Laser Vaporization.** *J Reprod Med* 1993,
      38:362–364.

80. Hohenleutner U, Landthaler M: **Laser Therapy of Verrucous Epider-**
•   **mal Naevi.** *Clin Exp Dermatol* 1993, **18**:124–127.
The argon laser effectively treated soft verrucous epidermal nevi. The CO_2 laser
worked for both soft and more hyperkeratotic lesions, but with a higher incidence of hypertrophic scarring.

81. Ashinoff R: **Linear Nevus Sebaceus of Jadassohn Treated With the
      Carbon Dioxide Laser.** *Pediatr Dermatol* 1993, **10**:189–191.

82. Rabbin PE, Baldwin HE: **Treatment of Porokeratosis of Mibelli With
      CO_2 Laser Vaporization Versus Surgical Excision With Split-Thickness
      Skin Graft: A Comparison.** *J Dermatol Surg Oncol* 1993, **19**:199–202.

83. Marsili M, Cockerell CJ, Lyde CB: **Hemangioma-Associated Rhino-**
•   **phyma: Report of a Case With Successful Treatment Using Carbon
      Dioxide Laser Surgery.** *J Dermatol Surg Oncol* 1993, **19**:206–212.
CO_2 laser excision followed by laser abrasion successfully treated both the
vascular and stromal components of the rhinophyma.

84. Olbricht SM: **Treatment of Malignant Cutaneous Tumors.** *Clin Plast
      Surg* 1993, **20**:167–180.

85. Hill S, Thomas JM: **Treatment of Cutaneous Metastases From Malig-**
•   **nant Melanoma Using the Carbon-Dioxide Laser.** *Eur J Surg Oncol*
      1993, **19**:173–177.
Cutaneous maetastatic melanoma lesions were successfully controlled with
three or fewer treatments with CO_2 laser vaporization in 18 of 32 patients.
The authors suggest that this method be offered as the first line of treatment
for nonnodal regional recurrence, and that isolated limb perfusion can be offered at a later stage.

Suzanne Linsmeier Kilmer, MD, 6620 Coyle Avenue, Suite 300,
Carmichael, CA 95608, USA.

Cosmetic dermatologic surgery

William P. Coleman III, MD

Tulane University, New Orleans, Louisiana, USA

Cosmetic dermatologic surgery continues to enjoy the development of new techniques. Tumescent liposuction has now become the standard for liposuction. Electronic pumps are available to facilitate the infiltration of the tumescent anesthetic fluid. The superficial liposuction technique remains controversial. The use of the Ultrapulse carbon dioxide laser (Coherent, Palo Alto, CA) may represent a compromise between grafting with round plugs and the slit method of hair transplantation. Scalp reductions can now be done much more rapidly with the Frechet extender (MXM, Antibes, France). The use of glycolic acid for superficial peels has become quite popular. Glycolic acid can also be used in conjunction with trichloroacetic acid to induce a medium-depth peel. This technique has been studied histologically and induces injury through the papillary dermis. Autologous fat transplantation continues to increase in popularity. Fat can be broken down into a less viscous material that has been termed autologous collagen. Although this material contains very little collagen, it does induce new collagen formation at the site of the injection.

Current Opinion in Dermatology 1995:162–166

Liposuction

Tumescent local anesthesia is being increasingly affirmed as the standard of care for liposuction. Although this technique has been well described in the dermatologic literature since 1988 [1–4], its acceptance by other specialties has been somewhat slower. In 1993, Klein [5••], the inventor of the tumescent technique, compared this technique with older approaches emphasizing general anesthesia. The Klein paper was designed to mirror a 1992 article by Courtiss et al. [6]. Courtiss et al. studied the effects of liposuction after minimal infiltration with lidocaine and epinephrine relying primarily on general anesthesia. This study revealed that one third of the aspirate obtained was blood. Klein's study of liposuction with the tumescent technique revealed only 1% blood in the aspirate.

The use of tumescent anesthesia significantly reduces bleeding from liposuction, largely eliminating the need for transfusions. Furthermore, it provides excellent anesthesia and eliminates or reduces the need for general anesthesia and intravenous sedation. Liposuction can now be easily and safely performed using local anesthesia with little or no sedation.

Mainly because of the development of the tumescent technique, liposuction has evolved from a hospital procedure to an office-based one in just over 10 years during its evolution in the United States. Patients can now have this procedure performed privately and ambulate immediately after surgery. Furthermore, they can recover comfortably in their own homes. All of these changes reduce the cost of the procedure and make it more widely available to more patients. They also make the procedure more attractive to an increasing number of office-based dermatologic surgeons.

Rapid infiltration of tumescent anesthetic

The infiltration of several liters of tumescent anesthetic fluid has remained a technical problem for dermatologic surgeons relying on this technique [7]. Using pneumatic devices such as blood pumps and blood pressure cuffs to force the fluid from an intravenous bag through intravenous tubing and a cannula into the fatty layer takes a minimum of 20 min/L. In areas that were previously operated on or that are fibrotic (eg, male flanks), this process often takes much longer. Typically, infiltration of the tumescent anesthetic fluid may require more time than the liposuction procedure itself.

Recently, a number of electric pumps have been developed that are capable of more rapidly instilling tumescent fluid [7,8]. These pumps can delivery approximately 1 L in 5 minutes through intravenous tubing. Clinically, when the fluid is pumped through a cannula into resistant fat, this rate slows to 6 or 7 min/L. This method is vastly more efficient that the old pneumatic systems and saves both the physician and the patient a great deal of time.

There is some concern, however, that more rapid instillation of tumescent anesthetic fluid may alter the dynamics of lidocaine absorption into the plasma [9]. With the use of slow infiltration methods, the plasma absorption of this material has been shown to be delayed and peaks approximately 14 hours postoperatively [10]. Total doses of 35 mL/kg or less have also been documented to result in minimal rises in lidocaine levels, far below the toxic threshold of 5 μg/mL [10]. Recent studies using the rapid instillation method with a motor-driven pump have cleared up this concern [8]. Plasma lidocaine levels measured at 30 minutes, 1 hour, and 12 hours after infiltration have been well within the safe range. The absorption dynamics are apparently similar to those measured when tumescent anesthesia is injected more slowly.

Superficial liposuction

Gasporotti [11•] has proposed the use of very small cannulas to extend liposuction into the superficial fat near the dermis. Proponents of this technique claim that they obtain a smoother result with minimal skin dimpling [12]. This approach is successful only if it is performed with small instruments in a thorough manner throughout the subdermal area to avoid obvious dimpling.

This technique is controversial because it removes the "buffer layer" of fat that has been used for years to disguise the effects of aggressive liposuction deeper in the fat (Fig. 1). Conventional wisdom has always held that leaving this buffer zone intact provided a smoother result [13]. This thin layer of superficial fat is found throughout the body and is a discrete zone. Any attempt to remove it may alter the appearance of the overlying skin. This fact has been used to advantage for years for liposuction in the neck area, where tightening of the dermis is often desirable [14]. Here, superficial liposuction near the dermis creates fibrosis and subsequent retraction of looser skin. This technique is used in an attempt to create a more pleasing neck appearance without face lifting.

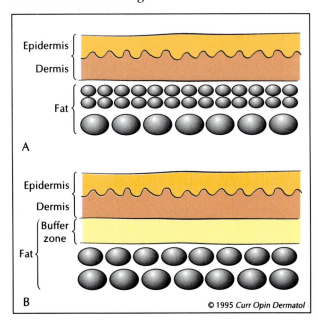

Fig. 1. A, Superficial liposuction. **B,** Standard liposuction.

Experience with the neck has shown that superficial liposuction generates a long-lasting inflammatory response with retraction and fibrosis of the skin, which may take many months to resolve. Using this approach elsewhere risks significant surface changes of the skin, some of which may be permanent. This is especially true on the arms and the inner thighs, where the skin is thin. There is also a risk of impairing the blood supply of the dermis, which may lead to tissue loss.

Mainstream dermatologic surgical theory still emphasizes aggressive liposuction in the deeper fat, with a buffer layer of superficial fat left intact. The use of larger cannulas in deeper planes and of increasingly smaller cannulas more superiorly is still recommended by most experienced dermatologic surgeons. Peripheral feathering with smaller cannulas continues to be performed to minimize contour changes between the suctioned tissues and the immediately adjacent non-treated tissues.

Hair transplantation

Unger (Paper presented at the American Academy of Cosmetic Surgery Annual Meeting, Palm Springs, CA, 1994) and others have studied the use of the Ultrapulse carbon dioxide laser (Coherent, Palo Alto, CA) for hair transplantation. This device is used to generate slits in the recipient area before the insertion of hair-bearing grafts. Although the slit method of hair transplantation avoids the disadvantages of tufting and temporary thinning associated with the use of round plugs, this technique has been criticized for producing linear compression of the grafts (Fig. 2) [15]. With the progressive loss of surrounding hairs, this defect can be quite noticeable, and additional grafting may be needed to correct it. Conversely, slit grafts are less detectable than round grafts during the early phases of healing and are especially appealing for use in younger men who have some remaining hair in the recipient area. Slit grafts can be placed between and used to supplement the existing hair follicles with very little damage to them.

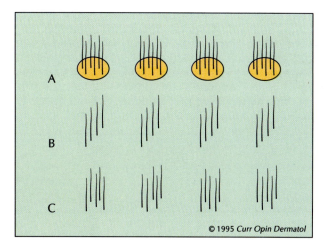

Fig. 2. Methods of hair grafting. **A,** Tufting with round grafts. **B,** Graft compression in slits. **C,** Laser grafting gives a more natural appearance.

The use of the Ultrapulse carbon dioxide laser is conceptually a compromise between these two methods. The laser creates a slit approximately 2 mm wide that provides ample room for small minigrafts. This avoids the compression problems associated with scalpel slits. Theoretically, heat energy extending to the surrounding tissues should impair support for graft growth.

However, early indications have shown that the laser grafts grow normally. This finding is thought to be due to the minimal energy transmitted to the surrounding skin by the Ultrapulse carbon dioxide laser. Studies are continuing on an international basis to verify the effectiveness of this approach. The cost of the laser, which is more than $100,000, currently restricts its use to a few experimental locations.

Scalp reduction

Scalp reduction has become a controversial subject in the 1990s [16]. Hair restoration surgeons seem to be divided into two camps: those who perform reductions and those who do not. The proponents of reduction claim that the focus of this technique is to "reduce" the area of baldness to minimize the need for future transplantation. Consequently, graft donor tissue can be preserved for its most efficacious distribution, primarily in the frontal scalp. Reducing vertex baldness minimizes the need for transplantation in this area.

Surgeons who do not perform scalp reduction complain that this technique increases the width of the temporal and the temporooccipital fringe areas [17], which diminishes the size of the safe donor area. Furthermore, they cite the incidence of "stretchback" and visible scars. The antireduction camp favors using diffuse transplantation in the vertex or restricting hair transplantation to the frontal area when the donor area is not sufficient to cover the entire extent of hair loss.

This argument may be null and void with the development of the Frechet extender (MXM, Antibes, France) [18•]. This silicone elastomer (Silastic; Dow Corning Corp., Midland, MI) device is installed under the galea across the portion of the vertex to be reduced during a normal scalp reduction. The silicone elastomer has a significant memory and gradually pulls the opposing sides of the vertex together, stretching the skin (Fig. 3). This allows increased amounts of tissue to be removed by scalp reduction during a second scalp re-

duction procedure 30 to 40 days later, when the extender is removed. Users have claimed reductions of up to 11 cm within only 6 weeks. If this device continues to be successful in widespread use, it will allow rapid reduction of the bald vertex area. Stretchback is apparently minimized, and the need for multiple procedures or tissue expanders would be obviated. These innovations may make scalp reduction more palatable even to the nonreduction camp and allow better use of the donor tissue for more dense transplantation in the frontal areas of the scalp.

Chemical peeling

Chemical peeling continues to interest physicians and patients alike. Glycolic acid has increasingly been incorporated into skin rejuvenation programs, both as a home product and as a superficial peeling agent used by the physician [19]. This substance is also found in low concentrations in dozens of cosmetics and moisturizers.

However, there is scant evidence that this acid is truly efficacious. Some studies do indicate that the regular use of glycolic acid on an at-home basis may enhance the effects of tretinoin against photoaging [20]. Superficial chemical peels with glycolic acid may help to reduce hyperpigmentation and surface signs of photoaging as well [21•]. However, α-hydroxy acids may not live up to the expectations of patients, who have seen them overglorified in consumer magazines.

Medium-depth chemical peels are those that extend into the dermis [22]. To make significant changes in the appearance of wrinkles, hyperpigmentation, and photoaging, the peeling injury must extend at least to this depth. A number of techniques have been developed for achieving medium-depth peels [23,24]. However, a novel approach has recently been studied [25••]. This method involves the application of 70% glycolic acid for 2 minutes to achieve epidermolysis. This step is followed by the application of 35% trichloroacetic acid, whose penetration into the dermis is augmented by the

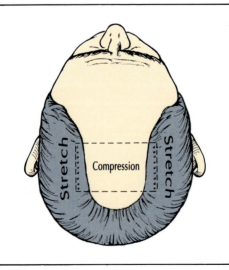

Fig. 3. Left, A Frechet extender (MXM, Antibes, France), shown in its unstretched position, is made up of a rectangular sheet of silicone elastomer with a row of hooks at either end. **Right**, Extender with its stretchback effect on the hair-bearing areas and shrinkback effect on bald areas. (*From* Frechet [18•]; with permission.)

previous glycolic acid treatment. This glycolic acid and trichloroacetic acid peel has been shown histologically to cause alterations of collagen in the papillary dermis (Fig. 4). This effect of altered collagen is similar to that seen after the application of Jessner's solution followed by 35% trichloroacetic acid [23]. Clinically, fine wrinkles, pigmentation, and other signs of photoaging are much reduced. This convenient approach using readily available compounds will expand the armamentarium of the dermatologic surgeon using chemical peels.

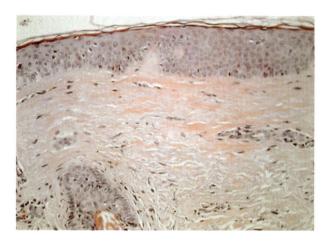

Fig. 4. Sixty days after a glycolic acid–trichloroacetic acid peel of the dermis of a 47-year-old white woman, a histologic stain shows epidermal acanthosis and rete effacement. The upper dermis is fibrotic and expanded by a thin band of rigid, streaked collagen bundles that are parallel to the skin surface. (*From* Coleman and Futrell [25••]; with permission.)

Fat transplantation

The microlipoinjection of aspirated fat continues to grow in popularity. Fat transplantation has become simplified and can easily be done under local anesthesia. Fat can be harvested from the central body using tumescent anesthetic infiltration. After gravity separates the fat from tissue and injectate fluids, these substances can be evacuated from the harvesting syringe, leaving only pure fat. With the same sterile syringe, this material can be injected into the donor area after a local anesthetic field block.

This approach has proved to be successful in improving areas of lipodystrophy throughout the body [26,27]. It has also been used to plump up the thin skin of the dorsal hand caused by aging changes.

Primarily, however, fat injection is used to augment depressions in the nasolabial and chin areas. Signs of central face aging are often not improved by face lifting [28]. Moreover, deep furrows are not efficiently plumped out with the use of commercially available fillers, such as Zyderm (Collagen Corp., Palo Alto, CA), collagen, and Fibrel (Serono, Norwell, MA). These products are too expensive to use in large quantities. Because patients usually have an abundant supply of

excess fat, large volumes can easily be obtained. Typically, 10 to 15 mL of fat is used for plumping up nasolabial and chin furrows.

Furthermore, fat has the advantage of being autologous. Worries persist about injecting foreign materials into human skin and about the potential for causing allergic reactions and possibly collagen vascular disorders [29,30]. The recent condemnation of silicone by the US Food and Drug Administration continues to frighten patients, and an autologous method of tissue augmentation is appealing to many individuals.

Fat can additionally be broken down into a less viscous form that can be injected through smaller-gauge needles into the dermis. This so-called autologous collagen can be prepared by rupturing fat cells with sterile distilled water and then centrifuging the mixture to separate the cell walls from intracellular triglycerides [31,32]. The remaining fibrous material can pass through a 23-gauge or smaller needle and be instilled into the dermis in a manner similar to Fibrel.

Although this material has been named autologous collagen, there is not much collagen in it [33••]; however, this popular term does not promise to change soon. It is more likely that the "collagen" associated with this technique results from collagen production at the site of injection. An inflammatory reaction results from the dermal injection of ruptured fat cells. This inflammatory reaction leads to the production of new collagen fibers, causing significant dermal thickening. Histologic studies have shown up to a threefold increase in dermal thickness 3 months after injection [33••].

An obvious advantage is gained by using one substance for both subcutaneous and dermal augmentation. The pure fat can be injected directly into the subcutaneous tissue and the autologous collagen used for dermal augmentation above. This layered approach gives satisfying cosmetic results, particularly in the nasolabial and chin areas.

References and recommended reading

Papers of particular interest, published within the annual period of review, have been highlighted as:
- Of special interest
- •• Of outstanding interest

1. Klein JA: **The Tumescent Technique for Liposuction Surgery**. *Am J Cosmetic Surg* 1987, 4:263–267.

2. Lillis PJ: **Liposuction Surgery Under Local Anesthesia: Limited Blood Loss and Minimal Lidocaine Absorption**. *J Dermatol Surg Oncol* 1988, 14:1145–1148.

3. Coleman WP III: **L'Anesthesie locale de la Lipo-suction**. *J Med Esthet* 1989, 16:241–243.

4. Lillis PJ: **The Tumescent Technique for Liposuction Surgery**. *Dermatol Clin* 1990, 8:439–450.

5. Klein JA: **Tumescent Technique for Local Anesthesia Improves Safety** •• **in Large Volume Liposuction**. *Plast Reconstr Surg* 1993, 92:1085–1098.
This major discussion of the tumescent anesthetic technique for liposuction is the first comprehensive review article on this subject published in the plastic surgery literature.

6. Courtiss EH, Choucair RJ, Donelan MB: **Large-Volume Suction Lipectomy: An Analysis of One Hundred New Patients**. *Plast Reconstr Surg* 1992, 89:1068–1079.

7. Coleman WP III, Badame A, Phillips H: **A New Technique for Injection of Tumescent Anesthetic Mixtures**. *J Dermatol Surg Oncol* 1991, 17:535–537.

8. Samdal F, Amland PF, Bugge JF: **Plasma Lidocaine Levels During Suction Assisted Lipectomy Using Large Doses of Dilute Lidocaine With Epinephrine.** *Plast Reconstr Surg* 1994, 93:1217–1223.

9. Piveral K: **Systemic Lidocaine Absorption During Liposuction.** *Plast Reconstr Surg* 1987, 80:643.

10. Klein JA: **Tumescent Technique for Regional Anesthesia Permits Lidocaine Doses of 35 mg/kg for Liposuction: Peak Plasma Lidocaine Levels Are Diminished and Delayed 12 Hours.** *J Dermatol Surg Oncol* 1990, 16:248–263.

11. Gasporotti M: **Superficial Liposuction: A New Application of the Technique for Aged and Flaccid Skin.** *Aesthetic Plast Surg* 1992, 16:141–146.
• This is the first article on this controversial technique in the English language.

12. Gasporotti M, Lewis CM, Toledo LS: *Superficial Liposculpture: Manual of Technique.* New York: Springer-Verlag; 1993.

13. Coleman WP, III: **Liposuction.** In *Cosmetic Surgery of the Skin.* Edited by Coleman WP III, Hanke CW, Asken S, Alt TH. Philadelphia: BC Decker; 1991:213–238.

14. Fodor P: **Where to Use Superficial Lipoplasty (Liposuction)?** [Letter]. *Plast Reconstr Surg* 1993, 92:769.

15. Coleman WP, III: **A Visit to the Office of Dr. Emanuel Marritt.** *J Dermatol Surg Oncol* 1993, 19: 664–668.

16. Norwood OT: **Scalp Reductions: Are They Necessary?** *Hair Transplant Forum* 1993, 3:1–2.

17. Marritt E: **Yes Virginia You Can Remove All the Baldness... But.** *Hair Transplant Forum* 1993, 3:3–7.

18. Frechet P: **Scalp Extension.** *J Dermatol Surg Oncol* 1993, 19:616–
• 622.
This article describes a new silicone device for rapid scalp reduction.

19. Moy LS, Muradtt, Moy RL, Murad H: **Use of AHA's Adds New Dimensions to Chemical Peeling.** *Cosmet Dermatol* 1990, 5:32–34.

20. Van Scott EJ: **Alphahydroxy Acids: Procedures for Use in Clinical Practice.** *Cutis* 1989, 43:222–228.

21. Moy LS, Moy RL: **Glycolic Acid Peels for the Treatment of Wrinkles and Photoaging.** *J Dermatol Surg Oncol* 1993, 19:243–246.
• This article provides a succinct discussion of the use of glycolic acid peels, a technique just gaining broad popularity.

22. Brody HJ: **Chemical Peeling.** St. Louis: Mosby Year Book; 1992.

23. Monheit GD: **The Jessner's and TCA Peel: A Medium Depth Chemical Peel.** *J Dermatol Surg Oncol* 1989, 15:945–950.

24. Brody HJ: **Variations and Comparison in Medium Depth Chemical Peeling.** *J Dermatol Surg Oncol* 1989, 15:953–963.

25. Coleman WP III, Futrell JM: **The Glycolic Acid Trichloracetic Acid Peel.**
•• *J Dermatol Surg Oncol* 1994, 20:76–80.
A new medium-depth peeling technique is described and histologic studies are performed to validate its depth of penetration.

26. Skouge JW: **Autologous Fat Transplantation in Facial Surgery.** In *Cosmetic Surgery of the Skin.* Edited by Coleman WP III, Hanke CW, Asken S, Alt TH. Philadelphia: BC Decker; 1991:239–249.

27. Pinski KS, Roenigk HH: **Autologous Fat Transplantation: Long Term Follow-up.** *J Dermatol Surg Oncol* 1992, 18:179–184.

28. Fournier PF: **Facial Recontouring With Fat Grafting.** *Dermatol Clin* 1990, 8:523–537.

29. DeLustro F, Fries J, Kang A, Katz, Kaye R, Reichlin M: **Immunity to Injectable Collagen and Autoimmune Disease: A Summary of Current Understanding.** *J Dermatol Surg Oncol* 1988, 14(suppl):57–65.

30. Sergott TJ, Limoli JP, Baldwin CM, Laub DR: **Human Adjuvant Disease, Possible Autoimmune Disease After Silicone Implantation: A Review of the Literature, Case Studies, and Speculation for the Future.** *Plast Reconstr Surg* 1988, 78:104–114.

31. Fournier PF: **Collagen Autologue.** In *Liposculpture: ma Technique.* Paris: Arnette; 1989:277–279.

32. Zocchi M: **Methode de Production de Collagene autologue par Traitement du Tissu graisseaux.** *J Esthet Chir Dermatol* 1990, 17:105–114.

33. Coleman WP, III, Lawrence N, Sherman RN, Reed RJ, Pinski KS: **Au-**
•• **tologous Collagen? Lipocytic Dermal Augmentation: A Histopathologic Study.** *J Dermatol Surg Oncol* 1993, 19:1032–1040.
This is the first histologic study of the autologous collagen technique for tissue augmentation with processed fat cells.

William P. Coleman III, MD, 4425 Conlin Drive, Metairie, LA 70006, USA.

Photobiology, photodermatoses, and photoaging

Edited by

John Hawk
St. Thomas's Hospital
London, UK

CURRENT SCIENCE

Novel approaches to tailoring psoralen use to phototherapeutic need

Francis P. Gasparro, PhD

Yale University School of Medicine, New Haven, Connecticut, USA

Empiricism has driven the development of and subsequent improvements in psoralen-based photochemotherapies from the initial application for psoriasis more than 20 years ago to the present diverse applications. Recent observations concerning the mode of drug administration and the optimal wavelength of irradiation may contribute to improving clinical efficacy and to reducing undesired side effects (nausea, pruritus, and skin cancer). Of the various psoralen photochemotherapeutic modalities currently employed, one may ultimately be determined to have superior therapeutic efficacy. However, this advance will occur only if laboratory studies can provide more information on the scientific basis for the mechanism or mechanisms underlying the responses by these photochemotherapies.

Current Opinion in Dermatology 1995:167–172

The remarkable success of psoralen photochemotherapy for several cutaneous diseases over the past 20 years can be attributed largely to its relative ease of administration and minimal short-term side effects. However, the continuing follow-up of patients who received psoralens and ultraviolet A (PUVA) therapy has now demonstrated an increased incidence of squamous cell carcinoma (SCC), especially in patients who were exposed to high cumulative ultraviolet A (UVA) doses [1•,2•,3••]. Similar long-term follow-up data have not been reported for vitiligo [4] and cutaneous T-cell lymphoma (CTCL) [5] patients who were also treated with PUVA. The increased incidence of PUVA-induced skin cancers has generated significant interest in designing new and improved PUVA modalities. In this update, the topics of drug bioavailability and mode of delivery, UVA dosing, and wavelength dependence are reviewed. In addition, recent articles providing some new insights into the mechanism underlying responses to psoralen photochemotherapies are discussed because the nature of the compound employed or the modality may have an impact on cellular mechanisms.

Psoralen bioavailability

A problem that has plagued PUVA photochemotherapy from its inception is drug bioavailability. Psoralens (typically 8-methoxypsoralen [MOP] in the United States and also 5-MOP in Europe) have very low aqueous solubilities (10 to 30 $\mu g/mL$), which leads to their very poor absorption and highly variable blood levels ($\approx 100 \pm 100$ ng/mL) (Fig. 1) [6]. Although these problems were documented early during the development of PUVA therapy, not until several years after its inception was the problem directly addressed. In 1979, Wagner et al. [7] demonstrated that poorly responding PUVA patients had consistently low plasma levels. Deviations from the expected 2-hour peak level were observed in 50% of problem cases and only 14% of control patients (responders). No correlation between ingested doses and 8-MOP plasma levels was observed for either group of patients. Three of 14 patients showed an improved therapeutic response when the time of UVA exposure was adjusted to coincide with the time of optimal plasma levels. In 1991, Walther and Haustein [8] also found abnormally low or "deviated" serum levels in seven of 11 PUVA problem patients. These two studies are cited because they indicate that plasma levels play an important role in the treatment of non–life-threatening disease (psoriasis) in which a facile determination of patient response can be made. It is also likely that suboptimal plasma levels may affect the outcome in CTCL patients being treated with photopheresis. However, the relatively slow response to CTCL makes it difficult to attribute suboptimal response solely to low 8-MOP levels.

Two different approaches have been employed to circumvent the psoralen bioavailability problem. In the treatment of psoriasis, drug delivery to the skin has been achieved by topical administration using either a lotion [9] or bath immersion [10]. Patchy results with the former led to the use of the latter, which has been

---

Abbreviations

CTCL—cutaneous T-cell lymphoma; **FDA**—Food and Drug Administration; **MOP**—methoxypsoralen; **PUVA**—psoralens and ultraviolet A; **PUVB**—psoralens and ultraviolet B; **SCC**—squamous cell carcinoma; **UVA**—ultraviolet A; **UVB**—ultraviolet B.

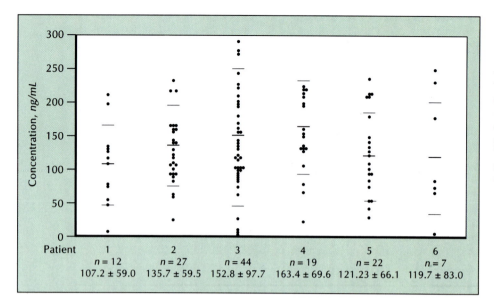

Fig. 1. 8-Methoxypsoralen levels in six cutaneous T-cell lymphoma patients. The overall average level in all of these patients was 122 ng/mL (±76). The *bold bars* indicate the average level for each patient (*light bars* indicate SD); *n* indicates the number of analyses performed for each patient. The individual patient average ±SD is also indicated. (*From* Gasparro [6]; with permission.)

repeatedly demonstrated to result in optimal and reproducible levels of psoralen in the skin [7]. It also eliminates nausea, the major short-term side effect of psoralen ingestion, and reduces the incidence of SCC (*see* later discussion). However, it has one logistical drawback: the patient must be immersed in a bath and then be exposed to the UVA radiation within 30 minutes. Thus, the patient must live relatively close to the treatment facility, or the facility must have tubs available for immersion.

For photopheresis, the ideal 8-MOP formulation would be a sterile aqueous solution that could be injected directly into the leukocyte plasma fraction just before UVA exposure. Considerably smaller amounts of drug would be required (100 to 200 µg in 740 mL, as compared with an average oral dose of ≈40 mg). A formulation of this type has been described by Knobler *et al.* [11••], who compared its bioavailability with that obtained with standard oral ingestion in a series of 16 patients. Oral ingestion of 8-MOP (0.6 mg/kg) led to an average 8-MOP plasma level of 99±49 ng/mL (91 treatments; range, 4 to 224 ng/mL). In six patients, 8-MOP levels were below the minimum considered effective (≈60 ng/mL). With the injectable formulation in the same series of patients, the average plasma level was 126±24 ng/mL (108 treatments; range, 66 to 178 ng/mL). No patients had a level of less than 60 ng/mL.

Is ultraviolet A radiation the optimal wavelength for the activation of psoralens in skin?

Why is UVA radiation used to activate psoralens? In 1958, Lerner (Paper presented at Brook Lodge Invitational Symposium, Kalamazoo, MI, 1958) recorded the fluorescence excitation spectra of several psoralen derivatives. Each showed a major excitation band near 360 nm. At the time, commercial lamps with sufficient output at these wavelengths were not available. How-

ever, the potential efficacy was demonstrated, and in early 1970s, the availability of higher-out UVA lamps was a crucial factor in the widespread implementation of PUVA therapy for psoriasis. Although action spectra studies then demonstrated that the most effective wavelengths for clearing psoriasis did not match the output of these lamps, being significantly shifted to shorter wavelengths (330 to 340 nm) [12], UVA lamps continued to be a convenient source for the photoactivation of psoralens. In 1993, Ortel *et al.* [13•] and Sakhuntabhai *et al.* [14•] demonstrated that ultraviolet B (UVB) radiation could also be used to activate psoralens. After bath water psoralen exposure, patients were exposed to narrow-band UVB radiation from Philips TL01 lamps (Philips NV, Eindhoven, Netherlands), which emit a narrow band of radiation at a wavelength of 311 nm (±2 nm) (Fig. 2). Doses were determined using standard minimal phototoxic dose testing to ensure that patients were not burned. Significantly lower doses were requires at 311 nm than with standard therapy employing broad-band UVA radiation.

Often, PUVA therapy and psoralens and ultraviolet B (PUVB) therapy are used sequentially to treat psoriasis. Although the idea has never been directly tested, it has been assumed that UVA radiation would induce the formation of psoralen DNA photoadducts and that UVB radiation would induce the formation of a separate population of DNA photoproducts (*eg*, thymine dimers), which might lead to a synergistic therapeutic effect. As a result of the apparent efficacy of PUVB therapy, we examined the photochemistry of UVB-activated 8-MOP and found that the same type of psoralen DNA photoadducts were induced (Fig. 3) (Gasparro *et al.*, Unpublished data). However, significantly lower doses of UVB radiation are required to photoactivate the 8-MOP because it has a much greater extinction coefficient at the shorter ultraviolet wavelengths (9350 and 918 M⁻¹cm⁻¹ at 311 and 365 nm, respectively) [15]. The distribution of photoadducts is also different. With UVA radiation, the major photoadduct was the inter-

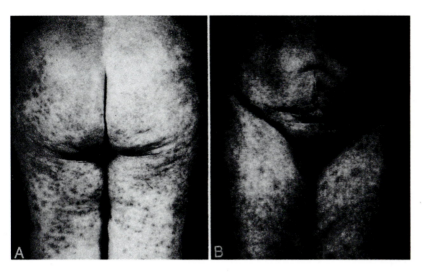

Fig. 2. Comparison of 311-nm ultraviolet A irradiation (*right body side*) with same dose of 311 nm after oral psoralen sensitization (*left body side*). **Left**, Increased erythemogenicity on psoralen-sensitized side after four exposures. **Right**, More intense pigmentation after nine exposures. (*From* Ortel *et al.* [13•]; with permission.)

strand cross-link (61%) [16•], whereas with UVB radiation, the extent of cross-link formation was much lower (29%). At this time, it is not known which combination of photoadducts is most efficacious, nor whether one type of adduct (monoadduct or cross-link) might pose a greater risk of skin cancer.

New psoralen derivatives

Other psoralens (5-MOP and trimethylpsoralen) are also used in photochemotherapies (5-MOP in Europe for psoriasis and trimethylpsoralen for vitiligo). A new drug application for 5-MOP in the United States is now pending at the US Food and Drug Administra-

tion (FDA). The results of a short-term clinical trial comparing 5-MOP and 8-MOP as therapy for psoriasis have been reported [17]. Despite the apparent therapeutic superiority of 8-MOP, interest in 5-MOP remains high, primarily because of the much lower incidence of pruritus and nausea after its ingestion. However, 5-MOP suffers from bioavailability problems similar to if not worse than those of 8-MOP. In addition, studies on the genotoxicity of 5-MOP have been performed only in Chinese hamster ovary cells [18]. Before the widespread implementation of 5-MOP, its relative mutagenicity (as compared with 8-MOP) should be determined in human cells in order to assess the risk associated with each and thus provide additional guidance to the clinician.

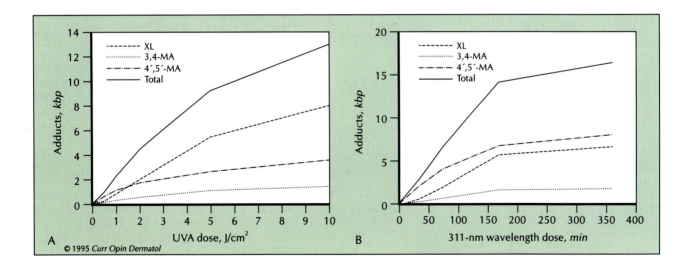

Fig. 3. 8-Methoxypsoralen (8-MOP) photoadduct formation and distribution in calf thymus DNA (77 μmol/L bp) and 8-MOP (180 μmol/L). **A,** Ultraviolet A (UVA) doses were delivered from standard UVA fluorescent bulbs. Radiometry was used to determine the incident UVA dose. **B,** Radiation (311 nm) was delivered by a monochromator (2-nm bandpass, mimicking Philips TL01 lamps [Philips NV, Eindhoven, the Netherlands]). Doses of 311 nm were chosen so that the number of adducts formed would be comparable to the number of adducts formed when UVA was employed. Note the different pattern of photoadduct distribution. For UVA the major photoadduct is the cross-link (XL), whereas for 311 nm the major photoadduct is the 4′,5′-monoadduct (MA).

Reducing the risks of psoralen photochemotherapy

Dermatologists have long been concerned about the potential risk of skin cancer induction by PUVA therapy. In the most recent follow-up study by Stern [1•] of the patients from the original US multicenter PUVA trial, a statistically significant increase in the incidence of SCC was observed. A comparative analysis of the incidence of SCC in US and European trials was also recently reported on [3••]. Although earlier comparisons appeared to show differences in the European and US experiences with the PUVA-induced incidence of SCC, the ongoing periodic reanalysis of each set of data with a longer follow-up period has now indicated comparable findings [3••]. The lower incidence of SCC in the European group was attributed to the more aggressive treatment schedule employed in Europe, which yields clearing with much lower cumulative UVA doses (800 vs 1500 J/cm², respectively). Recently, a correlation between SCC incidence (in non-PUVA patients) and mutations in the *p53* tumor suppressor gene has been reported [19••]. Similar studies have not been performed on SCC from PUVA patients.

The molecular basis for the efficacy of photochemotherapies

In 1966, photoactivated psoralens were shown to be capable of forming interstrand cross-links in DNA (*in vitro*) [20]. This observation appeared to provide a molecular rationale for how psoralen photoadducts could attenuate the proliferation of the hyperproliferative keratinocytes characteristic of psoriasis. It was later shown, however, that monofunctional compounds that could not form cross-links were also efficacious [21]. The efficacy of psoralen photochemotherapy may simply be derived from the induction of antiproliferative photoadducts. Thus, any psoralen that can induce the requisite damage may be efficacious. However, another possibility is that some genes are affected in a particular way (downregulated, as might be expected intuitively, or perhaps even upregulated [22]), resulting in the inhibition or stimulation of a particular gene product that attenuates the proliferation of keratinocytes. It is important to determine whether different psoralens induce a different distribution of photoadducts (monoadducts vs cross-links) at or not at mutagenic hot spots so that the most efficacious therapeutic regimen with the least risk can be employed in patient treatment.

It may be surprising that after 20 years more is not known about the cellular impact of psoralen photoadducts (other than their effects on proliferation and repair). However, it is easy to understand. The two major psoralen photochemotherapies (PUVA therapy and photopheresis) received FDA approval despite their known genotoxic effects (in bacteria and yeast) because the short-term side effects were minimal, being limited mainly to nausea in 15% to 20% of patients. Although PUVA therapy was considered to be an experimental therapy for many years after its inception (it received FDA approval in the mid-1980s), it gained widespread acceptance because of the response of patients in whom previous therapies have failed. In the mid-1980s, private-practice dermatologists began administering PUVA treatments. Approximately at this time, the first reports of an increased incidence of skin cancer became apparent in the United States [23]. Because of concerns about the mutagenicity of PUVA therapy and its potential carcinogenicity, patients who receive high doses of UVA radiation are now carefully monitored.

In the mid-1980s, when photopheresis became available, it was nearly a forgone conclusion that all that needed to be known about psoralens was known. However the remarkable efficacy of photopheresis, in which only a small fraction of the patient's malignant cells are treated before reinfusion, fueled a new interest in psoralens. It has been suggested that the extracorporeal phototreatment of malignant cells leads to an autovaccination on reinfusion, which serves to stimulate the patient's previously unresponsive immune system so that untreated malignant cells are also recognized and removed from the circulation [24]. As attractive a hypothesis as this is, no clinical data support it. Furthermore, most of the animal models that have been employed are far removed from photopheresis and CTCL in terms of the mode of administration of 8-MOP and UVA radiation and in terms of the end-point selected for analysis [25–27].

Several recent reports from diverse research areas, however, may provide a hint of a novel mechanism underlying the efficacy of psoralen photochemotherapies. Borroni *et al.* [28••] observed an upregulation of CD8+ T cells in PUVA patients up to 1 year after the suspension of therapy. The CD8+ T cells are suppressor cells that participate in the cytolysis of cells that display target antigens in the context of class I major histocompatibility complex molecules. In elegant studies over the past 15 years, Boon [29•] has demonstrated that DNA-damaging agents (*eg*, *N*-methyl-*N*-nitro-*N*-nitrosoguanidine) can alter the display of class I–restricted antigens on malignant murine cells, making them susceptible to CD8+-mediated lysis. Similar observations have been reported with the use of 8-MOP and UVA radiation [30•]. In another study, Vowels *et al.* [31•] showed that photopheresis upregulated tumor necrosis factor-α in patient cells, and Muramatsu *et al.* [32•] showed that the 8-MOP plus UVA treatment of human skin explants induced a 72-kD heat shock protein. These observations may be indicative of a more fundamental response to the DNA damage induced by psoralens and UVA radiation. In a recent review, Holbrook and Fornace [22] showed that several different DNA-damaging agents led to the upregulation of 40 different genes, but only one, β-polymerase, was involved in DNA repair. Several of the induced genes have a role in host defense mechanisms (*eg*, genes for acute-phase reactant proteins such as tumor necrosis factor-α, interleukin-1, and metallothionein). Many are general transcription regulators that fall in the class of "immediate early" genes (c-*fos*, c-*jun*, *JUNB*, c-*myc*, and *EGR1*). These genes are rapidly induced in response to growth-stimulatory signals and have been shown to be important players in signal transduction during proliferation and differentiation. They may activate the transcription of other genes (secondary DNA damage-response genes) that are sometimes induced over a slower time course (collagenase and plasminogen activator). Such events may be induced by psoralen photochemotherapies and could be responsible for their efficacy. Experiments in this area that examine the effects of wavelength (UVA or UVB radiation), the type of psoralen (8-MOP or 5-MOP), and the mode of delivery will yield much new information that could be the basis for the rational re-designing of psoralen photochemotherapies and the recognition that one compound or modality is superior.

Conclusions

The clinical utility of psoralen photochemotherapies can be greatly improved by advances in our understanding of the underlying mechanisms for therapeutic efficacy. In addition, the mode of drug administration (*ie*, oral, topical, or bath) needs to be evaluated for both short-term efficacy and long-term complications. Can the drug delivery be improved so that each phototherapy session is conducted with optimal levels of 8-MOP present in the target tissue? Is there a clear superiority of one type of radiation (*ie*, UVA or UVB)? Does the distribution of monoadducts and cross-links affect therapeutic efficacy or the risk of skin cancer? Delving into these questions should be a major goal of photobiology research groups.

References and recommended reading

Papers of particular interest, published within the annual period of review, have been highlighted as:
- •   Of special interest
- ••   Of outstanding interest

1. Stern RS: **Risks of Cancer Associated With Long-Term Exposure to**
•   **PUVA in Humans: Current Status. 1991.** *Blood Cells* 1992, 18:91–99.
This is the most recent article in a series of important publications on the follow-up of PUVA patients and an analysis of the incidence of skin cancers. This article provides an excellent summary of Stern's findings on nonmelanoma skin cancer, melanoma and pigmentary changes, and noncutaneous cancer in these patients.

2. Lindelöf B, Sigurgeirsson B, Tegner E, Larkö O, Berne B: **Comparison**
•   **of the Carcinogenic Potential of Trioxsalen Bath PUVA and Oral Methoxsalen PUVA.** *Arch Dermatol* 1992, 128:1341–1344.
This report compares the incidence of skin cancers in patients treated with either bath immersions PUVA or oral PUVA (4799 PUVA patients from the Swedish Cancer Registry). In this preliminary report, the authors show that bath immersion PUVA appears to be less carcinogenic.

3. Studniberg HM, Weller P: **PUVA, UVB, Psoriasis and Nonmelanoma**
••   **Cancer.** *J Am Acad Dermatol* 1993, 29:1013–1022.
This excellent summary compares analyses of the incidence of skin cancers in PUVA patients treated in US and European trials. Studniberg analyzes the initial statistics and accounts for the differences. Recommendations for safe application of PUVA therapy to minimize risks to patients are included.

4. Wildfang IL, Jacobsen FK, Thestrup-Pedersen K: **PUVA Treatment of Vitiligo: A Retrospective Study of 59 Patients.** *Acta Derm Venereol (Stockh)* 1992, 72:305–306.

5. Heald P, Rook A, Perez M, Wintroub B, Knobler R, Jegasothy B, Gasparro F, Berger C, Edelson R: **Treatment of Erythrodermic Cuta-**
neous T-Cell Lymphoma With Extracorporeal Photochemotherapy. *J Am Acad Dermatol* 1992, 27:427–433.

6. Gasparro FP: **Psoralen DNA Interactions.** In *Psoralen-DNA Photobiology,* vol 1. Edited by Gasparro FP. Boca Raton: CRC Press; 1988: 5–36.

7. Wagner G, Hofmann C, Busch U, Schmid J, Plewig G: **8-MOP Plasma Levels in PUVA Problem Cases in Psoriasis.** *Br J Dermatol* 1979, 101:285–292.

8. Walther T, Haustein UF: **8-Methoxypsoralen Serum Levels and Poor Response to Photochemotherapy: Importance of Drug Formulation and Individual Factors** *Int J Dermatol* 1991, 30:516–518.

9. Pham CT, Koo JY: **Plasma Levels of 8-Methoxypsoralen After Topical Paint PUVA.** *J Am Acad Dermatol* 1993, 28:460–466.

10. Collins P, Rogers S: **Bath-Water Compared With Oral Delivery of 8-Methoxypsoralen PUVA Therapy for Chronic Plaque Psoriasis.** *Br J Dermatol* 1992, 127:392–395.

11. Knobler RM, Trautinger F, Graninger W, Macheiner W, Gruenwald
••   C, Neumann R, Ramer W: **Parenteral Administration of 8-Methoxypsoralen in Photophoresis.** *J Am Acad Dermatol* 1993, 28:580–584.
These authors demonstrated the feasibility of delivering 8-MOP to an extracorporeal suspension of cells. This mode of administration can eliminate the problems associated with oral ingestion (pruritus and nausea) and may improve the clinical outcome of reproducibly achieving reproducible drug levels in the irradiated target cells.

12. Gasparro FP, Berger CL, Edelson RL: **Effect of Monochromatic UVA Light and 8-Methoxypsoralen on Human Lymphocyte Response to Mitogen.** *Photodermatology* 1984, 1:10–17.

13. Ortel B, Perl S, Kinaciyan T, Calzavara-Pinton PG, Hönigsmann H:
•   **Comparison of Narrow-Band (311 nm) UVB and Broad-Band UVA After Oral or Bathwater 8-Methoxypsoralen in the Treatment of Psoriasis.** *J Am Acad Dermatol* 1993, 29:736–740.
These authors examined the action spectrum for response to psoriasis and noted that shorter wavelengths of ultraviolet radiation appeared to be comparable to the long-wavelength UVA lights that are commonly employed in PUVA therapy. By performing half-body irradiation (one half UVA, one half narrow-band UVB), they demonstrated that the narrow-band UVB irradiation was efficacious. These studies are only preliminary; however, they indicate that a new light source (narrow-band UVB) may be more efficacious than the currently used source (UVA). A note about Lerner's observation in 1958 (Paper presented at Brook Lodge Invitational Symposium, Kalamazoo, MI, 1958) that led to the use of UVA lamps: although these measurements were accurate with respect to the technology available at that time, the data were not corrected for the variations in lamp output at different wavelengths. Today, photon-counting fluorescence measurements would show an exact correlation between the ultraviolet absorption spectra and the fluorescence excitation spectra of these compounds. This may have been fortuitous. Although Ortel *et al.* showed that narrow-band UVB irradiation can be effective, we do not know if it will be superior to, or even equivalent to, the UVA-based therapy in long-term studies.

14. Sakhuntabhai A, Diffey BL, Farr PM: **Response of Psoriasis to**
•   **Psoralen-UVB Photochemotherapy.** *Br J Dermatol* 1993, 128:296–300.
This report describes results similar to those of Ortel *et al.* (*J Am Acad Dermatol* 1993, 29:736–740). The narrow-band UVB dose required for the clearance of psoriatic lesions was one quarter that was found in earlier studies using UVA radiation.

15. Gasparro FP, Gattolin P, Olack GA, Deckelbaum LI, Sumpio BE: **Visible Excitation of 8-Methoxypsoralen: HPLC Quantitation of Monoadducts and Crosslinks.** *Photochem Photobiol* 1993, 57:1007–1010.

16. Olack GA, Gattolin P, Gasparro FP: **Improved HPLC Analysis of**
•   **8-Methoxypsoralen Monoadducts and Crosslinks in Polynucleotide, DNA and Cellular Systems: Analysis of Split-Dose Protocols.** *Photochem Photobiol* 1993, 57:941–949.
This paper describes methods for the analysis of 8-MOP photoadducts under conditions comparable to those used to treat patients. The analysis of photoadducts (monoadducts and cross-links) may provide valuable information for assessing which source (UVA or narrow-band UVB) is most suitable for the activation of 8-MOP. However, these data can be interpreted only if concurrent studies on photoadduct mutagenesis are performed.

17. Calzavara-Pinton PG, Ortel B, Carlino AM, Hönigsmann H, DePanfilis G: **Reappraisal of the Use of 5-Methoxypsoralen in the Therapy of Psoriasis.** *Exp Dermatol* 1992, 1:46–51.

18. Papdopoulo D, Averbeck D: **Genotoxic Effects and DNA Photoadducts Induced in Chinese Hamster V79 Cells by 5-Methoxypsoralen and 8-Methoxypsoralen.** *Mutat Res* 1985, 151:281–291.

19. Ziegler A, Leffell DJ, Kunala S, Sharma HW, Gailini M, Simon JA,
••   Halperin JA, Baden HP, Shapiro PE, Bale AE, Brash DE: **Mutation Hotspots Due to Sunlight in the *p53* Gene of Nonmelanoma Skin Cancers.** *Proc Natl Acad Sci U S A* 1993, 90:4216–4220.

Ziegler *et al.* showed that *p53* genes from SCCs contain a UVB mutation fingerprint. Patients who receive PUVA treatments two to three times per week until clearing with maintenance follow-up can reach these threshold levels in 2 to 3 years. Long before this time, however, as a result of repetitive exposure to PUVA, critical mutations (*eg*, in *p53*) might already have occurred. It might be useful for the clinician to know the *p53* mutational status of patients receiving long-term PUVA therapy. The accumulation of threshold levels of *p53* mutations may precede the clinical development of SCC.

20. Dall'Acqua F, Marciani S, Ciavatta L, Rodighiero G: **Formation of Interstand Crosslinkings in the Photoreaction Between Furocoumarins and DNA.** *Z Naturforsch* 1971, 26:561–569.

21. Recchia G, Cristofolin M, Bordin F, Dall'Acqua F, Rodighiero P: **Methylangelicin in the Topical Treatment Photochemotherapy of Psoriasis: Preliminary Report.** *Med Biol Environ* 1983, 11:471–481.

22. Holbrook NK, Fornace AJ: **Response to Adversity: Molecular Control of Gene Activation Following Genotoxic Stress.** *New Biol* 1991, 3:825–833.

23. Stern RS, Laird N, Melski J, Parrish JA, Fitzpatrick TB, Bleich HL: **Cutaneous Squamous-Cell Carcinoma in Patients Treated With PUVA.** *N Engl J Med* 1984, 310:1156–1161.

24. Edelson RL: **Photopheresis: A Clinically Relevant Immunobiologic Response Modifier.** *Ann N Y Acad Sci* 1991, 636:154–164.

25. Berger CL, Perez M, LaRoche L, Edelson RL: **Inhibition of Murine Autoimmune Disease by Reinfusion of Syngeneic Lymphocytes Inactivated With Psoralen and Ultraviolet A Light.** *J Invest Dermatol* 1990, 94:52–57.

26. Perez M, Lobo FM, Yamane Y, John L, Edelson RL: **Inhibition of Antiskin Allograft Immunity Induced by Infusions With Photoinactivated Effector T Lymphocytes (PET Cells): Is In Vitro Cell Transferable?** *Ann N Y Acad Sci* 1991, 636:95–112.

27. LaRoche L, Edelson RL, Perez M, Berger CL: **Antigen-Specific Tolerance Induced by Autoimmunization With Photoinactivated Syngeneic Effector Cells.** *Ann N Y Acad Sci* 1991, 636:113–123.

28. •• Borroni G, Zaccone C, Vignati G, Fietta A, Merlini C, Rabbiosi G: **Evidence for CD8+ Cell Increase in Long-Term PUVA-Treated Psoriatic Patients After PUVA Discontinuation.** *Dermatology* 1992, 185:69–71.

The authors describe an increase in CD8+ T cells in patients who received long-term PUVA therapy up to 1 year after the suspension of therapy. These cells may play a role in preventing the recurrence of psoriasis.

29. • Boon T: **Towards a Genetic Analysis of Tumor Rejection Antigens.** *Adv Cancer Res* 1992, 58:177–210.

It has been shown that CD8+ T cells can be induced by treating cells with mutagenic agents. Boon employed *N*-methyl-*N*-nitro-*N*-nitrosoguanidine, a very potent mutagen, to create tumor-negative cell lines, which were capable of protecting animals from challenge with the original tumor-positive cell line. The mutagenized cells were shown to express new antigens that are recognized by CD8+ T cells.

30. • Gasparro FP, Malane MS, Maxwell VM, Tigelaar RE: **8-Methoxypsoralen and Long Wavelength Ultraviolet Radiation Enhances the Immunogenicity of P815 Mastocytoma Cells.** *Photochem Photobiol* 1993, 58:682–688.

Using the Boon model (*Adv Cancer Res* 1992, 58:177–210), these authors demonstrated that similar effects (cross-protection and adoptive transfer) could be obtained with 8-MOP and UVA radiation.

31. • Vowels BE, Cassin M, Boufal MH, Walsh LJ, Rook AH: **Extracorporeal Photochemotherapy Induces the Production of Tumor Necrosis Factor-α by Monocytes: Implications for the Treatment of Cutaneous T Cell Lymphoma and Systemic Sclerosis.** *J Invest Dermatol* 1992, 98:686–692.

The enhanced production of tumor necrosis factor-α may play a role in the response of photopheresis patients (with lymphoma and scleroderma). In lymphoma patients, tumor necrosis factor-α could mediate antitumor effects, and in scleroderma, it could suppress collagen synthesis and induce collagenase production.

32. • Muramatsu T, Yamashida Y, Tada H, Kobayashi M, Yamaji M, Ohno H, Shirai T, Takahashi A, Ohnishi T: **8-Methoxypsoralen Plus UVA Induces the 72kDa Heat Shock Protein in Organ-Cultured Normal Human Skin.** *Photochem Photobiol* 1993, 58:809–812.

Heat shock protein may be just one example of an agent induced by 8-MOP plus UVA treatment. Other DNA-damaging agents (*see* Holbrook and Fornace, *New Biol* 1991, 3:825–833) are known to induce the expression of other genes. Other than those found in this study and that of Vowels *et al.* (*J Invest Dermatol* 1992, 98:686–692), no molecular species have been reported to be inducible by photoactivated psoralens.

Francis P. Gasparro, PhD, Yale University Photobiology Laboratory, Department of Dermatology, 333 Cedar Street, New Haven, CT 06510, USA.

Advances in sunscreen technology: choosing the sunscreen to suit

Rik Roelandts, MD

University Hospital, Leuven, Belgium

Technological developments and a change in the perception of consumers have increased the importance of protection against sunlight. A market for sunscreens with high protection factors has developed, and additional ultraviolet A protection has become necessary. These developments have been made possible by the newer ultraviolet A filters and micronized powders. The skin can now be protected not only against solar erythema but also against some of the long-term side effects of solar exposure. The protection of abnormally photosensitive skin has also improved. Nevertheless, guidelines for sunscreen use need to be adhered to, or the degree of protection actually afforded may be much less than expected or claimed.

Current Opinion in Dermatology 1995:173–177

A major revolution in sunscreen technology has taken place in the past few years. Once restricted to ultraviolet B (UVB) filters, sunscreen manufacturers can now use ultraviolet A (UVA) filters and also UVA-reflecting micronized powders. Sunscreens have been used mainly to protect the skin from erythema. Because sunscreens with high sun protection factors (SPFs) allow very long irradiation times, and UVA may also play role in the formation of solar erythema, additional UVA protection has become necessary. In addition, some people started to use sunscreens to protect their skin from the long-term effects of solar exposure.

The availability of broad-spectrum sunscreens with increasingly acceptable cosmetic qualities also makes them suitable for the protection of some patients with UVA-induced photodermatoses. We may now expect this increasing public demand for sun-protection measures to be matched by an increasing sophistication of the products.

Sunscreen ingredients

Ultraviolet B absorbers

Almost all sunscreens contain one or more UVB filters to eliminate the erythemogenic part of the ultraviolet spectrum. Today, many different kinds of UVB absorbers are used, such as para-aminobenzoic acid and its derivatives, camphor derivatives, cinnamates, benzophenones, salicylates, and other compounds such as 2-phenylbenzimidazol-5-sulfonic acid, 2-phenyl-5-methylbenzoxazol, sodium 3, 4-dimethoxyphenylglyoxylate, dibenzalazine, and digalloyl trioleate. Most of these UVB filters are now used in lotions or creams, a trend that started in the 1970s when the less protective oil preparations became less popular. The types of UVB filters preponderantly used in sunscreen preparation varies somewhat from one country to another. Although the benzophenones have an absorption spectrum that extends into the UVA range, they may not be considered true UVA filters.

Ultraviolet A absorbers

More and more sunscreen products contain not only UVB filters but also UVA filters. This has been possible since the dibenzoylmethane derivatives became available in 1979. Two such derivatives have been commercially marketed. The first is 4-isopropyldibenzoylmethane (Eusolex 8020; Merck, Darmstadt, Germany); the second is 4-tert-butyl-4'-methoxydibenzoylmethane (Parsol 1789; Givaudan, Vernier, Switzerland). Both filters have been used in 1.5% to 4% concentrations and have about the same UVA absorption from 320 to 330 nm to about 370 to 380 nm. Because of their lack of UVB absorption, both of these filters have to be combined with UVB filters when used in sunscreen preparations. Unfortunately, because of the high incidence of contact and photocontact allergy with Eusolex 8020 compared with Parsol 1789 due to its specific chemical structure, Eusolex 8020 was withdrawn from the market in 1993.

A new UVA filter was introduced in 1993 for use in sunscreen preparations: 3,3'-(1.4 phenylenedimethylidyne) bis (7.7 dimethyl-2-oxobicyclo [2.2.1]) heptane-1-methanesulfonic acid (Mexoryl SX; L'Oréal, Clichy, France). It has been shown in hairless mice that Mex-

---

Abbreviations

SPF—sun protection factor; UVA—ultraviolet A; UVB—ultraviolet B.

oryl SX is an efficient photoprotector against chronic UVA irradiation [1]. This filter is derived from the UVB filter benzylidene camphor, which has been used mainly for its high level of photostability. It is usually used in 1% to 4% concentrations and absorbs not only UVA up to about 370 nm but also UVB, with maximum absorption at 345 nm. Mexoryl SX can thus be considered a combined UVB-UVA filter, unlike Eusolex 8020 or Parsol 1789. However, Eusolex 8020 and Parsol 1789 absorb more of the longer-wavelength UVA. Mexoryl SX is water-soluble and can be combined with lipophilic filters to increase ultraviolet absorption. Combining Mexoryl SX with Parsol 1789, for example, augments the UVA protection of a sunscreen in this way. Protection against the longest UVA wavelength is possible to some extent by combining UVB and UVA filters with powders or by using dihydroxyacetone in combination with lawsone [2].

Inorganic powders

Some powders, such as zinc oxide, titanium oxide, and ferric oxide, are used as ultraviolet-scattering agents and have been combined with UVB and UVA absorbers to obtain wide-spectrum protection. The main problem with such powders in sunscreens is cosmetic acceptability. To overcome this problem, mica-based pigments can be used, particles of the mica being coated with a metal oxide such as titanium dioxide; depending on the thickness of the coating, different colors are possible. Another possibility is the use of micronized powders. The smaller the particle diameter, the better the cosmetic acceptability and the more scattering, and thus the greater efficacy. Therefore, both the concentration and the particle size of the inorganic powder are critical.

One of the best micronized titanium dioxides presently available is Tioveil (Tioxide Specialties, Billingham Cleveland, UK), which has been used in sunscreens since 1989. Because its maximal absorption is at a wavelength of 308 nm, this preparation can be used without other ultraviolet absorbers as the only active ingredient in sunscreen preparations to prevent solar erythema. To obtain adequate UVB filtering, a concentration of about 5% titanium dioxide is necessary, whereas in concentrations over 10% the white color again becomes readily visible. Micronized titanium dioxide also partly absorbs UVA between 320 and 340 nm, but it is much less effective at wavelengths between 340 and 400 nm. While micronized titanium dioxide provides much better UVB and UVA protection up to 370 nm than does nonmicronized pigmentary titanium dioxide, the latter gives better albeit still limited protection above 370 nm and further into the visible range. Standard pigmentary titanium dioxide with a crystal size of 200 to 500 nm scatters visible light. Micronized titanium dioxide usually has a crystal size of less than 60 nm, which scatters ultraviolet light and transmits visible light.

In 1992, micronized zinc oxide became available as Spectraveil (Tioxide Specialties, Billingham Cleveland,

UK) and is now also being used in sunscreen preparations. For UVB protection, zinc oxide is markedly inferior to titanium dioxide, but it does have advantages for UVA protection. For maximum UVA protection, a crystal size of 60 to 80 nm is necessary.

Micronized zinc oxide and micronized titanium dioxide can be used individually or in combination. They can also be combined with the UVB and UVA absorbers discussed above. Such absorbers act by absorbing ultraviolet rays to convert the residual energy into innocuous longer-wave radiation, whereas powders act by reflecting and scattering, not by absorbing ultraviolet light (Fig. 1).

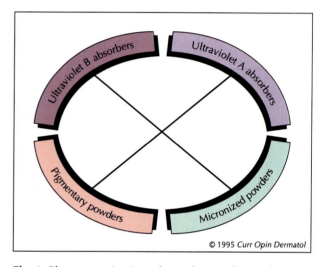

Fig. 1. Photoprotective ingredients that can be used in sunscreen preparations.

Making the right choice

The choice of a sunscreen will depend on the effect against which one wants to protect the skin. If a sunscreen preparation is used to prevent solar erythema, the preparation should contain one or more UVB filters, possibly combined with a UVA filter in products offering very high UVA protection. If a sunscreen is used to prevent the long-term effects of solar irradiation, such as skin aging and cancers, broad-spectrum sunscreens must be used because of the role UVA plays in these effects. However, the chronic use of UVB and UVA filters on the skin very likely increases the risk of contact sensitization. This risk may be avoided by using the newer micronized powders such as titanium dioxide and zinc oxide, provided that no other side effects become apparent with their long-term use. When sunscreens are used to protect patients against UVA-induced photodermatoses, the preparation should contain UVB filters, one or two UVA filters, and powders. Such patients need not just UVA protection but the maximum UVA protection available. It has been shown that the best UVA protection is provided by the combination of UVA absorbers and scattering powders and that the efficacy of such a combination appears to be cumulative (Table 1) [3].

The use of sunscreens

As important as the choice of a sunscreen product is the way it is used. A major portion of the total lifetime ultraviolet dose received by the skin is due to childhood exposure. In addition, the sun protection habits of adults are often based on the practices learned in childhood. Therefore, protection against ultraviolet radiation should start in early childhood to avoid the long-term cutaneous effects of solar exposure. Because there is some evidence that solar exposure before the age of 20 years is associated more strongly with malignant melanoma than exposure later in life, special care to avoid excessive sunlight and sunburn is necessary for children. A recent study undertaken in the southern United States revealed that only half the children under 12 years of age on a particular beach were protected with sunscreens [4]. A similar survey among college students showed that only about half of them

used sunscreens when sunbathing [5]; frequent sunbathers were more likely to be women. Another study from South Africa gave similar results: only half of the beach-goers used a sunscreen [6]. In addition, only 5% of the population used a sunscreen with an SPF of 15 or more. Other studies confirm that the overall level of protection used in children and adolescents is low [7–9,10•,11]. Therefore, sunscreens are clearly not being used in optimal fashion; many people fail to apply a sunscreen regularly enough, even if they expect painful results the day after. However, it would be even more difficult to motivate people to apply a sunscreen daily from infancy so as to avoid potential side effects in the distant future, especially in a society in which it is still fashionable to have a tan and to keep it as long as possible [12].

Sunscreen preparations can very efficiently prevent solar erythema even in extreme circumstances. This does not automatically mean, however, that they offer adequate protection against other acute or chronic side effects of solar exposure. Nevertheless, animal experiments have demonstrated the possibility of preventing

Table 1. Protection against ultraviolet A radiation from six sunscreen preparations tested on 20 subjects[*]

Preparation	Active components	Mean UVA sun PF ± SEM	Mean PUVA PF ± SEM
I	Vehicle UVB filter[†] UVB/UVA filter[‡] UVA filter[§] Physical agents[¶]	6.68±0.93	40.18±5.24
II	Vehicle UVB filter[†] UVB/UVA filter[‡] UVA filter[§]	2.80±0.37	26.85±4.19
III	Vehicle UVB filter[†] UVA filter[§]	2.91±0.32	17.64±2.21
IV	Vehicle UVB filter[†] UVB/UVA filter[‡]	1.77±0.19	4.23±0.29
V	Vehicle UVB filter[†] Physical agents[¶]	2.26±0.28	3.28±0.20
VI	Vehicle	1.16±0.08	1.32±0.06

[*]*From* Roelandts [3]; with permission.
[†]3.20% 3-(4-methylbenzylidene)-dl-camphor (Eusolex 6300; Merck, Darmstadt, FRG).
[‡]3% 2-hydroxy-4-methoxybenzophenone (Eusolex 4360; Merck, Darmstadt, FRG).
[§]1.80% 4-isopropyl dibenzoylmethane (Eusolex 8020; Merck, Darmstadt, FRG).
[¶]1.12% ferric oxide, 2% titanium oxide, 2% mica/titanium.
PF—protection factor; PUVA—psoralens and ultraviolet A; UVA—ultraviolet A; UVB—ultraviolet B.

collagen changes and solar elastosis by means of sunscreens [1,12]. The regular use of sunscreens can also prevent the development of solar keratoses in human skin; the amount of the sunscreen preparation used is related both to the development of new lesions and to the remission of existing ones with a dose-response relationship [13••].

Convincing evidence that sunscreens also offer protection against skin cancers comes from animal studies using hairless mice. However, there are clearly differences between the mouse model and what happens in human skin; the life span of a mouse is only 2 years, and the animal also has an increased susceptibility to ultraviolet-induced skin tumors. In addition, the mice are exposed to very high daily doses of artificial ultraviolet radiation and not solar radiation [14]. A further problem is that sunscreens seem to protect better against ultraviolet-induced epidermal DNA damage (ie, initiator effect) than against ultraviolet-induced immunosuppression (ie, the promotor effect); the immunoprotective ability of sunscreens is apparently limited [15] and less than their ability to protect against erythema [16•].

It is becoming common practice to add sunscreening agents to cosmetics to provide protection against ultraviolet-induced erythema, sunburn cell formation, and Langerhans cell damage, as demonstrated by the exposure of cosmetic-protected human skin to a 1.5 minimal erythema dose daily for 4 consecutive days [17•]. However, such sun protection is easier to use for women than men.

If sunscreens are used daily, other problems may arise. The greater the number of ingredients, the longer the product is used, and the higher the concentration of filters, the greater will be the possibility of irritant, allergic, or photoallergic reactions [18–21]; a recent Australian study revealed an adverse reaction in about 20% of the daily sunscreen users. Most of these adverse responses were consistent with an irritant reaction, and many of the people who had such a reaction were atopic [22•]. Similarly, allergic reactions are more frequently seen in patients with chronic actinic dermatitis as compared with control subjects, the benzophenone group of sunscreens being the most frequent sensitizers [23].

The effect that sunscreens may have on sun-exposure behavior is also very important [24]; apparently, some people believe incorrectly that highly protective sunscreens will eliminate all danger from sun exposure. Sunscreens should be used to protect the skin and not to prolong the sun-exposure time, and sunscreen users should preferentially at noon and wear appropriate clothing as much as possible [25].

It has been shown that the amount of sunscreen applied to the skin of volunteers to determine the SPF of a sunscreen product (2 μL/cm^2 or 2 mg/cm^2) is higher than generally worn by sunscreen users, and because the degree of protection is determined by the amount of sunscreen applied, the real SPF in practice is presumably less than advertised. Sunscreen users should

therefore be instructed to apply enough of the product. The SPF may also depend somewhat upon the skin type of the test subjects, because subjects with lower minimal erythema doses may show higher SPFs [26].

Other problems arise if the sunscreen is easily removed by water or perspiration. The substantivity of the sunscreen can thus influence the overall protection offered [27]. It must therefore be realized that an SPF can be misleading or even have no real value at all if the product is not waterproof or water-resistant. Hence, an important requirement is always to reapply the sunscreen after swimming or perspiration. A final problem is the photostability of the different filters used in the vehicle, which can also reduce the SPF to less than the stated value.

Conclusions

Improved sunscreen technology has led to the development of products offering very good protection against UVA radiation. The choice of sunscreen depends on the kind of skin damage one wishes to prevent, and the way the sunscreen is used is of utmost importance in determining the efficacy of protection.

References and recommended reading

Papers of particular interest, published within the annual period of review, have been highlighted as:
•   Of special interest
••   Of outstanding interest

1.   Fourtanier A, Labat-Robert J, Kern P, Berrebi C, Gracia AM, Boyer B: **In Vivo Evaluation of Photoprotection Against Chronic Ultraviolet-A Irradiation by a New Sunscreen Mexoryl SX.** *Photochem Photobiol* 1992, **55**:549–560.

2.   Johnson JA, Fusaro RM: **Therapeutic Potential of Dihydroxyacetone.** *J Am Acad Dermatol* 1993, **29**:284–286.

3.   Roelandts R: **Which Components in Broad-Spectrum Sunscreens Are Most Necessary For Adequate UVA Protection?** *J Am Acad Dermatol* 1991, **25**:999–1004.

4.   Maducdoc LR, Wagner RF, Wagner KD: **Parents' Use of Sunscreen on Beach-Going Children.** *Arch Dermatol* 1992, **128**:628–629.

5.   Vail-Smith K, Felts WM: **Sunbathing: College Students' Knowledge, Attitudes, and Perceptions of Risks.** *J Am Coll Health* 1993, **42**:21–26.

6.   von Schirnding Y, Strauss N, Mathee A, Robertson P, Blignaut R: **Sunscreen Use and Environmental Awareness Among Beach-Goers in Cape Town, South Africa.** *Public Health Rev* 1991-1992, **19**:209–217.

7.   Mermelstein RJ, Riesenberg LA: **Changing Knowledge and Attitudes About Skin Cancer Risk Factors in Adolescents.** *Health Psychol* 1992, **11**:371–376.

8.   Grob JJ, Guglielmina C, Gouvernet J, Zarour H, Noé C, Bonerandi JJ: **Study of Sunbathing Habits in Children and Adolescents: Application to the Prevention of Melanoma.** *Dermatology* 1993, **186**:94–98.

9.   Banks BA, Silverman RA, Schwartz RH, Tunnessen WW JR: **Attitudes of Teenagers Toward Sun Exposure and Sunscreen Use.** *Pediatrics* 1992, **89**:40–42.

10.   Fritschi L, Green A, Solomon PJ: **Sun Exposure in Australian Ado-**
•   **lescents.** *J Am Acad Dermatol* 1992, **27**:25–28.
Adolescents spend long periods on summer weekends in the sun and do not follow recommended sun-protection guidelines.

11.   Jarrett P, Sharp C, McLelland J: **Protection of Children By Their Mothers Against Sunburn.** *BMJ* 1993, **306**:1448.

12.   Roelandts R: **Aging and Photoaging.** In *Cosmetic Dermatology.* Edited by Baran R, Maibach H. London: Martin Dunitz; in press.

13.   Thompson SC, Jolley D, Marks R: **Reduction of Solar Keratoses by**
••   **Regular Sunscreen Use.** *N Engl J Med* 1993, **329**:1147–1151.

Regular use of sunscreens can prevent the development of solar keratoses and thus may possibly reduce the risk of skin cancer later on.

14. Drolet BA, Connor MJ: Sunscreens and the Prevention of Ultraviolet Radiation–Induced Skin Cancer. *J Dermatol Surg Oncol* 1992, **18**:571–576.

15. van Praag MCG: Clinical and Fundamental Aspects of Photodamage and Photoprotection [Thesis]. Leiden: University of Leiden; 1994.

16. Wolf P, Donawho CK, Kripke ML: Analysis of the Protective Effect
•   of Different Sunscreens on Ultraviolet Radiation–Induced Local and Systemic Suppression of Contact Hypersensitivity and Inflammatory Responses in Mice. *J Invest Dermatol* 1993, **100**:254–259.
Sunscreens are shown to be less effective in protecting against the immunosuppressive effects of ultraviolet radiation than against the inflammatory effects. Protection against inflammation does not necessarily imply prevention of immunologic alterations.

17. Elmets CA, Vargas A, Oresajo C: Photoprotective Effects of Sun-
•   screens in Cosmetics on Sunburn and Langerhans Cell Photodamage. *Photodermatol Photoimmunol Photomed* 1992, **9**:113–120.
Incorporation of some photoprotective agents into cosmetic preparations can provide protection against the adverse effects of acute ultraviolet irradiation.

18. Pons-Guiraud A, Jeanmougin M: Allergie et Photo-allergie de Contact aux Crèmes de Photoprotection. *Ann Dermatol Venereol* 1993, **120**:727–731.

19. Buckley DA, O'Sullivan D, Murphy GM: Contact and Photocontact Allergy to Dibenzoylmethanes and Contact Allergy to Methylbenzylidene Camphor. *Contact Dermatitis* 1993, **28**:47.

20. Goldermann R, Vardarman E, Neumann N, Scharffetter-Kochanek K, Goerz G: Contact Dermatitis From UV-A and UV-B Filters in a Patient With Erythropoietic Protoporphyria. *Contact Dermatitis* 1993, **28**:300–301.

21. Urbach F: Risk of Contact Dermatitis From UV-A Sunscreens. *Contact Dermatitis* 1993, **29**:220–221.

22. Foley P, Nixon R, Marks R, Frowen K, Thompson S: The Frequency
•   of Reactions to Sunscreens: Results of a Longitudinal Population-Based Study on the Regular Use of Sunscreens in Australia. *Br J Dermatol* 1993, **128**:512–518.
Presents results of a 7-month study of 603 people who applied a broad-spectrum sunscreen cream or its cream base. Of these subjects, 18.9% developed an adverse reaction to the cream, but only a small proportion of the eruptions were allergic in nature.

23. Bilsland D, Ferguson J: Contact Allergy to Sunscreen Chemicals in Photosensitivity Dermatitis/Actinic Reticuloid Syndrome (PD/AR) and Polymorphic Light Eruption (PLE). *Contact Dermatitis* 1993, **29**:70–73.

24. Stiller MJ, Davis IC, Shupack JL: A Concise Guide to Topical Sunscreens: State of the Art. *Int J Dermatol* 1992, **31**:540–543.

25. Diffey BL, Cheeseman J: Sun Protection With Hats. *Br J Dermatol* 1992, **127**:10–12.

26. Kawada A, Noda T, Hiruma M, Ishibashi A, Arai S: The Relationship of Sun Protection Factor to Minimal Erythema Dose, Japanese Skin Type, and Skin Color. *J Dermatol* 1993, **20**:514–516.

27. Patel HP, Highton A, Moy RL: Properties of Topical Sunscreen Formulations. A Review. *J Dermatol Surg Oncol* 1992, **18**:316–320.

Rik Roelandts, MD, University of Leuven, Photodermatology Unit, Kapucijnenvoer 33, B-3000 Leuven, Belgium.

Therapy

Edited by

Ralph Coskey
Wayne State School of Medicine
Detroit, Michigan, USA

CURRENT SCIENCE

Recent advances in antimicrobial therapy of bacterial infections of the skin

Yelena Mirensky, MD, Lawrence Charles Parish, MD, and Joseph A. Witkowski, MD

School of Hygiene and Public Health, Johns Hopkins University, Baltimore, Maryland, Jefferson Medical College of Thomas Jefferson University, and University of Pennsylvania School of Medicine, Philadelphia, Pennsylvania, USA

This article reviews current research on a number of oral and topical antimicrobial agents used in dermatologic practice. Clarithromycin is a macrolide effective against atypical mycobacteria. Azithromycin can be administered once a day. Photosensitivity and the emergence of resistant strains of staphylococci are of concern regarding the quinolones. In addition to being effective against mycobacteria and gram-positive organisms, rifampin may be useful in alleviating pruritus associated with primary biliary cirrhosis and psoriasis. Propionibacteria are less resistant to minocycline than to the other tetracyclines. Fusidic acid and mupirocin seem to be equally effective in treating superficial skin infections. The treatment of contact dermatitis with neomycin continues to be documented.

Current Opinion in Dermatology 1995:179–184

Antimicrobial agents (Table 1) continue to play a significant role in dermatologic practice, not only because of their active role in the treatment of bacterial infections of the skin and skin structure, but also because of their side effects. Adverse reactions are accentuated in immunocompromised patients.

Older agents have been reassessed for their possible use in other diseases. For example, one of the rifamycin drugs has been successful in the treatment of leishmaniasis. Newer drugs are proving to be highly versatile. A new macrolide, clarithromycin, is being studied in a variety of diseases, including mycobacterial infections and peptic ulcer disease. More attention is also being directed toward topical agents with clinical trials of fusidic acid.

Resistance patterns of staphylococcal strains are creating some problems with the quinolones, as is awareness of the photodermatitis that occurs with their administration. Whether the former will be overcome with the introduction of newer quinolones and whether the latter can be avoided in the future by the use of new techniques employed in animal model test-

Table 1. Oral antimicrobials of interest to the dermatologist

Cephalosporins	Macrolides	Quinolones	Rifamycins	Tetracyclines
Cefaclor	Azithromycin	Ciprofloxacin	Rifampin	Demeclocycline
Cefadroxil	Clarithromycin	Enoxacin		Doxycycline
Cefdinir	Dirithromycin	Fleroxacin		Minocycline
Cefixime	Erythromycin	Lomefloxacin		Oxytetracycline
Cefotaxime		Norfloxacin		Tetracycline
Cefpodexime		Ofloxacin		
Cefprozil				
Cefuroxime axetil				
Cephalexin				
Cephradine				
Lorocarbef				

ing remain to be seen. Regardless, these agents are extremely valuable in contemporary dermatologic practice (Fig. 1).

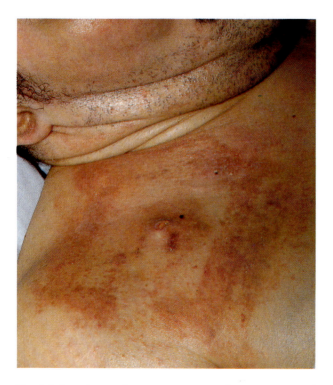

Fig. 1. Infected central venous pressure catheter site required intravenous vancomycin therapy. The staphylococci recovered were resistant to most oral agents.

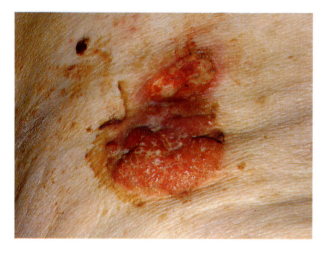

Fig. 2. Infected surgical site responded to an oral cephalosporin.

Finally, there is a trend toward once-a-day administration of oral an antimicrobials. Several oral penicillins and augmented synthetic penicillins were initially studied at dosages of three and four times a day. Trials have now been conducted to determine the possibility of reducing the frequency without sacrificing efficiency.

Azithromycin, one of the newer macrolides, is administered once a day.

Cephalosporins

The cephalosporins, β-lactam bactericidal antimicrobial agents, are widely used in dermatologic practice (Fig. 2). A number of serum sickness cases associated with cefaclor reported in 1992 initially caused new awareness of this type of drug reaction [1,2,3•]. With further use of these compounds, additional cases of serum sickness appear to be exceedingly rare.

More cephalosporins are reaching the clinical arena. In Japan, cefditoren pivoxil is being studied. It is effective against streptococci, staphylococci, and *Hemophilus influenzae*. A major attribute is its safety in children [4,5].

Macrolides

Erythromycin, the original cell wall synthesis inhibitor, has been used for over 40 years to combat gram-positive and gram-negative infections. Clarithromycin, an acid-stable analogue of erythromycin, appears to be a particularly promising new macrolide. In two recent multicenter studies, clarithromycin (250 mg twice daily) was shown to be equally as safe and effective as erythromycin and cefadroxil in treating skin and soft tissue infections. The most common side effect, nausea, occurred in 5% to 7% of the patients [6•]. Clarithromycin is also uniquely effective against the atypical mycobacteria, including *Mycobacterium chelonae*, *Mycobacterium avium-intracellulare*, *Mycobacterium marinum*, *Mycobacterium simiae*, *Mycobacterium scrofulaceum*, *Mycobacterium kansasii*, *Mycobacterium szulgai*, *Mycobacterium gordonae*, and *Mycobacterium nonchromogenicum* [6•]. Case reports of clarithromycin's effectiveness in eradicating *M. chelonae* [7] were recently confirmed in an open trial of 14 patients with *M. chelonae* infections. Cure was achieved in 11 of 14 patients after 6 months of treatment with clarithromycin (500 mg twice daily). Of the remaining three patients, two died from other causes, and one was noncompliant [8]. Twice-a-day dosing makes clarithromycin a convenient agent to administer, especially in patients with β-lactam allergy.

Azithromycin, another new macrolide, is concentrated in the tissues. It can be administered once a day for a short period of time. Azithromycin was shown to be as effective as dicloxacillin in treating 60 adults with skin and soft tissue infections. *Staphylococcus aureus*, streptococci, and coagulase-negative staphylococci were isolated from the lesions. Azithromycin given for 3 days resulted in 90% bacteriological eradication; dicloxacillin, given for 7 days, had an eradication rate of 87% [9•]. A study of 118 children resulted in similar data [10]. Another investigation showed it to be equal to doxycycline in the treatment of Lyme borreliosis in 55 adults [11].

Antibiotics are not used exclusively for their antibacterial action. Potent anti-inflammatory properties of some of the newer macrolides confirm the importance of not categorizing a drug. For example, FK 506 was recently shown to be superior to corticosteroids when applied topically to mice and pigs with allergic contact dermatitis [12].

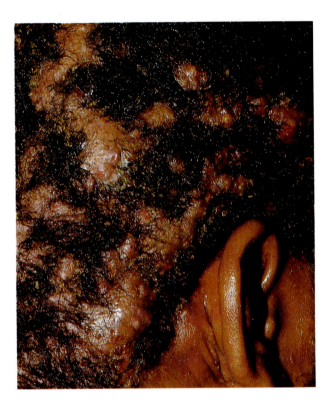

Fig. 3. Perifolliculitis capitis abscedens et suffodiens was due to gram-negative as well as gram-positive organisms. Quinolone therapy was used.

Quinolones

Potent gram-positive and gram-negative coverage allows the new fluoroquinolones to be used orally, often in place of intravenous agents, to treat serious infections (Fig. 3). The convenient once- to twice-daily dosing combined with mild side effects has made these compounds uniquely popular. Two recent concerns, however, have been the increasing development of resistant staphylococcal strains [13] and photosensitivity reactions in outpatients. The latter problem is significant in dermatologic practice, because patients often undergo significant light exposure. Since the release of a drug alert by G.D. Searle & Co. (Chicago, IL) in 1993 describing a study in which 92% of hairless mice developed well-differentiated squamous cell carcinomas after being exposed to lomefloxacin and high dose ultraviolet A radiation [14], this subject has aroused particular interest. Incidence of phototoxic reactions, reported to be 0.4% to 2.4%, is higher in compounds with longer half-lives and those with more bioavailability [15]. A re-

cent case report described an exaggerated sunburn on the face of a 25-year-old skier taking lomefloxacin [16]. While this reaction was most likely phototoxic in nature, rare photoallergic reactions to lomefloxacin [17] and enoxacin [18,19] have also been reported. It is not always possible to determine which type of reaction has taken place.

In a randomized trial of 37 young men, another new quinolone, ofloxacin, was found to be equally as phototoxic as naproxen, the active control substance. The ultraviolet A flux used in this investigation was 10 times greater than solar ultraviolet A. The most severe reactions consisted of erythema and edema [20]. There have been no studies to date comparing all of the fluoroquinolones. With presently available data, an empirical hierarchy of photosensitivity among the quinolones, in descending order, would be fleroxacin, lomefloxacin, pefloxacin, ciprofloxacin, enoxacin, norfloxacin, and ofloxacin [20].

Rifamycins

Rifampin has been a useful antimicrobial agent since 1966. Inhibiting protein synthesis, it is bactericidal against mycobacteria and gram-positive organisms. Although effective in treating pyodermas, it continues to be most commonly used to treat cutaneous tuberculosis and leprosy. Rifampin has also been shown effective in alleviating the pruritus associated with primary biliary cirrhosis and severe psoriasis, particularly *Streptococcus*-associated psoriasis [21••]. Cutaneous leishmaniasis seems to respond to this agent as well [22]. Topical rifampin can be used on postoperative wounds, burns, eschars, impetigo, and abscesses, but it is not available in the United States.

Tetracyclines

A growing problem in the treatment of acne is the increasing resistance of propionibacteria. When erythromycin, doxycycline, clindamycin, tetracycline, and trimethoprim were tested on isolates from 468 patients with acne, 78 (38%) of the isolates proved resistant to one of the antibiotics *in vitro*. There was no resistance against minocycline [23]. Because propionibacteria seem to be more sensitive to minocycline than to either tetracycline or doxycycline, it may be the antibiotic of choice for acne. In one study, the most effective dosage of minocycline was 100 mg orally twice a day [24]. The extent of laboratory monitoring necessary for patients receiving this or any long-term oral antibiotic for acne remains unclear [25••].

Topical antimicrobials

When effective, topical antibiotics have a number of obvious advantages over the oral agents in treating localized skin infections. They usually have fewer side effects and less drug interactions. The agent can be directed to the site of infection and applied in high concentrations. Several new compounds are soon to be investigated, such as a synthetic magainin derived from frogs (Figs. 4 and 5).

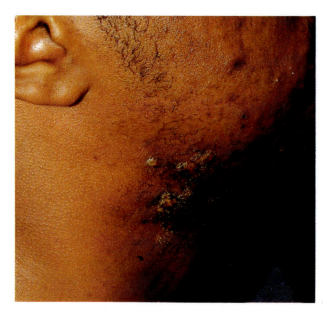

Fig. 4. Folliculitis is superficial enough to permit topical antimicrobial therapy.

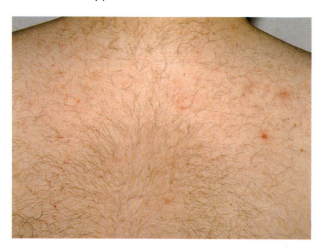

Fig. 5. Folliculi on the back may be treated with topical antimicrobial agents.

Fusidic acid

New to the United States and currently under study, fusidic acid has been successfully used in Europe for over 20 years. This antibiotic inhibits protein synthesis in both procaryotic and eukaryotic cells [26], impairs T-cell proliferation, and acts as an immunosuppressive agent [27]. Fusidic acid is used to treat superficial skin infections and is particularly effective in eradicating *S. aureus* [28]. It may also be an alternative to circumcision in treating plasma cell balanitis. The disease was cured in three of eight patients in one trial and suppressed in another two [29]. Three patients with folliculitis decalvans were apparently cured after treatment with a combination of oral and topical fusidic acid and oral zinc sulfate [30]. Side effects associated with topical fusidic acid are rare and usually eczematous in appearance. In one report, acanthosis nigricans–like lesions appeared in a 4-year-old girl after application of fusidic acid; the lesions cleared with appropriate treatment [31].

Gentamicin

Topical gentamicin (0.1%) is now available as an ointment or as a sponge made from cattle tendons. The sponge has been shown to be effective in treating infected bone cavities [32].

Mupirocin

Mupirocin binds to esoleucyl transfer RNA synthetase and thereby inhibits bacterial protein synthesis. It is used to treat a number of primary and secondary superficial skin infections. It has been shown to be as effective as oral agents, and it provides a topical alternative in treating streptococcal and staphylococcal impetigo [33,34•,35•,36••]. It is also effective in eradicating *S. aureus* from the nares of patients undergoing peritoneal dialysis [37,38]. In one study, *S. aureus* was eradicated in 100% of the patients treated with mupirocin and 40% of the patients treated with neomycin [39]. Although possibly capable of eradicating staphylococci and streptococci present in exudative venous ulcers [40,41], it is probably not a good choice for empirical use, as it is ineffective against *Pseudomonas aeruginosa* [42]. Mupirocin and fusidic acid seem to be similarly effective in treating superficial skin infections [43,44], but mupirocin was shown to be slightly better (96% vs 88%) in eliminating *S. aureus* and β-hemolytic streptococci of group A [44]. Mupirocin can be mixed with a variety of other creams, lotions, and ointments, except for betamethasone valerate lotion, with which it is physically incompatible [45•].

Neomycin

Despite a varied incidence of associated contact dermatitis, reported to be up to 20% in past studies, neomycin continues to be a widely used topical antibiotic. In a recent study, the incidence of contact dermatitis in patients receiving neomycin for postoperative wound care was shown to be 5% [46].

Conclusions

The advent of newer agents and advances in the understanding of currently available antimicrobial agents will permit better patient care. Unwanted side effects may prove to be beneficial in selected patients.

References and recommended reading

Papers of particular interest, published within the annual period of review, have been highlighted as:
- • Of special interest
- •• Of outstanding interest

1. Parra FM, Igea JM, Martin JA, Alonso MD, Lezaun A, Sainz T: Serum Sickness-like Syndrome Associated With Cefaclor Therapy. *Allergy* 1992, 47:439–440.

2. Vial T, Pont J, Pham E, Rabilloud M, Descotes J: Cefaclor-Associated Serum Sickness-like Disease: Eight Cases and Review of the Literature. *Ann Pharmacother* 1992, 26:910–914.

3. Stricker BH, Tijssen JG: Serum Sickness-like Reactions to Cefaclor. *J*
• *Clin Epidemiol* 1992, 45:1177–1184.
In this example of epidemiologic methodology, the relative risk of developing serum sickness from cefaclor and amoxicillin was found to be 15.1 and 5.5, respectively.

4. Toyonaga Y, Ishihara T, Sano T, Tezuka T, Nakamura H: Bacteriological, Pharmacokinetic and Clinical Studies of Cefditoren Pivoxil in the Pediatric Field [in Japanese]. *Jpn J Antibiot* 1993, 46:406–428.

5. Nishimura T, Tabuki K, Aoki S, Takagi M: Clinical Studies of Cefditoren Pivoxil in Pediatric Field [in Japanese]. *Jpn J Antibiot* 1993, 46:629–636.

6. Parish LC: Clarithromycin in the Treatment of Skin and Skin Structure
• Infections: Two Multicenter Clinical Studies. *Int J Dermatol* 1993, 32:528–531.
A thorough report describing two multicenter studies in which clarithromycin was compared to cefadroxil and erythromycin in a total of 1239 patients.

7. Franck N, Cabie A, Villette B, Amor B, Lessana-Leibowitch M, Escande JP: Treatment of *Mycobacterium chelonae*-Induced Skin Infection With Clarithromycin. *J Am Acad Dermatol* 1993, 28:1019–1021.

8. Wallace RJ Jr, Tanner D, Brennan PJ, Brown BA: Clinical Trial of Clarithromycin for Cutaneous (Disseminated) Infection Due to *Mycobacterium chelonae*. *Ann Intern Med* 1993, 119:482–486.

9. Amaya-Taipa G, Aquirre-Avalos J, Andrade-Villanueva G, Peredo-
• Gonzalez G, Morfin-Otero R, Esparza-Ahumada S, Rodreguez-Noriega E: Once-Daily Azithromycin in the Treatment of Adult Skin and Skin-Structure Infections. *J Antimicrob Chemother* 1993, 31(suppl E):129–135.
In a well-designed, randomized, blinded study, azithromycin was equally as effective and as safe as dicloxacillin in treating 60 patients with mostly abscesses and cellulitis. *S. aureus*, streptococci, and coagulase-negative staphylococci were the most common isolates.

10. Rodriguez-Solares A, Perez-Gutierrez F, Prosperi J, Milgram E, Martin A: A Comparative Study of the Efficacy, Safety and Tolerance of Azithromycin, Dicloxacillin and Flucloxacillin in the Treatment of Children With Acute Skin and Skin-Structure Infections. *J Antimicrob Chemother* 1993, 31(suppl E):103–109.

11. Strle F, Preac-Mursic V, Cimperman J, Ruzic E, Maraspin V, Jereb M: Azithromycin Versus Doxycycline for Treatment of Erythema Migrans: Clinical and Microbiological Findings. *Infection* 1993, 21:830–888.

12. Meingassner JG, Stutz A: Anti-inflammatory Effects of Macrophilin-Interacting Drugs in Animal Models of Irritant and Allergic Contact Dermatitis. *Int Arch Allergy Immunol* 1992, 99:486–489.

13. Parish LC, Witkowski JA, Mirensky YM: Recent Advances in Antimicrobial Therapy of Bacterial Infections of the Skin. *Curr Opin Dermatol* 1994, 1:263–270.

14. *Important Drug Information for Maxaquin.* Chicago: GD Searle & Co.; 1993.

15. Mirensky YM, Parish LC: Photosensitivity and the Quinolones. In
• press.
A comprehensive review of current information on photosensitivity associated with the quinolones.

16. Poh-Fitzpatrick MB: Lomefloxacin Photosensitivity. *Arch Dermatol* 1994, 130:261.

17. Kurumaji Y, Shon M: Scarified Photopatch Testing in Lomefloxacin Photosensitivity. *Contact Dermatitis* 1992, 26:5–10.

18. Kawabe Y, Mizuno N, Shigeru S: Photoallergic Reaction Caused by Enoxacin. *Photodermatology* 1989, 6:58–60.

19. Kang JS, Kim TH, Park KB, Chung BH, Youn JI: Enoxacin Photosensitivity. *Photodermatol Photoimmunol Photomed* 1993, 9:159–161.

20. Scheife RT, Cramer WR, Decker EL: Photosensitizing Potential of Ofloxacin. *Int J Dermatol* 1993, 32:413–416.

21. Tsankov NK, Kamarashev JA: Rifampin in Dermatology. *Int J Der-*
•• *matol* 1993, 32:401–406.
An excellent review of rifampin indications, pharmacology, and side effects.

22. Joshi RK, Nambiar PMK: Dermal Leishmaniasis and Rifampicin. *Int J Dermatol* 1989, 28:612–614.

23. Eady EA, Jones CE, Tipper JL, Cove JH, Cunliffe WJ, Layton AM: Antibiotic Resistant Propionibacteria in Acne: Need for Policies to Modify Antibiotic Usage. *BMJ* 1993, 306:555–556.

24. Eady EA, Jones CE, Gardner KJ, Taylor JP, Cove JH, Cunliffe WJ: Tetracycline-Resistant Propionibacteria From Acne Patients Are Cross-Resistant to Doxycycline, but Sensitive to Minocycline. *Br J Dermatol* 1993, 128:556–560.

25. Driscoll M, Rothe M, Abrahamian L, Grant-Kels JM: Long Term Oral
•• Antibiotics for Acne: Is Laboratory Monitoring Necessary? *J Am Acad Dermatol* 1993, 28:595–602.
This excellent article provides results of a survey and reviews the literature dealing with the value of routine laboratory monitoring in patients receiving oral antibiotics for acne. According to the survey, 29% of the dermatologists questioned routinely test the patients, 64% do some laboratory monitoring, and 35% test only under special circumstances.

26. Von Dachne W, Godtfredsen WO, Rasmussen PR: Structure-Activity Relationships in Fusidic Acid-Type Antibiotics. *Adv Appl Microbiol* 1979, 25:95–146.

27. Bendtzen K, Diamant M, Faber V: Fusidic Acid: An Immunosuppressive Drug With Functions Similar to Cyclosporin A. *Cytokine* 1990, 2:423–429.

28. Godtfredsen WO, Jahnsen S, Lork H, *et al.*: Fusidic Acid: A New Antibiotic. *Nature* 1962, 193:987.

29. Petersen CS, Thomsen K: Fusidic Acid Cream in the Treatment of Plasma Cell Balanitis. *J Am Acad Dermatol* 1992, 27:633–634.

30. Abeck K, Korting HC, Braun-Falco O: Folliculitis Decalvans: Long-Lasting Response to Combined Therapy With Fusidic Acid and Zinc. *Acta Derm Venereol (Stockh)* 1992, 72:143–145.

31. Teknetzis A, Lefaki I, Joannides D, Minas A: Acanthosis Nigricans-like Lesions After Local Application of Fusidic Acid. *J Am Acad Dermatol* 1993, 28:501–502.

32. Boda A, Muhsammer M: First Experience in Hungary With the Use of a Garamycin Sponge in the Treatment of Suppurative Bone and Joint Wounds. *Magy Traumatol Orthop Helyreallito Sebesz* 1991, 34:133–140.

33. Leyden JJ: Review of Mupirocin Ointment in the Treatment of Impetigo. *Clin Pediatr (Phila)* 1992, 31:549–553.

34. Rice TD, Duggan AK, De Angeles C: Cost-Effectiveness of Ery-
• thromycin Versus Mupirocin for the Treatment of Impetigo in Children. *Pediatrics* 1992, 89:210–214.
An interesting article. Although mupirocin was more expensive, it was associated with fewer side effects and fewer disruptions in the daily activities of working parents of the children being treated.

35. Dagan R, Bar-David Y: Double-Blind Study Comparing Erythromycin
• and Mupirocin for Treatment of Impetigo in Children: Implications of a High Prevalence of Erythromycin-Resistant *Staphylococcus aureus* Strains. *Antimicrob Agents Chemother* 1992, 366:287–290.
Mupirocin was better than oral erythromycin in treating 102 patients in a community with high rates (28%) of *S. aureus* resistant to erythromycin.

36. Booth JH, Shalom IB: Mupirocin in the Treatment of Impetigo. *Int*
•• *J Dermatol* 1992, 31:1–9.
An excellent review and critique of trials conducted from 1984 to 1990.

37. Watanakunakorn C, Brandt J, Durkin P, Santore S, Bota B, Stahl CJ: The Efficacy of Mupirocin Ointment and Chlorhexidine Body Scrubs in the Eradication of Nasal Carriage of *Staphylococcus aureus* Among Patients Undergoing Long-Term Hemodialysis. *Am J Infect Control* 1992, 20:138–141.

38. Boelaert JR, Van Landuyt HW, Godard CA, Daneels RF, Schurgers ML: Nasal Mupirocin Ointment Decreases the Incidence of *Staphylococcus aureus* Bacteraemias in Haemodialysis Patients. *Nephrol Dial Transplant* 1993, 8:235–239.

39. Perez-Fontan M, Rosales M, Rodriguez-Carmona A, Moncalian J, Fernandez-Revera C, Cao M, Valdes F: Treatment of *Staphylococcus aureus* Nasal Carriers in CAPD With Mupirocin. *Adv Perit Dial* 1992, 8:242–245.

40. Mehtar S, Fox D: A Double-Blind Comparative Study With Mupirocin Versus Placebo Base in the Treatment of Chronic Leg Ulcers. *Br J Clin Pract* 1988, 42:324–328.

41. Dahl MG, Bint AJ: Bacterial and Clinical Effects of Bactroban Ointment in Infected Ulcerated Skin Lesions. In *Bactroban (Mupirocin): Proceedings of an International Symposium, Nassau, May 21–22,*

1984. Edited by Dobson RL, Leyden JJ, Noble WC, Price JD. Amsterdam: Elsevier Science Publishers (Excerpta Medica); 1985: 91–95. [Current Clinical Practice Series, **16.**]

42.   Pardes JB, Carson PA, Eaglstein WH, Falanga V: **Mupirocin Treatment**
•   **of Exudative Venous Ulcers.** *J Am Acad Dermatol* 1993, 29:497–498.
Thirty-seven patients with exudative venous ulcers were evaluated. *P. aeruginosa,* present in 49% of the patients, was eliminated by mupirocin only 29% of the time, versus 21% for placebo.

43.   Gilbert M: **Topical 2% Mupirocin Versus 2% Fusidic Acid Ointment in the Treatment of Primary and Secondary Skin Infections.** *J Am Acad Dermatol* 1989, **20:**1083–1087.

44.   White DG, Collins PO, Rowsell RB: **Topical Antibiotics in the Treatment of Superficial Skin Infections in General Practice: A Comparison of Mupirocin With Sodium Fusidate.** *J Infect* 1989, **18:**221–229.

45.   Jagota NK, Stewart JT, Warren FW, John PM: **Stability of Mupirocin**
•   **Ointment (Bactroban) Admixed With Other Proprietary Dermatological Products.** *J Clin Pharm Ther* 1992, 17:181–184.
A descriptive study. Mupirocin was mixed with various other commonly used preparations and stored at 37° C for 60 days. Hibiclens (Stuart Pharmaceuticals, Wilmington, DE) and Lotrimin (Schering Corp., Kenilworth, NJ) lotion mixtures remained homogeneous for the entire 60 days.

46.   Gette MT, Marks JG, Maloney ME: **Frequency of Postoperative Allergic Contact Dermatitis to Topical Antibiotics.** *Arch Dermatol* 1992, 128:365–367.

Lawrence Charles Parish, MD, 1819 JFK Boulevard, Philadelphia, PA 19103, USA.

The use of interferon in dermatology

R. Kenneth Landow, MD

University of Southern California School of Medicine, Los Angeles, California, USA

Currently, the only Food and Drug Administration–approved indications for interferon therapy in dermatology are resistant or recalcitrant genital warts and Kaposi's sarcoma. Although unresolved questions still exist regarding the efficacy of this treatment, it offers a novel and intellectually appealing approach in these previously difficult areas. However, interferons have generated the most excitement in the field of cutaneous neoplasia. Benign and malignant tumors appear highly susceptible to the antiproliferative and immunomodulating effects of these drugs. Because the cosmetic results associated with this therapy regularly exceed those of radiation or surgery, this novel application warrants further evaluation. Newborn children with hemangiomas, adults with cutaneous T-cell lymphoma, and those with a variety of infectious diseases may receive considerable benefits from interferon. Severe atopic dermatitis also frequently responds to this treatment.

Current Opinion in Dermatology 1995:185–192

Expanding interest coupled with novel applications portends a bright future for interferon therapy in the field of cutaneous medicine. After an initial phase of unbridled enthusiasm followed by one of unwarranted disillusionment, a mature attitude now appears to be developing in regard to the use of these compounds. Insight into the molecular biology of these cytokines provides a rational basis for their use in a wide array of diseases ranging from anogenital warts and cutaneous neoplasia to immune dysregulatory syndromes and connective tissue diseases (Table 1). Genetic recombinant engineering currently offers an almost unlimited, relatively inexpensive supply of these chemicals.

Two broad categories of interferons exist (Tables 2 and 3). Type I consists of at least 15 variants of interferon alfa together with a single form of interferon beta. A newly isolated species, interferon omega, remains to be more fully evaluated. Interferon gamma currently constitutes the sole member of the type II classification. This protein arises on a different chromosome, binds to its own cell surface receptor, and seems uniquely capable of attacking such microorganisms as *Toxoplasma gondii*, *Listeria monocytogenes*, and *Staphylococcus aureus* [1,2••,3•].

Human papillomavirus infections

Interferons have generated substantial interest in the field of venereology—specifically, the treatment of anogenital warts. Except in the most unusual situations, initial therapy should continue to employ the traditional approach with podophyllin, electrodesicca-tion, or cryosurgery. These methods usually provide an economical approach and a satisfactory outcome [4]. For resistant or recurrent cases, injections of interferon, especially when coupled with one of the more destructive approaches, provide a satisfactory although still controversial alternative. While treatment schedules lack standardization, experts agree that intralesional injections rather than subcutaneous, intramuscular, or topical administration offer the greatest potential for reward with the least likelihood of toxicity. Unfortunately, treatment with interferon requires two or three office visits each week for a minimum of nine visits. Condyloma acuminata begin to involute after 2 or 3 weeks of therapy and often reach their maximum level of resolution 4 to 8 weeks after commencement of therapy [1].

While monotherapy with intralesional injections of interferon alfa has received the imprimatur of the Food and Drug Administration, most current investigators advocate a multidimensional approach. To limit toxicity, no more than five lesions should be treated during any one session. As a single agent, interferon causes approximately 60% of injected lesions to resolve eventually, a number consistent with any standard monotherapy [3•]. Whether genetically engineered products provide a superior outcome compared with the natural varieties remains to be established (Figs. 1 and 2) [3•] . Even an immunocompromised host with lesions demonstrating bowenoid features and changes suggestive of early carcinoma may benefit from an intensive regimen of interferon alfa therapy [5].

In a review of four studies involving 86 patients treated with interferon alfa, the complete response rate averaged slightly in excess of 60%, but the subsequent

Table 1. Interferon mechanisms of action and activities*

Mechanisms of action
  Alteration of gene function
  Regulation of gene transcription and translation
  Activation or inactivation of gene or protooncogene
  Regulation of enzyme expression
  Alteration of endothelial cell function
  Immunomodulation
  Expression of cell surface antigens
  Expression of Fc receptors
  Expression of class I or class II major histocompati-
    bility complex antigens
  Stimulation of macrophage function
  Stimulation of natural killer cell activity
  Cell differentiation
  Stimulation of production of other cytokines
Summary of activities
  Antiviral
  Antiproliferative
  Antitumor
  Immunomodulatory

*Data from Browder et al. [1], Stadler and Ruszczak [2••], and Steinmann et al. [3•].

Table 2. Sites of natural interferon production*

Interferon	Sites	Gene location
Type I		Chromosome 9
Alfa	Leukocytes, endothelial cells, macrophages, tumor cells, keratinocytes, mesenchymal cells	
Beta	Fibroblasts, epithelial cells	
Omega	T lymphocytes	
Type II		Chromosome 12
Gamma	T lymphocytes	

*Data from Stadler and Ruszczak [2••] and Steinmann et al. [3•].

Table 3. Commercially available interferon preparations

Roferon-A*
  Interferon alfa-2a
  Recombinant
  FDA-approved indications
    Hairy-cell leukemia
    AIDS-related Kaposi's sarcoma
Intron A†
  Interferon alfa-2b
  Recombinant
  FDA-approved indications
    Hairy-cell leukemia
    Condyloma acuminata
    AIDS-related Kaposi's sarcoma
    Chronic hepatitis C
    Chronic hepatitis B
Alferon N injection ‡
  Interferon alfa-n3
  Natural
  FDA-approved indication
    Refractory or recurring external condyloma acuminata
Actimmune§
  Interferon gamma-1b
  Recombinant
  FDA-approved indication
    Chronic granulomatous disease

*Roche Laboratories, Nutley, NJ.
†Schering Laboratories, Kenilworth, NJ.
‡Purdue Frederick Co., Norwalk, CT.
§Genentech, South San Francisco, CA.
FDA—Food and Drug Administration.

relapse rate was at least 25%. Approximately 13% of patients discontinued therapy owing to systemic toxicity [6••]. Whereas early reports detailed the promise of dual therapy, more recent investigations cast some doubt on the role of this approach. The most recent data from the Condylomata International Collaborative Study Group [7•] dealt with a multicenter, double-blind, placebo-controlled investigation in which all visible lesions were ablated with a carbon dioxide laser. This was followed by injections of interferon alfa-2a into the deltoid area three times each week for 4 weeks. With this questionable approach, neither the response rate nor the recurrence rate differed between those receiving the active injections and those receiving the placebo therapy. By all accounts, however, this method involved a route of administration acknowledged to be less active than the standard intralesional injections.

A somewhat smaller study evaluated cryotherapy for genital warts followed by subcutaneous injections of interferon alfa-2a into the thigh, abdominal fat pad, and deltoid area. A 6-month review of these patients revealed no significant differences between those receiving interferon therapy and others treated with placebo injections, but the same objections can be raised to subcutaneous therapy at sites far removed from the involved skin [8]. Still another open, uncontrolled investigation utilized destructive therapy with podophyllin or trichloroacetic acid followed by systemic administration of interferon alfa-2a. The recurrence rate after 1 year exceeded 50% [9]. Finally, doctors in Berlin treated 20 patients with recalcitrant anogenital warts with a combination of electrocautery or carbon dioxide laser followed by subcutaneous injections of interferon gamma into the thigh. No significant differences separated the group receiving placebo from that receiving active injections at 3, 6, 9, or 12 months [10].

In spite of these negative reports and comments that interferon therapy offers "no demonstrable advantages over other treatments" for condyloma acuminata [4], enthusiasts remain undaunted. Arguments remain to be evaluated involving variable results on the basis of circadian timing of the injections [11], immune status of the patient, the type of interferon employed, the presence of neutralizing antibodies, the mode of administration, and even the dose of therapy [12]. Unfortunately, many of the investigations into treatment of warts with interferon fail to conform to the scientific model and cannot be used either to support or to reject the use of these drugs.

In uncontrolled investigations, interferon therapy proved useful in a patient with verruca vulgaris located on the glabrous skin. Biweekly injections with the Dermojet needleless injector (Robbins Instruments, Chatham, NJ) [13] proved highly satisfactory in several patients. In other patients, subcutaneous injections of natural interferon beta were rewarded with a complete involution of previously recalcitrant warts on the hands and feet [14].

Cutaneous neoplasia

More consistent results and less controversy surround other applications of the interferons. These drugs may prove to be a valuable asset in treating skin tumors. As an example, Swedish investigators evaluated 15 patients with deeply infiltrating, morphea-like or recurrent basal cell carcinomas [15••]. These aggressive lesions, located on the face, measured 7 to 25 mm in diameter. Treatment consisted of three weekly intralesional injections each containing 1.5 MU of interferon alfa-2b. After receiving a total of nine injections, patients were evaluated for 2 months before the treated areas underwent surgical excision. At this dose, only 27% of the patients were cured, but another 33% manifested shrinkage of their lesions by more than 75%. A higher dose of interferon appeared to boost the rate of complete response substantially. Recurrences were infrequent after up to 2.5 years of posttreatment observation. Although the cure rate appeared independent

of tumor size, a sufficient quantity of the material was necessary to permeate the entire lesion.

Data regarding involution of squamous cell carcinomas following interferon treatment suggest an even better response [16••]. A multicenter collaborative study evaluated 48 healthy volunteers with actinically induced tumors. These patients received the same dose and type of interferon as those in the study of basal cell carcinoma. After 18 weeks, the involved sites were excised and evaluated microscopically. Subsequent histologic review determined that only 27 of these tumors were invasive squamous cell carcinomas with another seven falling under the heading of carcinoma *in situ*; 11 were actinic keratoses, and one was an atypical fibroxanthoma. Ninety-seven percent of the invasive and *in situ* lesions disappeared with intralesional therapy. In the majority of tumors, this resolution occurred within 12 weeks after the initiation of therapy. Both patients and doctors rated the cosmetic results as very good to excellent in 94% of cases.

Six patients with histologically confirmed giant keratoacanthomas received three weekly injections of either 3 or 6 MU of interferon alfa-2a while the lesions were still in their rapid growth phase [17•]. A complete response ensued in all five patients who completed at least 4 weeks of therapy. During the follow-up period, which lasted as long as 3 years, no recurrences were noted. Cosmetic results were rated as excellent in four of these five patients. The fifth patient opted for surgery to correct a small defect in the nasal skin.

A series of patients with metastatic breast cancer involving the chest wall was reported on from Columbia University [18]. Patients received injections of natural interferon alfa or gamma or a combination of the two

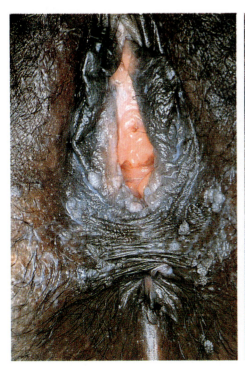 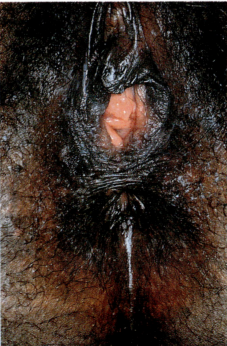

Fig. 1. Left, A 24-year-old black woman with evidence of condyloma acuminata for 6 months. She had received 10 previous treatments with podophyllin and trichloroacetic acid. **Right,** For 6 weeks, the patient received parenteral interferon therapy as the only form of treatment. Photograph was taken 2 weeks after discontinuation of treatment. (*From* Greenberg [48]; with permission.)

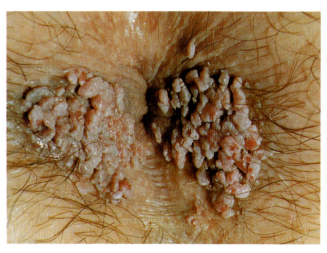 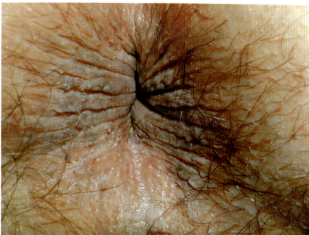

Fig. 2. Left, Perirectal condylomata before treatment with Alferon (Purdue Frederick Co., Norwalk, CT). **Right,** Six weeks post-treatment. (*Courtesy of* R. J. Brodell, Warren, OH.)

forms. For reasons yet to be fully elucidated, dual therapy provided superior results. After an initial three to five injections, the lesions began to involute. In the group receiving the combined therapy, 70% (five of seven) underwent a complete local remission, while the others showed a partial response. Overall, those treated with natural interferon alfa did only slightly worse, with fewer patients enjoying a complete response and more responding only partially.

Hemangiomas

Large, troublesome hemangiomas and an unusual condition, diffuse neonatal hemangiomatosis, also seem to respond, albeit slowly, to intralesional injections of interferon alfa-2a. In one case, a 3.5-month-old girl had an enlarging vascular lesion extending from the buttock and vulva to the lower extremity. Treatment with the tunable dye laser proved ineffective. This patient received injections in the evening in order to minimize toxicity with common flulike symptoms, the most frequent complication. At a daily maintenance dosage of 3 MU/m², these subcutaneous injections were associated with a decrease in size that persisted during the entire year of therapy [19].

After corticosteroid therapy proved ineffective, another girl was started on a prolonged course of interferon alfa-2a for a lifelong history of small but innumerable hemangiomas on the face, scalp, trunk, and extremities, as well as in the liver. At a daily intramuscular dosage of 3 MU, the lesions faded and finally disappeared when the child was 24 months old [20]. In the absence of effective treatment, death occurs during the first 6 months of life in 60% to 95% of patients with diffuse neonatal hemangiomatosis.

Doctors in Boston reported on their experience with interferon therapy for the treatment of life- or vision-threatening hemangiomas. Twenty patients unrespon-

sive to corticosteroids were treated for 1 to 13 months with daily injections of subcutaneous interferon alfa-2a at dosages of up to 2 MU/m². Treatment was initiated in patients between the ages of 3 weeks and 2 years. One child died within 1 month of the beginning of therapy, but this individual's disease was thought to represent a malignant variant more closely resembling Kaposi's sarcoma than a typical hemangioma. Eighteen patients experienced at least a 50% regression in their lesions after 2 to 13 months (mean 7.8 months) of therapy. Children with the Kasabach-Merritt syndrome demonstrated a remarkable improvement, except for patient who died shortly after the initiation of therapy. Typically, within 1 week after beginning treatment, children with consumptive coagulopathy demonstrated an improved blood profile, which occurred prior to any change in the size of their vascular lesions [21••].

The medical literature details the cases of at least 20 pediatric patients [22] with hemangiomas who received subcutaneous injections with interferon after the failure of corticosteroids. Partial remissions were noted in at least 90% of these patients.

Kaposi's sarcoma

Kaposi's sarcoma, especially of the epidemic or AIDS-related variety, poses considerable obstacles to therapy. Standard antiretroviral therapy with zidovudine fails to control the cutaneous lesions even early in their course. In one study, Spanish investigators [23] combined 500 to 800 mg/d of zidovudine with daily subcutaneous injections of interferon alfa-2b. Patients remained on the therapy for at least 3 months at a daily dosage of 10 or 20 MU; subsequently, the therapy was reduced to three times weekly. When patients were otherwise well, without poor prognostic indicators, the response rate approached 100%. Remissions persisted for an average of 14 months with a range of 3 to 27 months. On the other hand, a combination of constitutional symptoms (fever, fatigue, weight loss), a history of previous opportunistic infections, or a CD4+ count of less than 300 predicted a bleak outcome. For all patients, the 3-month response rate averaged 45%. Ninety-two percent of responders were still in remission 6 months after therapy (Fig. 3).

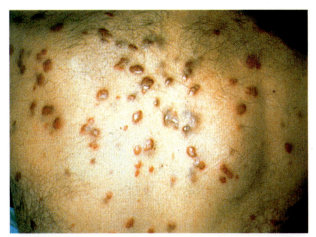
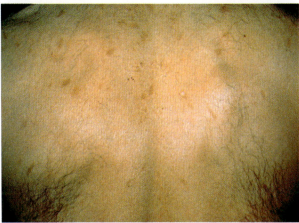

Fig. 3. Top, Typical AIDS-related Kaposi's sarcoma lesions in a patient before treatment with interferon alfa-2a. **Bottom,** Lesions in the same patient after treatment. (*Courtesy of* Roche Laboratories, Nutley, NJ.)

Another study examined the merits of zidovudine combined with intralesional interferon alfa-2b in HIV-positive individuals with Kaposi's sarcoma. Patients received 1 MU injected into each lesion three times each week for 6 weeks. No more than five lesions were treated. Depending on the response, a boost was allowed of up to 2.5 MU of interferon, and the total duration of therapy was extended to 10 weeks [24]. The response rate following interferon treatment averaged 85%, while in the placebo group, an amazingly high response rate exceeding 50% was found.

Several patients treated for endemic Kaposi's sarcoma, *ie,* the non–AIDS associated disease, responded within 6 to 8 weeks [25]. They were treated with injections of interferon alfa-2b administered subcutaneously for 5 days each week at a dose of 1 MU. After discontin-

uation of therapy, several patients were noted to have recurrence of their disease but they responded rapidly to the reinstitution of therapy.

Atopic dermatitis

In the largest trial to date involving patients with severe atopic dermatitis, Hanifin *et al.* [26••] conducted a multicenter study of interferon. Encouraged in part by reports in the literature of patients either with or without HIV infection and an atopic-like state who responded to interferon therapy, these investigators began a double-blind, placebo-controlled study. Patients received either placebo or daily subcutaneous injections of interferon gamma at a dosage of 50 $\mu g/m^2$. Seventy-eight individuals in four centers completed 12 weeks of therapy. These individuals were severely affected by atopic dermatitis, as exemplified by an average severity score of 12 out of a possible 18 points. Skin involvement averaged 60% of the body surface area. More than 50% improvement occurred in about 50% of interferon-treated patients compared with only 21% of those who received placebo. Among patients treated with interferon, stratification by age revealed more than 50% clearing in 67% of those aged 3 to 20 years, 56% of those aged 21 to 40 years, and 44% of those aged 41 to 65 years. The response in the placebo groups was 20%, 35%, and 0%, respectively. In the active therapy group, erythema, pruritus, and excoriations responded better than induration, dryness, and lichenification. Serum IgE levels rose in both interferon- and placebo-treated patients.

Another study, this one from Germany, evaluated the response of 14 patients unresponsive to topical corticosteroids and oral antihistamines and who suffered at least three severe exacerbations of atopic dermatitis during the previous year [27]. These patients received a slightly different regimen of interferon gamma. They were originally treated with 100 $\mu g/d$ for 5 days, and then their schedule called for three weekly injections and finally two injections each week for the last 2 weeks. Nearly 60% of the patients achieved at least a 50% reduction in their severity score by the termination of therapy. Three months after the discontinuation of therapy, four patients maintained stable improvement, while three relapsed. As with the previous report, IgE levels actually rose.

Several reports detail the less than optimal response of atopic dermatitis to interferon alfa. In one report, seven patients with severe disease were treated with 3 MU of interferon alfa-2b three times each week for 3 months. While transient improvement in this skin disease occurred, five of the seven patients suffered bacterial superinfection of their dermatitis, which required antibiotic therapy [28]. Another study evaluated the response of eight patients with atopic dermatitis to interferon alfa-2b at doses ranging from 9 to 15 MU each week [29]. Among these patients, one discontinued therapy owing to an adverse reaction, three dropped out after 4 weeks owing to worsening of the skin disease, another unexpectedly flared after 5 weeks of therapy, and only one of the three remaining patients who completed the trial was improved.

Table 4. Interferon therapy side effects*
Frequent
Fever
Flulike symptoms
Pain
Fatigue
Myalgia
Headache
Less common
Chills
Nausea
Vomiting
Anorexia
Diarrhea
Abdominal cramps
Weight loss
Impaired concentration
Depression
Confusion
Hair loss
Uncommon
Hypocalcemia
Hyperkalemia
Adrenal insufficiency
Bone marrow suppression
Leukopenia
Thrombocytopenia
Altered liver function tests
Induction of neutralizing antibodies
Renal toxicity
Cardiac changes
Supraventricular tachycardia
*Data from Browder et al. [1], Stadler and Ruszczak [2••], and Steinmann et al. [3•].

Leishmania

Interferon also seems to offer significant advantages in case reports of patients resistant to standard therapy for American mucocutaneous leishmaniasis [30] and visceral and diffuse cutaneous leishmaniasis [31]. Experimental treatment proved rewarding with interferon gamma at a daily dosage of 100 µg in combination with pentavalent antimony.

Herpes simplex

For patients suffering from AIDS and severe nonhealing cutaneous herpes simplex infections resistant to both acyclovir and foscarnet, a topical preparation of interferon gamma combined with trifluorothymidine (Viroptic; Burroughs Wellcome Co., Research Triangle Park, NC) seems to offer rather striking benefits [32].

Immune abnormalities and connective tissue disease

Other novel applications of interferon include the treatment of patients with progressive systemic sclerosis. In one report from Germany, nine patients with generalized involvement completed a 12-month trial of subcutaneous interferon gamma at an initial daily dosage of 50 µg that was later decreased to two to three injections each week. Five of these nine patients demonstrated modest improvement in their skin symptoms, while three others displayed minimal response, and one patient actually deteriorated. Lung function improved slightly [33]. In an English study, 19 patients were begun on intramuscular interferon alfa-2a at a dose of 3 MU three times each week with a subsequent increase to 9 MU. Although several patients were unable to tolerate the highest dose, 70% of those receiving treatment showed either improvement or stabilization of their skin disease. Unfortunately, neither grip strength nor digital contractures demonstrated favorable alterations [34].

A patient with Behçet's disease [35] noted complete relief with interferon alfa-2b injections at a dosage schedule of 3 MU administered subcutaneously three times each week for 3 months. Thirteen patients with severe pruritus [36] due to polycythemia vera that was in remission received interferon alfa in a typical regimen. A majority of these individuals experienced dramatic improvement of their symptoms within 2 to 8 weeks.

Cutaneous T-cell lymphoma

Interferon, especially when used in combination with another agent, seems to offer significant, long-lasting benefits to patients with early cutaneous T-cell lymphoma. A review of the literature [37•] reported a complete response rate, after interferon alfa treatment, of 10% to 27% in patients with mycosis fungoides who failed or relapsed from previous therapy, compared with a 20% to 40% response rate in patients without any previous intervention. These authors report on a series of five of their own patients with stage I mycosis fungoides resistant to psoralen and ultraviolet A treatment. Their patients subsequently received interferon alfa-2a at a dose of 3 MU for 1 week followed by 6 MU during the 2nd week and until a complete response occurred, after which the drug was tapered while the patients continued psoralen and ultraviolet A therapy. All patients achieved a complete response after an average of 3 months. This therapy markedly reduced the amount of ultraviolet A radiation necessary to bring about relief and hasten the resolution of the abnormality.

A group of patients with mycosis fungoides or Sezary syndrome refractory to standard treatment was evaluated with a new chemotherapeutic agent, pentostatin (deoxycoformycin), which was employed in conjunction with interferon alfa-2a at a dose of 10 MU on day 22 and 50 MU administered intramuscularly on days 23 to 26. Of the 42 patients who entered the trial, 5% enjoyed a complete response, while 36% achieved a partial response, for an overall improvement rate of 41%. Another 24% of these patients stabilized, while 34% progressed [38•]. A survival advantage occurred in those patients who responded favorably to this combination.

Most dermatologists recognize the sign of Leser-Trélat as a marker for internal neoplasia, but few realize the second most frequent association of this condition is with hematologic malignancies. In one case, a patient presented with both eruptive seborrheic keratoses and cutaneous T-cell lymphoma, both of which remitted with interferon alfa therapy [39].

Unusual side effects

Numerous mild side effects occur with therapy (Table 4), and a series of novel complaints associated with interferon therapy have been documented during the past several years. These latter include cutaneous flushing [40], arthritis in a patient with psoriasis [41], leukocytoclastic vasculitis in a patient with mixed cryoglobulinemia and hepatitis C [42], lichen planus in a patient with hepatitis C [43], and a bullous eruption resembling pemphigus or pemphigoid in two patients with the nonepidemic form of Kaposi's sarcoma [44]. A patient with hepatitis C developed an eruption consistent with Reiter's syndrome while on therapy with interferon [45], and 60% of patients with either borderline or lepromatous leprosy developed changes of erythema nodosum leprosum while receiving interferon gamma [46]. Several patients with colorectal malignancies evidenced skin abnormalities suggestive of graft-versus-host disease after receiving chemotherapy consisting of 5-fluorouracil, folinic acid, and interferon alfa-2b [47].

Conclusions

Many unanswered questions exist regarding the role of interferon in curing or palliating a variety of dermatologic diseases. Despite initial optimism regarding its role in controlling anogenital condylomata, recent trials raise questions about the drug's future. Nevertheless, clinical experience provides a basis for continued investigation and therapy. Of even greater interest, interferon seems to be well established in the treatment of both basal cell carcinomas and squamous cell carcinomas. In this age of cost control and heightened cosmetic consciousness, a short course of interferon may prove superior to a $2000 Mohs procedure coupled with a $3000 repair of the area by a plastic surgeon. Treatment for cutaneous T-cell lymphoma and

Kaposi's sarcoma palliates rather than cures these lesions but certainly offers significant benefits.

References and recommended reading

Papers of particular interest, published within the annual period of review, have been highlighted as:
- • Of special interest
- •• Of outstanding interest

1. Browder JF, Araujo OE, Myer NA, Flowers FP: **The Interferons and Their Use in Condyloma Acuminata.** *Ann Pharmacother* 1992, 26:42–45.

2. Stadler R, Ruszczak Z: **Interferons: New Additions and Indications**
•• **for Use.** *Dermatol Clin* 1993, 11:187–199.
A valuable, in-depth assessment of the molecular biology of interferons. This article provides a comprehensive evaluation of interferon therapy in dermatology with special attention to malignant melanoma.

3. Steinmann GG, Rosenkaimer F, Leitz G: **Clinical Experience With**
• **Interferon-Alpha and Interferon-Gamma.** *Int Rev Exp Pathol* 1993, 34B:193–207.
A good survey of the toxicities associated with interferon therapy. This article introduces a fourth variety of these compounds.

4. **Drugs for Sexually Transmitted Diseases.** *Med Lett Drugs Ther* 1994, 36:1–6.

5. Lebbe C, Rybojad M, Ochonisky S, Miclea JM, Verola O, Cordoliani F, Ablon G, Morel P: **Extensive Human Papillomavirus–Related Disease (Bowenoid Papulosis, Bowen's Disease, and Squamous Cell Carcinoma) in a Patient With Hairy Cell Leukemia: Clinical and Immunologic Evaluation After an Interferon Alpha Trial.** *J Am Acad Dermatol* 1993, 29:644–646.

6. Ling MR: **Therapy of Genital Human Papilloma Virus Infections: Part**
•• **II. Methods of Treatment.** *Int J Dermatol* 1992, 31:769–776.
With the burgeoning number of available options for genital warts, it becomes necessary to prioritize the various treatments. This article provides a rather extensive evaluation of the interferons in this area. Additionally a cost comparison is presented comparing these drugs to the more standard options as well as to laser therapy.

7. Condylomata International Collaborative Study Group: **Random-**
• **ized Placebo-Controlled Double-Blind Combined Therapy With Laser Surgery and Systemic Interferon-Alpha 2a in the Treatment of Anogenital Condylomata Acuminata.** *J Infect Dis* 1993, 167:824–829.
This International Collaborative Study Group provides the largest evaluation to date of systemic interferon therapy compared with placebo as an adjunctive approach in patients treated with laser surgery. Although the results seem rather unremarkable, many would argue that interferon must be injected intralesionally for successful therapy in herpesvirus infections.

8. Eron LJ, Alder MV, O'Rourke JM, Rittweger K, DePamphilis J, Pizzuti DJ: **Recurrences of Condyloma Acuminata Following Cryotherapy Is Not Prevented by Systemically Administered Interferon.** *Genitourin Med* 1993, 69:91–93.

9. Hopfl RM, Sandbichler M, Zelger BWH, Conrad FG, Fritsch PO: **Adjuvant Treatment of Recalcitrant Genitoanal Warts With Systemic Recombinant Interferon Alpha-2c.** *Acta Derm Venereol (Stockh)* 1992, 72:383–386.

10. Zouboulis CC, Buttner P, Orfanos C: **Systemic Interferon Gamma as Adjuvant Therapy for Refractory Anogenital Warts: A Randomized Clinical Trial and Meta-analysis of the Available Data.** *Arch Dermatol* 1992, 128:1413–1414.

11. Srecko K, Elbert W, Fleishmann WR: **Circadian Dependence of Interferon Antitumor Activity in Mice.** *J Natl Cancer Inst* 1993, 85:1927–1932.

12. Gross GE: **Current Dermatologic Therapy: Use of Interferon in Genital Warts.** *J Am Acad Dermatol* 1993, 29:665.

13. Naples SP, Brodell RT: **Verruca Vulgaris: Treatment With Natural Interferon Alfa Using a Needleless Injector.** *Arch Dermatol* 1993, 129:698–700.

14. Beissert S, Koch U, Sunderkotter C, Luger T, Schwarz T: **Successful Treatment of Disseminated Verruca Vulgares With Interferon Beta.** *J Am Acad Dermatol* 1993, 29:1041–1042.

15. Stenquist B, Wennberg AM, Gisslen H, Larko O: **Treatment of Aggres-**
•• **sive Basal Cell Carcinoma With Intralesional Interferon: Evaluation of Efficacy by Mohs Surgery.** *J Am Acad Dermatol* 1992, 27:65–69.
Fifteen patients were treated with nine injections of interferon alfa-2b over a 3-week period. Sixty percent had either complete resolution of their tumors or greater than 75% reduction in tumor size. This novel approach to cutaneous tumors offers the potential to simplify therapy for patients with tumors

in difficult-to-treat locations. Increasing the dose above the standard level increases the ultimate cure rate.

16. Edwards L, Berman B, Rapini RP, Whiting DA, Tyring S, Greenway
•• HT, Eyre SP, Tanner DJ, Taylor EL Peets E, Smiles KA: **Treatment of Cutaneous Squamous Cell Carcinomas by Intralesional Interferon Alfa 2b Therapy.** *Arch Dermatol* 1992, 128:1486–1489.
Forty-eight healthy patients with squamous cell carcinomas and bowenoid actinic keratoses underwent therapy with nine intralesional injections of interferon alfa-2b over a 3-week period. This treatment provided a 97% response rate with only minor side effects. Cosmetic results were excellent and seemed to exceed those likely to be associated with surgery or radiation.

17. Grob JJ, Suzini F, Richard MA, Weiller M, Zarour H, Noe C, Munoz
• MH, Bonerandi JJ: **Large Keratoacanthomas Treated With Intralesional Interferon Alfa-2a.** *J Am Acad Dermatol* 1993, 29:237–241.
Management of keratoacanthomas creates concern, because at times it appears impossible to eliminate completely the possibility that these lesions actually represent malignancies. Treatment with injectable interferon offers the potential for rapid resolution without the need to intervene surgically.

18. Ozzello L, Habif DV, DeRosa CM, Cantell K: **Cellular Events Accompanying Regression of Skin Recurrence of Breast Carcinomas Treated with Intralesional Injections of Natural Interferons Alpha and Gamma.** *Cancer Res* 1992, 52:4571–4581.

19. Blei F, Orlow SJ, Geronemus RS: **Interferon Alpha 2a Therapy for Extensive Perianal and Lower Extremity Hemangioma.** *J Am Acad Dermatol* 1993, 29:98–99.

20. Spiller JC, Sharma V, Woods GM, Hall JC, Seidel FG: **Diffuse Neonatal Hemangiomatosis Treated Successfully With Interferon Alfa-2a.** *J Am Acad Dermatol* 1992, 27:102–104.

21. Ezekowitz RAB, Mulliken JB, Folkman J: **Interferon Alfa-2a Therapy**
•• **for Life Threatening Hemangiomas of Infancy.** *N Engl J Med* 1992, 326: 1456–1463.
Sometimes referred to as "alarming hemangiomas," lesions that pose a treat to life or vision constitute a particularly troublesome area. Corticosteroid therapy causes regression of no more than one third of these lesions. Until recently, attempts to find an alternative therapy have proven ineffective. It now appears that daily injections of interferon alfa-2a provide a safe and effective alternative to corticosteroids. This article presents a protocol from the Boston Children's Hospital and Harvard Medical School.

22. Davis A, Krafchik BR: **New Drugs in Pediatric Dermatology.** *Curr Opin Pediatr* 1993, 5:212–215.

23. Podzamczer D, Bolao F, Clotet B, Garcia P, Casanova A, Pagerols X, Gudiol F: **Low Dose Interferon Alpha Combined With Zidovudine in Patients With AIDS-Associated Kaposi's Sarcoma.** *J Intern Med* 1993, 233:247–253.

24. Dupuy J, Price M, Lynch G, Bruce S, Scwartz M: **Intralesional Interferon Alpha and Zidovudine in Epidemic Kaposi's Sarcoma.** *J Am Acad Dermatol* 1993, 28:966–972.

25. Tur E, Brenner S, Michalencz R: **Low Dose Recombinant Interferon Alpha Treatment for Classic Kaposi's Sarcoma.** *Arch Dermatol* 1993, 129:1297–1300.

26. Hanifin JM, Schneider LC, Leung DYM, Ellis CN, Jaffe HS, Izu AE,
•• Bucalo LR, Hirabayashi SE, Tofte SJ, Cantu-Gonzales G, *et al.*: **Recombinant Interferon Gamma Therapy for Atopic Dermatitis.** *J Am Acad Dermatol* 1993, 28:189–197.
Atopic dermatitis remains one of the most important challenges in cutaneous medicine. Severely affected patients suffer lifelong disease, often requiring extensive topical corticosteroid therapy or potentially dangerous oral medication. Injectable interferon therapy improves a considerable number of these patients. This review examines the outcome of 78 patients treated with either interferon or placebo during a 12-week trial. While the patients did not experience complete involution of their disease, more than half obtained major improvement.

27. Reinhold U, Kukel S, Bazoska J, Kreysel H: **Systemic Interferon Gamma Treatment in Severe Atopic Dermatitis.** *J Am Acad Dermatol* 1993, 29:58–63.

28. Gruschwitz M, Peters KP, Heese A, Stosiek N, Koch HU, Horstein OP: **Effects of Interferon-Alpha-2b on the Clinical Course, Inflammatory Skin Infiltrates and Peripheral Blood Lymphocytes in Patients With Severe Atopic Eczema.** *Int Arch Allergy Immunol* 1993, 101:20–30.

29. Jullien D, Nicolas JF, Frappaz A, Thivolet J: **Alpha Interferon Treatment in Atopic Dermatitis.** *Acta Derm Venereol (Stockh)* 1993, 73:130–132.

30. Bottasso O, Cabrini J, Falcoff R, Falcoff E: **Successful Treatment of an Antimony-Resistant American Mucocutaneous Leishmaniasis: A Case Report.** *Arch Dermatol* 1992, 128:996–997.

31. Badaro R, Johnson WD: **The Role of Interferon Gamma in the Treatment of Visceral and Diffuse Cutaneous Leishmaniasis.** *J Infect Dis* 1993, 167(suppl 1):13–17.

32. Birch CJ, Tyssen DP, Tachedjian G, Doherty R, Hayes K, Mijch A, Lucas CR: **Clinical Effects and In Vitro Studies of Trifluorothymidine Combined With Interferon-Alpha for Treatment of Drug Resistant and Sensitive Herpes Simplex Virus Infections.** *J Infect Dis* 1992, 166:108–112.

33. Hein R, Behr J, Hundgen M, Hunzelmann N, Meurer M, Braun-Falco O, Urbanski A, Krieg T: **Treatment of Systemic Sclerosis With Gamma Interferon.** *Br J Dermatol* 1992, 126:496–501.

34. Stevens W, Vancheeswaren R, Black CM: **Alpha Interferon-2a (Roferon-A) in the Treatment of Diffuse Cutaneous Systemic Sclerosis: A Pilot Study UK Systemic Sclerosis Study Group.** *Br J Rheumatol* 1992, 31:683–689.

35. Durand JM, Kaplanski G, Telle H, Soubeyrand J, Paulo F: **Beneficial Effects of Interferon-Alpha 2b in Behçet's Disease.** *Arthritis Rheum* 1993, 36:1025–1026.

36. Finelli C, Gugliotta L, Gamberi B, Vianelli N, Visani G, Tura S: **Relief of Intractable Pruritus in Polycythemia Vera With Recombinant Interferon Alfa.** *Am J Hematol* 1993, 43:316–318.

37. Mostow EN, Neckel SL, Oberhelman L, Anderson DJ, Cooper K:
• **Complete Remissions in Psoralen and UV-A (PUVA)–Refractory Mycosis Fungoides–Type Cutaneous T-Cell Lymphoma With Combined Interferon Alpha and PUVA.** *Arch Dermatol* 1993, 129:747–752.
Fortunately, cutaneous T-cell lymphomas are relatively uncommon. Therapeutic options include psoralen and ultraviolet A, topical nitrogen mustard, or electron beam therapy. Many of these patients will not improve. Interferon in combination with psoralen and ultraviolet A therapy seems to offer significant rewards.

38. Foss FM, Ihde DC, Breneman DL, Phelps RM, Fischmann AB,
• Schechter GP, Linnoila I, Breneman JC, Cotelingam JD, Bhosh BC, *et al.*: **Phase II Study of Pentostatin and Intermittent High-Dose Recombinant Interferon Alfa-2a in Advance Mycosis Fungoides/Sezary's Syndrome.** *J Clin Oncol* 1992, 10:1907–1913.
Combining interferon therapy with a novel chemotherapeutic agent, pentostatin, offers a relatively safe method of achieving a long-term remission in mycosis fungoides and Sezary's syndrome. Partial responses outnumbered complete responses, but among patients previously untreated, the survival rate was doubled.

39. Cohen J, Lessin SK, Vowels BR, Benoit B, Witmer WK, Rook AH: **The Sign of Leser-Trelat in Association With Sezary Syndrome: Simultaneous Disappearance of Seborrheic Keratoses and Malignant T Cell Clone During Combined Therapy With Photopheresis and Interferon Alfa [Letter].** *Arch Dermatol* 1993, 129:1213–1215.

40. Wilkin JK: **Flushing Reactions in the Cancer Chemotherapy Patient.** *Arch Dermatol* 1992, 19:1387–1389.

41. O'Connell PG, Gerber LH, Digiovanna JJ, Peck GL: **Arthritis in Patients With Psoriasis Treated With Gamma-Interferon.** *J Rheumatol* 1992, 19:80–82.

42. Zimmerman R, Konig V, Bauditz S, Hopf U: **Interferon Alfa in Leukocytoclastic Vasculitis, Mixed Cryoglobulinemia and Chronic Hepatitis C.** *Lancet* 1993, 341:561–562.

43. Agner T, Fogh H, Weisman K: **The Relation Between Lichen Planus and Hepatitis C: A Case Report.** *Acta Derm Venereol* 1992, 72:380.

44. Parodi A, Semino M, Gallo R, Rebora A: **Bullous Eruption With Circulating Pemphigus-like Antibodies Following Interferon-Alpha Therapy.** *Dermatology* 1993, 186:155–157.

45. Cleveland MG, Mallory SB: **Incomplete Reiter's Syndrome Induced by Systemic Interferon Alpha Treatment.** *J Am Acad Dermatol* 1993, 29:788–789.

46. Sampaio EP, Moreira AL, Sarno EN, Malta AM, Kaplan G: **Prolonged Treatment With Recombinant Interferon Gamma Induces Erythema Nodosum Leprosum in Lepromatous Leprosy Patients.** *J Exp Med* 1992, 175:1729–1737.

47. Beard J, Smith K, Shelton H: **Combination Chemotherapy With 5-Fluorouracil, Folinic Acid and Alpha Interferon Producing Histologic Features of Graft-Versus-Host Disease.** *J Am Acad Dermatol* 1993, 29:325–330.

48. Greenberg M: *Management of Condyloma Acuminatum: Clinical Images.* New York: World Health Communications.

R. Kenneth Landow, MD, Department of Dermatology, Los Angeles County–University of Southern California Medical Center, Room 8441, General Hospital, 1200 N. State Street, Los Angeles, CA 90033, USA.

Topical glucocorticoids in dermatology

Roger C. Cornell, MD

Scripps Clinic and Research Foundation, La Jolla, California, USA

Topical glucocorticosteroids remain among the most widely prescribed medications for many of the dermatoses seen by the practicing physician. With the advent of superpotent agents, topical agents exist with great potential to rapidly control such dermatoses. However, such agents increase the risk of side effects, both topical and systemic. To date, the ideal agent that provides outstanding clinical effectiveness with minimal side effects does not exist. This review summarizes some of the literature over the past year regarding side effects, suggestions for new usage, alternative treatment strategies, and current status of vasoconstriction and bioequivalency. Contact allergy to corticosteroids, an area of increasing importance, is also considered.

Current Opinion in Dermatology 1995:193–197

Chemistry and pharmacology

There is a need for congeners with an increased benefit-risk ratio. Some new glucocorticoids, especially the nonfluorinated double-ester type such as prednicarbate, appear promising, in that they may affect fibroblast growth *in vitro* as well as skin thickness *in vivo* less than equipotent conventional glucocorticosteroids [1].

The development of nonfluorinated double esters such as hydrocortisone aceponate and prednicarbate ointment suggests that an increased therapeutic index may exist with nonfluorinated double esters; in a trial using A and B mode images, neither induced significant reduction in skin thickness. Table 1 shows mean values of skin thickness after 6 weeks' application of four treatment modalities [2]. This work is preliminary, and additional confirmatory studies are in order.

Aalto-Korte and Turpeinen [3] report a highly significant correlation between the postapplication rise of plasma cortisol levels and the mean transepidermal water loss in nine patients with widespread dermatitis treated with 1% hydrocortisone cream. They suggest the measurement of transepidermal water loss affords a simple, noninvasive method for assessing the systemic effects of hydrocortisone.

Vasoconstriction and bioequivalence

Anderson *et al.* [4•], studying the cutaneous corticosteroid vasoconstriction assay, have demonstrated that steroid-induced vasoconstriction is caused predominantly by decreased venous deoxygenated hemoglobin components and that only the most potent corticosteroids cause a significant decrease in arterial oxygenated components. Results obtained using reflectance spectroscopy allowed separation of cutaneous hemoglobin into oxygenated and deoxygenated components and correlated well with visual assessment. A simple method using a commercially available synthetic membrane and diffusion cell assembly has been described and established to measure the release rate of steroids from cream formulations. Preliminary data indicate that the release rate (flux) of betamethasone valerate was higher for the higher blanching formulation that was used and was statistically different from the other betamethasone valerate cream, which caused significantly less blanching [5]. Tristimulus color

Table 1. Mean values of skin thickness after 6 weeks' application of four corticosteroid treatment modalities*

Day	Skin thickness, $\mu m \pm SD$			
	Hydrocortisone aceponate	Corresponding base	Prednicarbate	Betamethasone 17-valerate
0	1189±149	1201±106	1209±127	1193±122
42	1038±134	1091±125	1072±106	979±96

*From Kerscher and Korting [2]; with permission.

analysis using a chromometer may have promise in the interpretation of skin blanching; the method involves only one investigator and may have applicability as an internationally accepted color measurement [6]. Animal models testing the potency of topical corticosteroids by measuring their effects on induced conditions that are analogous to human skin disease have been reviewed. Such models can examine the anti-inflammatory, antiallergic, antiproliferative and atrophogenic effects of topical corticosteroids. While animal models are currently relatively imprecise, innovations using newly available histologic, autoradiographic, and biochemical techniques have great potential for precisely quantitating the effects of corticosteroids in animal model systems [7•]. Human experimental models of inflammation would be useful in screening topical steroids for potency and efficacy, but none are reliable enough at this time to warrant their general use. Potential pitfalls to be avoided in planning such studies include the use of occlusion of test agents and the use of topical steroids to prevent rather than to moderate inflammation. Uniform production of mild, as opposed to severe, reactions that may show responsiveness to topical steroids and the choice of models that are easy to duplicate are both important in developing safe, inexpensive, reproducible, and reliable assays [8•]. In addition, other aspects of bioequivalence of topical steroids were a subject of a round-table discussion in October 1992. Regulatory perspectives, pharmacokinetic evaluation, the problem of bioequivalent studies of topical preparations, quality control considerations, and recent developments in vasoconstrictor assays were also reviewed in detail [9••].

Use

The use of superpotent topical steroids for patients with vulvar lichen sclerosis has been recently reviewed. The authors note that sustained treatment of this condition for 3 months with a very potent topical agent controlled symptoms and resulted in marked clinical and histologic improvement. Relatively small amounts of topical steroids were then required for subsequent control. Faster and better control of disease activities may reduce the risk of scarring and the development of squamous cell carcinoma and justify the cautious use of a superpotent agent for this condition [10].

Two patients with inflammatory linear verrucous epidermal nevi benefited from topical fluorinated steroids under occlusion [11]. Shapiro [12••] reviews the use of topical intralesional corticosteroids for alopecia areata. In addition to topical steroids, intradermal injection of corticosteroids remains one of the mainstays of therapy for this condition. Most dermatologists favor the use of triamcinolone acetonide rather than the more atrophogenic agent triamcinolone hexacetonide.

The treatment of nummular psoriasis with a clobetasol propionate stick, 0.05%, was evaluated. No signif-

icant difference was found between two sites treated with the stick vehicle and conventional clobetasol propionate ointment. Patients may have had a preference for the stick formulation and required less of it than the ointment, but additional studies are necessary [13]. The synergistic effect of reduction of ultraviolet B–induced erythema and skin blood flow when an oral nonsteroidal anti-inflammatory agent was used in combination with topical betamethasone dipropionate has been studied in 24 patients. This synergistic effect could have implications for the therapy of conditions such as sunburn in humans, in that the nonsteroidal anti-inflammatory agent in combination with a topical corticosteroid provided the greatest reduction in skin blood flow [14].

Treatment strategies

Specific two-phase strategies in the treatment of chronic inflammatory skin disorders using a steroid preparation followed by a nonsteroid preparation have been reviewed. In psoriasis, for example, the use of potent topical steroids plus salicylic acid for 5 to 7 days followed by dithranol plus tar or calcipotriol cream is recommended. Another strategy involves the use of a midstrength topical steroid for 5 to 7 days followed by occlusive hydrocolloid dressings (Duoderm; Convatec, Princeton, NJ). Similar strategies are proposed for eczematous conditions; topical steroids are used for 5 to 7 days followed by capsaicin cream. Individualization of therapy in patients with the use not only of topical steroids, but also of nonsteroid products is important [15••]. In general, patients on intermittent therapy do best when the psoriatic lesions are clear or nearly clear before the same or other agents are initiated on an intermittent basis. One might expect that one should commence with intermittent therapy to reduce the risk of tachyphylaxis, but such is not the case. The ideal agent is rapidly absorbed, exhibits a strong but short activity, and is rapidly inactivated after reaching the circulation [16].

The once-daily application of a superpotent agent with the application 12 hours later of a simple water-in-oil emollient has been shown to be equivalent in efficacy to twice-daily application of the same corticosteroid alone and superior to once-daily application of the corticosteroid alone. The use of water-in-oil emollients as steroid-sparing agents has also been discussed [17].

Combination therapy

Some dermatoses may be suited to treatment with combination therapy in which the corticosteroid is combined with an antimicrobial agent. In the treatment of dermatophyte and monilial infection, isoconazole 1% in combination with diflucortolone 0.1% appears to be more effective than isoconazole alone with regard not only to regression of signs and symptoms but also to mycological cure. Giannotti and Pimpinelli [18] postulate that this superiority may be due to the greater bioavailability of the antifungal agent in the epidermis because of the local vasoconstrictive activity of the corticosteroid, which allows a less rapid "wash out" of the antifungal drug by the dermal microcirculation.

Side effects

Adverse effects of topical corticosteroids continue to be an area of interest in the dermatologic literature. Litt [19] describes steroid-induced rosacea ("iatrosacea") in a series of eight patients ranging in age from 9 months to 80 years. All but one of the patients were women who had used midstrength to potent topical agents on the face for varying periods of time. Treatment consisted of discontinuation of the agent, initiation of appropriate oral antibiotics, and the use of various local nonsteroidal remedies. In this report, all of the offending agents were fluorinated corticosteroids, but it must be pointed out that steroid-induced rosacea may occur with midstrength nonfluorinated corticosteroids as well. Figure 1 illustrates corticosteroid-induced rosacea in a 38-year-old woman.

The importance of psychological support and dermatologic therapy to break the habit of applying corticosteroids to the face and the difficulty of educating the patient who depends on such agents have been reviewed by Wells and Brodell [20•]. The patient may need to accept a transient flare-up of the disease when the treatment is discontinued; the importance of edu-

cating the patient cannot be overemphasized. Although tapering the dose of corticosteroids or prescribing less potent agents may reduce the flare-up, such a course may delay the patent's full recovery.

Extensive visual loss after this use of topical facial corticosteroids in five cases is discussed by Aggawal *et al.* [21•], who review the phenomenon of steroid-induced glaucoma in certain patients who are "steroid responders" and develop an increase in intraocular pressure. Patients so predisposed may have chronic open-angle glaucoma, a positive family history of steroid responsiveness, diabetes, and connective tissue disorders. In four of five cases, the intraocular pressure returned to normal after discontinuation of the topical agent. In one case involving a 23-year-old man, one eye failed to respond to discontinuation of the topical steroid and required a trabeculectomy to control the intraocular pressure [21•].

A comparison of clobetasol 17-propionate cream and betamethasone 17-valerate cream with methylprednisolone aceponate cream with and without occlusion suggests that the latter agent, while highly potent, may have a lower potential for suppression of the adrenal function. The authors postulate that this lower potential may result from rapid metabolism in the liver and that esterhydrolysis in the skin may contribute to its metabolism [22]. Walsh *et al.* [23] confirm and extend their previous finding that significant hypothalamic-pituitary-adrenal axis suppression can occur in pa-

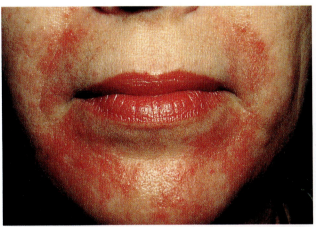

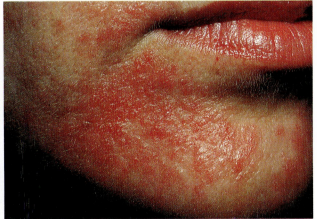

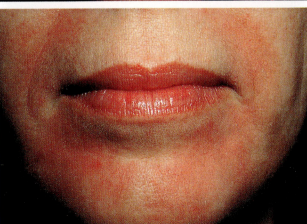

Fig. 1. Corticosteroid-induced acne rosacea and perioral dermatitis in a 38-year-old woman who had been using desoximetasone for 1 year. **Upper left,** Perioral papules and pustules on broad areas of blanching erythema at initial presentation. **Upper right,** Flaring erythema and papules and fine scaling 4 days after withdrawal of desoximetasone. **Bottom,** Complete clearing of active inflammation and only mild residual comedonal acne and blanching erythema after 1 month of treatment with topical clindamycin and oral tetracycline. (*From* Wells and Brodell [20•]; with permission.)

tients using superpotent agents such as optimized be-tamethasone dipropionate and halobetasol propionate and is greatest during the first 7 days before healing of the skin lesions occurs.

High-dose inhaled corticosteroids are an important therapeutic advance in the treatment of asthma. How-ever, such agents seem to parallel systemic topical corticosteroids in their effects on the hypothalamic-pituitary-adrenal axis and in the causation of dermal atrophy and purpura. The onset of moderately severe acne in four patients, aged 35 to 56 years, on the trunk as well as the face following use of inhaled corticos-teroids strongly suggests a causative factor. Dermatol-ogists must be aware of the potential side effects of inhaled corticosteroids, but it must be stressed that asthma is a serious and potentially life-threatening dis-order, and treatment should not be abruptly withdrawn without expert advice [24].

Contact allergy to corticosteroids

In most cases, contact allergy is detected by the use of tixocortol pivalate as a marker. Reports have shown corticosteroids to be the seventh most common al-lergen. The incidence of contact allergies to corticos-teroids has increased. In 1991, 5.4% of a group of pa-tients had positive skin tests for topical glucocorticos-teroids. Issues that are not yet completely resolved in-clude the manner of testing (patch testing versus in-tradermal testing), test concentration, test vehicle, ap-propriate time to read the test, and whether different patterns of cross sensitivity occur. The importance of reading patch tests not only after 24 and 48 hours but also after 6 to 7 days is stressed because the anti-inflam-matory effect of corticosteroids can suppress a posi-tive skin reaction for a period of time [25••]. A sepa-rate corticosteroid patch test series and the inclusion of corticosteroid preparations in standard patch tests to enhance allergy detection have been recommended.

Patch test series should include as many topical agents as possible that are used in the respective area where the patient is being treated [26]. In 59 cases of hydro-cortisone sensitivity, patients with stasis dermatitis and leg ulcerations were significantly more likely to be al-lergic to hydrocortisone. Patients with hand eczema were less sensitive. Duration of the dermatitis seems not to be important in determining the presence of hy-drocortisone allergy [27].

The advantages of intradermal testing for corticos-teroids allergy include the fact that delivery of the hap-ten to the skin is ascertained. Disadvantages include the fact that the application is more complicated and more painful than in patch testing and the possibil-ity of anaphylactic or anaphylactoid reactions. The use of a prick test first, followed by intradermal testing af-ter a wait of approximately 30 minutes, during which time flares should appear in immediate type hyper-sensitivity, is suggested. Without systemic studies with intradermal tests, important contact allergens can re-main underappreciated [28•]. The negative association of HLA-B8 and -DR3 in contact hypersensitivity to hy-drocortisone has been described. Both HLA-B8 and -DR3 may be potentially important in contact hyper-sensitivity to hydrocortisone [29]. Cross sensitization to mometasone furoate occurs in patients with corticos-teroid contact allergy, but it seems to be rare; this com-pound may serve as an alternative for the topical treat-ment of corticosteroid-sensitive patients [30]. In routine patch testing in over 2000 patients, Dooms-Goossens and Morren [31••] find corticosteroids to be the seventh most frequent allergen. In their series, budesonide was the most common allergen and often gave simultane-ous reactions with other corticosteroids. Table 2 shows results of testing with corticosteroids in their standard series. Allergic contact dermatitis from budesonide has been reported in multiple short communications [32]. Findings of positive intradermal reactions to several corticosteroids in patients who had negative patch tests for the same material suggest that intradermal tests may be extremely useful to confirm or refute positive patch

Table 2. Results of patch testing for corticosteroid allergy*

Substance	Vehicle	Patients tested, n†	Positive reactions, n(%)
Tixocortol pivalate	1% petrolatum	2073	22(1.1)
Hydrocortisone 17-butyrate	1% ethanol	2073	20(1)
β-Dexamethasone	1% ethanol	1960	1(<0.1%)
Amcinonide	1% ethanol	1960	10(0.5)
Fluocortinbutyl ester	1% ethanol	1960	8(0.4)
Clobetasol propionate	1% ethanol	1960	4(0.2)
Triamcinolone acetonide	1% ethanol	1747	6(0.3)
Hydrocortisone alcohol	0.5% ethanol and DMSO	1150	17(1.5)
Budesonide	1% ethanol	710	21(3)

*From Dooms-Goossens and Morren [31•]; with permission.
†Not all the corticosteroid contact allergy markers were present from the outset.
DMSO—dimethyl sulfoxide.

test reactions to topical agents. The use of patch testing as the sole investigative method in patients with suspected allergies is to be discouraged [33].

Prospective patch and intradermal testing on 105 consecutive patients to determine the optimum method of screening for corticosteroid hypersensitivity showed that patch tests with tixocortol pivalate, 1%, and a corticosteroid series (all 1% in ethanol) detected all patients with steroid sensitivity. However, intradermal tests were essential to exclude false-positive reactions and detect all relevant steroid allergies in any individual patient [34].

References and recommended reading

Papers of particular interest, published within the annual period of review, have been highlighted as:
- Of special interest
- • Of outstanding interest

1. Korting HC, Kerscher MJ, Schäfer-Korting M: **Topical Glucocorticoids With Improved Benefit/Risk Ratio: Do They Exist?** *J Am Acad Dermatol* 1992, 27:87–92.

2. Kerscher JR, Korting HC: **Topical Glucocorticoids of the Non-fluorinated Double-Ester Type.** *Acta Derm Venereol (Stockh)* 1992, 72:214–216.

3. Aalto-Korte K, Turpeinen M: **Transepidermal Water Loss and Absorption of Hydrocortisone in Widespread Dermatitis.** *Br J Dermatol* 1993, 128:633–635.

4. Anderson P, Milioni K, Maibach H: **The Cutaneous Corticosteroid**
• **Vasoconstriction Assay: A Reflectance Spectroscopic and Laser Doppler Flowmetric Study.** *Br J Dermatol* 1993, 128:660–665.
An interesting evaluation of corticosteroids of different potency in alcoholic solution applied under occlusion with cutaneous blanching evaluated using visual scoring, reflectance spectroscopy, and laser-doppler flowmetry.

5. Shah VP, Elkins J, Skelly JP: **Relationship between In Vivo Skin Blanching and In Vitro Release Rate for Betamethasone Valerate Creams.** *J Pharm Sci* 1992, 81:104–106.

6. Chan SY, Po ALW: **Quantitative Skin Blanching Assay of Corticosteroid Creams Using Tristimulus Colour Analysis.** *J Pharm Pharmacol* 1992, 44:371–378.

7. Penneys NS: **Animal Models for Testing Topical Corticosteroids Po-**
• **tency: A Review and Some Suggested New Approaches.** *Int J Dermatol* 1992, 31(suppl 1):6–8.
A review of animal models that allow the potency of topical corticosteroids to be tested by measuring their effects on induced conditions analogous to human skin disease.

8. Olsen EA: **Human Test Models for Bioequivalence of Topical Corti-**
• **costeroids: A Review.** *Int J Dermatol* 1992, 31(suppl 1):9–13.
A review of existing human test systems noting their strengths and weaknesses.

9. Maibach H, ed: **Bioequivalence of Topical Corticosteroids.** *Int J Der-*
•• *matol* 1992, 31(suppl 1):1–41.
A comprehensive scientific round table in which animal and human models for testing topical corticosteroids were reviewed. Virtually all aspects of bioequivalency were addressed, including regulation, measurement of percutaneous absorption, vasoconstrictor assay, statistical considerations, and quality control considerations.

10. Dalziel KL, Wojnarowska F: **Long-Term Control of Vulval Lichen Sclerosis After Treatment With a Potent Topical Steroid Cream.** *J Reprod Med* 1993, 38:25–27.

11. Cerio R, Wilson Jones E, Eady RAJ: **ILVEN Responding to Occlusive Potent Topical Steroid Therapy.** *Clin Exp Dermatol* 1992, 17:279–281.

12. Shapiro J: **Alopecia Areate: Update on Therapy.** *Dermatol Clin* 1993,
•• 11:35–46.
A comprehensive review of therapy for alopecia areate.

13. Bergstedt C, Gamborg Nielsen P, Karlsson L, Strömberg L: **Treatment of Nummular Psoriasis With a Clobetasol Propionate Stick.** *Dermatology* 1992, 184:51–53.

14. Hughes GS, Francom SF, Means LK, Bohan DF, Caruana C, Holland M: **Synergistic Effects of Oral Nonsteroidal Drugs and Topical Corticosteroids in the Therapy of Sunburn in Humans.** *Dermatology* 1992, 184:54–58.

15. Panconesi E, Lotti T: **Steroids Versus Nonsteroids in the Treatment**
•• **of Cutaneous Inflammation: Therapeutic Modalities for Office Use.** *Arch Dermatol Res* 1992, 284(suppl 1):S37–S41.
A short but succinct review of vehicles and carriers, combination therapy, and alternatives to topical corticosteroids over the long term.

16. Sterry W: **Therapy With Topical Corticosteroids.** *Arch Dermatol Res* 1992, 284(suppl 1):S27–S29.

17. Watsky KL, Freije L, Leneveu MC, Wenck HA, Leffell DJ: **Water-in-Oil Emollients as Steroid Sparing Adjunctive Therapy in the Treatment of Psoriasis.** *Cutis* 1992, 50:383–386.

18. Giannotti B, Pimpinelli N: **Topical Corticosteroids: Which Drug and When?** *Drugs* 1992, 44:65–71.

19. Litt JZ: **Steroid Induced Rosacea.** *Am Fam Physician* 1993, 48:67–71.

20. Wells K, Brodell RT: **Topical Corticosteroid "Addiction".** *Postgrad*
• *Med* 1993, 93:225–230.
A good discussion of this condition and the psychological support often necessary to break the habit of habitual use of corticosteroids on the face.

21. Aggarwal RK, Potamitis T, Chong NHV, Guarro M, Shah P, Kheterpol S: **Extensive Visual Loss With Topical Facial Steroids.** *Eye* 1993,
• 7:664–666.
Dermatologists often use topical corticosteroids near the eyes. This paper reviews the risk to patients of developing advanced glaucoma and discusses screening of such patients.

22. Kecskes A, Jahn P, Matthes H, Kleine Kuhlmann R, Lange L: **Systemic Effects of Topically Applied Methylprednisolone Aceponate in Healthy Volunteers.** *J Am Acad Dermatol* 1993, 28:789–792.

23. Walsh P, Aeling JL, Huff L, Weston WL: **Hypothalmic-Pituitary-Adrenal Axis Suppression by Superpotent Topical Steroids.** *J Am Acad Dermatol* 1993, 29:501–503.

24. Monk B, Cunliffe WJ, Layton AM, Rhodes DJ: **Acne Induced by Inhaled Corticosteroids.** *Clin Exp Dermatol* 1993, 18:148–150.

25. Degreef H, Dooms-Goossens A: **The New Corticosteroids: Are They**
•• **Effective and Safe?** *Dermatol Clin* 1993, 11:155–160.
The authors review properties of new corticosteroids, including their structure. They include the clinical picture of contact allergy to topical corticosteroids, the propensity of allergic patients to react to other substances, and the clinical course of such patients.

26. Lauerma AI, Reitamo S: **Contact Allergy to Corticosteroids.** *J Am Acad Dermatol* 1993, 28:618–622.

27. Wilkinson SM, English JSC: **Hydrocortisone Sensitivity: Clinical Features of Fifty-Nine Cases.** *J Am Acad Dermatol* 1992, 27:683–687.

28. Herbst RA, Lauerma AI, Maibach HI: **Intradermal Testing in the Di-**
• **agnosis of Allergic Contact Dermatitis: A Reappraisal.** *Contact Dermatitis* 1993, 29:1–5.
The authors concisely review the advantages and disadvantages of intradermal testing.

29. Wilkinson SM, Morrey K, Hollowood K, Heagerty AH, English JSC: **HLA-A, -B and -DR Antigens in Hydrocortisone Contact Hypersensitivity.** *Contact Dermatitis* 1993, 28:295–297.

30. Räsänen L, Tuomi ML: **Cross Sensitization to Mometasone Furoate in Patients With Corticosteroid Contact Allergy.** *Contact Dermatitis* 1992, 27:323–325.

31. Dooms-Goossens A, Morren M: **Results of Routine Patch Testing**
• **With Corticosteroid Series in 2073 Patients.** *Contact Dermatitis* 1992, 26:182–191.
An in-depth review of patch test results of 61 patients allergic to at least one corticosteroid molecule. Corticosteroids were the seventh most frequent allergen, positive results being obtained in 2.9% of all patients referred to their contact dermatitis unit.

32. Veraldi S, Fallahdar O, Riboldi A: **Allergic Contact Dermatitis from Budesonide.** *Contact Dermatitis* 1993, 28:116.

33. Wilkinson SM, English JSC: **Patch Tests Are Poor Predictors of Corticosteroid Allergy.** *Contact Dermatitis* 1992, 26:67–68.

34. Wilkinson SM, Heagerty AHM, English JSC: **A Prospective Study Into the Value of Patch and Intradermal Tests in Identifying Topical Corticosteroid Allergy.** *Br J Dermatol* 1992, 127:22–25.

Roger C. Cornell, MD, Department of Dermatology, Scripps Clinic, mail code MS112, 10666 North Torrey Pines Road, La Jolla, CA 92037, USA.

The use of vitamin D_3 analogues in dermatology

Knud Kragballe, MD, PhD

Marselisborg Hospital, University of Aarhus, Aarhus, Denmark

The physiologically active metabolite of vitamin D_3, 1,25-dihydroxy-vitamin D_3 (1,25[OH]$_2D_3$, calcitriol) has achieved the status of a hormone. It is believed to mediate its effects by binding to a specific receptor that belongs to a superfamily of nuclear receptors. 1,25(OH)$_2D_3$ has the ability to regulate growth and differentiation in many cell types, including cancer cells, epidermal keratinocytes, and activated lymphocytes. The recognition of this ability has set the stage for the development of a new class of vitamin D_3 derivatives. Ideally, such agents should possess potent effects as regulators of cell proliferation and differentiation at concentrations well below those that may induce side effects related to the classic vitamin D activity on calcium absorption and bone mineralization. In addition to 1,25(OH)$_2D_3$, the synthetic vitamin D_3 analogues calcipotriol and 1,24(OH)$_2D_3$ have undergone clinical evaluation. Calcipotriol has been studied extensively. Compared with 1,25(OH)$_2D_3$, calcipotriol is about 200 times less potent in its effect on calcium metabolism, although similar in receptor affinity. In double-blind, placebo-controlled multicenter studies, topical calcipotriol has been shown to be both efficacious and safe for the short- and long-term treatment of plaque-type psoriasis. The novel vitamin D analogues may also be of potential interest for the treatment of ichthyoses, cancer, and autoimmune diseases.

Current Opinion in Dermatology 1995:198–203

The therapeutic effect of the natural, biologically active form of vitamin D_3, 1,25-dihydroxyvitamin D_3 (1,25[OH]$_2D_3$, calcitriol) and its synthetic analogues has been assessed for a number of skin diseases (Table 1). So far, only one of these vitamin D_3 analogues, calcipotriol (calcipotriene), has reached the market, and it is registered only for the topical treatment of psoriasis.

Table 1. Vitamin D_3 analogues used in the treatment of psoriasis

Topical
    1,25-Dihydroxyvitamin D_3 (calcitriol)
    Calcipotriol (calcipotriene)
    1,24-Dihydroxyvitamin D_3 (tacalcitol)
Oral
    1,25-Dihydroxyvitamin D_3
    1,α-Hydroxyvitamin D_3

Vitamin D_3 is a major regulator of calcium and bone metabolism. In the classic target organs, the intestine and bone, vitamin D_3 enhances calcium transport and mineral mobilization through a receptor-coupled process. Hypervitaminosis D, therefore, results in increased urinary calcium excretion, in elevated serum calcium levels, and ultimately in soft tissue calcifications. Recently, a specific vitamin D_3 receptor (VDR) has been detected in a variety of tissues not previously regarded as targets for vitamin D, such as normal human skin and cultures of human epidermal keratinocytes and human dermal fibroblasts. It has been suggested that vitamin D_3 is involved in the regulation of epidermal proliferation and differentiation. At physiologic concentrations, 1,25(OH)$_2D_3$ causes a decrease in proliferation and an increase in the morphologic and biochemical differentiation of cultured keratinocytes. Studies with human keratinocytes grown on deepidermized dermis indicate that 1,25(OH)$_2D_3$ stimulates specifically the last steps of epidermal differentiation (reviewed in Kragballe [1]).

1,25(OH)$_2D_3$ is also recognized to have immunoregulatory properties. Defined actions of the hormone on human peripheral blood mononuclear cells include the inhibition of mitogen- and antigen-stimulated proliferation and the inhibition of immunoglobulin production. There is experimental evidence that the specific target of 1,25(OH)$_2D_3$ is the T-helper inducer lymphocyte and that a significant portion of the vitamin D effect

---

Abbreviations
PUVA—psoralens and ultraviolet A; **VDR**—vitamin D_3 receptor.

is mediated by inhibition of interleukin-2 production. 1,25(OH)₂D₃ also modulates the ability of monocytes to provide signals important in T-lymphocyte activation.

Therapeutic use of 1,25-dihydroxyvitamin D₃

Because of its calciotropic effects, the natural form of vitamin D₃, 1,25(OH)₂D₃ (Fig. 1), has been applied in low concentrations and to limited skin areas. Application of 1,25(OH)₂D₃ ointment at a concentration of 3 µg/g over a skin surface area of up to 300 cm² twice daily for 6 weeks produced clearance or considerable improvement in 72% of the lesions compared with 31% of the vehicle-treated lesions in 29 psoriatic patients [2]. Using a similar trial design, the same investigators assessed the efficacy of 1,25(OH)₂D₃ ointment, 15 µg/g, in 32 patients, the only difference being that 1,25(OH)₂D₃ ointment was applied over a skin surface area of up to 1200 cm². Clearance or considerable improvement was obtained in 75% of the lesions treated with 1,25(OH)₂D₃ and in 44% of the lesions treated with vehicle. In patients treated with 1,25(OH)₂D₃, 3 µg/g [3••], there were no changes in serum calcium levels or 24-hour urinary calcium excretion. However, 3 patients treated with 15 µg/g developed hypercalcemia; two had transient hypercalcemia at week 1 (treated area between 450 and 600 cm²), and one had asymptomatic hypercalcemia at week 6 (treated area 1000 cm²). In this case, serum calcium normalized 3 days after therapy was stopped. Furthermore, patients treated over a skin surface area of 600 to 1200 cm² showed an increase in mean urinary calcium excretion, although it remained within the normal range.

The safety of the 1,25(OH)₂D₃ concentration of 15 µg/g was recently assessed in an uncontrolled study [4]. A total of 30 psoriatic patients were treated once daily for 6 weeks: 12 patients with treated areas of 300 to 600 cm², 10 with treated areas of 600 to 1200 cm², and 8 with treated areas of 1200 to 2400 cm². In the 2 groups

with the largest treatment areas, urinary calcium excretion increased, particularly in the beginning, although not to a statistically significant degree. Because of the uncontrolled study design, it is impossible to draw any definitive conclusions from this particular study.

From the available results, it can be concluded that 1,25(OH)₂D₃ at concentrations of 3 µg/g and 15 µg/g is effective for the short-term treatment of plaque-type psoriasis. Applied to limited skin areas, a concentration of 3 µg/g is well tolerated and safe. However, calcium metabolism may be affected when the concentration is raised to 15 µg/g.

Therapeutic use of calcipotriol

Calcipotriol (calcipotriene, MC 903) (Fig. 1) is a synthetic vitamin D analogue with potent cell-regulating properties but with a lower risk of inducing calcium-related side effects. As a consequence of a modification of the side chain, it is rapidly transformed into inactive metabolites. Therefore, calcipotriol is about 200 times less potent than 1,25(OH)₂D₃ in producing hypercalcemia and hypercalcuria after oral and intraperitoneal administration in rats. In contrast, calcipotriol and 1,25(OH)₂D₃ are equipotent in their affinity for the VDR and in their *in vitro* effects [5].

The antipsoriatic effect of calcipotriol ointment, 50 µg/g, has been documented in a number of clinical trials. Calcipotriol ointment, 50 µg/g, is manufactured by Leo Pharmaceutical Products, Ballerup, Denmark, and marketed for the treatment of plaque-type psoriasis vulgaris under the trade names Daivonex, Dovonex (Westwood-Squibb Pharmaceuticals, Buffalo, NY), and Psorcutan. A cream formulation of calcipotriol has recently also become available, but a solution for scalp psoriasis has still not reached the market. In a double-blind, right-left comparative double-blind study, calcipotriol ointment (25, 50, and 100 µg/g) and vehicle were compared in 50 patients with psoriasis vulgaris [6]. After treatment for 8 weeks calcipotriol, 50 µg/g, had a significantly greater antipsoriatic effect than vehicle. Calcipotriol, 50 µg/g, was more effec-

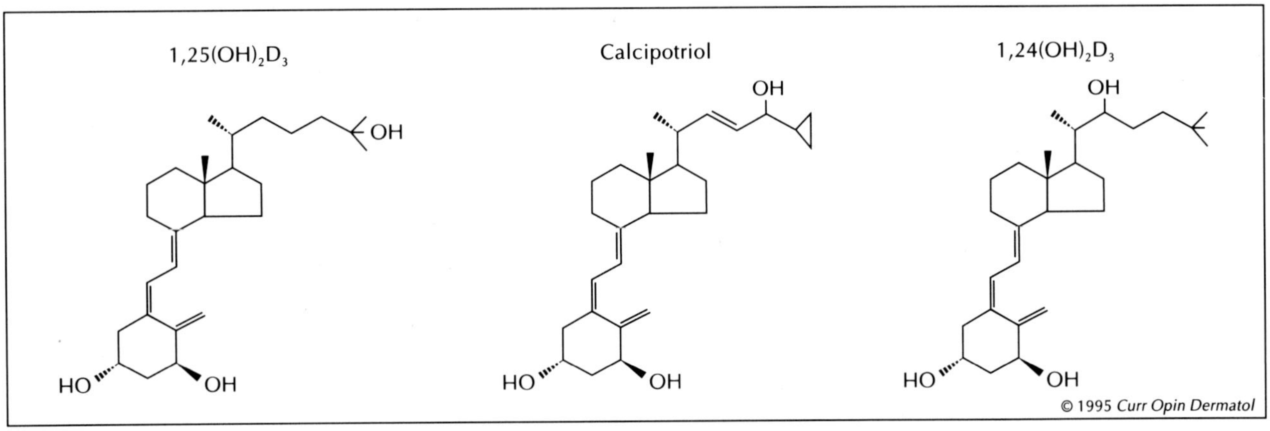

Fig. 1. Chemical structures of 1,25(OH)₂D₃ (calcitriol), calcipotriol (calcipotriene), and 1,24(OH)₂D₃ (tacalcitol).

tive than calcipotriol ointment 25 µg/g, whereas no difference was found between concentrations of 50 µg/g and 100 µg/g. From this study, it was concluded that a calcipotriol concentration of 50 µg/g in an ointment is optimal for the treatment of psoriasis. Treatment with this concentration induced a significant improvement after only 1 week, and a marked improvement was observed in about two thirds of the patients after 6 weeks (Fig. 2). The efficacy and safety of calcipotriol ointment, 50 µg/g, was later confirmed in a multicenter, double-blind, placebo-controlled, right-left comparative study including 66 psoriatic patients [7].

Calcipotriol ointment, 50 µg/g, was compared with betamethasone 17-valerate ointment, 0.1%, in a multicenter, randomized, double-blind, right-left comparison (*n* = 345) [8] and in a parallel group comparison (*n* = 409) [9••]. Taken together, these two studies showed that calcipotriol was superior to betamethasone after treatment for 6 weeks, and although the superiority was slight, it was statistically significant. Because betamethasone 17-valerate is a medium-strength corticosteroid, the results document that treatment with calcipotriol ointment, 50 µg/g, is efficacious for psoriasis.

Calcipotriol ointment, 50 µg/g, was compared with anthralin in a multicenter, open, randomized parallel-group comparison. Patients were treated for 8 weeks with either calcipotriol ointment, 50 µg/g applied twice daily, or Dithrocreme (American Dermal Corp., Plumsteadville, PA) applied once daily for 30 minutes according to a short-contact regimen [10••]. At the end of treatment, both the percentage reduction and the absolute reduction of the psoriasis area and severity index were significantly greater in the calcipotriol group (58.1%) than in the anthralin group (41.6%). These results show that calcipotriol ointment is more efficacious

than Dithrocreme, the most widely prescribed anthralin formulation in the United Kingdom, for treating patients with mild to moderate psoriasis vulgaris.

Because psoriasis is a chronic and relapsing disease, it becomes important to determine whether the beneficial effect of calcipotriol seen in the short-term studies can be maintained when patients are treated on a long-term basis. This question has been assessed in two prospective, noncomparative, open studies with calcipotriol ointment, 50 µg/g. Included were patients who had a good clinical response without significant adverse events to calcipotriol in previous calcipotriol studies. In the first study, 15 patients were treated with calcipotriol ointment, 50 µg/g twice daily (maximally 100 g ointment per week) for at least 6 months [11]. One of the 15 patients dropped out after 3 months because of lack of efficacy. Assessment of efficacy by the investigator at month 6 showed a mild improvement in two (13%), a moderate improvement in four (27%), a marked improvement in five (33%), and clearance in three (20%). These long-term results have been confirmed in a larger but still unpublished multicenter study. Although calcipotriol usually decreases infiltration rather fast, some residual infiltration does persist. Therefore, it may be necessary to supplement calcipotriol therapy (Table 2). If a limited number of plaques persist, calcipotriol can be successfully occluded with a hydrocolloid dressing. After treatment for 12 days (ointment applied three times for 4 days under a hydrocolloid dressing), most lesions cleared completely, and the therapeutic response was similar to that of occlusive therapy with clobetasol ointment [12].

In a bilateral comparative study, calcipotriol was combined with ultraviolet B phototherapy in 20 patients with more widespread lesions [13]. Patients were

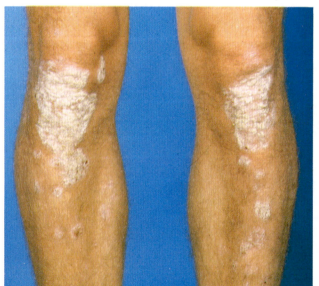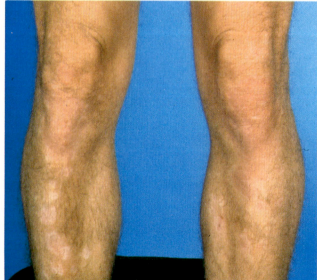

Fig. 2. Psoriatic plaques before (*left panel*) and after (*right panel*) treatment with calcipotriol ointment, 50 µg/g twice daily for 6 weeks.

Table 2. Therapeutic efficacy of calcipotriol

Monotherapy
    Calcipotriol > placebo
    Calcipotriol > betamethasone
    Calcipotriol > anthralin
Combination therapy
    Hydrocolloid occlusion plus calcipotriol > calciportriol
    Ultraviolet B plus calcipotriol > ultraviolet B
    Psoralens and ultraviolet A plus calcipotriol >
       psoralens and ultraviolet A
    Cyclosporine plus calcipotriol > cyclosporine

> Indicates greater effectiveness of therapy.

treated with calcipotriol ointment on both sides (twice daily application) and with ultraviolet B irradiation on one side (suberythemogenic doses three times weekly) for 8 weeks. The investigator's overall assessment at the end of treatment showed that calcipotriol had resulted in marked improvement in 12 (66%) of the patients and in clearance in two (17%). Combination of calcipotriol ointment with ultraviolet B radiation resulted in marked improvement in nine (50%) of the patients and in clearance in five (39%). In this small study, the difference between monotherapy and combination therapy did not reach statistical significance. In a multicenter study, however, the combination of calcipotriol and ultraviolet B phototherapy was found to be superior to calcipotriol alone (Unpublished data). In these studies, conventional broad-band (290 to 320 nm) ultraviolet B light sources were used. In a recent, preliminary report it was found that narrow-band ultraviolet B (311 nm) phototherapy combined with calcipotriol was much more effective than calcipotriol alone [14•]. These results might indicate that photocombination with narrow-band ultraviolet B is superior to combination with broad-band ultraviolet B.

Moreover, it has been found that calcipotriol improves the response to psoralens and ultraviolet A (PUVA). In a bilateral comparison of calcipotriol and ointment vehicle (*n* = 13), topical treatment was commenced on the first day of PUVA therapy [15•]. Lesions treated with calcipotriol cleared earlier or were consistently judged to improve better than those treated with vehicle alone. In a larger, multicenter study, calcipotriol or vehicle treatment was started 2 weeks before PUVA therapy was initiated. The combination of calcipotriol and PUVA reduced the cumulative ultraviolet A dose and the number of PUVA treatments required for clearance of psoriasis (Unpublished data). Finally, in a placebo-controlled study, low-dose cyclosporin A (2 mg/kg per day) given together with calcipotriol was more efficacious than cyclosporine alone (Unpublished data).

Skin irritation is the only important local side effect seen with calcipotriol therapy. Skin atrophy and photosensitization do not occur, and the development of skin allergy is extremely rare. A lesional or perilesional irritation is seen in 4% to 20% of the treated patients. The lesional or perilesional irritation is in most cases mild,

consisting of a burning or stinging sensation. It is, in general, transient and has no clinical consequence. In more severe cases, erythema and scaling are present. The face is particularly sensitive to calcipotriol ointment. Facial irritation may be seen not only after local application, but also after transfer of calcipotriol ointment applied elsewhere. Facial irritation can almost be avoided if the face is not treated and if the patients are instructed to wash their hands after applying the ointment. Mild skin irritation (*ie*, burning or stinging) disappears spontaneously within a few days after therapy is stopped and may even resolve during continued therapy. There are two reported cases of suspected delayed-type contact allergy to calcipotriol [16,17]. Clinically it is difficult to differentiate allergic contact dermatitis from irritant contact dermatitis, which is much more common with calcipotriol treatment.

In the clinical trials with calcipotriol ointment, no significant changes of serum calcium were detected, except in one patient [9••]. This patient applied approximately 400 g of calcipotriol ointment, 50 μg/g, during 10 days, *ie*, about three times the amount permitted under the protocol. During the first 10 days of treatment, the serum calcium rose from 2.29 mmol/L to 3.40 mmol/L (normal range, 2.10 to 2.70 mmol/L). The calcipotriol was stopped, and 5 days later serum calcium had normalized. No clinical symptoms or signs of hypercalcemia were reported in this patient. There is another case of hypercalcemia during excessive use of calcipotriol ointment [18]. This psoriatic patient had a "moderate" degree of renal impairment. After applying approximately 200 g of calcipotriol ointment to her extensive disease over the first week of treatment, she developed nausea, muscle weakness, and abdominal pain, and the serum calcium rose from 2.44 mmol/L to 3.51 mmol/L. After calcipotriol therapy was stopped, serum calcium normalized within 1 week. No sequelae were reported. In addition, there were two cases of hypercalcemia after application of 150 g/w and 200 g/w, respectively (Data on file at the manufacturer).

Although serum calcium levels were unchanged when calcipotriol ointment was used according to the recommendations (maximum 100 g/wk), the 4 cases of hypercalcemia that developed after excessive use of calcipotriol raise the question of whether changes of bone and calcium metabolism can take place even when serum calcium remains unchanged. This question has been assessed in a randomized, double-blind, placebo-controlled, parallel group comparison [19]. Thirty-four psoriatic patients were randomly assigned to receive treatment with either calcipotriol ointment, 50 μg/g, or placebo ointment for 3 weeks. Calcipotriol-treated patients (*n* = 17) used on average 40.3 g of ointment per week. During treatment, there was no difference between the calcipotriol group and the placebo group in urinary calcium excretion or in the other biochemical indices assessed. The absence of an effect of calcipotriol treatment on bone and calcium metabolism has been confirmed in a similar study, in which patients applied approximately 80 g of ointment per week (Unpublished data) and in an open noncomparative study involving 12 psoriatic patients, who were treated for 4 weeks with an average of 100 g of ointment per week [20]. Contrary to the results of these 3 studies, it was reported that the application of calcipotriol ointment, 100 g/w for 4 weeks, induced a slight but statistically significant increase in urinary calcium excretion [21]. Furthermore, there were two cases of slight hypercalcemia after application of 70 g/wk and 80 g/wk, respectively [22]. When these sporadic cases of slight hypercalcemia are considered, it should be remembered that such elevations of serum calcium were equally distributed among patients treated with calcipotriol and patients receiving the control treatment. Therefore, the available data seem to suggest that calcipotriol ointment, 50 µg/g, in amounts up to 100 g/wk is safe for the treatment of psoriasis.

Patients included in the clinical trials with calcipotriol were all adults with plaque-type psoriasis vulgaris. Studies in psoriatic children have been completed but not yet reported. In generalized pustular psoriasis, calcipotriol treatment was evaluated in three consecutive patients [23]. In all three cases, topical calcipotriol was found to be effective, well tolerated, and safe in the short-term management of this severe form of psoriasis. Patients with HIV-related psoriasis are often refractory to conventional therapy. An erythrodermic psoriasis patient with advanced HIV disease responded well to calcipotriol therapy [24]. If such results are confirmed in other similar patients, calcipotriol may prove to be a useful option in these conditions.

Although the clinical studies with calcipotriol and other vitamin D_3 analogues have focused almost exclusively on psoriasis, there are no reasons to believe that this class of compounds is beneficial only in this disease. So far, there are case reports of calcipotriol improving pityriasis rubra pilaris [25] and disseminated superficial actinic porokeratosis [26]. The results obtained in other dyskeratotic disorders are more mixed. While topical $1,25(OH)_2D_3$ (0.1 µg/g) [27] and oral 1-α(OH)D_3, 1 µg/d [28] were ineffective, a higher concentration of calcipotriol (50 µg/g) was both effective and well tolerated in congenital ichthyosis, X-linked ichthyosis, and ichthyosis vulgaris [29] In the same study, keratosis pilaris and palmoplantar keratoderma were found to be unresponsive, and Darier's disease even worsened during calcipotriol therapy. There is a limited experience with calcipotriol in other skin diseases. Alopecia areata does not improve during calcipotriol therapy [30]. It is, however, of considerable interest that T-cell lymphoma of the skin was improved, both clinically and histologically, by calcipotriol [31].

Clinical use of tacalcitol

Tacalcitol (1,24[OH]$_2D_3$) (Fig. 1) is another synthetic vitamin D analogue developed for topical use in psoriasis. It is equipotent with $1,25(OH)_2D_3$ in its affinity for the VDR and in its capacity to inhibit keratinocyte proliferation and to stimulate keratinocyte differentiation *in vitro* [32]. Its advantage over $1,25(OH)_2D_3$ is that

it induces a smaller increase of serum calcium levels after a single intravenous dose to rats. However, the doses inducing hypercalcemia are similar for tacalcitol and $1,25(OH)_2D_3$ [32].

In a preliminary study with tacalcitol, a concentration of 4 µg/g, applied with or without 12-hour occlusion, was superior to vehicle (petrolatum) in two patients [33]. The optimal concentration of tacalcitol was examined in a randomized, double-blind trial. Tacalcitol ointment containing either 1, 2, or 4 µg/g was applied to a single lesion on one side, and hydrocortisone butyrate, 0.1%, or betamethasone 17-valerate ointment, 0.1%, to a similar lesion on the contralateral side in 92 psoriatic patients. After treatment twice daily for 4 weeks, 1, 2, and 4 µg/g of tacalcitol had produced a moderate to marked improvement in 55%, 52% and 54% of the patients, respectively. However, a marked improvement was more frequently noted in patients treated with 2 and 4 µg/g than with 1 µg/g. For comparison, the improvement rates were 64% for betamethasone valerate and 52% for hydrocortisone butyrate [34].

In a subsequent placebo-controlled, double-blind study in 106 psoriatic patients, tacalcitol ointment, 2 µg/g, was compared with vehicle (petrolatum). Compared with placebo, tacalcitol induced significant improvement after only 1 week, but the difference was greater after 4 weeks (*ie*, the end of treatment) [35].

Conclusions

Vitamin D_3 and its derivatives represent a new class of compounds that are becoming available for the treatment of skin diseases. Ideally, such compounds should have strong effects on cell proliferation and differentiation as well as on immunocompetent cells, but they should lack calciotropic action. These criteria are partially fulfilled by the synthetic analogues calcipotriol (calcipotriene) and tacalcitol. Only calcipotriol has been studied extensively. When used according to established guidelines, topical calcipotriol appears to be efficacious, well tolerated, and safe for both the short- and long-term treatment of plaque-type psoriasis vulgaris. Vitamin D analogues may also be beneficial in certain disorders of keratinization.

References and recommended reading

Papers of particular interest, published within the annual period of review, have been highlighted as:
* Of special interest
•• Of outstanding interest

1. Kragballe K: **Treatment of Psoriasis With Calcipotriol and Other Vitamin D Analogues.** *J Am Acad Dermatol* 1992, 27:1001–1008.

2. Langner A, Verjans H, Stapor V, Mol M, Elzerman J: **Treatment of Chronic Plaque Psoriasis by 1-Alpha,25-Dihydroxyvitamin D₃ Ointment.** In *Vitamin D: Gene Regulation Structure-Function Analysis and Clinical Application.* Edited by Norman AW, Bouillon R, Thomasset M. Berlin: Walter de Gruyter; 1983:430–431.

3. Langner A, Verjans H, Stapor V, Mol M, Fraczykowska M: **Topical**
•• **Calcipotriol in the Treatment of Chronic Plaque Psoriasis: A Double-Blind Study.** *Br J Dermatol* 1993, 128:566–571.

Assessment of the efficacy and safety of 1,25(OH)₂D₃.

4. Wishart JM: **Calcitriol (1,25-Dihydroxyvitamin D₃) Ointment in Psoriasis: A Safety Tolerance and Efficacy Multicentre Study.** *Dermatology* 1994, 188:135–139.

5. Binderup L, Kragballe K: **Origin of the Use of Calcipotriol in Psoriasis Treatment.** *Rev Contemp Pharmacother* 1992, 3:401–409.

6. Kragballe K: **Treatment of Psoriasis by the Topical Application of the Novel Cholecaliferol Analogue Calcipotriol (MC 903).** *Arch Dermatol* 1989, 125:1647–1652.

7. Dubertret L, Wallach D, Souteyrand P, Perusell M, Maynadiet J, Chevtrant-Breton J, Beylot C, Basex JA, Jurgensen HJ: **Efficacy and Safety of Calcipotriol (MC 903) Ointment in Psoriasis Vulgaris.** *J Am Acad Dermatol* 1992, 27:983–988.

8. Kragballe K, Gjertsen BT, De Hoope D, Karlsmark T, van der Kerkhof P, Larko P, Nieboer C, Roed-Petersen J, Strand A, Tikjöb G: **Double-Blind, Right-Left Comparison of Calcipotriol and Betamethasone Valerate in Treatment of Psoriasis Vulgaris.** *Lancet* 1991, 337:193–196.

9. Cunliffe WJ, Claudy A, Fairiss G, Goldin D, Gratton D, Holden CA,
•• Berth-Jones J, Maddin WS, Ortonne J-P, Henderson CA, Young M: **A Multicentre Comparative Study of Calcipotriol and Betamethasone 17-Valerate in Patients With Psoriasis Vulgaris.** *J Am Acad Dermatol* 1992, 26:736–743.
Comparative study of calcipotriol and the medium-strength corticosteroid betamethasone 17-valerate.

10. Berth-Jones J, Chu AC, Dodd WAH, Ganpule M, Griffiths WAD,
•• Haydey RP, Klaber MR, Murray SJ, Rogers S, Jurgensen HJ: **A Multicentre Parallel-Group Comparison of Calcipotriol Ointment and Short-Contact Dithranol Therapy in Chronic Plaque Psoriasis.** *Br J Dermatol* 1992, 127:266–271.
Comparative study of calcipotriol and short-contact dithranol (anthralin) therapy in psoriasis.

11. Kragballe K, Fogh K: **Long-Term Efficacy and Tolerability of Topical Calcipotriol in Psoriasis.** *Acta Derm Venereol (Stockh)* 1991, 71:475–478.

12. Gamborg Nielsen P: **Calcipotriol or Clobetasol Propionate Occluded With a Hydrocolloid Dressing for Treatment of Nummular Psoriasis [Letter].** *Acta Derm Venereol (Stockh)* 1993, 73:394.

13. Kragballe K: **Combination of Topical Calcipotriol (MC 903) and UVB Radiation for Psoriasis Vulgaris.** *Dermatologica* 1990, 181:211–214.

14. Kerscher M, Volkenandt M, Plewig G, Lehmann P: **Combination Pho-
• totherapy of Psoriasis With Calcipotriol and Narrow-Band UVB [Letter].** *Lancet* 1993, 342:923.
Preliminary report on combined effects of topical calcipotriol and PUVA. Only a small number of patients were included, however.

15. Speight EL, Farr PM: **Calcipotriol Improves the Response of Psoriasis
• to PUVA.** *Br J Dermatol* 1994, 130:79–82.
Report on combination therapy using topical calcipotriol and PUVA. Only a small number of patients were included, however.

16. Yip J, Goodfield M: **Contact Dermatitis From MC 903, a Topical Vitamin D₃ Analogue.** *Contact Dermatitis* 1991, 25:139–140.

17. Bruynzel DP, Hol CW, Nieboer C: **Allergic Contact Dermatitis to Calcipotriol.** *Br J Dermatol* 1992, 126:66.

18. Dwyer C, Chapman RS: **Calcipotriol and Hypercalcemia.** *Lancet* 1991, 338:764–765.

19. Mortensen L, Kragballe K, Wegmann E, Schifter S, Risteli J, Charles P: **Treatment of Psoriasis Vulgaris With Topical Calcipotriol Has No Short-Term Effect on Calcium or Bone Metabolism.** *Acta Derm Venereol (Stockh)* 1993, 73:300–304.

20. Gumowski-Sunek D, Rizzoli R, Saurat J-J: **Effects of Topical Calcipotriol on Calcium Metabolism in Psoriatic Patients: Comparison With Oral Calcitriol.** *Dermatologica* 1991, 183:275–279.

21. Berth-Jones J, Bourke JF, Iqbal SJ, Hutchinson PE: **Urine Calcium Excretion During Treatment of Psoriasis With Topical Calcipotriol.** *Br J Dermatol* 1993, 129:411–414.

22. Hardman KH, Heath DA: **Hypercalcaemia Associated With Calcipotriol (Dovonex) Treatment [Letter].** *BMJ* 1993, 306:896.

23. Berth-Jones J, Bourke J, Bailey K, Graham-Brown RAC, Hutchinson PE: **Generalised Pustular Psoriasis: Response to Topical Calcipotriol.** *BMJ* 1992, 305:868–869.

24. Gray JD, Bottomley E, Layton AM, Cotterill JA, Monteiro E: **The Use of Calcipotriol in HIV-Related Psoriasis.** *Clin Exp Dermatol* 1992, 17:342–343.

25. van de Kerkhof PCM, De Jong EMGJ: **Topical Treatment With the Vitamin D₃ Analogue MC 903 Improves Pityriasis Rubra Pilaris: Clinical and Immunohistochemical Observations.** *Br J Dermatol* 1992, 125:293–294.

26. Harrison PV, Stollery N: **Disseminated Superficial Actinic Porokeratosis Responding to Calcipotriol.** *Clin Exp Dermatol* 1994, 19:95.

27. Okano M: **1α,25(OH)₂D₃ Use on Psoriasis and Ichthyosis.** *Int J Dermatol* 1991, 30:62–64.

28. Masaki O, Kitano Y, Yoshikawa K: **A Trial of Oral 1-Alpha-Hydroxyvitamin D₃ for Ichthyosis.** *Dermatologica* 1988, 177:23.

29. Kragballe K, Steijlen PM, Ibsen HH, Van de Kerkhof PCM, Esmann J, Sørensen LH, Axelsen MS: **Efficacy, Tolerability and Safety of Calcipotriol Ointment in Disorders of Keratinization: Results of a Randomized, Double-Blind, Vehicle-Controlled, Right/Left Comparative Study.** *Arch Dermatol,* in press.

30. Berth-Jones J, Hutchinson PE: **Alopecia Totalis Does Not Respond to the Vitamin D₃ Analogue Calcipotriol.** *J Dermatol Treatment* 1991, 1:293–294.

31. Scott-Mackie P, Hickish T, Mortimer P, Sloane J, Cunningham D: **Calcipotriol and Regression in T-Cell Lymphoma of Skin [Letter].** *Lancet* 1993, 342:172.

32. Matsunaga T, Yamamoto M, Mimura H, Ohta T, Kiyoki M, Onba T, Naruchi T, Hosoi J, Kuroki T: **1,24R-Dihydroxyvitamin D₃: A Novel Active Form of Vitamin D₃ With High Activity for Inducing Epidermal Differentiation but Decreased Hypercalcemia Activity.** *J Dermatol* 1990, 17:135–142.

33. Kato T, Rokugo M, Teuri T, Tagami H: **Successful Treatment of Psoriasis With Topical Application of the Active Vitamin D₃ Analogue, 12,4-Dihydroxycholecalciferol.** *Br J Dermatol* 1986, 115:431–433.

34. TV-02 Ointment Research Group: **A Dose-Finding Study for the TV-02 Ointment [in Japanese].** *Nishinibon J Dermatol* 1989, 51:310–316.

35. TV-02 Ointment Research Group: **A Placebo-Controlled Double-Blind, Right-Left Comparison Study on the Efficacy of TV-02 Ointment for the Treatment of Psoriasis [in Japanese].** *Nishinibon J Dermatol* 1991, 53:1252–1561.

Knud Kragballe, MD, PhD, Department of Dermatology, Marselisborg Hospital, DK-8000 Aarhus, Denmark.

Antimalarial therapy for skin diseases

Jeffrey P. Callen, MD

University of Louisville, Louisville, Kentucky, USA

Antimalarial drugs have been used for treatment of dermatologic diseases since the early 1950s. While it is still not known how these drugs work, there are data that suggest that they have immunosuppressive and anti-inflammatory effects. Effective use in selected patients with lupus erythematosus, dermatomyositis, sarcoidosis, porphyria cutanea tarda, and polymorphous light eruption has been documented. Newer uses include prophylaxis against thrombosis, treatment of oral lichen planus, and adjunctive therapy for pemphigus foliaceus. The safe use of chloroquine or hydroxychloroquine in patients with psoriatic arthritis has been documented. Although multiple toxic effects are possible, the most important issue remains the possibility of irreversible retinopathy. The use of antimalarials during pregnancy may be safe, but their use in lactating women remains controversial.

Current Opinion in Dermatology 1995:204–209

The antimalarial drugs that have been used for the treatment of dermatologic disorders include chloroquine, hydroxychloroquine, and quinacrine. Quinacrine has recently become difficult to obtain; however, it is still considered in this review because it may become widely available again in the near future. The antimalarials are 4-aminoquinolones (Fig. 1) and derivatives of quinine, a naturally occurring substance. Quinine is an alkaloid derived from the bark of the South American cinchona tree [1]. This bark is believed to have been used initially for its antipyretic effects, and thus the cinchona tree has also become known as the "fever" tree. In the 1800s, quinine became popular as an effective antimalarial agent.

The First World War provided the impetus for the synthetic production of antimalarials. Quinacrine hydrochloride was synthesized in 1930, chloroquine phosphate in 1934, and hydroxychloroquine sulfate in 1946. The dermatologic use of antimalarials is attributed to Payne's [2] use in lupus erythematosus (LE) in 1894. In 1951, Page [3] used quinacrine to treat cutaneous LE.

Mechanism of action

The exact mechanism by which antimalarials act to affect disease is not fully understood. Among the postulates for the mechanism of action are effects on light filtration, immunosuppressive actions, anti-inflammatory actions, and DNA binding. Antimalarials inhibit ultraviolet–induced cutaneous reaction in LE and polymorphous light eruption, perhaps through effects on prostaglandin metabolism, the inhibition of superoxide production, or their ability to bind to DNA [4].

Antimalarial compounds raise intracytoplasmic pH levels, which can result in a decreased ability of macrophages to express major histocompatibility complex antigens on its cell surface. In a recent experiment, Fox and Kang [5•] demonstrated a dose-dependent inhibition of the release of interleukin-2 from a CD4+ T-cell clone by both chloroquine and hydroxychloroquine. Antimalarials may inhibit the formation of antigen-antibody complexes. They have also been shown to decrease lymphocyte responsiveness to mitogens *in vitro* [6].

Anti-inflammatory effects of antimalarials may also be an important factor in their action. Antimalarials have been noted to decrease lysosomal size and might possibly inhibit their function [7]. They also impair chemotaxis [8].

An additional effect that may be of importance is the ability of antimalarials to inhibit platelet aggregation and adhesion and thrombus formation [9]. Wallace *et al.* [10•] recently found that thromboembolic events are decreased in hydroxychloroquine-treated systemic LE (SLE) patients. They also observed decreases in cholesterol and, after 6 weeks of therapy, decreased interleukin-2 and soluble CD8 levels.

Abbreviations
LE—lupus erythematosus; **PCT**—porphyria cutanea tarda; **SLE**—systemic lupus erythematosus.

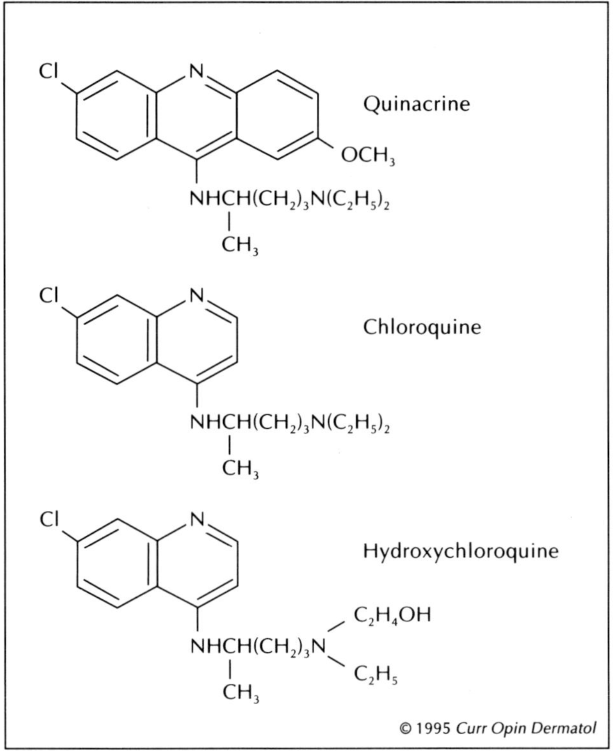

Fig. 1. Structural formulae of antimalarial agents used in dermatology.

Clinical uses

Lupus erythematosus

One double-blind trial of hydroxychloroquine therapy for discoid LE demonstrated that it was more effective than placebo at 3 months and 1 year and that at crossover it was more effective than the placebo at 3 months [11]. Antimalarials are used in patients who fail to respond well to topical measures such as sun protection, sunscreens, and topical corticosteroids. In large, open, clinical studies, 70% of patients with chronic cutaneous LE have responded to antimalarials with a good to excellent response [12]. Certain subsets seem to respond less well: those patients with widespread involvement, those with hypertrophic or verrucous lesions, and those who have SLE with prominent discoid LE lesions. Similar excellent results in patients with subacute cutaneous LE have been observed in open trials. Anecdotal information has suggested that when hydroxychloroquine is not effective, a switch to chloroquine may result in control of the process. Prior to its removal from the market, quinacrine could be added to either chloroquine or hydroxychloroquine or used alone to control LE in some patients. The onset of action for cutaneous LE is between 4 and 8 weeks. Cessation of therapy during the winter months is possible with some patients.

The usefulness of antimalarials in SLE was less well documented until the Canadian Hydroxychloroquine Study Group recently published their data [13]. It had been generally accepted that arthritis, pleuritis, pericarditis, and lethargy respond to antimalarials [14]. The Canadian group found that the risk of a clinical flare of SLE was significantly greater in patients on placebo as compared with hydroxychloroquine. In the accompanying editorial, Lockshin [15] pointed out that although these data are significant, they do not address the usefulness of hydroxychloroquine in acutely ill SLE patients, nor do they address whether all patients with SLE should have hydroxychloroquine prescribed. In a recent report, Esdaile [16] reviewed the existing data on the use of antimalarials in SLE. While only two controlled studies exist, it appears that patients with mild to moderate SLE can benefit from antimalarial therapy. Esdaile also discussed a study of lupus arthritis in which objective benefits were not noted, but subjective, patient-reported benefits were statistically associated with hydroxychloroquine therapy. In addition, he discussed studies that have demonstrated a corticosteroid-sparing role for antimalarials.

Porphyria cutanea tarda

Antimalarials are not the first choice of therapy for patients with porphyria cutanea tarda (PCT). After exogenous exacerbating factors are removed or discontinued, phlebotomy remains the primary therapy. In patients who are anemic or who fail to respond to phlebotomy, antimalarial therapy may be attempted. The mechanism of antimalarials is their effect on hepatocytes with release of porphyrins into the circulation and eventual excretion. The observation that antimalarials are useful was made when they were used to treat patients with LE, who may occasionally have subclinical PCT [17]. When given hydroxychloroquine or chloroquine in usual doses, such patients developed fever, nausea, vomiting, abdominal pain, and elevated liver function tests [18]. Recovery from this acute toxic reaction could result in a prolonged remission of the PCT. To avoid the toxic reaction, low dosages of antimalarials (chloroquine, 125 mg twice weekly, or hydroxychloroquine, 100 mg twice weekly) have been found to be safe and effective [19]. This therapy cannot be used in patients with renal failure on hemodialysis. Petersen and Thomsen [20] used high-dose hydroxychloroquine, 250 mg three times daily for 3 days, in hospitalized patients and thus induced prolonged remission in a majority of them. Some remission lasted as long as 4.5 years.

Photodermatoses

Photosensitivity diseases such as polymorphous light eruption and solar urticaria and photoaggravated diseases such as dermatomyositis and reticulated erythematosus mucinosis have been successfully treated with antimalarials. Polymorphous light eruption can be treated intermittently with hydroxychloroquine, 200 to 400 mg daily. This treatment has been shown in a placebo-controlled trial to reduce the eruption and its attendant symptoms [21]. Only anecdotal cases of solar urticaria treated with antimalarials have been reported. Some patients with reticulated erythematous mucinosis, a rare condition, have been successfully treated with hydroxychloroquine.

In patients with dermatomyositis, cutaneous lesions may be present long after the myositic component resolves. These lesions may be extremely difficult to treat despite the use of potent topical corticosteroids, sunscreens, systemic corticosteroids, and various immunosuppressives. In an effort to reduce the corticosteroid dosage, I treated several patients with cutaneous dermatomyositis with oral hydroxychloroquine (Fig. 2). After noting a favorable response, we used hydroxychloroquine in an open-labeled trial in seven patients [22]. In all of our patients, improvement was noted with consequent lowering of the corticosteroid dosage in two patients, and in three a complete response occurred. Subsequently, other reports on both adults [23] and children [24] have appeared that detail similar results.

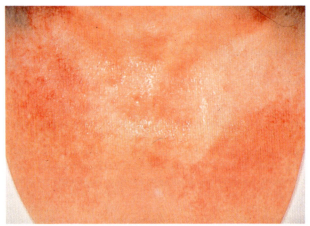

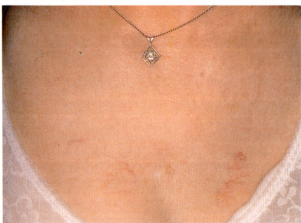

Fig. 2. Before (*top panel*) and approximately 2 months after (*bottom panel*) hydroxychloroquine therapy for dermatomyositis.

Other dermatoses

Antimalarials have been used to treat various manifestations of sarcoidosis. Jones and I [25] recently reported on our experience with 17 patients with cutaneous sarcoidal granulomas treated with hydroxychloroquine.

Patients were treated with 200 to 400 mg per day and began to note improvement after 4 to 12 weeks (Fig. 3). Higher initial dosages were not noted to result in a more rapid response. Twelve patients were able to discontinue other therapy. Relapse was noted in six patients who had a complete response when the dosage was lowered or stopped. Maintenance therapy with hydroxychloroquine, 200 mg three times per week, was used in three patients. Hydroxychloroquine may therefore be a useful adjunctive therapy for patients with sarcoidosis.

Oral lichen planus is a common disorder. Although topical or intralesional corticosteroids are effective, there are numerous patients in whom the response is incomplete or in whom secondary candidal infection may occur. Eisen [26••] reported an open trial of 10 patients with oral lichen planus, seven of whom had erosive disease. Nine of the 10 patients had an excellent response, with the onset of effect occurring as early as 1 to 2 months after therapy began. Erosions took 3 to 5 months to heal. None of his patients had cutaneous LP. Moreover, none of the patients had an adverse reaction, but this was a short-term study.

The most recent addition to the list of conditions that may benefit from antimalarial therapy (Table 1) is pemphigus foliaceus. Hymes and Jordon [27•] noted benefits and corticosteroid-sparing effects in two patients. The effects were noted within 2 months of therapy.

Psoriatic arthritis

The use of antimalarials in patients with psoriasis has been reported to increase the severity of psoriasis, and in some cases to lead to an exfoliative erythroderma [28,29]. In addition, patients without skin disease can have the initial onset of psoriasis during therapy [30]. However, large series of patients with psoriatic arthritis have been treated successfully with hydroxychloroquine [31] or chloroquine [32•]. In Kammer *et al.*'s [31] report on hydroxychloroquine therapy, there were no patients whose psoriasis flared. Similarly, Gladman *et al.* [32•] reported that the psoriasis worsened in six of 32 patients treated with chloroquine as well as in six of 24 control patients. None of these patients had an exfoliative erythroderma.

Toxicity

Antimalarials may produce a wide array of adverse reactions, some of which may be serious (Table 2). With the exception of retinopathy, most of the side effects are reversible upon discontinuation of the antimalarial agent. Several differences pertaining to the risk of certain reactions exist between the antimalarials. Yellow pigmentation is limited to quinacrine therapy. Hematologic side effects may be more common with quinacrine, but ocular toxicity is not seen with quinacrine. Whereas both chloroquine and hydroxychloroquine have been associated with retinopathy, it appears that chloroquine is more toxic than hydroxychloroquine.

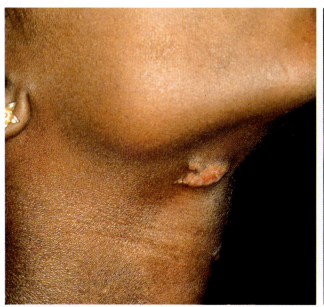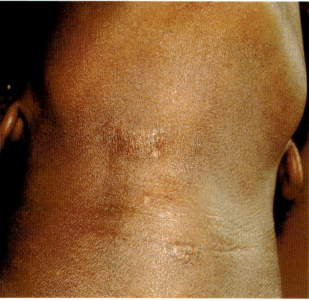

Fig. 3. Before (*left panel*) and approximately 3 months after (*right panel*) hydroxychloroquine therapy for cutaneous sarcoidosis.

Table 1. Effectiveness of antimalarials in dermatologic disease

Strong evidence for effectiveness
 Lupus erythematosus
  Cutaneous
  Discoid
  Subacute cutaneous
  Systemic
 Lupus panniculitis
 Porphyria cutanea tarda
 Sarcoidosis (cutaneous and pulmonary)
 Prophylaxis against deep venous thrombosis and
  pulmonary embolism following surgery
Effective in small, open-label clinical trials
 Polymorphous light eruption
 Solar urticaria
 Dermatomyositis (cutaneous disease only)
 Antiphospholipid antibody syndrome
 Oral lichen planus
Anecdotal evidence of effectiveness
 Benign lymphocytic infiltrate
 Granuloma annulare
 Lichen sclerosus et atrophicus
 Panniculitis
 Atopic dermatitis
 Vasculitis (small vessel)
 Reticulated erythematous mucinosis syndrome
 Pemphigus foliaceus

The issue of most concern to physicians who use antimalarials often is that of ophthalmologic toxicity. Three types of ocular side effects may develop: corneal deposits, neuromuscular eye toxicity, and retinopathy. Only retinopathy is potentially nonreversible. It has been divided into two forms: true retinopathy and premaculopathy. Premaculopathy is defined as changes on visual field or funduscopic examination that are not associated with visual loss. It is believed that premaculopathy would progress if the antimalarial agent is continued, and that it is potentially reversible when the agent is discontinued [33•]. Rynes and Bernstein [33•] recommended that the patient be evaluated for retinopathy at baseline, then reevaluated every 6 months by an ophthalmologist. They suggested that testing visual acuity and visual fields and performing a funduscopic examination are acceptable, and that the results of tests such as serial photography, fluorescein angiography, and electrooculogram may remain normal even in the presence of retinopathy. Further, they point out that patient-administered Amsler grid testing has not been established as a method of screening. An interesting study from Indiana University evaluated the recommendations of rheumatologists and ophthalmologists in Indiana [34•]. In a review of 24 patients on hydroxychloroquine therapy, most of the physicians recommended follow-up every 6 months, although there were seven in whom no record of an ophthalmologic evaluation could be found. Fortunately, the risk of true retinopathy is very low, with chloroquine believed to be more risky than hydroxychloroquine [35].

Two special situations are worthy of discussion: the use of antimalarial drugs in children and in pregnant or lactating women. Until 1984, most reviews of antimalarials suggested that they were contraindicated in children. In a careful review of the literature, however, Rasmussen [36] pointed out that the risk of chronic toxicity was no greater than for adults. Furthermore, the main concern for children is acute toxicity usually resulting from accidental or intentional overdosage. Recently, Ziering *et al.* [37•] examined this issue further. They pointed out that antimalarials have been used safely and successfully in the treatment of children with LE, juvenile rheumatoid arthritis, dermatomyositis, panniculitis, morphea, and PCT. They concluded that antimalarials could be safely used in children. For young children, the issue of administration may be important. Neither hydroxychloroquine nor chloroquine comes in

Table 2. Potential side effects of antimalarials

Gastrointestinal
  Nausea
  Vomiting
  Diarrhea
Cutaneous
  Pruritus
  Pigmentation
  Bleaching of hair
  Morbilliform drug eruption
  Lichenoid drug eruption
  Exacerbation of psoriasis
Neuromuscular
  Vertigo
  Headache
  Psychosis
  Seizure
  Neuropathy
  Myopathy
Ophthalmologic
  Keratopathy
  Retinopathy
  Neuromuscular toxicity
Hematologic
  Aplastic anemia
  Leukopenia
  Hemolytic anemia
  Agranulocytosis

a syrup. Ziering *et al.* suggested that the capsules can be pulverized, weighed, and put into packets or gelatin capsules containing the desired dosage. The powder can then be mixed with jam, jelly, or applesauce to mask the bitter taste.

Almost all reviews suggest that chloroquine and hydroxychloroquine are contraindicated in pregnancy. However, women of childbearing age may take chloroquine or hydroxychloroquine prior to pregnancy and then become pregnant. In a study of 24 women exposed to hydroxychloroquine or chloroquine during the first trimester of 27 pregnancies, there were no congenital abnormalities observed [38]. The use throughout pregnancy was not recommended by these authors since they believed that deposition in the eyes of the fetus could result in toxicity at a later date. On the other hand, Parke [39•] who followed up into their teenage years some of the infants born to mothers on antimalarials without noting toxicity, recommended that the antimalarial not be discontinued.

The issue of lactation is controversial [39•]. Chloroquine is probably expressed in greater quantities in breast milk than hydroxychloroquine, but the data are scanty. The issue of safety relates to the effects of antimalarials on infants. While in small doses antimalarials are safe in children, it is not clear how large the doses would be in breast milk. Thus, at the current time, either the patient should refrain from breast feeding, or the antimalarial should be discontinued.

References and recommended reading

Papers of particular interest, published within the annual period of review, have been highlighted as:
• Of special interest
•• Of outstanding interest

1. Isaacson D, Elgart M, Turner ML: Antimalarials in Dermatology. *Int J Dermatol* 1982, 21:379–395.
2. Payne JF: A Post-graduate Lecture on Lupus Erythematosus. *Clin J* 1894, 4:223–229.
3. Page F: Treatment of Lupus Erythematosus With Mepacrine. *Lancet* 1951, ii:755–758.
4. Bickers DA, Hazen PG, Lynch WS: Antimalarials. In *Clinical Pharmacology of Skin Disease*. New York: Churchill Livingstone; 1984:189–199.
5. Fox RI, Kang HI: Mechanism of Action of Antimalarial Drugs: Inhibition of Antigen Processing and Presentation. *Lupus* 1993, 2(suppl 1):S9–S12.
These authors review the steps involved in the association of antigenic peptides with major histocompatibility complex–encoded proteins. Antimalarial compounds may act to prevent autoimmunity by stabilizing intracytoplasmic peptides, which normally aggregate, forming α-β complexes that migrate to the cell surface. There is a decreased presentation of autoantigenic peptides by macrophages, which results in a downregulation of autoimmune CD4+ cells and a diminished release of cytokines.
6. Dijkmans BA, deVriese E, deVreede TM, Cats AL: Effects of Antirheumatic Drugs on In Vitro Mitogenic Stimulation of Peripheral Blood Mononuclear Cells. *Transplant Proc* 1988, 20(suppl 2):253–258.
7. Norris DA, Weston WL, Sams WM Jr: The Effect of Immunosuppressive and Anti-inflammatory Drugs on Monocyte Function In Vitro. *J Lab Clin Med* 1977, 90:569–580.
8. Ward PA: The Chemosuppression of Chemotaxis. *J Exp Med* 1964, 7:302–307.
9. London JR: Hydroxychloroquine and Postoperative Thromboembolism After Total Hip Replacement. *Am J Med* 1988, 85(suppl 4A):57–61.
10. Wallace DJ, Linker-Israeli M, Metzger AL, Stecher VS: The Release of Antimalarial Therapy With Regard to Thrombosis, Hypercholesterolemia and Cytokines in SLE. *Lupus* 1993, 2(suppl 1):S13–S15.
These authors analyzed their data on 464 patients with SLE. They found that thromboembolic events were statistically less frequent in patients treated with antimalarials. Further, those with anticardiolipin antibodies who took antimalarials (ie, hydroxychloroquine) had fewer thromboembolic events than those who never took hydroxychloroquine. They also found that treated patients had lower cholesterol, and that after 6 weeks of therapy with 400 mg of hydroxychloroquine, there was a decrease in soluble CD8 levels and interleukin-2 levels.
11. Kraak JH, VaKetel WG Prakken, Van Zwet WR: The Value of Hydroxychloroquine (Plaquenil) for the Treatment of Chronic Discoid Lupus Erythematosus: A Double-Blind Trial. *Dermatologica* 1965, 130:293–305.
12. Callen JP: Chronic Cutaneous Lupus Erythematosus. *Arch Dermatol* 1982, 118:412–416.
13. The Canadian Hydroxychloroquine Study Group: A Randomized Study of the Effect of Withdrawing Hydroxychloroquine Sulfate in Systemic Lupus Erythematosus. *N Engl J Med* 1991, 324:150–154.
14. Wallace DJ, Dubois EL, eds: *Dubois' Lupus Erythematosus*. Philadelphia: Lea & Febiger; Philadelphia, 1987.
15. Lockshin MD: Therapy for Systemic Lupus Erythematosus [Editorial]. *N Engl J Med* 1991, 324:189–191.
16. Esdaile JM: The Efficacy of Antimalarials in Systemic Lupus Erythematosus. *Lupus* 1993, 2(suppl):S3–S8.
17. Cram DL, Epstein JH, Tuffanelli DL: Lupus Erythematosus and Porphyria. *Arch Dermatol* 1973, 108:779–784.
18. Linden IH: Development of Porphyria During Chloroquine Therapy for Chronic Discoid Lupus Erythematosus. *California Med* 1954, 51:235–238.
19. Malkinson FD, Levitt L: Hydroxychloroquine Treatment of Porphyria Cutanea Tarda. *Arch Dermatol* 1980, 116:1147–1150.
20. Petersen CS, Thomsen K: High-Dose Hydroxychloroquine Treatment of Porphyria Cutanea Tarda. *J Am Acad Dermatol* 1992, 26:614–619.
21. Murphy GM, Hawk JLM, Magnus IA: Hydroxychloroquine in Polymorphic Light Eruption: A Controlled Trial With Drug and Visual Sensitivity Monitoring. *Br J Dermatol* 1987, 116:379–386.

22. Woo TY, Callen JP, Voorhees JJ, Bickers DR, Hanno R, Hawkins C: **Cutaneous Lesions of Dermatomyositis Are Improved by Hydroxychloroquine.** *J Am Acad Dermatol* 1984, 10:592–600.

23. James WD, Dawson N, Rodman OG: **The Treatment of Dermatomyositis With Hydroxychloroquine.** *J Rheumatol* 1985, 12:1214–1216.

24. Olson NY, Lindsley CB: **Adjunctive Use of Hydroxychloroquine in Childhood Dermatomyositis.** *J Rheumatol* 1989, 16:1545–1547.

25. Jones EM, Callen JP: **Hydroxychloroquine Is Effective Therapy for Control of Cutaneous Sarcoidal Granulomas.** *J Am Acad Dermatol* 1990, 23:487–490.

26. Eisen D: **Hydroxychloroquine Sulfate (Plaquenil) Improves Oral**
•• **Lichen Planus: An Open Trial.** *J Am Acad Dermatol* 1993, 28:609–612.
Nine of 10 patients with oral lichen planus improved with hydroxychloroquine, 200 to 400 mg/d. Response was observed in 1 to 2 months, but erosive disease took 3 to 6 months to control.

27. Hymes SR, Jordon RE: **Pemphigus Foliaceus: Use of Antimalarial**
• **Agents As Adjuvant Therapy.** *Arch Dermatol* 1992, 128:1462–1464.
These authors used antimalarial therapy in two patients successfully to reduce corticosteroid dosage.

28. Cornbleet T: **Action of Synthetic Antimalarial Drugs on Psoriasis.** *J Invest Dermatol* 1956, 26:435–436.

29. Luzar MJ: **Hydroxychloroquine in Psoriatic Arthropathy: Exacerbations of Psoriatic Skin Lesions.** *J Rheumatol* 1982, 9:462–464.

30. Gray RG: **Hydroxychloroquine Provocation of Psoriasis.** *J Rheumatol* 1985, 12:391.

31. Kammer GM, Soter NA, Gibson DJ, Schur PH: **Psoriatic Arthritis: A Clinical Immunologic and HLA Study of 100 Patients.** *Semin Arthritis Rheum* 1979, 9:75–95.

32. Gladman DD, Blake R, Brubacher B, Farewell VT: **Chloroquine Therapy in Psoriatic Arthritis.** *J Rheumatol* 1992, 19:1724–1726.
•
These authors treated 32 patients with psoriatic arthritis with chloroquine, 250 mg/d. They were compared with 24 age- and sex-matched control subjects with similar psoriasis and arthritis. There was statistically significant benefit from the therapy. Six patients in each group had worsening of their psoriasis

during this 6-month study. Therefore, chloroquine is an effective and reasonably safe agent for psoriatic arthritis.

33. Rynes RI, Bernstein HN: **Ophthalmic Safety Profile of Antimalarial**
• **Drugs.** *Lupus* 1993, 2(suppl 1):S17–S19.
This is an excellent review of the current status of ocular toxicity with chloroquine or hydroxychloroquine.

34. Mazzuca ST, Yung R, Brandt KD, Urowitz MB, Koren G: **Current**
• **Practices for Monitoring Ocular Toxicity Related to Hydroxychloroquine (Plaquenil) Therapy.** *J Rheumatol* 1994, 21:59–63.
These authors surveyed the practice and recommendations of ophthalmologists and rheumatologists. Although the physicians recommended administration every 6 months, when they reviewed the patients seen in their clinic, they found that for seven of 24 cases there were no documented examinations.

35. Finbloom DS, Silver K, Newsome DA, Gunkel R: **Comparison of Hydroxychloroquine and Chloroquine Use and the Development of Retinal Toxicity.** *J Rheumatol* 1985, 12:692–694.

36. Rasmussen JE: **Antimalarials: Are They Safe to Use in Children?** *Pediatr Dermatol* 1985, 1:89–91.

37. Ziering CL, Rabinowitz LG, Esterly NB: **Antimalarials for Children:**
• **Indications, Toxicities and Guidelines.** *J Am Acad Dermatol* 1993, 28:764–770.
This is an excellent review of the current status of antimalarial therapy in children.

38. Levy M, Buskila D, Gladman DD, Urowitz MB, Koren G: **Pregnancy Outcome Following First Trimester Exposure to Chloroquine.** *Am J Perinatol* 1991, 8:174–178.

39. Parke AL: **Antimalarial Drugs, Pregnancy and Lactation.** *J Rheumatol*
• 1993, 2(suppl 1):S21–S23.
This review summarizes the current knowledge of antimalarial use during pregnancy and lactation.

Jeffrey P. Callen, MD, Division of Dermatology, University of Louisville, School of Medicine, Louisville, KY 40292, USA.

Clinical research

Edited by

Mark Pittelkow
Mayo Clinic
Rochester, Minnesota, USA

CURRENT SCIENCE

Analysis, diagnosis, and molecular genetics of keratin disorders

Joseph A. Rothnagel, PhD, and Dennis R. Roop, PhD

Baylor College of Medicine, Houston, Texas, USA

The recent identification of keratin mutations in certain genodermatoses has revealed the extent to which the epidermis depends on an intact intermediate filament cytoskeleton. The number of reported mutations has increased exponentially over the past year, and mutations have now been described in six keratin genes in four distinct epidermal diseases. Molecular genetic diagnosis of these disorders is not yet routine in clinical practice but has already been used for prenatal diagnosis. In addition to improving the differential diagnosis of keratin disorders, these studies have greatly contributed to our understanding of the biology of keratins and the structures they form.

Current Opinion in Dermatology 1995:211–218

Keratinization is the term given to the process of keratinocyte differentiation, which involves the progressive and orderly maturation of the major epidermal cell type from a basal cell with proliferative potential to a lifeless flattened squame of the stratum corneum. During the course of epidermal differentiation, certain genes are activated while others are downregulated, leading to changes not only in the structural proteins, but also in the expression and activation of enzymes involved in posttranslational modifications, metabolic changes, and lipid synthesis. In the normal epidermis, these changes are tightly regulated, with a balance between the processes of proliferation and desquamation resulting in complete renewal of the epidermis every 12 to 14 days [1]. A malfunction in any one of the structural components of enzymatic processes has the potential to cause disease. In the clinical literature, disorders of keratinization are those manifested by an abnormal stratum corneum that is sometimes accompanied by gross morphologic changes. Although there is no universally accepted schema for the classification of these disorders, most generally include the ichthyoses, the follicular keratoses, and the keratodermas. For a complete listing, see the excellent reviews by Griffiths *et al.* [2] and Goldsmith and Thomas [3]. Of these disorders, the causative genetic defect has been identified only in X-linked ichthyosis, epidermolytic hyperkeratosis (EHK), and palmoplantar keratoderma (PPK). The latter of two disorders, together with epidermolysis bullosa simplex (EBS), are examples of keratin disorders, which are the focus of this review.

Keratin expression during differentiation

Keratins are the major gene product of the most abundant cell type of the epidermis, and changes in their expression correlate with changes in the morphology of the keratinocyte, particularly in the early stages of differentiation. It is also readily apparent from recent studies that the integrity of these proteins, and of the filament network that they form, is essential to the function of the keratinocyte and in turn to the vitality of the epidermis. Epidermal keratinocytes express a distinct subset of genes that are characteristic for each stage of differentiation, and these are often referred to as "marker" proteins [1,4,5]. Keratinocytes in the basal cell layer express keratins K5 and K14 as their major products [6,7]. Whereas K5 and K14 gene transcription is tightly restricted to the basal layer, their protein products persist, although in a modified form [8], into the suprabasal layers. In response to as yet unidentified signals, basal layer cells cease their mitotic activity and begin to differentiate. As they do so, they downregulate the genes for K5 and K14 and induce the expression of the differentiation-specific keratins K1 and K10 [9–11]. The expression of these keratins is one of the earliest markers of differentiation and can be observed in the occasional prespinous layer cell prior to its migration away from the basement membrane [12]. In the spinous cell, the K1/K10 filament network eventually replaces the preexisting K5/K14 network to produce a thicker, more dense cytoskeleton. In the late spinous–early granular cell, yet another keratin is expressed, K2e [13]. It is not known if K2 simply replaces

Abbreviations

EBS—epidermolysis bullosa simplex; EHK—epidermolytic hyperkeratosis;
IF—intermediate filament; PPK—palmoplantar keratoderma.

K1 in the K1/K10 network or if it dimerizes with another, as yet undiscovered, type I keratin. As spinous cells mature into granular layer cells, they cease expression of K1 and K10 and induce expression of the late differentiation markers such as filaggrin and loricrin [14,15]. The other major keratins found in the epidermis and its appendages are K6, K16, and K9. The expression of K6 and K16 is normally limited to the outer root sheath of the hair follicle [16] and to the palmar and plantar epidermis [17]. When the epidermis is stressed, however, as occurs in certain skin disorders such as psoriasis, cancer, or wounding, the expression of these keratins is induced in the interfollicular epidermis [18]. The expression of keratin K9 is limited to the suprabasal layers (late spinous and early granular cells) of the palmar and plantar epidermis [19]. The functional significance of the expression of different keratin gene pairs in proliferating, differentiating, and hyperproliferating keratinocytes, as well as in differential expression at different body sites, remains to be elucidated.

Keratin intermediate filaments

Keratins belong to a multigene family of structural proteins called intermediate filaments (IFs), which have been the subject of numerous recent reviews [20,21•–23•]. Two types of keratin subunits have been described based on their physicochemical properties. In general, type I subunits are smaller, with an acidic pI, and include keratins K9 through K21, while type II subunits are larger and more basic and include keratins K1 through K8 [24]. Functional keratin genes have been found clustered with the type I keratins located on chromosome 17 and the type II keratins on chromosome 12 [25]. One feature that distinguishes keratin IFs from the other classes is that they are heterodimeric, and one member of each type is required to form the two-chain coiled coil, which is the basic building block of the filament [26,27]. The coiled coil results from the interaction of the α helical rod domains of neighboring subunits. The α helical structure of the rod domain is conferred by a repeating unit of seven amino acids (a,b,c,d,e,f,g)$_n$, where the "a" and "d" residues are generally apolar and positioned on one face of the helix. The other residues alternate in charge and present a hydrophilic face that is important for higher-order interactions. The hydrophobic interactions between the apolar faces of neighboring subunits drives the self-assembly process and stabilizes the two-chain coiled-coil heterodimer. The α helical rod domain is not continuous and is interrupted by three nonhelical regions that have been described as "linkers" and denoted as L1, L12, and L2. These linker peptides separate the rod domain into four helical segments, termed 1A, 1B, 2A, and 2B [20]. Another discontinuity also occurs within the 2B segment and has been termed the "stutter." The ends of the rod domain are demarcated by a region of highly conserved residues that are relatively invariant in all IF types and have been variously referred to as helix capping or helix initiating-terminating motifs. While the rod domain is a common feature of all IFs,

the flanking nonhelical sequences exhibit wide variations in composition and size. For a given IF type, however, they show remarkable sequence conservation between species, which suggests that they have evolved to mediate specialized functions. A conserved substructure has been observed within these nonhelical domains, which have been denoted as the end (E1, E2), variable (V1, V2), and homologous (H1, H2) domains (Fig. 1) [20].

The first step in the assembly of keratin IF is the formation of the heterodimer, which consists of two keratin subunits aligned in the same orientation and in exact axial register [26,27]. Subsequent steps involve the formation of a tetrameric unit, which polymerizes both laterally and longitudinally to form the mature IF. The orientation and alignment of subunits within the tetramer have not been unequivocally established [22•]. However, Steinert et al. [28••,29••] have proposed four possible modes for the alignment of two heterodimer molecules based on cross-linking experiments. Their data predict several important regions of overlap between neighboring molecules: H1 and the beginning of 1A with the end of 2B and H2; and H1 with L2 and H2 and L2 (Fig. 1). Significantly, mutations have been found within three of these regions (ie, H1, 1A, and 2B) in the keratin genes of EBS, EHK and PPK patients.

Molecular analysis of keratin disorders

In 1991, a number of studies were performed that ultimately resulted in the identification of the first keratin mutations associated with a disease. Ultrastructural analysis of keratinocytes from EBS patients and expression of a mutant K14 gene in transgenic mice suggested the involvement of the basal cell keratins in the etiology of this disease [30,31]. Gene linkage data showed that the disorder mapped to the keratin gene cluster on chromosome 12, and shortly thereafter, mutations were identified in K14 by direct gene sequencing [32,33]. Since these initial studies, there have been many more reports of mutations in both K5 and K14 in EBS patients, amounting to a total of 17 incidences (Fig. 2, bottom).

With the identification of mutations in K5 and K14 in patients with EBS, it became clear that mutations in other keratin genes would be found in patients with related skin diseases. We and others focused on EHK, because ultrastructural studies had shown keratin filament abnormalities together with cell lysis of the suprabasal keratinocytes in these patients [30]. By direct sequencing of the differentiation-specific genes, we identified mutations within the 1A region of K10 and 2B region of K1 [34]. Almost simultaneously, mutations were found by Cheng et al. [35] in K10 and by Chipev et al. [36] within the H1 region of K1. Another 18 incidences of K1 or K10 mutations in EHK patients have since been identified (Fig. 2, bottom). In addition, we have recently identified mutations within the conserved sequence at the end of the 2B region of K2e in patients presenting a variant of EHK, ichthyosis bullosa of Siemens (Rothnagel et al., Unpublished data). These

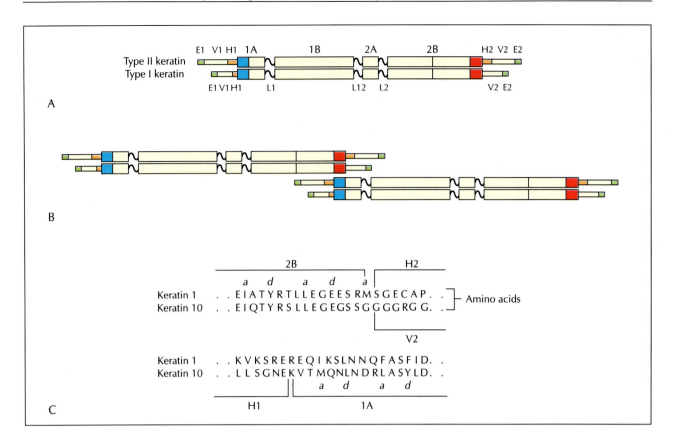

Fig. 1. The alignment of the heterodimer and one of the possible modes of interaction at the four-molecule level of structure. **A,** The heterodimer consists of one type I subunit and one type II subunit aligned in the same orientation and in exact axial register. Each subunit consists of four helical segments (1A, 1B, 2A, 2B) separated by linker peptides (L1, L2, L12). **B,** The A_{CN} mode (*ie,* end-to-end overlap) of alignment between similarly directed molecules. **C,** The predicted overlap defined by the A_{CN} mode of alignment between similarly directed molecules. The letters *a* and *d* refer to the first and forth positions, respectively, of the heptad repeat within the α helical rod domain. E1, E2—end domains; H1, H2—homologous domains; V1, V2—variable domains. (*Adapted from* Steinert *et al.* [29••]; with permission.)

patients show keratin filament clumping and cytolysis typical of EHK but confined to the granular layer [37], consistent with the expression of K2e [13]. Mutations have also been identified within the 1A region of the palmoplantar-specific keratin K9 in patients with PPK [38••,39••], bringing the total number of mutations identified to date in keratin genes to 34 out of 57 separate incidences of disease (Fig. 2, *bottom*).

Except for one report of a 3-bp deletion within the 2B region of K14 [40••], all of the mutations identified to date are due to single base substitutions. As is evident from Figure 2, these mutations are clustered at the end of the rod domains, and even if some degree of ascertainment bias is allowed for, they underscore the lack of tolerance to change in these sequences. The arginine residue at position 10 of the 1A segment of type 1 keratins is the most frequently substituted, with 50% of all reported mutations mapping to this site (Fig. 2, *top*). It has already been noted that this codon (CGC or CGG) is a hot spot for mutation [41••,42••], most likely because of the sensitivity of methylated cytosines to deamination and conversion to thymidine [35]. These studies have also revealed a striking correlation of the site of the mutation with disease severity and the de-

gree of perturbation of the keratin IF (Fig. 2, *bottom*). Generally, mutations within the conserved sequences at the beginning of the 1A segment or at the end of the 2B segment are found in patients with the most severe form of disease, such as Dowling-Meara EBS. In contrast, mutations within the H1 segment of type II keratins (K1, K5) or in the L12 region of both keratin types are associated with the mildest form of disease, such as Weber-Cockayne EBS. It is clear, however, that the type of substitution also contributes to the severity of the phenotype, as is evident from the two mutations identified within the L12 region of K14 (Mutations 8 and 9, Fig. 2, *bottom*) [43••,44••].

Assessment of mutations for causality

How do researchers verify that a mutation is the etiological agent for a given disease? There are a number of "tests" that can be applied, and no one test is unequivocal. The first step is to ascertain whether the mutated residue is invariant in all IF types, invariant in only a subset of them, such as the type I keratins, or invariant in at least the same keratin in all species (*ie,* an

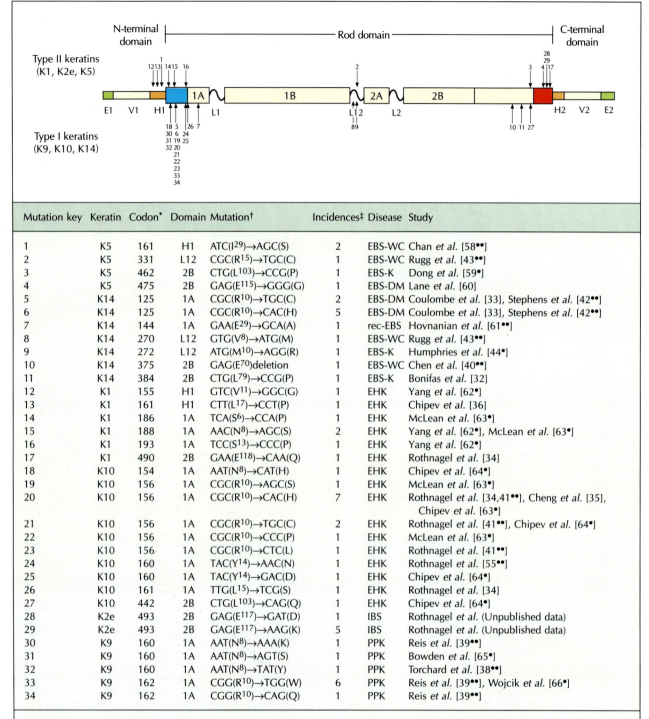

Mutation key	Keratin	Codon*	Domain	Mutation†	Incidences‡	Disease	Study
1	K5	161	H1	ATC(I^{29})→AGC(S)	2	EBS-WC	Chan et al. [58••]
2	K5	331	L12	CGC(R^{15})→TGC(C)	1	EBS-WC	Rugg et al. [43••]
3	K5	462	2B	CTG(L^{103})→CCG(P)	1	EBS-K	Dong et al. [59•]
4	K5	475	2B	GAG(E^{115})→GGG(G)	1	EBS-DM	Lane et al. [60]
5	K14	125	1A	CGC(R^{10})→TGC(C)	2	EBS-DM	Coulombe et al. [33], Stephens et al. [42••]
6	K14	125	1A	CGC(R^{10})→CAC(H)	5	EBS-DM	Coulombe et al. [33], Stephens et al. [42••]
7	K14	144	1A	GAA(E^{29})→GCA(A)	1	rec-EBS	Hovnanian et al. [61••]
8	K14	270	L12	GTG(V^8)→ATG(M)	1	EBS-WC	Rugg et al. [43••]
9	K14	272	L12	ATG(M^{10})→AGG(R)	1	EBS-K	Humphries et al. [44•]
10	K14	375	2B	GAG(E^{70})deletion	1	EBS-WC	Chen et al. [40••]
11	K14	384	2B	CTG(L^{79})→CCG(P)	1	EBS-K	Bonifas et al. [32]
12	K1	155	H1	GTC(V^{11})→GGC(G)	1	EHK	Yang et al. [62•]
13	K1	161	H1	CTT(L^{17})→CCT(P)	1	EHK	Chipev et al. [36]
14	K1	186	1A	TCA(S^6)→CCA(P)	1	EHK	McLean et al. [63•]
15	K1	188	1A	AAC(N^8)→AGC(S)	2	EHK	Yang et al. [62•], McLean et al. [63•]
16	K1	193	1A	TCC(S^{13})→CCC(P)	1	EHK	Yang et al. [62•]
17	K1	490	2B	GAA(E^{118})→CAA(Q)	1	EHK	Rothnagel et al. [34]
18	K10	154	1A	AAT(N^8)→CAT(H)	1	EHK	Chipev et al. [64•]
19	K10	156	1A	CGC(R^{10})→AGC(S)	1	EHK	McLean et al. [63•]
20	K10	156	1A	CGC(R^{10})→CAC(H)	7	EHK	Rothnagel et al. [34,41••], Cheng et al. [35], Chipev et al. [63•]
21	K10	156	1A	CGC(R^{10})→TGC(C)	2	EHK	Rothnagel et al. [41••], Chipev et al. [64•]
22	K10	156	1A	CGC(R^{10})→CCC(P)	1	EHK	McLean et al. [63•]
23	K10	156	1A	CGC(R^{10})→CTC(L)	1	EHK	Rothnagel et al. [41••]
24	K10	160	1A	TAC(Y^{14})→AAC(N)	1	EHK	Rothnagel et al. [55••]
25	K10	160	1A	TAC(Y^{14})→GAC(D)	1	EHK	Chipev et al. [64•]
26	K10	161	1A	TTG(L^{15})→TCG(S)	1	EHK	Rothnagel et al. [34]
27	K10	442	2B	CTG(L^{103})→CAG(Q)	1	EHK	Chipev et al. [64•]
28	K2e	493	2B	GAG(E^{117})→GAT(D)	1	IBS	Rothnagel et al. (Unpublished data)
29	K2e	493	2B	GAG(E^{117})→AAG(K)	5	IBS	Rothnagel et al. (Unpublished data)
30	K9	160	1A	AAT(N^8)→AAA(K)	1	PPK	Reis et al. [39••]
31	K9	160	1A	AAT(N^8)→AGT(S)	1	PPK	Bowden et al. [65•]
32	K9	160	1A	AAT(N^8)→TAT(Y)	1	PPK	Torchard et al. [38••]
33	K9	162	1A	CGG(R^{10})→TGG(W)	6	PPK	Reis et al. [39••], Wojcik et al. [66•]
34	K9	162	1A	CGG(R^{10})→CAG(Q)	1	PPK	Reis et al. [39••]

*Numbered from from the ATG codon using the published sequences for K1 (Johnson et al. [67]), K2e (Collin et al. [13]), K5 (Eckert and Rorke [68]), K9 (Langbein et al. [19]), K10 (Rieger and Franke [69]), and K14 (Marchuk et al. [70]).
†The position of the residue within each respective domain is indicated.
‡Number of unrelated incidences.
DM—Dowling-Meara; EBS—epidermolysis bullosa simplex; EHK—epidermolytic hyperkeratosis; IBS—ichthyosis bullosa of Siemens; K—Koebner; PPK—palmoplantar keratoderma; rec—recessive; WC—Weber-Cockayne.

Fig. 2. Top, The distribution of mutations along a keratin chain. Mutations in the type I keratins (K9, K10, K14) are shown below the diagram, and mutations in the type II keratins (K1, K2e, K5) are shown above. The helix initiation and termination motifs are denoted by the *blue box* and the *red box*, respectively. The *numbers* refer to the *mutation key*. Bottom, Catalogue of gene mutations, including *mutation key* for diagram. 1A, 1B, 2A, 2B—helical segments of rod domain; E1, E2—end domains; H1, H2—homologous domains; L1, L2, L12—linker peptides; V1, V2—variable domains.

interspecies comparison). Finally, it is necessary to ascertain whether this residue is invariant in the human population. A survey of the recent literature shows that most researchers are willing to exclude the possibility of benign polymorphic variation if 100 normal individuals have the identical sequence at this position. Although sequence comparison analysis can indicate the likelihood of a given mutation causing a phenotype, it is not definitive. Its biggest shortcoming is in predicting the effect of conservative substitutions. Therefore, it is often necessary to confirm the effect of a mutation with a functional assay. Four assays have been used to date: 1) peptide disassembly assay, 2) expression of mutant keratins in cultured cells, 3) expression of mutant keratins in bacteria and assessment of their assembly *in vitro*, and 4) expression of mutant keratins in transgenic mice.

The peptide disassembly assay is based on the observation that synthetic peptides encoding certain IF sequences are able to interact with wild-type IF subunits and compete with them in the assembly process. Because filaments are dynamic structures, these peptides are able to disassemble preformed filaments in an *in vitro* assay, and the extent of filament unraveling can be visualized by electron microscopy [36,45] or quantitated by measuring the reduction in light scattering due to changes in filament length [36,46•]. Peptides that bear mutations have a reduced capacity for disassembling preformed filaments, presumably due to an impaired ability to interact with specific IF sequences. The peptide disassembly assay was used by Hatzfeld and Weber [45] to define the role or critical amino acids at the end of the 2B domain in keratin filament assembly, and later by Steinert *et al.* [28••,29••] to ascertain the function of the various keratin filament domains. These researchers have also adopted this assay to extrapolate the effect of mutations on filament assembly *in vivo* [36,46•]. The assay is limited, however, to those regions on a keratin molecule that are capable of interacting with neighboring molecules and are thought to involve the principal overlap regions of keratin type I and type II subunits, namely the H1 and 1A domains and the end of the 2B segment. Mutations that lie in more internal regions of the rod domain can not be assessed by this methodology [46•]. Secondly, the technique depends on the solubility of the synthetic peptide, and some sequences such as the H2 domain of the K1 keratin may be excluded on this basis [36]. The researcher should also be aware of nonspecific effects caused by molar excess of synthetic peptides on IF integrity and control for them accordingly.

The expression of mutant proteins in transfected cultured keratinocytes has also been used to assess the contribution of mutation to a phenotype. Earlier studies have shown that truncated keratins, expressed in cultured cells, even in small amounts, can cause dominant phenotypic changes and perturb the cytoskeletal architecture [47,48]. Once the mutation has been introduced into the complementary DNA of interest, the mutant construct is inserted into a mammalian expression vector, and transfected into a keratinocyte cell line.

Transfected cells are later analyzed for perturbation of their IF cytoskeleton by fluorescent microscopy. It has been suggested that because keratinocytes in culture express large amounts of the hyperproliferative keratins, the K6/K16 filament network may support the cell and ameliorate the effects of any introduced mutant keratins, so that a weakened or compromised IF network may not be readily apparent [36]. It has also been noted that cells in culture lack the stresses and strains that impinge on cells in, for example, the epidermis of the palms or soles. Nevertheless, this assay has been successfully used to analyze point mutations in K5 and K14 [33,49,50]. However, we and others [35] have been unable to use the assay reliably for the suprabasal keratins. In fact, in our hands, transfection of SV40-driven wild-type K1 and K10 constructs into murine keratinocytes resulted in filament network abnormalities [51]. One way to overcome these limitations is to produce the mutant keratin in a bacterial-bacculovirus expression system and to assess its effect on filament assembly and structure *in vitro* [49,50]. These effects are often subtle, however, requiring the use of ultrastructural techniques for their observation [49,50]. The interpretation of these data can be difficult, and consideration should be given to analyzing mutant filaments using biophysical methods [52].

Finally, the expression of the mutant gene in transgenic animals offers the prospect of investigating the contribution of a particular mutation to a given phenotype in the context of the entire organism. This method has been successfully used to generate mice exhibiting an EBS-like phenotype due to the expression of a truncated K14 protein [31] and a EHK-like phenotype due to the expression of K10 [53] and K1 [54] mutant constructs. However, attempts to produce mice expressing keratin genes with point mutations has so far failed to generate a phenotype. We speculate that hair follicles may support the surrounding epidermis, as well as protect the epidermal cells from incidental trauma, thus preventing cell lysis and blister formation and other secondary events in these animals. It may be that the introduction of mutant keratin constructs into the germline of "hairless" mice will create models more representative of the human disease. We are currently introducing these point mutations directly into the endogenous genes, using homologous recombination technology, so that the mutant protein can achieve a higher relative concentration over the wild-type proteins within these cells and thereby produce a phenotype more readily.

Prospects

The availability of keratin gene sequences together with an ever-increasing catalogue of inconsequential polymorphisms and disease associated mutations has made it practical to diagnose keratin disorders at the genetic level. The application of this technology for the prenatal diagnosis of EHK using chorionic villus samples has already been demonstrated [55••]. Rapid polymerase chain reaction–based protocols can now be used to screen *in vitro* fertilized embryos from affected couples for keratin mutations prior to implantation [56], thus eliminating the need for risky diagnostic procedures later in pregnancy.

In the immediate term the application of these technologies is limited to improved diagnosis, but in the future these studies will likely lead to improved therapeutic approaches. Gene therapy has been widely touted as an attractive approach for the amelioration of skin diseases, because the epidermis is readily accessible, and many of the adjunct techniques, such as cell culture and grafting, are well established [57]. Because most keratin mutations are dominant, it is necessary only to abrogate or diminish the expression of the mutant allele. This might be achieved through the use of ribozymes or other antisense technologies that specifically target the mutant RNA transcript. It may also be possible to modulate pharmacologically the expression of the mutant gene together with the upregulation of another keratin gene. Progress in this area awaits an improvement of our understanding on the regulation of individual keratin genes.

Conclusions

Considerable progress has been made in identifying mutations and inconsequential polymorphisms occurring in keratins K1, K2e, K5, K9, K10, and K14. The data have already identified codons (residues) that are prone to mutation and likely to cause disease. Moreover, it is apparent that mutations that occur within the highly conserved sequences at the end of the rod domain are more likely to be deleterious in terms of filament disruption and phenotype severity than those occurring at other sites within the rod domain, which in turn are more deleterious than those occurring with the H1 region. It is clear, however, that the type of mutation also influences the severity of the phenotype, and the acquisition of more data will enhance our understanding on the impact of individual mutations on IF assembly and function. Furthermore, an expanded data base will allow diagnoses based on mutational data to be made with greater confidence.

Future endeavors will likely be directed towards the search for causative mutations in other epidermal keratins, notably K6, K16 and K17. It has already been noted that in about one third of EBS and EHK patients, a mutation has not been identified in the respective basal cell or differentiation-specific keratins, suggesting the possibility of mutations in other keratins (some yet to be discovered), or perhaps in regions outside of the rod and H1 domains, such as the end domains. Another possibility is that proteins that associate or otherwise interact directly with keratin filaments may bear mutations that could impair these alliances and thereby perturb keratin filament function. Potential candidates from this group of proteins include the classic IF-associated proteins, proteins of the desmosome complex, proteins of the nuclear lamina, and modifying enzymes such as kinases, phosphatases, and glycosylases. Given the intensity of research in this area, the identification

of disease causing mutations in these proteins cannot be far off.

Acknowledgments

We thank J. Laminack for the preparation of this manuscript. Dr. Rothnagel is the recipient of the Dermatology Foundation Career Development Award. Studies summarized from our laboratory were supported by National Institutes of Health grant HD25479.

References and recommended reading

Papers of particular interest, published within the annual period of review, have been highlighted as:
- • Of special interest
- •• Of outstanding interest

1. Eckert RL: Structure, Function and Differentiation of the Keratinocyte. *Physiol Rev* 1989, 69:1316–1346.

2. Griffiths WAD, Leigh IM, Marks R: Disorders of Keratinization. In *Textbook of Dermatology*. Edited by Champion RH, Burton JL, Ebling FJG. Oxford: Blackwell Scientific Publications; 1992:1325–1390.

3. Goldsmith LA, Thomas NE: Disorders of Cornification. In *Dermatology*. Edited by Moschella SL, Hurley HJ. Philadelphia: WB Saunders Co.; 1992:1383–1417.

4. Roop DR, Nakazawa H, Mehrel T, Chen C, Chung R, Rothnagel JA, Steinert PM, Yuspa SH, Roop DR: Sequential Changes in Gene Expression During Epidermal Differentiation. In *The Biology of Wool and Hair*. Edited by Rogers GE, Reis PJ, Ward KA, Marshall RC. New York: Chapman and Hall; 1988:311–324.

5. Fuchs E: Epidermal Differentiation: The Bare Essentials. *J Cell Biol* 1990, 111:2807–2814.

6. Fuchs E, Green H: Changes in Keratin Gene Expression During Terminal Differentiation of the Keratinocyte. *Cell* 1980, 19:1033–1042.

7. Woodcock-Mitchell JR, Eichner R, Nelson WG, Sun T-T: Immunolocalization of Keratin Polypeptides in Human Epidermis Using Monoclonal Antibodies. *J Cell Biol* 1982, 95:580–588.

8. Bowden PE, Stark HJ, Breitkreutz D, Fusenig NE: Expression and Modification of Keratins During Terminal Differentiation of Mammalian Epidermis. *Curr Top Dev Biol* 1987, 22:35–68.

9. Roop DR, Hawley-Nelson P, Cheng CK, Yuspa SH: Keratin Gene Expression in Mouse Epidermis and Cultured Epidermal Cells. *Proc Natl Acad Sci U S A* 1983, 80:716–720.

10. Schweizer J, Kinjo M, Furstenberger G, Winter H: Sequential Expression of mRNA Encoded Keratin Sets in Neonatal Mouse Epidermis: Basal Cells With Properties of Terminally Differentiating Cells. *Cell* 1984, 37:159–170.

11. Regnier M, Vaigot P, Darmon M, Prunieras M: Onset of Epidermal Differentiation in Rapidly Proliferating Basal Keratinocytes. *J Invest Dermatol* 1986, 87:472–476.

12. Huitfeld HS, Heyden A, Clausen OPF, Vibeke-Thrane E, Roop DR, Yuspa SH: Altered Regulation of Growth and Expression of Differentiation-Associated Keratins in Benign Mouse Skin Tumors. *Carcinogenesis* 1991, 12:2063–2067.

13. Collin C, Moll R, Kubicka S, Ouhayoun JP, Franke WW: Characterization of Human Cytokeratin 2, an Epidermal Cytoskeletal Protein Synthesized Late During Differentiation. *Exp Cell Res* 1992, 202:132–141.

14. Rothnagel JR, Mehrel T, Idler WW, Roop DR, Steinert PM: The Gene for Mouse Epidermal Filaggrin Precursor: Its Potential Characterization, Expression, and Sequence of a Repeating Unit. *J Biol Chem* 1987, 262:15643–15648.

15. Mehrel T, Hohl D, Rothnagel JA, Longley MA, Bundman DS, Cheng C, Lichti U, Bisher ME, Steven AC, Steinert PM, Yuspa SH, Roop DR: Identification of a Major Keratinocyte Cell Envelope Protein, Loricrin. *Cell* 1990, 61:1103–1112.

16. Stark H-J, Breitkreutz D, Limat A, Bowden P, Fusenig NE: Keratins of the Human Hair Follicle: "Hyperproliferative" Keratins Consistently Expressed in Outer Root Sheath Cells *In Vivo* and *In Vitro*. *Differentiation* 1987, 35:236–248.

17. Quinlan RA, Schiller DL, Hatzfeld M, Achstätter T, Moll R, Jorcano JL, Magin TM, Franke WW: Patterns of Expression and Organization

of Cytokeratin Intermediate Filaments. *Ann N Y Acad Sci* 1985, 455:282–306.

18. Weiss RA, Eichner R, Sun T-T: **Monoclonal Antibody Analysis of Keratin Expression in Epidermal Diseases: A 48- and 56-KDalton Keratin as Molecular Markers for Hyperproliferative Keratinocytes.** *J Cell Biol* 1984, 98:1397–1406.

19. Langbein L, Heid HW, Moll I, Franke WW: **Molecular Characterization of the Body Site-Specific Human Epidermal Cytokeratin 9: cDNA Cloning, Amino Acid Sequence, and Tissue Specificity of Gene Expression.** *Differentiation.* 1993, 55:57–71.

20. Steinert PM, Roop DR: **Molecular and Cellular Biology of Intermediate Filaments.** *Annu Rev Biochem* 1988, 57:593–625.

21. Coulombe PA: **The Cellular and Molecular Biology of Keratins: Be-**
• **ginning of a New Era.** *Curr Opin Cell Biol* 1993, 5:17–29.
A comprehensive, well-balanced review on keratin filament function and biology.

22. Stewart M: **Intermediate Filament Structure and Assembly.** *Curr Opin*
• *Cell Biol* 1993, 5:3–11.
A comprehensive review on the structure and assembly of IFs.

23. Steinert PM: **Structure, Function, and Dynamics of Keratin Interme-**
• **diate Filaments.** *J Invest Dermatol* 1993, 100:729–734.
Reviews the recent progress made in keratin IF biology and model building.

24. Moll R, Franke WW, Schiller D, Geiger B, Krepler R: **The Catalog of Human Cytokeratins: Patterns of Expression in Normal Epithelia, Tumors and Cultured Cells.** *Cell* 1982, 31:11–24.

25. Epstein EH: **Molecular Genetics of Epidermolysis Bullosa.** *Science* 1992, 256:799–804.

26. Hatzfeld M, Weber K: **The Coiled-Coil of *In Vitro* Assembled Keratin Filaments Is a Heterodimer of Type I and Type II Keratins: Use of Site-Specific Mutagenesis and Recombinant Protein Expression.** *J Cell Biol* 1990, 110:1199–1210.

27. Steinert PM: **The Two-Chain Coiled-Coil Molecule of Native Epidermal Keratin Intermediate Filaments Is a Type I-Type II Heterodimer.** *J Biol Chem* 1990, 265:8766–8774.

28. Steinert PM, Parry DAD: **The Conserved H1 Domain of the Type II**
•• **Keratin 1 Chain Plays an Essential Role in the Alignment of Nearest Neighbor Molecules in Mouse and Human Keratin 1/Keratin 10 Intermediate Filaments at the Two-to-Four-Molecule Level of Structure.** *J Biol Chem* 1993, 268:2878–2887.
This study predicts a critical role for the H1 domain in filament assembly. See Steinert *et al.* (*J Mol Biol* 1993, 230:436–452).

29. Steinert PM, Marekov LN, Fraser RDB, Parry DAD: **Keratin Inter-**
•• **mediate Filament Structure: Crosslinking Studies Yield Quantitative Information on Molecular Dimensions and Mechanism of Assembly.** *J Mol Biol* 1993, 230:436–452.
The contribution of the various subdomains of the keratin subunit to filament structure and assembly was investigated by the combined analysis of inter-chain cross-linked amino acids between neighboring molecules and by the addition of defined synthetic peptides in an *in vitro* assembly assay. These studies predict a number of regions likely to produce filament perturbation due to mutation.

30. Anton-Lamprecht I: **Genetically Induced Abnormalities of Epidermal Differentiation and Ultrastructure in Ichthyoses and Epidermolysis: Pathogenesis, Heterogeneity, Fetal Manifestation, and Prenatal Diagnosis.** *J Invest Dermatol* 1983, 81:149s–156s.

31. Vassar R, Coulombe PA, Degenstein L, Albers K, Fuchs E: **Mutant Keratin Expression in Transgenic Mice Causes Marked Abnormalities Resembling a Human Genetic Skin Disease.** *Cell* 1991, 64:365–380.

32. Bonifas JM, Rothman AL, Epstein EH: **Epidermolysis Bullosa Simplex: Evidence in Two Families for Keratin Gene Abnormalities.** *Science* 1991, 254:1202–1205.

33. Coulombe PA, Hutton ME, Letai A, Hebert A, Paller A, Fuchs E: **Point Mutations in Human Keratin 14 Genes of Epidermolysis Bullosa Simplex Patients: Genetic and Functional Analysis.** *Cell* 1991, 66:1301–1311.

34. Rothnagel JA, Dominey AM, Dempsey LD, Longley MA, Greenhalgh DA, Gagne TA, Huber M, Frenk E, Hohl D, Roop DR: **Mutations in the Rod Domains of Keratins 1 and 10 in Epidermolytic Hyperkeratosis.** *Science* 1992, 257:1128–1130.

35. Cheng J, Syder AJ, Yu Q-C, Letai A, Paller AS, Fuchs E: **The Genetic Basis of Epidermolytic Hyperkeratosis: A Disorder of Differentiation-Specific Epidermal Keratin Genes.** *Cell* 1992, 70:811–819.

36. Chipev CC, Korge BP, Markova N, Bale SJ, DiGiovanna JJ, Compton JG, Steinert PM: **A Leucine→Proline Mutation in the H1 Subdomain of Keratin 1 Causes Epidermolytic Hyperkeratosis.** *Cell* 1992, 70:821–828.

37. Traupe H, Kolde G, Hamm H, Happle R: **Ichthyosis Bullosa of Siemens: A Unique Type of Epidermolytic Hyperkeratosis.** *J Am Acad Dermatol* 1986, 14:1000–1005.

38. Torchard T, Blanchet-Bardon C, Serova O, Langbein L, Narod S,
•• Janin N, Goguel AF, Bernheim A, Franke WW, Lenoir GM, Feunteun J: **Epidermolytic Palmoplantar Keratoderma Cosegregates With a Keratin 9 Mutation in a Pedigree With Breast and Ovarian Cancer.** *Nature Genet* 1994, 6:106–110.
This study documents an asparagine (N[8]) to tyrosine substitution within the 1A region of K9. See Reis *et al.* (*Nature Genet* 1994, 6:174–179).

39. Reis A, Hennies HC, Langbein L, Digweed M, Mischke D, Drech-
•• sler M, Schröck E, Royer-Pokora B, Franke WW, Sperling K, Küster W: **Keratin 9 Gene Mutations in Epidermolytic Palmoplantar Keratoderma (EPK).** *Nature Genet* 1994, 6:174–179.
This is the first report, together with that of Torchard *et al.* (*Nature Genet* 1994, 6:106–110) of mutations within the palmar-plantar–specific keratin K9. It is noteworthy that substitution of the arginine residue (R[10]) within the 1A region was the most prevalent mutation found, as was the case for the other type I keratins, K10 and K14. See Rothnagel *et al.* (*Hum Mol Genet* 1993, 2:2147–2150) and Stephens *et al.* (*J Invest Dermatol* 1993, 101:240–243).

40. Chen MA, Bonifas JM, Matsumura K, Blumenfeld A, Epstein EH: **A**
•• **Novel Three-Nucleotide Deletion in the Helix 2B Region of Keratin 14 in Epidermolysis Bullosa Simplex ΔE375.** *Hum Mol Genet* 1993, 2:1971–1972.
This study is the first report of a deletion mutation within the rod domain of a keratin gene. Surprisingly, this mutation was found in a patient with the mildest form of the disease.

41. Rothnagel JA, Fisher MP, Axtell SM, Pittelkow MR, Anton-Lamprecht
•• I, Huber M, Hohl D, Roop DR: **A Mutational Hot Spot in Keratin 10 (KRT10) in Patients With Epidermolytic Hyperkeratosis.** *Hum Mol Genet* 1993, 2:2147–2150.
This study documents four new incidences of mutation at the arginine residue (R[10]) of the 1A domain of K10. Genetic analysis of these patients and other reported incidences of mutation at this position suggests that the R[10] codon is a mutational hot spot and that the prevalence of R[10] mutations is not due to founder effects or ascertainment bias.

42. Stephens K, Sybert VP, Wijsman EM, Ehrlich P, Spencer A: **A Ker-**
•• **atin 14 Mutational Hot Spot for Epidermolysis Bullosa Simplex, Dowling-Meara: Implications for Diagnosis.** *J Invest Dermatol* 1993, 101:240–243.
This study documents the prevalence of mutations at the arginine residue (R[10]) within the 1A segment of K14. Mutations at this position account for 50% of all mutations identified to date.

43. Rugg EL, Morley SM, Smith FJD, Boxer M, Tidman MJ, Navsaria H,
•• Leigh IM, Lane EB: **Missing Links: Weber-Cockayne Keratin Mutations Implicate the L12 Linker Domain in Effective Cytoskeletal Function.** *Nature Genetics* 1993, 5:294–300.
This study defines the genetic basis of Weber-Cockayne EBS. See Chen *et al.* (*Hum Mol Genet* 1993, 2:1971–1972) and Chan *et al.* (*Proc Natl Acad Sci U S A* 1993, 90:7414–7418).

44. Humphries MM, Sheils DM, Farrar GJ, Kumar-Singh R, Kenna PF,
• Mansergh FC, Jordon SA, Young M, Humphries P: **A Mutation (Met → Arg) in the Type I Keratin (K14) Gene Responsible for Autosomal Dominant Epidermolysis Bullosa Simplex.** *Hum Mutat* 1993, 2:37–42.
This is the first report of a disease-associated mutation within the L12 region of a keratin rod domain.

45. Hatzfeld M, Weber K: **A Synthetic Peptide Representing the Consensus Sequence Motif at the Carboxy-Terminal End of the Rod Domain Inhibits Intermediate Filament Assembly and Disassembles Preformed Filaments.** *J Cell Biol* 1992, 116:840–848.

46. Steinert PM, Yang J-M, Bale SJ, Comptom JG: **Concurrence Between**
• **the Molecular Overlap Regions in Keratin Intermediate Filaments and the Locations of Keratin Mutations in Genodermatosis.** *Biochem Biophys Res Commun* 1993, 197:840–848.
A comprehensive *in vitro* analysis of keratin mutations reported in EBS and EHK patients using the peptide disassembly assay. The authors were able to confirm that most of the reported mutations affect filament assembly. An important exception was the E[118] → Q mutation found in the 2B region of K1 (Mutation 17, Fig. 2, *bottom*).

47. Albers K, Fuchs E: **Expression of Mutant Keratin cDNAs in Epithelia Cells Reveal Possible Mechanisms for Initiation and Assembly of Intermediate Filaments.** *J Cell Biol* 1989, 108:1477–1493.

48. Lu X, Lane EB: **Retrovirus-Mediated Transgenic Keratin Expression in Cultured Fibroblasts: Specific Domain Functions in Keratin Stabilization and Filament Formation.** *Cell* 1990, 62:681–696.

49. Letai A, Coulombe PA, Fuchs E: **Do the Ends Justify the Mean? Proline Mutations at the Ends of the Keratin Coiled-Coil Rod Segment Are More Disruptive Than Internal Mutations.** *J Cell Biol* 1992, 116:1181–1195.

50. Letai A, Coulombe PA, McCormick MB, Yu Q-C, Hutton E, Fuchs E: **Disease Severity Correlates With Position of Keratin Point Mutations in Patients With Epidermolysis Bullosa Simplex.** *Proc Natl Acad Sci U S A* 1993, 90:3197–3201.

51. Kartosova T, Roop DR, Holbrook KA, Yuspa SH: **Mouse Differentiation Keratins 1 and 10 Require a Pre-existing Keratin Scaffold to Form a Filament Network.** *J Cell Biol* 1993, 120:1251–1261.

52. Janmey PA, Euteneuer U, Traub P, Schliwa M: **Viscoelastic Properties of Vimentin Compared With Other Filamentous Biopolymer Networks.** *J Cell Biol* 1991, 113:155–160.

53. Fuchs E, Esteves RA, Coulombe PA: **Transgenic Mice Expressing a Mutant Keratin 10 Gene Reveal the Likely Genetic Basis for Epidermolytic Hyperkeratosis.** *Proc Natl Acad Sci U S A* 1992, 89:6906–6910.

54. Rothnagel JA, Greenhalgh DA, Wang X-J, Sellheyer K, Bickenbach JR, Dominey AR, Roop DR: **Transgenic Models of Skin Disease.** *Arch Dermatol* 1993, 129:1430–1436.

55. Rothnagel JA, Longley MA, Holder RA, Küster W, Roop DR: **Prenatal
•• Diagnosis of Epidermolytic Hyperkeratosis by Direct Gene Sequencing.** *J Invest Dermatol* 1994, 102:13–16.
This study is the first report of a prenatal diagnosis by the direct gene sequencing of a keratin disorder.

56. Handyside AH, Lesko JG, Tavin JJ, Winston RM, Hughes MR: **Birth of a Normal Girl After *In Vitro* Fertilization and Preimplantation Diagnostic Testing for Cystic Fibrosis.** *N Engl J Med* 1992, 327:905–909.

57. Greenhalgh DA, Rothnagel JA, Roop DR: **The Epidermis: An Attractive Target Issue for Gene Therapy.** *J Invest Dermatol* 1994, in press.

58. Chan Y-M, Yu Q-C, Fine J-D, Fuchs E: **The Genetic Basis of Weber-
•• Cockayne Epidermolysis Bullosa Simplex.** *Proc Natl Acad Sci U S A* 1993, 90:7414–7418.
This study defines the genetic basis of Weber-Cockayne EBS. See also Chen *et al.* (*Hum Mol Genet* 1993, 2:1971–1972) and Rugg *et al.* (*Nature Genetics* 1993, 5:294–300).

59. Dong W, Ryynänen M, Uitto J: **Identification of a Leucine-to-Pro-
• line Mutation in the Keratin 5 Gene in a Family With Generalized Köber Type of Epidermolysis Bullosa Simplex.** *Human Mutation* 1993, 2:94–102.
This study reports of a mutation of leucine residue (L[103]) at the end of the 2B domain of K5.

60. Lane EB, Rugg EL, Navsaria H, Leigh IM, Heagerty AHM, Ishida-Yamamoto A, Eady RAJ: **A Mutation in the Conserved Helix Termination Peptide of Keratin 5 in Hereditary Skin Blistering.** *Nature* 1992, 356:244–246.

61. Hovnanian A, Pollock E, Hilal L, Rochat A, Prost C, Barrandon Y,
•• Goossens M: **Missense Mutation in the Rod Domain of Keratin 14 Associated With Recessive Epidermolysis Bullosa Simplex.** *Nature Genetics* 1993, 3:327–332.

This study is the first report of a recessive mutation in a keratin gene.

62. Yang J-M, Chipev CC, DiGiovanna JJ, Bale SJ, Marekov LN, Steinert
• PM, Compton JG: **Mutations in the H1 and 1A Domains in the Keratin 1 Gene in Epidermolytic Hyperkeratosis.** *J Invest Dermatol* 1994, 102:17–23.
This study documents mutations of the K1 gene in three separate incidences of EHK.

63. McLean WHI, Eady RAJ, Dopping-Hepenstal PJC, McMillan JR, Leigh
• IM, Navsaria HA, Higgins C, Harper JI, Paige DG, Morley SM, Lane EB: **Mutations in the Rod 1A Domain of Keratins 1 and 10 in Bullous Congenital Ichthyosiform Erythroderma (BCIE).** *J Invest Dermatol* 1994, 102:24–30.
This study identifies mutations in the differentiation-specific keratins in four incidences of EHK.

64. Chipev CC, Yang J-M, DiGiovanna JJ, Steinert PM, Marekov L, Comp-
• ton JG, Bale SJ: **Preferential Sites in Keratin 10 That Are Mutated in Epidermolytic Hyperkeratosis.** *Am J Hum Genet* 1994, 54:179–190.
This study documents mutations of the K10 gene in six separate incidences of disease.

65. Bowden PE, Watts CE, Marks R: **Mutation of Human Keratin 9 (HK9)
• Gene in Epidermolytic Tylosis.** *J Invest Dermatol* 1994, 102:576.
This study reports on an asparagine (N[8]) to serine substitution within the 1A region of K9.

66. Wojcik S, Rothnagel JA, Hohl D, Roop DR: **Mutation of a Critical
• Arginine Residue Within the 1A Segment of Keratin 9 in Epidermolytic Palmoplantar Keratoderma.** *J Invest Dermatol* 1994, 102:541.
This study documents an arginine (R[10]) to tryptophan substitution in K9.

67. Johnson LD, Idler WW, Zhou X-M, Roop DR, Steinert PM: **Structure of a Gene for the Human Epidermal Keratin of 67,000 Da.** *Proc Natl Acad Sci U S A* 1985, 82:1896–1900.

68. Eckert RL, Rorke EA: **The Sequence of the Human Epidermal 58-kD (#5) Type II Keratin Reveals an Absence of 5' Upstream Sequence Conservation Between Coexpressed Epidermal Keratins.** *DNA* 1988, 7:337–345.

69. Rieger M, Franke WW: **Identification of an Orthologous Mammalian Cytokeratin Gene.** *J Mol Biol* 1988, 204:841–856.

70. Marchuk D, McCrohon S, Fuchs E: **Complete Sequence of a Gene Encoding a Human Type 1 Keratin: Sequences Homologous to Enhancer Elements in the Regulatory Region of the Gene.** *Proc Natl Acad Sci U S A* 1985, 82:1609–1613.

Joseph A. Rothnagel, PhD, and Dennis R. Roop, PhD, Departments of Cell Biology and Dermatology, Baylor College of Medicine, One Baylor Plaza, Houston, TX 77030, USA.

The molecular genetics of erythropoietic protoporphyria

Robert P. E. Sarkany, MBBS, MRCP

University of Cambridge, Cambridge, UK

Erythropoietic protoporphyria is an inherited disorder of heme biosynthesis characterized by lifelong photosensitivity and occasionally by severe liver disease. The gene responsible for this disorder has been characterized, and molecular analysis of the ferrochelatase gene has now identified a number of mutations causing the disease. Investigations into the molecular genetics of erythropoietic protoporphyria promise insights into its mode of inheritance, which should ultimately improve genetic counseling. Advances in the understanding of the potentially fatal hepatic complications of the disease could make it possible to identify which patients are at risk, so that preventive measures could be taken. For the future, gene therapy offers the hope of definitive treatment for this disabling and occasionally fatal condition.

Current Opinion in Dermatology 1995:219–224

On October 14, 1912, Dr. Friedrich Meyer-Betz [1], senior physician at one of the major hospitals in Königsberg, injected himself with 200 mg of hematoporphyrin and documented his severe photosensitive skin reaction over the following weeks (Fig. 1). Since then, no one has doubted that porphyrins cause photosensitivity. In erythropoietic protoporphyria (EPP), the porphyrin causing sensitivity to long-wavelength ultraviolet light is protoporphyrin [2], the last intermediate in the biosynthesis of heme. When photoactivated in the skin, it probably causes a reaction by damaging endothelial cells, activating the complement cascade, and causing mast cell degranulation [3]. In EPP, protoporphyrin accumulates because of an inherited deficiency of ferrochelatase [4]. This enzyme is embedded in the inner membrane of the mitochondrion [5] and catalyzes the insertion of ferrous iron into the protoporphyrin molecule to form heme. Because most heme is synthesized for hemoglobin formation, the erythroid cells of the bone marrow are the main source of the excess porphyrin in this disorder [6].

Although the metabolic defect is well understood, unresolved problems remain for the management of patients with EPP. The lifelong painful photosensitivity can be very disabling, and patients often wish to know whether their children will have the disease. It is not possible to provide genetic counseling, however, because the mode of inheritance of the disease is not fully understood. Analysis of the ferrochelatase gene in affected families is the obvious starting point for investigating this problem of disease transmission.

Another difficulty involves the hepatic complications of EPP. About 5% of patients die of rapidly progressive hepatic failure [7], but it is not possible to identify those at risk. If molecular analysis revealed factors predisposing individuals to severe liver disease, prophylactic therapy could be provided before liver damage occurred.

The ferrochelatase gene

Clearly, analysis of the gene encoding ferrochelatase is central to the molecular investigation of EPP. The gene (actually the complementary DNA [cDNA], a copy of the messenger RNA [mRNA]) was cloned from the mouse [8] using an antibody to the enzyme, and the human cDNA was then isolated by virtue of its similarity to the murine sequence [9]. The ferrochelatase gene maps to the long arm of chromosome 18 [10] (Fig. 2) and directs formation of a precursor of ferrochelatase in the cytosol [11]. The characterization of the cDNA has shown that the precursor protein contains 423 amino acid residues, and the 54 residues at the N-terminal probably constitute the hydrophobic signal sequence [9], which targets the enzyme to the mitochondrion [12].

So far, investigations in affected families have used the techniques of reverse transcription and the polymerase chain reaction to facilitate sequence analysis of the mRNA that encodes ferrochelatase [13•]. Once a mutation has been identified in a patient, genomic

---

Abbreviations

cDNA—complementary DNA; EPP—erythropoietic protoporphyria; mRNA—messenger RNA.

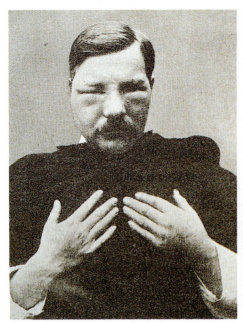 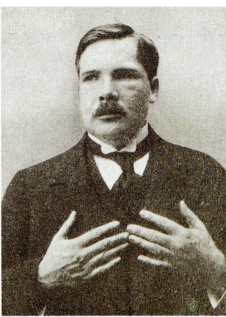

Fig. 1. The photosensitization of Dr. Meyer-Betz. **Left**, Two days after injecting himself with porphyrin, he intentionally exposed his left hand and the right side of his face when the sun came out unexpectedly during a train journey. The other hand and rest of the face served as unexposed controls. **Right**, The swelling and pain had almost resolved 3 days later. (*From* Meyer-Betz [1].)

DNA from other individuals can readily be examined for it with various detection systems including restriction enzyme digestion of amplified DNA and selective hybridization to mutation-specific oligonucleotide probes.

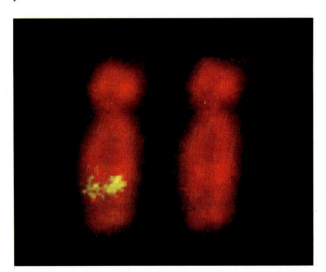

Fig. 2. Localization of the ferrochelatase gene to chromosome 18 by fluorescent *in situ* hybridization. A yellow fluorescent clone from the ferrochelatase gene hybridizes specifically on the long arm of human chromosome 18 (*left*) at band 18q22. (Chromosome on *right* is a control.)

Genetic defects

Eleven ferrochelatase mutations have now been identified in patients with EPP (Table 1). So far, almost all the mutations have been found only in single families, which is perhaps not unexpected, because biochemical studies have previously indicated genetic heterogeneity in this disease [22]. The only one found in more than one family was the deletion 40ΔG [19•]. It occurred in Northern Ireland, where founder effects or genetic drift may cause clustering of rare mutations in inherited diseases [23].

Most of the mutations reported either cause amino acid substitutions in the enzyme or are associated with defective processing of the ferrochelatase RNA. The effects of all the mutations are probably complicated, because ferrochelatase proteins normally pair up to form a dimeric enzyme. Thus, heterodimers would occur that contain normal subunits with mutant ones, as well as both mutant and normal homodimers.

Mutations causing substitutions of amino acids in the enzyme

Two of these missense mutations have been studied in protein expression systems. Substitution of the phenylalanine at residue 417 by serine profoundly reduces the enzyme's activity [18•]. In contrast, the substitution of the methionine at residue 267 by isoleucine [17] causes a very subtle abnormality. The enzyme's catalytic properties are not altered, but its thermostability is marginally decreased [24••].

Mutations causing defective ferrochelatase RNA splicing

Many of the mutations cause defective splicing of the ferrochelatase RNA. The ferrochelatase gene is normally copied or "transcribed" into RNA. Processing or "splicing" of the RNA (Fig. 3A) is then required to remove the noncoding sections (ie, introns) to form a mature mRNA molecule containing the protein-coding sections only (ie, exons) [25]. A critical role in this process is played by the "donor" and "acceptor" splice sites at the boundaries between exons and in-

Table 1. Ferrochelatase gene defects identified in patients with erythropoietic protoporphyria

Study	Patients	Mutation	Effect on messenger RNA	Effect on enzyme
No hepatic involvement				
Sarkany *et al.* [13•]	1 heterozygote	Exon 3 donor site mutation (t(+2)→g)	Exclusion of exon 3	Absent stretch of 40 amino acids
Nakahashi *et al.* [14•]	1 heterozygote	Exon 7 donor site mutation (g(+1)→a)	Exclusion of exon 7	Absent stretch of 33 amino acids
Wang *et al.* [15•]	1 heterozygote	Exon 10 donor site mutation (A(−3)→T)	Exclusion of exon 10	Absent stretch of 20 amino acids
Nakahashi *et al.* [16]	1 heterozygote	Intron 1 mutation (c→t 23 bp 5′ of exon 2)	Exclusion of exon 2	Truncated protein (29 amino acids)
Lamoril *et al.* [17]	1 compound heterozygote	163 G→T		Glycine→cysteine at amino acid 55
		801 G→A		Methionine→isoleucine at amino acid 267: normal enzyme activity but reduced thermal stability
Brenner *et al.* [18•]	1 heterozygote	1250 T→C		Phenylalanine→serine at residue 417: reduced enzyme activity
Todd *et al.* [19•]	3 heterozygotes (unrelated)	40ΔG		Truncated protein (79 residues)
Severe hepatic involvement				
Nakahashi *et al.* [20•]	1 heterozygote	Exon 9 donor site mutation (g(+1)→a)	Exclusion of exon 9	Absent stretch of 55 residues
Sarkany *et al.* [21••]	2 compound heterozygotes	Exon 10 donor site mutation (a(+3)→g)	Exclusion of exon 10	Absent stretch of 20 residues
		Exon 10 mutation (1088 T→G, 8 bp from acceptor site)	Exclusion of exon 10	Absent stretch of 20 residues and valine→glycine at residue 363

trons because they must be recognized by the cellular splicing apparatus. Mutations within the donor site in a number of these cases disrupt splicing of the preceding exon, so that it is mistakenly excluded from mature mRNA molecules [13•–15•,20•,21••] (Fig. 3). A mutation within an exon near an acceptor site (1088T →G) [19•] also causes the same defect of splicing. These splice-site mutations cause the formation of grossly abnormal ferrochelatase enzymes missing large blocks of amino acids.

Implications for clinical practice

The problem of inheritance

An understanding of the mode of inheritance of the disease is required to provide genetic counseling for affected families. The transmission of EPP is often stated to be autosomal dominant, so that individuals with a single ferrochelatase gene defect should have the disease. This is clearly not the case, because the parent-to-offspring transmission of disease characteristic of simple dominant inheritance occurs in fewer than 10% of affected families [26]. This situation is sometimes described as dominant inheritance with "incomplete penetrance," but this term merely reiterates that one defective ferrochelatase gene is not sufficient of itself to cause symptoms, and that additional factors are required for the disease to occur. Without an understanding of all the factors involved in disease transmission, useful genetic counseling with predictive power is not possible.

Analyses of families at the molecular level have confirmed that the inheritance is not simply autosomal dominant. Although only one defective ferrochelatase allele has been identified in most of the patients, close analysis reveals the complexity of the situation. A patient heterozygous for the exon 9 splice site mutation [20•] died of hepatic complications of the disease, but

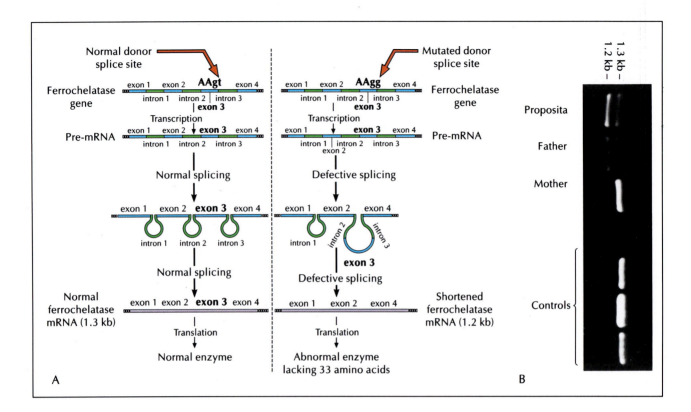

Fig. 3. An example of defective splicing of ferrochelatase RNA in erythropoietic protoporphyria. **A**, A mutation at the exon 3 donor splice site causes abnormal exclusion of that exon from the mature messenger RNA (mRNA), because the site is no longer recognizable to the cellular splicing apparatus. This results in an abnormal shortened enzyme. **B**, Gel electrophoresis of amplified ferrochelatase complementary DNA shows that a father and daughter heterozygous for the exon 3 donor site mutation possess the abnormal 1.2-kb ferrochelatase mRNA lacking exon 3. The patient's mother and normal control subjects did not have the mutation and possessed only the normal 1.3-kb mRNA. *Lengths* are of the protein-coding portion of the mRNA only. (*Panel B from* Sarkany *et al.* [13•]; with permission.)

four of his relatives heterozygous for the same mutation were quite asymptomatic. Similarly, a patient heterozygous for an exon 3 donor site mutation [13•] had profound enzymatic deficiency and severe photosensitivity, while her father, who was also a heterozygote, was asymptomatic with a milder biochemical abnormality. These cases confirm that inheritance of a severe ferrochelatase defect may not be enough to cause the disease and that some additional factor is necessary.

Ten years ago, Went and Klasen [26] proposed that the "additional factor" contributing to disease expression was a less severe defect of the other ferrochelatase gene. In their large survey of affected families, very few of the patients had a parent with clinical symptoms, but abnormalities in the metabolism of protoporphyrin were detected in one parent of almost every patient. They proposed that the disease resulted from inheritance of a severe ferrochelatase defect from the biochemically abnormal parent with a second, subtler defect from the other parent. It is very interesting that the findings of Lamoril *et al.* [17] are in agreement with this concept. The patient in that study inherited a different ferrochelatase missense mutation on each allele, one of which was of the subtle type postulated by Went and

Klasen: the substitution of isoleucine for the methionine residue at position 267 does not affect enzyme activity and only marginally decreases its thermostability [24••].

Many mutations causing subtle ferrochelatase defects may prove impossible to identify by cDNA analysis alone, and other techniques will be necessary to identify mutations causing defective regulation of gene transcription. Clinical expression of a ferrochelatase defect could also be affected by abnormalities in a host of other proteins such as those mediating the enzyme's transport to the mitochondrion (for which there are precedents [27]) and any factors that might alter the protoporphyrin concentration (*eg*, the other enzymes of heme biosynthesis and the hepatic clearance of the porphyrin). Environmental factors (*eg*, type of sun exposure) may also play a part.

Molecular genetic studies are clearly indicating the complexity of the inheritance problem, and it remains to be seen how much will be accounted for by Went and Klasen's theoretical model. Clearly, it will not be possible to provide genetic counseling until this difficult question is resolved.

The prevention of hepatic disease

In 5% of all patients [6], a rapid onset of cholestatic jaundice may lead to hepatic failure within weeks [28] (Fig. 4). The only effective treatment in this situation is liver transplantation. It is a source of great frustration that measures to prevent hepatic damage cannot be taken because there are no means of identifying the patients at risk from this complication.

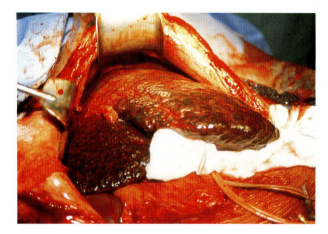

Fig. 4. Severe liver disease in erythropoietic protoporphyria. The liver is seen during transplantation surgery. There is macronodular cirrhosis with black staining due to massive protoporphyrin deposition.

The finding of families with severe hepatic disease occurring in more than one sibling [29] has suggested that there may be genetic factors predisposing to liver failure. It is therefore of interest that an autosomal recessive pattern of inheritance has recently been demonstrated in a family in which two siblings developed hepatic failure requiring liver transplantation in adolescence [21••]. The inheritance in this family was classically recessive, because the parents were asymptomatic carriers who each harbored a mutation that led to partial ferrochelatase deficiency, and the affected siblings had marked enzyme deficiency associated with inheritance of both mutations.

It remains to be seen how many patients with hepatic failure complicating EPP have this recessive form of the disease, but it is noteworthy that hereditary protoporphyria in mice is also recessive and causes liver failure [30]. If EPP with severe liver involvement proves to be a recessive disorder distinct from the purely dermatologic syndrome, investigation of inheritance in affected families might identify those at risk, so that prophylactic treatment could be given. For example, the ion-exchange resin cholestyramine could be used because it interrupts the enterohepatic circulation of protoporphyrin and so reduces hepatic exposure to the porphyrin [31].

Prospects for gene therapy

Although a variety of treatments, including sunscreens and β-carotene, may reduce photosensitivity in EPP, none is completely effective. Gene therapy directed to erythropoietic stem cells in the bone marrow may ultimately provide a definitive treatment.

For gene therapy, the normal ferrochelatase gene would be introduced into the patient's hematopoietic progenitor cells, which would then give rise to a self-perpetuating mass of erythroid cells in the marrow without the enzyme deficiency [32].

In many ways, EPP is a good candidate for gene therapy. Hematopoietic progenitor cells may be isolated from patients' marrow as a CD34+ population, and retroviral vectors can introduce new genes into them, because they are dividing cells. It should be possible to select cells in which the metabolic defect has been corrected by their resistance to exposure to ultraviolet light, and the mouse model of the disease [30] could be used to assess the effects of the treatment. However, there are formidable technical difficulties. The ferrochelatase gene, together with neighboring regions required for regulation of transcription, would be much too large to insert into a retroviral vector. Gene therapy for EPP will probably have to wait for the development of new vectors such as mammalian artificial chromosomes. The scarcity of progenitor cells may also be a problem, although the use of growth factors to induce the appearance of the cells in peripheral blood may provide a solution [33].

It has now been 4 years since the cDNA for ferrochelatase was isolated. In that time, analysis of the gene in a small number of families with EPP has provided a tantalizing glimpse into the nature of the inheritance of the disease and its hepatic complications. Gene therapy may eventually become available to treat this disabling, occasionally fatal condition.

Acknowledgment

I would like to thank Professor T. M. Cox (Department of Medicine, University of Cambridge) for helpful advice and discussion.

References and recommended reading

Papers of particular interest, published within the annual period of review, have been highlighted as:
• Of special interest
•• Of outstanding interest

1. Meyer-Betz F: Untersuchungen über die biologische (photodynamische) Wirkung des Hämatoporphyrins und anderer Derivate des Blut- und Gallenfarbstoffs. *Deutsch Arch Klin Med* 1913, 112:476–503.

2. Magnus IA, Jarrett A, Prankerd TAJ, Rimington C: Erythropoietic Protoporphyria: A New Porphyria Syndrome With Solar Urticaria Due to Protoporphyrinaemia. *Lancet* 1961, ii:448–451.

3. Brun A, Sandberg S: Mechanisms of Photosensitivity in Porphyric Patients With Special Emphasis on Erythropoietic Protoporphyria. *J Photochem Photobiol* 1991, 10:285–302.

4. Bottomley SS, Tanaka M, Everett MA: Diminished Erythroid Ferrochelatase Activity in Protoporphyria. *J Lab Clin Med* 1975, 86:126–131.

5. Jones MS, Jones OTG: The Structural Organisation of Haem Synthesis in Rat Liver Mitochondria. *Biochem J* 1969, 113:507–514.

6. Samuel D, Boboc B, Bernau J, Bismuth H, Benhamou JP: Liver Transplantation for Protoporphyria: Evidence for the Predominant

Role of the Erythropoietic Tissue in Protoporphyrin Overproduction. *Gastroenterology* 1988, **95**:816–819.

7. Doss MO, Frank M: **Hepatobiliary Implications and Complications in Protoporphyria: A 20-Year Study.** *Clin Biochem* 1989, **22**:223–229.

8. Taketani S, Nakahashi Y, Osumi T, Tokunaga R: **Molecular Cloning, Sequencing, and Expression of Mouse Ferrochelatase.** *J Biol Chem* 1990, **265**:19377–19380.

9. Nakahashi Y, Taketani S, Okuda M, Inoue K, Tokunaga R: **Molecular Cloning and Sequence Analysis of cDNA Encoding Human Ferrochelatase.** *Biochem Biophys Res Commun* 1990, **173**:748–755.

10. Whitcombe DM, Carter NP, Albertson DG, Smith SJ, Rhodes DA, Cox TM: **Assignment of the Human Ferrochelatase Gene (FECH) and a Locus for Protoporphyria to Chromosome 18q22.** *Genomics* 1991, **11**:1152–1154.

11. Karr SR, Dailey HA: **The Synthesis of Murine Ferrochelatase In Vitro and In Vivo.** *Biochem J* 1988, **254**:799–803.

12. Pfanner N, Hartl F-U, Neupert W: **Import of Proteins Into Mitochondria: A Multi-step Process.** *Eur J Biochem* 1988, **175**:205–212.

13. Sarkany RPE, Whitcombe DM, Cox TM: **Molecular Characterization**
• **of a Ferrochelatase Gene Defect Causing Anomalous RNA Splicing in Erythropoietic Protoporphyria.** *J Invest Dermatol* 1994, **102**:481–484.
A mutation at the ferrochelatase exon 3 donor splice sites causes defective RNA splicing and is associated with the enzyme deficiency in an affected family.

14. Nakahashi Y, Miyazaki H, Kadota Y, Naitoh Y, Inoue K, Yamamoto
• M, Hayashi N, Taketani S: **Human Erythropoietic Protoporphyria: Identification of a Mutation at the Splice Donor Site of Intron 7 Causing Exon 7 Skipping of the Ferrochelatase Gene.** *Hum Mol Genet* 1993, **2**:1069–1070.
A mutation at the exon 7 donor splice site causes defective RNA splicing and is associated with the enzyme deficiency in an affected family.

15. Wang X, Poh-Fitzgerald M, Carriero D, Ostasiewicz L, Chen T, Taketani S, Piomelli S: **A Novel Mutation in Erythropoietic Protoporphyria: An Aberrant Ferrochelatase mRNA Caused by Exon Skipping During RNA Splicing.** *Biochim Biophys Acta* 1993, **1181**:198–200.
A mutation near the exon 10 donor splice site is associated with defective RNA splicing in two patients with EPP.

16. Nakahashi Y, Fujita H, Taketani S, Ishida N, Kappas A, Sassa S: **The Molecular Defect of Ferrochelatase in a Patient With Erythropoietic Protoporphyria.** *Proc Natl Acad Sci U S A* 1992, **89**:281–285.

17. Lamoril J, Boulechfar S, de Verneuil H, Grandchamp B, Nordmann Y, Deybach J-C: **Human Erythropoietic Protoporphyria: Two Point Mutations in the Ferrochelatase Gene.** *Biochem Biophys Res Commun* 1991, **181**:594–599.

18. Brenner DA, Didier JM, Frasier F, Christensen SR, Evans GA, Dailey
• HA: **A Molecular Defect in Human Protoporphyria.** *Am J Hum Genet* 1992, **50**:1203–1210.
Indentification of a missense mutation in a patient with EPP, and protein studies showing that the mutation reduces enzyme activity.

19. Todd DJ, Hughes AE, Ennis KT, Ward AJ, Burrows D, Nevin NC:
• **Identification of a Single Base Pair Deletion (40ΔG) in Exon 1 of the Ferrochelatase Gene in Patients With Erythropoietic Protoporphyria.** *Hum Mol Genet* 1993, **2**:1495–1496.

Indentification of the same ferrochelatase in more than one affected family.

20. Nakahashi Y, Miyazaki H, Kadota Y, Naitoh Y, Inoue K, Yamamoto
• M, Hayashi N, Taketani S: **Molecular Defect in Human Erythropoietic Protoporphyria With Fatal Liver Failure.** *Hum Genet* 1993, **91**:303–306.
Identification of an exon 9 donor site mutation causing defective RNA splicing in a patient with severe hepatic involvement.

21. Sarkany RPE, Alexander GJMA, Cox TM: **Recessive Inheritance of**
•• **Erythropoietic Protoporphyria With Liver Failure.** *Lancet* 1994, in press.
Finding of an association between recessive inheritance and the development of hepatic failure in adolescence in two siblings with EPP.

22. Norris PG, Nunn AV, Hawk JLM, Cox TM: **Genetic Heterogeneity in Erythropoietic Protoporphyria: A Study of the Enzymatic Defect in Nine Affected Families.** *J Invest Dermatol* 1990, **95**:260–263.

23. Cutting GR, Curristin SM, Nash E, Rosenstein BJ, Lerer T, Abeliovich D, Hill A, Graham C: **Analysis of Four Diverse Population Groups Indicates That a Subset of Cystic Fibrosis Mutations Occur in Common Among Caucasians.** *Am J Hum Genet* 1992, **50**:1185–1194.

24. Dailey HA, Sellers VM, Dailey TA: **Mammalian Ferrochelatase: Expres-**
•• **sion and Characterization of Normal and Two Human Protoporphyric Ferrochelatases.** *J Biol Chem* 1994, **269**:390–395.
Detailed investigation of the effects of two ferrochelatase missense mutations (F417S and M267I) with protein expression studies. Protein engineering to study structure-function relationships in the enzyme.

25. Sharp PA: **RNA Splicing and Genes.** *JAMA* 1988, **260**:3035–3041.

26. Went LN, Klasen EC: **Genetic Aspects of Erythropoietic Protoporphyria.** *Ann Hum Genet* 1984, **48**:105–117.

27. Schapira AHV, Cooper JM, Morgan-Hughes JA, Landon DN, Clark JB: **Mitochondrial Myopathy With a Defect of Mitochondrial-Protein Transport.** *N Engl J Med* 1990, **323**:37–42.

28. Bloomer JR: **The Liver in Protoporphyria.** *Hepatology* 1988, **8**:402–407.

29. Thompson RPH, Molland EA, Nicholson DC, Gray CH: **"Erythropoietic" Protoporphyria and Cirrhosis in Sisters.** *Gut* 1973, **14**:934–938.

30. Tutois S, Montagutelli X, Da-Silva V, Joualt II, Rouyet-Fessard P, Leroy-Viard K, Guénet JL, Nordmann Y, Beuzard Y, Deybach JCL: **Erythropoietic Protoporphyria in the House Mouse: A Recessive Inherited Ferrochelatase Deficiency With Anemia, Photosensitivity, and Liver Disease.** *J Clin Invest* 1991, **88**:1730–1736.

31. Bloomer JR: **Pathogenesis and Therapy of Liver Disease in Protoporphyria.** *Yale J Biol Med* 1979, **52**:39–48.

32. Levine F: **Gene Therapy.** *Am J Dis Child* 1993, **147**:1167–1174.

33. Turner ML: **Human Haematopoietic Progenitors as a Target for Gene Therapy.** *Scott Med J* 1993, **38**:131–133.

Robert P. E. Sarkany, MBBS, MRCP, Department of Medicine, Level 5, Addenbrook's Hospital, Hills Road, Cambridge CB2 2QQ, UK.

Cutaneous biologic responses to ultraviolet radiation

Stephen E. Ullrich, PhD

MD Anderson Cancer Center, Houston, Texas, USA

Ultraviolet radiation is the primary cause of nonmelanoma skin cancer. Ultraviolet radiation is also immunosuppressive, and studies of both experimental animals and patients with biopsy-proven skin cancer have suggested a link between the carcinogenic and the immunosuppressive effects of ultraviolet radiation. The effects of ultraviolet radiation on molecular and cellular targets within the skin are reviewed here. The presence of unique "ultraviolet signature" mutations in the genes that encode for p53 suggest that mutations in this tumor suppressor gene early during carcinogenesis are essential for the development of skin cancer. In addition, ultraviolet radiation alters the type of immune response generated by modulating antigen-presenting cell function (locally or systemically) so that T helper 1 cells are rendered inactive and T helper 2 cells proliferate. The result, tumor cell transformation corresponding with immunomodulation, permits the outgrowth of ultraviolet-induced skin cancers.

Current Opinion in Dermatology 1995:225–230

Ultraviolet radiation is a ubiquitous environmental agent that adversely affects human health and well-being. Ultraviolet irradiation can result in sunburn, premature aging of the skin, cataract formation, damage to the immunocompetent cells of the skin, systemic immunosuppression, and the induction of skin cancer. Ultraviolet radiation is the primary cause of nonmelanoma skin cancer in the world today. Moreover, ultraviolet radiation is also a potent immunosuppressive agent. After exposure to ultraviolet radiation, a person's ability to generate T cell–mediated immune reactions, such as delayed-type hypersensitivity, is severely suppressed. The ability of ultraviolet radiation to induce immunosuppression has been linked to its carcinogenic potential [1,2].

Exposure to this environmental carcinogen appears to be on the rise. Changes in recreational activities, increases in leisure time, and clothing styles that provide less protection are all factors that may contribute to increased ultraviolet exposure. The seasonal thinning of the ozone layer over Antarctica and more recently over the northern latitudes [3,4] also suggests that exposure to this environmental carcinogen will certainly increase. Obviously, this carcinogen cannot be removed from the environment, and attempts to decrease exposure to ultraviolet radiation, such as using sunscreens and wearing protective clothing, are not always successful (as evidenced by the estimated 700,000 new cases of skin cancer in the United States in 1993).

The ultraviolet radiation present in sunlight is divided into three regions (Fig. 1): short-wave ultraviolet C radiation (200 to 280 nm), midrange ultraviolet B (UVB) radiation (280 to 320 nm), and long-wave ultraviolet A (UVA) radiation (320 to 400 nm). Although ultraviolet C radiation is a potent mutagen and can induce immunosuppression, all of the ultraviolet C radiation present in solar radiation is absorbed by the stratospheric ozone layer, so its role in pathogenesis is minimal. UVB radiation is also mutagenic, and extensive epidemiologic evidence has indicated that midrange ultraviolet radiation is responsible for inducing skin cancer [5]. Moreover, wavelengths within the UVB portion of the spectrum are responsible for sunburn and immunosuppression. Until recently, UVA radiation, the major component of the ultraviolet portion of the solar spectrum, was thought to be relatively benign. However, UVA radiation causes premature aging of the skin, can suppress some immunologic functions (*ie*, the activity of natural killer cells [6]), and is carcinogenic by itself (although at much higher doses than UVB radiation [7]). Perhaps what is more important is the observation that UVA radiation can act in an additive manner to enhance the carcinogenic potential of UVB radiation [8•].

The target organ of ultraviolet radiation is the skin. Ultraviolet exposure appears to promote the induction of skin cancer by two mechanisms. The first involves direct mutagenesis of epidermal DNA, which promotes the induction of neoplasia. The second is associated with immunosuppression, which allows the

---

Abbreviations

IL—interleukin; T$_H$—T helper; TNF-α—tumor necrosis factor-α; UVA—ultraviolet A; UVB—ultraviolet B.

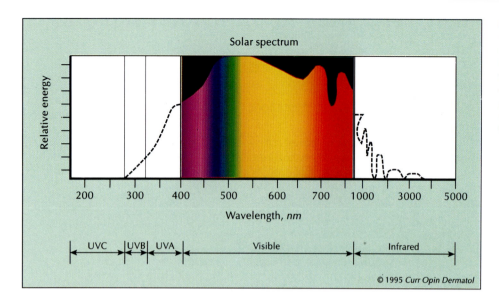

Fig. 1. The ultraviolet (UV) solar spectrum. The component wavebands of UV, visible, and infrared light are plotted against the relative energy of each. The *dashed line* depicts that percentage of energy in each waveband that reaches the earth's surface.

© 1995 *Curr Opin Dermatol*

developing tumor to escape immunosurveillance and grow progressively.

Molecular targets in the skin

The lesions found in DNA after ultraviolet exposure (cyclobutane-type pyrimidine dimers and the pyrimidine (6-4) pyrimidone lesions [Fig. 2]) are unique. Only ultraviolet radiation, no other carcinogen, induces these types of lesions. These "signature mutations" (C→T, CC→TT), which occur at dipyrimidine sites, provide useful biomarkers of ultraviolet exposure and allow investigators to trace the path of tumorigenic transformations caused by ultraviolet radiation. To date, much attention has focused on the potential role of oncogenes and tumor suppressor genes in the development of ultraviolet-induced skin cancers. Mutations in the *ras* gene family (H-*ras*, K-*ras*, and N-*ras*) have been found in human skin cancers isolated from sun-exposed body sites. Most of the mutations occur at pyrimidine-rich sequences, suggesting that they resulted from ultraviolet radiation–induced damage [9,10]. Similarly, up to 58% of human skin cancers were reported to have ultraviolet signature mutations in the *p53* tumor suppressor gene [11]. These observations were confirmed with murine skin tumors induced by ultraviolet sunlamp use. In this case, 100% of the tumors had ultraviolet signature mutations in the *p53* tumor suppressor gene [12••]. Perhaps even more interesting is the finding that *p53* mutations (CC→TT) occur at a high frequency (74%) in samples of non–tumor-bearing skin taken from sun-exposed sites. No mutations were found when non–sun-exposed skin was examined [13••]. These findings strongly suggest that ultraviolet-induced mutations in *p53* are involved in the induction of skin cancer, occur early during carcinogenesis, and may serve as biomarkers for ultraviolet exposure.

Cellular targets in the skin

Ultraviolet radiation also affects elements of the immune system that reside within the skin. Ultraviolet radiation alters the morphology and function of epidermal Langerhans cells, the epidermal antigen-presenting cells. Sensitization with contact allergens through ultraviolet-irradiated skin results in immunosuppression rather than immunostimulation. Recent studies have indicated that the antigen-presenting cell function of Langerhans cells is targeted by ultraviolet exposure. When "FACS [fluorescence-activated cell sorter]–purified," hapten-conjugated, ultraviolet-irradiated Langerhans cells were injected into mice, immunosuppression, not immunostimulation, resulted [14]. Subsequently, it was discovered that ultraviolet exposure modulates Langerhans cells' antigen-presenting cell function so that only certain subsets of T helper (T$_H$) cells are activated. Ultraviolet-irradiated Langerhans cells presented antigen only to the T cells that help B cells to produce antibody (T$_H$2 cells); ultraviolet exposure rendered Langerhans cells incapable of presenting antigen to the T cells that activate cellular immune responses (T$_H$1 cells). The ultraviolet-irradiated Langerhans cells not only fail to stimulate T$_H$1 cells but also induce tolerance, so that the next time these cells encounter antigen, they fail to respond [15]. Ultraviolet irradiation also perturbs the function of a second antigen-presenting cell in the skin. In human skin, ultraviolet damage is quickly followed by an influx of macrophages that preferentially stimulate cells that suppress immunity [16,17•].

Another important target of ultraviolet radiation in the skin is the keratinocyte. After ultraviolet exposure, keratinocytes secrete various immunomodulatory cytokines [18••]. These cytokines act locally and systemically to suppress the immune response. Much attention has been focused on the roles of tumor necrosis factor-α (TNF-α) and interleukin (IL)–10 in ultraviolet-induced immunosuppression. TNF-α is released by

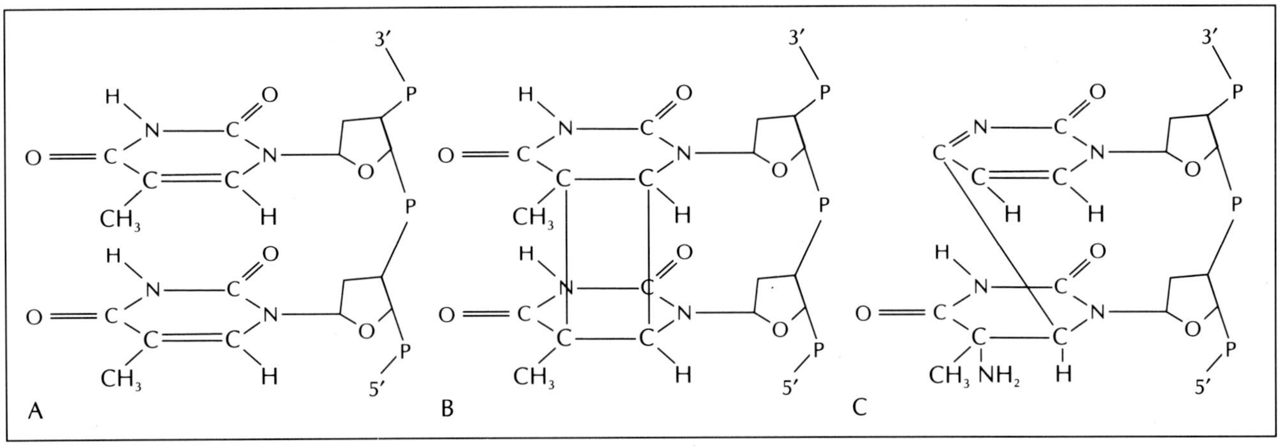

Fig. 2. Structures of the major ultraviolet (UV)–induced photoproducts in DNA. **A**, Two adjacent thymine molecules in non–UV-irradiated DNA. **B**, A thymine-thymine cyclobutane dimer. **C**, A thymine-cytosine (6-4) photolesion. (*From* Kanjilal *et al.* [38]; with permission.)

ultraviolet-irradiated keratinocytes [19], and injecting antibodies to TNF-α can block the immunosuppressive effects of ultraviolet radiation [20]. The intracutaneous injection of TNF-α mimics the effect of ultraviolet exposure and alters the skin so that epicutaneous application of a hapten leads to nonresponsiveness rather than immunity. Moreover, TNF-α alters the morphology of epidermal Langerhans cells. Within 1 to 2 minutes after the intradermal injection of TNF-α, Langerhans cells withdraw their dendrites and take on a globular appearance [21,22•].

Ultraviolet-irradiated keratinocytes also secrete IL-10, and antibodies to IL-10 can block the induction of immunosuppression after ultraviolet exposure. IL-10 is found in the serum of ultraviolet-irradiated mice and alters splenic antigen-presenting cell function so that the ability of these cells to stimulate T_H1 cells is suppressed but the stimulation of T_H2 cells is enhanced [23••,24••]. In addition, recent findings in my laboratory have suggested that the "suppressor T cells" induced by ultraviolet radiation are antigen-activated T_H2 cells that downregulate the immune response by secreting anti-inflammatory cytokines such as IL-4 and IL-10 (Rivas and Ullrich, Unpublished data).

Keratinocyte-derived IL-10 apparently contributes to the ultraviolet-induced modulation of epidermal Langerhans cells' antigen-presenting cell function in the skin because Langerhans cells have been shown to be susceptible to the inhibitory effects of IL-10. Similar to what was described previously, IL-10–treated Langerhans cells present antigen to T_H2 cells but tolerize T_H1 clones [25••]. These findings suggest that a major effect of ultraviolet radiation on the immune system is to modify antigen-presenting cell function so that only certain subclasses of T cells are stimulated. This results either from direct irradiation of the antigen-presenting cell *in situ* or from the effects of epidermal cytokines, such as TNF-α and IL-10, on the function of antigen-presenting cells. We suggest that activated T_H2 cells, by

producing immunomodulatory cytokines such as IL-4 and IL-10, can limit the induction of cell-mediated immune reactions in ultraviolet-irradiated mice (Fig. 3).

The photoreceptor for ultraviolet B radiation in the skin

What is the photoreceptor in the skin that initiates the cascade of events leading to immunosuppression? Because the action spectrums for the photoisomerization of urocanic acid, the absorption of UVB radiation by DNA, and ultraviolet-induced immunosuppression are almost identical, urocanic acid and DNA are the two most likely candidates. Because early studies demonstrated that the removal of the stratum corneum before ultraviolet exposure abrogated the ability of ultraviolet radiation to induce immunosuppression, urocanic acid, which is found in the superficial layers of the skin and is isomerized from the *trans* form to the *cis* form by ultraviolet exposure, was identified as a photoreceptor. Subsequently, it was demonstrated that injecting *cis*-urocanic acid into mice suppressed immunity, in a manner similar to that seen after ultraviolet exposure [26•].

Findings by others, however, have questioned whether urocanic acid is actually the photoreceptor. The superficial location of the photoreceptor has been questioned [27], and the *in vivo* action spectrum for the photoisomerization of urocanic acid does not correlate with the action spectrum for immunosuppression [28]. Other studies support a role for DNA as the photoreceptor. Immunosuppression in marsupials were reversed when visible light was used to activate the photoreactivating pyrimidine dimer repair enzyme [29]. Moreover, when liposomes containing an excision repair enzyme, T4 endonuclease V, which is specific for pyrimidine dimers, were used to deliver the endonuclease to epidermal cells, ultraviolet-induced immunosuppression was reversed [30•]. Thus, the identity of the

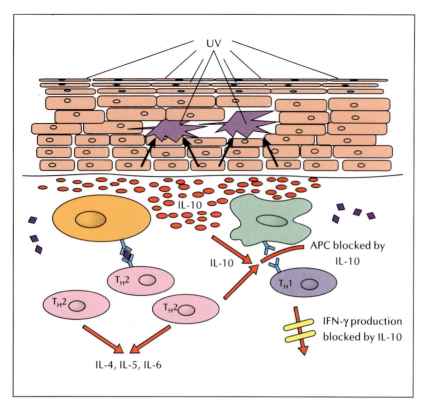

Fig. 3. A working model for ultraviolet (UV)–induced immune suppression. UV irradiation alters the function of epidermal Langerhans cells either directly or through the action of keratinocyte-derived cytokines (*ie*, tumor necrosis factor-α and interleukin [IL]–10). This alteration interferes with antigen presentation to T-helper (T$_H$) 1 cells, inhibiting interferon gamma (IFN-γ) production and cell-mediated immune reactions. Keratinocyte-derived cytokines, such as IL-10, can also have systemic effects. Circulating IL-10 also interferes with antigen presentation to T$_H$1 clones. Because the antigen-presenting cells for T$_H$1 and T$_H$2 cells differ, and because IL-10 does not affect all antigen-presenting cells (APCs) to the same degree, we suggest that T$_H$2 cells expand and proliferate in UV-irradiated individuals. Upon subsequent exposure to antigen, these cells are activated to secrete IL-4 and IL-10, which further limits the generation of cell-mediated immune responses (delayed-type hypersensitivity and tumor rejection). We suggest that the CD4+ "suppressor T cells" previously described in this system are antigen-activated T$_H$2 cells. (*From* Rivas and Ullrich [39]; with permission.)

photoreceptor for ultraviolet-induced immunosuppression still appears to be open to question.

Limiting the harmful effects of ultraviolet radiation

How can the harmful effects of ultraviolet exposure be modulated? Approaches have included changing ones' lifestyle to limit ultraviolet exposure by avoidance, wearing protective clothing, and using sunscreens. Studies by Wolf *et al.* [31•,32•] have suggested that although sunscreens are quite effective at limiting erythema induced by ultraviolet exposure, they may not be as effective at blocking the immunosuppression. Their use may induce a false sense of security that ultimately leads to more, not less, harmful exposure. It is important to keep in mind, however, that these investigators employed artificial fluorescent light in their studies. Recently, Roberts and Beasley [33•], who used a "solar simulator" whose output more closely mimics the radiation produced by sunlight, reported that sunscreens do afford protection against ultraviolet-induced immunosuppression. Obviously, more research is required to resolve this issue.

Data have also suggested that including antioxidants in the diet or limiting the dietary intake of polyunsaturated lipids, which can provide a source of free radicals, can limit ultraviolet-induced skin cancer formation [34,35]. In addition, topically applying retinoic acid or supplementing the diets of ultraviolet-irradiated mice with the retinoid temarontene blocked the ability of

ultraviolet radiation to prevent Langerhans cell depletion [36]. Similarly, treating mice with a gel extract from *Aloe barbadensis* after ultraviolet exposure blocked the induction of immunosuppression [37]. These observations suggest that it may be possible to alleviate some of the harmful effects of ultraviolet radiation, thereby lessening its effect on human health.

Conclusions

Although exposure to ultraviolet radiation is associated with a multitude of harmful effects, perhaps the most damaging effects of exposure from the perspective of human health are the induction of skin cancer and immunosuppression. Moreover, the mutagenic and immunosuppressive effects of ultraviolet radiation appear to work in concert to induce skin cancer and prevent its rejection by the immune system. Although impressive gains have been made in the past few years in identifying molecular targets of ultraviolet radiation and in determining the type of immune defects induced after ultraviolet exposure, much remains to be done, at both the cellular and the molecular levels, to understand how ultraviolet radiation modifies homeostatic mechanisms and induces skin cancer and immunosuppression.

Acknowledgment

This work was supported by grant AR 40824 from the National Institutes of Arthritis and Musculoskeletal and Skin Disease.

References and recommended reading

Papers of particular interest, published within the annual period of review, have been highlighted as:
- •   Of special interest
- ••   Of outstanding interest

1.   Kripke ML: **Photoimmunology.** *Photochem Photobiol* 1990, 52:919–924.

2.   Yoshikawa T, Rae V, Bruins-Slot W, vand den Berg JW, Taylor JR, Streilein JW: **Susceptibility to Effects of UVB Radiation on Induction of Contact Hypersensitivity as a Risk Factor for Skin Cancer in Humans.** *J Invest Dermatol* 1990, 95:530–536.

3.   Coldiron BM: **Thinning of the Ozone Layer: Facts and Consequences.** *J Am Acad Dermatol* 1992, 27:653–662.

4.   Kerr JB, McElroy CT: **Evidence for Large Upwards Trends of Ultraviolet-B Radiation Linked to Ozone Depletion.** *Science* 1993, 262:1032–1034.

5.   Urbach F: **Evidence and Epidemiology of UV-Induced Carcinogenesis in Man.** *Natl Cancer Inst Monogr* 1978, 50:5–10.

6.   Hersey P, MacGrath H, Wilkinson F: **Development of an In Vitro System for the Analysis of UV Radiation-Induced Suppression of Natural Killer Cell Activity.** *Photochem Photobiol* 1993, 57:279–284.

7.   Strickland PT: **Photocarcinogenesis by Near-Ultraviolet (UVA) Radiation in Sencar Mice.** *J Invest Dermatol* 1986, 87:272–275.

8.   Berg RJW, de Gruijl FR, van der Leun JC: **Interaction Between UVA**
•   **and UVB Radiation in Skin Cancer Induction in Hairless Mice.** *Cancer Res* 1993, 53, 4212–4217.
Demonstrates the additive effect of UVB and UVA radiation on skin cancer induction.

9.   Ananthaswamy HN, Pierceall WE: **Molecular Mechanisms of Ultraviolet Radiation Carcinogenesis.** *Photochem Photobiol* 1990, 52:1119–1136.

10.   Pierceall WE, Goldberg LH, Tainsky MA, Ananthaswamy HN: *Ras* **Gene Mutation and Amplification in Human Nonmelanoma Skin Cancer.** *Mol Carcinog* 1991, 4:196–202.

11.   Brash DE, Rudolf JA, Simon JA, Lin A, McKenna GJ, Baden HP, Halperin AJ, Ponten J: **A Role for Sunlight in Skin Cancer: UV-Induced *p53* Mutations in Squamous Cell Carcinoma.** *Proc Natl Acad Sci U S A* 1991, 88:10124–10128.

12.   Kanjilal S, Pierceall WE, Cummings K, Kripke ML, Ananthaswamy
••   HN: **High Frequency of *p53* Mutations in UV Radiation-Induced Murine Skin Tumors: Evidence for Strand Bias and Tumor Heterogeneity.** *Cancer Res* 1993, 53:2961–2964.
Identifies the molecular target for skin cancer induction. One hundred percent of skin tumors from these mice had mutations in dipyrimidine sites of the *p53* gene, most of which were ultraviolet signature mutations. This unprecedented frequency of *p53* mutations strongly suggests that this gene plays a fundamental role in the development of skin tumors after ultraviolet exposure.

13.   Nakazawa H, English D, Randell PL, Nakazawa K, Martel N, Arm-
••   strong BK, Yamasaki H: **UV and Skin Cancer: Specific *p53* Gene Mutation in Normal Skin as a Biologically Relevant Exposure Measurement.** *Proc Natl Acad Sci U S A* 1994, 91:360–364.
A high percentage (74%) of *p53* mutations in samples of normal sun-exposed skin was found. Ultraviolet radiation was also used to induce *p53* mutations in cultured human keratinocytes. Most of the *p53* mutations were ultraviolet signature mutations. The authors suggest that *p53* mutations may play a role early in the course of skin cancer induction (unlike that seen with internal malignancies). They also suggest that *p53* mutations in pyrimidine sites may serve as a biomarker for ultraviolet exposure.

14.   Cruz PD, Nixon-Fulton J, Tigelaar RE, Bergstresser PR: **Disparate Effects of In Vitro UVB Irradiation in Intravenous Immunization With Purified Epidermal Cell Subpopulations for the Induction of CHS.** *J Invest Dermatol* 1989, 92:160–165.

15.   Simon JC, Tigelaar RE, Bergstresser PR, Edelbaum D, Cruz PD: **Ultraviolet B Radiation Converts Langerhans Cells From Immunogenic to Tolerogenic Antigen-Presenting Cells: Induction of Specific Clonal Anergy in CD4+ T Helper 1 Cells.** *J Immunol* 1991, 146:485–491.

16.   Baadsgaard O, Salvo B, Mannie A, Dass B, Fox D, Cooper KC: **In Vivo Ultraviolet-Exposed Human Epidermal Cells Activate T Suppressor Cell Pathways That Involve CD4+CD45RA+ Suppressor-Inducer T Cells.** *J Immunol* 1990, 145:2854–2861.

17.   Cooper KD, Oberhelman L, Hamilton TA, Baadsgaard O, Terhune M,
•   Levee G, Anderson T, Koren H: **UV Exposure Reduces Immunization Rates and Promotes Tolerance to Epicutaneous Antigens in Humans: Relationship to Dose, CD1a⁻DR⁺ Epidermal Macrophage Induction,** and Langerhans Cell Depletion. *Proc Natl Acad Sci U S A* 1992, 89:8497–8501.
Clearly demonstrates the deleterious effects of ultraviolet radiation on the human immune system.

18.   Luger TA, Schwarz T, eds: *Epidermal Growth Factors and Cytokines.*
••   New York: Marcel Dekker; 1994.
This book provides an excellent, in-depth review of the cytokines produced by epidermal cells and their role in cutaneous biology.

19.   Kock A, Schwarz T, Kirnbauer R, Urbanski A, Perry P, Ansel JC, Luger TA: **Human Keratinocytes Are a Source for Tumor Necrosis Factor α: Evidence for Synthesis and Release Upon Stimulation With Endotoxin or Ultraviolet Light.** *J Exp Med* 1990, 172:1609–1614.

20.   Yoshikawa T, Streilein JW: **Tumor Necrosis Factor-α and Ultraviolet Light Have Similar Effects on Contact Hypersensitivity in Mice.** *Reg Immunol* 1990, 3:139–144.

21.   Streilein JW, Taylor JR, Yoshikawa T, Kurimoto I: **Immunology of Human Skin Cancer and Its Relationship to Skin Cancers.** *Cancer Bull* 1993, 45:225–231.

22.   Vincek V, Kurimoto I, Medema JP, Prieto E, Streilein JW: **Tumor**
•   **Necrosis Factor α Polymorphism Correlates With Deleterious Effects of Ultraviolet B Light on Cutaneous Immunity.** *Cancer Res* 1993, 53:728–732.
By correlating the genetic differences in the *TNFA* locus with susceptibility or resistance to the immunosuppressive effects of ultraviolet radiation, this paper provides additional strong evidence for the role of TNF-α in ultraviolet-induced immunosuppression.

23.   Rivas JM, Ullrich SE: **Systemic Suppression of DTH by Supernatants**
••   **From UV-Irradiated Keratinocytes: An Essential Role for Interleukin 10.** *J Immunol* 1992, 149:3865–3871.
Provides evidence of the upregulation of IL-10 messenger RNA and the secretion of biologically active IL-10 by ultraviolet-irradiated keratinocytes. Moreover, the data presented in this paper indicate that IL-10 released *in vivo* plays an essential role in the induction of systemic immunosuppression after ultraviolet exposure because injecting ultraviolet-irradiated mice with antibodies to IL-10 reverses the immunosuppression.

24.   Ullrich SE: **Mechanism Involved in the Systemic Suppression of**
••   **Antigen-Presenting Cell Function by UV Irradiation: Keratinocyte-Derived IL-10 Modulates Antigen-Presenting Cell Function of Splenic Adherent Cells.** *J Immunol* 1994, 152:3410–3416.
These data indicate that keratinocyte-derived IL-10 induces a systemic T$_H$1-to-T$_H$2 shift in ultraviolet-irradiated animals by affecting splenic antigen-presenting cell function. After ultraviolet exposure, antigen presentation to T$_H$1 cells is depressed, whereas the ability of spleen cells to present antigen to T$_H$2 cells is enhanced. Injecting the ultraviolet-irradiated mice with anti-IL-10 reverses these effects.

25.   Enk AH, Angeloni V, Udey MC, Katz SI: **Inhibition of Langerhans Cell**
••   **Antigen-Presenting Function by IL-10: A Role for IL-10 in Induction of Tolerance.** *J Immunol* 1993, 151:2390–2398.
Treating Langerhans cells with IL-10 blocked antigen presentation to T$_H$1 clones, with no measurable effect on the stimulation of T$_H$2 clones. In addition, when IL-10–treated Langerhans cells were used to present antigen to T$_H$1 clones, tolerance induction rather than proliferation resulted. These findings suggest that ultraviolet exposure activates a T$_H$1-to-T$_H$2 shift by inducing ultraviolet-irradiated keratinocytes to secrete IL-10, which then targets the function of epidermal Langerhans cells.

26.   Noonan FP, De Fabo EC: **Immunosuppression by Ultraviolet B Radiation:**
•   **Initiation by Urocanic Acid.** *Immunol Today* 1992, 13:250–254.
Summarizes the evidence for urocanic acid as the photoreceptor for UVB radiation.

27.   Morison WL, Kelly SP: **Urocanic Acid May Not Be the Photoreceptor of Contact Hypersensitivity.** *Photodermatology* 1986, 3:98–101.

28.   Gibbs NJ, Norval M, Traynor NA, Wolf M, Johnson BE, Crosby J: **Action Spectra for the Trans to Cis Photoisomerization of Urocanic Acid In Vitro and in Mouse Skin.** *Photochem Photobiol* 1993, 57:584–590.

29.   Applegate LA, Ley RD, Alcalay J, Kripke ML: **Identification of the Molecular Target for the Suppression of Contact Hypersensitivity by UV Radiation.** *J Exp Med* 1989, 170:1117–1131.

30.   Kripke ML, Cox PA, Alas LG, Yarosh DB: **Pyrimidine Dimers in**
•   **DNA Initiate Systemic Immunosuppression in UV-Irradiated Mice.** *Proc Natl Acad Sci U S A* 1992, 89:7516–7520.
Provides evidence of DNA as the photoreceptor by demonstrating that repair of pyrimidine dimers in ultraviolet-irradiated skin reverses the immunosuppressive effects of ultraviolet radiation.

31.   Wolf P, Donawho CK, Kripke ML: **Analysis of the Protective Effect**
•   **of Different Sunscreens on Ultraviolet-Radiation–Induced Local and Systemic Suppression of Contact Hypersensitivity and Inflammatory Responses in Mice.** *J Invest Dermatol* 1993, 100:254–259.
The data presented here indicate that although sunscreens efficiently block the erythema and inflammation induced by ultraviolet radiation, they do not block all the harmful effects of ultraviolet radiation on immunity.

32. Wolf P, Donawho CK, Kripke ML: **Effect of Sunscreens on UV**
• **Radiation-Induced Enhancement of Melanoma Growth in Mice.** *J Natl Cancer Inst* 1994, **86**:99–105.
The ability of sunscreens to block the enhanced growth of transplanted melanoma cells in ultraviolet-irradiated animals, which is a measurement of depressed immune function, was tested. Although the sunscreens applied blocked erythema, they did not block the ultraviolet-induced immune defects (*ie*, the melanoma grew faster in sunscreen-treated and ultraviolet-irradiated animals than in nonirradiated controls).

33. Roberts LK, Beasley DG: **Sunscreens Prevent Ultraviolet Radiation**
• **Induced Suppression of Contact Dermatitis in Mice: The Level of Protection Depends Upon the Energy Spectrum of the Light Source** [Abstract]. *J Invest Dermatol* 1993, **100**:597a.
The findings presented here suggest that the light source used to determine the efficacy of sunscreens is critical. When solar simulators were used, rather than fluorescent sunlamps, the ability of sunscreens to protect against immune damage increased dramatically.

34. Mukhtar H, Katiyar SK, Agarwal R: **Green Tea and Skin–Anti-carcinogenic Effects.** *J Invest Dermatol* 1994, **102**:3–7.

35. Fisher MA, Black HS: **Modification of Membrane Composition, Eicosanoid Metabolism, and Immunoresponsiveness by Dietary Omega-3 and Omega-6 Fatty Acid Sources, Modulators of Ultraviolet Carcinogenesis.** *Photochem Photobiol* 1991, **54**:381–387.

36. Halliday GM, McKay DA: **Topical Retinoic Acid Inhibits Changes in Langerhans Cell Density During Carcinogenesis.** *In Vivo* 1993, **7**:271–276.

37. Strickland FM, Pelley RP, Kripke ML: **Prevention of Ultraviolet Radiation-Induced Suppression of Contact and Delayed Hypersensitivity by** *Aloe barbadensis* **Gel Extract.** *J Invest Dermatol* 1994, **102**:197–204.

38. Kanjilal S, Pierceall WF, Ananthaswamy HN: **Ultraviolet Radiation in the Pathogenesis of Skin Cancers: Involvement of** *ras* **and** *p53* **Gene.** *Cancer Bull* 1993, **45**:205–211.

39. Rivas JM, Ullrich SE: **UV Band Skin Immunology.** In *Immunotoxicology and Immunopharmacology*, edn 2. Edited by Dean J, Luster M, Munson A, Kimber I. New York: Raven Press;in press.

Stephen E. Ullrich, PhD, Department of Immunology-178, The University of Texas, MD Anderson Cancer Center, 1515 Holcombe Boulevard, Houston, TX 77030, USA.

The long-term experience with isotretinoin treatment of acne

Victoria Goulden, MB, MRCP, and William J. Cunliffe, MB, FRCP

The General Infirmary at Leeds, Leeds, UK

Over the past 12 years, isotretinoin has become well established as a uniquely effective treatment for acne vulgaris. It is now the first-line treatment of nodular acne and is increasingly being used to treat moderate acne unresponsive to conventional antibiotic therapy. Patients who are likely to develop significant scarring or psychological problems associated with their acne should be considered for early treatment. This article reviews the long-term experience that has now been accumulated. This experience has confirmed the ability of isotretinoin to induce long-term remission of acne and has provided important information on optimal treatment regimens (a total cumulative dose of 120 mg/kg given at 1 mg/kg/d for 4 months) and patient selection. Repeated courses of treatment may be given with no increased risk of side effects, and no significant long-term side effects occur after treatment.

Current Opinion in Dermatology 1995:231–234

During the past 12 years, isotretinoin has become a well-established and uniquely effective treatment for acne vulgaris. It is now the first-line treatment for nodular acne and is increasingly being used to treat moderate acne unresponsive to conventional antibiotic therapy. This article reviews the literature of the past 2 years, with particular emphasis on the long-term experience that has now been accumulated. This experience has provided important information on patient selection, optimal treatment regimens, and long-term benefits.

The unique success of isotretinoin is related to its ability to influence the four major factors that are involved in the pathogenesis of acne. It dramatically reduces sebum production [1], comedogenesis [2], surface and ductal *Propionibacterium acnes* [3], and production of the inflammatory response inhibiting both neutrophil [4] and monocyte [5] chemotaxis.

Long-term outcome

Early studies confirmed the effectiveness of isotretinoin as a treatment for acne (Fig. 1) and predicted the possibility of long-term remission [6,7]. Until recently, however, data on its long-term benefits were limited. Two major long-term studies, published within the last 2 years, have provided clear evidence of isotretinoin's long-term benefits, as well as valuable information on optimal dosage regimens and patient selection.

Lehucher-Ceyrac and Weber-Buisset [8••] in France observed 188 patients treated with isotretinoin over a 9-year period. Ninety-five percent of the patients had achieved complete healing of their acne at the end of the treatment. The average treatment period was 7 months, and the average total dose received was 101 mg/kg. Sixty-two percent remained in stable long-term remission on follow-up (remission in this study was defined as complete cure or recurrence of acne to a maximum of grade 2 acne controlled by standard therapy). Recurrence of the acne was noted in 38% of patients; in the majority of these patients, it occurred within the first 12 months after stopping treatment. The most common site of recurrence was the face and neck. After further treatment with isotretinoin of the patients who had had relapses, 88% of the original treatment group achieved stable long-term remission. The dose-response curve obtained from these data suggests that a maximal effect is obtained with a total cumulative dose of 110 mg/kg (95 mg/kg in women and 125 mg/kg in men). This study also identified a threshold cumulative dose of 150 mg/kg, above which further therapeutic benefit is not achieved. The reason for this is not known. Among the patients who showed only a partial response to treatment or failed to obtain long-term remission, there was a higher proportion of women with symptoms suggestive of gynecoendocrinologic problems and of patients with microcystic acne. Lehucher-Ceyrac (Personal communication) indicated that the term *microcystic* was used to describe large comedones, usually whiteheads. This observation is in keeping with the findings of the Leeds group [9•], who observed that such lesions account for a proportion of subjects who show a slow response to isotretinoin therapy (>4 months of therapy at 1 mg/kg/d). The optimal treatment for macrocomedones

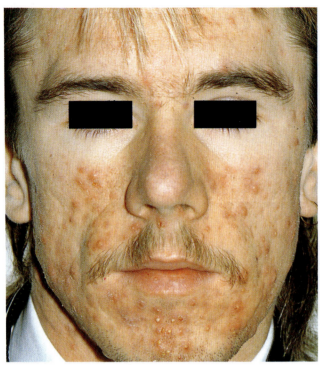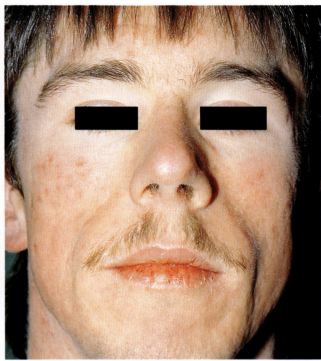

Fig. 1. Patient with severe facial acne before therapy (*left panel*) and at the end of 4 months' treatment with isotretinoin (*right panel*).

is light cautery under topical anesthesia [10]. An antiandrogenic agent such as cyproterone acetate combined with estrogen should be considered in women with a history suggestive of gynecoendocrinologic problems.

Layton *et al.* [11••] have carried out the longest followup study to date. Over a 10-year period, 88 patients were followed up for a mean period of 9 years after therapy. Results similar to those of the French study were obtained. Stable long-term remission was observed in 61% of patients after one course of isotretinoin. Thirty-nine percent of patients had relapses (*ie*, recurrence of the acne requiring systemic therapy, either antibiotics or a second course of isotretinoin). As in the French study, the majority of relapses occurred within the first 12 to 18 months after treatment. This study also confirms the importance of the total cumulative dose. A total dose of more than 120 mg/kg was associated with a significantly lower incidence of relapse. In contrast to the French study, however, a higher incidence of relapse was noted in patients with predominantly truncal acne (Fig. 2). Patient age and gender did not influence relapse.

A third recent long-term follow-up study of 116 patients with severe acne who were treated with isotretinoin showed similar rates of response to therapy and long-term remission. Ninety-two percent of the patients were completely healed or had marked improvement at the end of treatment (0.75 mg/kg/d for 6 months), and 81% remained in remission on follow-up 42 months later [12].

Factors that may predict the need for more than one course of isotretinoin have recently been investigated

[13]. Low-dose regimens were found to be an important cause of relapse. This finding had been clearly shown in several previous studies [6,14]. Patients with predominantly facial acne had a higher incidence of relapse. This finding contrasts with those of Layton *et al.* [11•] in their recent 10-year follow-up study and of several previous relapse studies [15,16], which have shown a greater incidence of relapse in truncal acne. Detailed analysis of the results of this retreatment study also showed that female patients older than 25 years of age required repeated courses of isotretinoin more frequently, possibly reflecting the greater concern about the cosmetic effect of acne in women. The presence of very severe acne at the start of treatment with isotretinoin was also a risk factor for relapse [13]. Younger patients were not found to have an increased incidence of relapse, in contrast to the results of several previous studies [15,16].

Current indications

In recent years, the indications for isotretinoin therapy have significantly altered: more patients with moderate acne unresponsive to systemic antibiotic therapy are being treated. Recent guidelines for the optimal use of isotretinoin in acne [9•] stress its use in both severe nodular acne and moderate acne that fails to respond to, or relapses rapidly after, three consecutive courses of conventional antibiotics. It is emphasized that patients who scar and those who are severely depressed or dysmorphobic should be treated early. Often a combination of reasons, such as an inadequate response to antibiotics and scarring, or a partial response and psy-

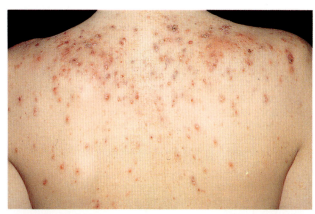

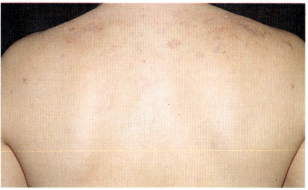

Fig. 2. Patient with truncal acne before therapy (*top panel*) and after treatment with isotretinoin (*bottom panel*).

chological disturbance, forms the indication for treatment. Data from the dermatology unit at The General Infirmary at Leeds (Leeds, UK) show that between 1984 and 1987, 65% of patients who received isotretinoin had severe acne, whereas 22% had moderate acne unresponsive to antibiotic therapy. More recent figures (from 1989 to 1992) show a reversal of prescribing habits: 60% of patients receiving isotretinoin had unresponsive moderate acne, whereas 23% had severe acne.

In addition to being used in acne vulgaris, isotretinoin is being employed as part of the treatment of unusual acne variants, including acne fulminans [17], gram-negative folliculitis [18], and rosacea faciale [19].

Side effects

Side effects that occur during treatment with isotretinoin are well recognized. They most commonly involve the skin, the mucous membranes, and the musculoskeletal system, and they are dose dependent. Biochemical side effects, including abnormalities of liver function and lipid levels, are also well recognized, and routine monitoring of patients receiving treatment is usual. A recent study, however, has questioned the need for repeated laboratory tests if initial normal values are obtained [20]. Repeated courses of treatment were not associated with increased incidence or severity of side effects or with acquired tolerance [13].

Teratogenicity remains a major clinical problem. A study reviewed the voluntary reports of exposure to isotretinoin during pregnancy that were received by Hoffmann-La Roche in the United States between 1982 and 1989 [21]. During this period, 433 spontaneous reports occurred. Among the 409 pregnancies in which the outcome was known, 54% ended in elective abortions, 7% in spontaneous or missed abortions, and 37% in live births (17.6% normal, 17.4% with congenital malformations, and 2% with abnormalities other than malformations). Thirty-three percent of the 396 patients in whom the timing of conception was known in relation to isotretinoin therapy were already pregnant at the start of treatment. This emphasizes the importance of obtaining a negative pregnancy test result before treatment is started. Very uncommon side effects occurring during treatment continue to be reported; they have recently included acute Achilles tendinitis [22]; enthesopathy of the patellar tendon insertion [23]; seronegative oligoarthritis [24]; pseudoporphyria [25]; median nail dystrophy [26]; decreased dark adaptation, persistent dry eye syndrome, and cataracts [27]; and severe hyperlipidemia associated with pancreatitis [28].

Acne fulminans [29] and severe flare of acne have been documented to occur during treatment with isotretinoin. Isotretinoin dramatically alters the local microenvironment within the pilosebaceous duct, creating a hostile environment for *P. acnes*. It is suggested that the sudden death of many *P. acnes* in the follicles releases antigens and inflammatory mediators producing a flare of the acne. The presence of macrocomedones has been reported as a risk factor for severe exacerbation of acne during treatment with isotretinoin [30]. Macrocomedones are thought to be colonized with *P. acnes*, the death of which will lead similarly to the release of inflammatory mediators.

The long-term safety of isotretinoin use in acne has recently been investigated [31]. Seven hundred and twenty patients were followed up for 9 years after therapy. Persistent symptoms were reported by 7.2% of the patients, but the relationship of many of these symptoms to previous treatment with isotretinoin was not clearly established. Probable long-term side effects included xeroderma, persistent dry eye syndrome, arthralgia, and possibly exacerbation of eczema in predisposed individuals. These effects occurred in fewer than 1% of the patients, and symptoms were mild in all cases, requiring little or no treatment.

Conclusions

Isotretinoin is now established as a uniquely effective treatment for acne vulgaris with the ability to induce long-term remission. Patients who should be considered for treatment are those with severe disease, those with moderate disease who respond poorly to adequate conventional therapy, and those who are likely to develop significant scarring or significant psychological problems associated with their acne. The optimal treatment regimen consists of a total cumulative dose of 120 mg/kg (*ie*, 1 mg/kg/d for 4 months). Repeated courses may be given with no increased risk of side effects. Teratogenicity remains a serious problem during treatment, but no serious long-term side effects occur after therapy with isotretinoin. Isotretinoin remains an expensive drug, but compared with prolonged treatment with systemic antibiotics, isotretinoin therapy can be judged cost-effective [32].

References and recommended reading

Papers of particular interest, published within the annual period of review, have been highlighted as:
- Of special interest
- • Of outstanding interest

1. Stewart ME, Benoit AM, Downing AT, Strauss JS: **Suppression of Sebum Secretion With 13-*cis* Retinoic Acid: Effect on Individual Skin Surface Lipids and Implications for the Anatomic Origins.** *J Invest Dermatol* 1984, 8:74–78.

2. Cunliffe WJ, Jones DH, Pritlove J, *et al.*: **Long Term Benefit of Isotretinoin in Acne.** In *Retinoids: New Trends in Research Therapy.* Basel: Karger; 1985:242–251.

3. King K, Jones DH, Daltrey DC, Cunliffe WJ: **A Double Blind Study of the Effect of 13-*cis*-Retinoic Acid on Acne, Sebum Excretion and Microbiological Population.** *Br J Dermatol* 1982, 107:583–590.

4. Pigatto PD, Fioroni A, Riva F, Brugo MA, Morandotti A, Altomare GF, Finzi AF: **Effects of Isotretinoin on Neutrophil Chemotaxis in Cystic Acne.** *Dermatologica* 1983, 167:16–18.

5. Falcon RH, Lee WL, Shalita AR, Sunthraralineam K, Fikrig SM: **In Vitro Effects of Isotretinoin on Monocyte Chemotaxis.** *J Invest Dermatol* 1986, 86:550–552.

6. Farrell LN, Strauss JS, Stranieri AM: **The Treatment of Severe Cystic Acne With 13-*cis* Retinoic Acid: Evaluation of Sebum Production and the Clinical Response in a Multiple Dose Trial.** *J Am Acad Dermatol* 1980, 3:602–611.

7. Strauss JS, Rapini RP, Shalita AR, Konecky E, Polchi PE, Comite H, Exner JH: **Isotretinoin Therapy for Acne: Results of a Multicenter Dose-Response Study.** *J Am Acad Dermatol* 1984, 10:490–496.

8. Lehucher-Ceyrac D, Weber-Buisset MJ: **Isotretinoin and Acne in Prac-**
•• **tice: A Prospective Analysis of 188 Cases Over 9 Years.** *Dermatology* 1993, 186:123–128.
Major long-term follow-up study.

9. Layton AM, Cunliffe WJ: **Guidelines for the Optimal Use of**
• **Isotretinoin in Acne.** *J Am Acad Dermatol* 1992, 2:S2–S7.
A comprehensive review of the guidelines for the optimal use of isotretinoin.

10. Pepall LM, Cosgrove MP, Cunliffe WJ: **Ablation of Whiteheads by Cautery Under Topical Anaesthesia.** *Br J Dermatol* 1991, 125:256–259.

11. Layton AM, Knaggs H, Taylor J, Cunliffe WJ: **Isotretinoin for Acne**
•• **Vulgaris: 10 Years Later, A Safe and Successful Treatment.** *Br J Dermatol* 1993, 129:292–296.
Major long-term follow-up study.

12. Falk ES, Stenvold SE: **Long Term Effects of Isotretinoin in the Treatment of Severe Nodulocystic Acne.** *Riv Eur Sci Med Farmacol* 1992, 14:215–220.

13. Stainforth JM, Layton AM, Taylor JP, Cunliffe WJ: **Isotretinoin for the Treatment of Acne Vulgaris: Which Factors May Predict the Need for More Than One Course.** *Br J Dermatol* 1993, 129:297–301.

14. Wokalek H, Hennes R, Schell H, *et al.*: **Relapse Rate of Acne Conglobata After Stopping Isotretinoin.** In *Retinoid Therapy.* Edited by Cunliffe WJ, Miller AJ. Lancaster: MTP Press; 1984:231–239.

15. Chivot M, Midoun H: **Isotretinoin and Acne: A Study of Relapses.** *Dermatologica* 1990, 175(suppl 1):133–137.

16. Harms M, Marouye I, Radeff B: **The Relapses of Cystic Acne After Isotretinoin Are Age Related: A Long Term Follow Up Study.** *Dermatologica* 1986, 172:148–153.

17. Choi EH, Bang D: **Acne Fulminans and 13-*cis* Retinoic Acid.** *J Dermatol* 1992, 19:378–383.

18. Amichai B, Grunwald MH, Halevy S: **Treatment of Gram-Negative Folliculitis With Isotretinoin.** *Harefuah* 1993, 124:200–201.

19. Plewig G, Jansen T, Kligman AM: **Pyoderma Faciale: A Review and Report of 20 Additional Cases. Is It Rosacea?** *Arch Dermatol* 1992, 128:1611–1617.

20. Barth JH, Macdonald Hull SP, Mark J, Jones RG, Cunliffe WJ: **Isotretinoin Therapy for Acne Vulgaris: A Reevaluation of the Need for Measurement of Plasma Lipids and Liver Function Tests.** *Br J Dermatol* 1993, 129:704–707.

21. Dai WS, Labraico JM, Stern RS: **Epidemiology of Isotretinoin Exposure During Pregnancy.** *J Am Acad Dermatol* 1992, 26:599–606.

22. Bottomley WW, Cunliffe WJ: **Acute Achilles Tendinitis Following Oral Isotretinoin Therapy for Acne Vulgaris.** *Clin Exp Dermatol* 1992, 17:250–251.

23. Schuderi AJ, Datz FL, Valdivia S, Morton KA: **Enthesopathy of the Patellar Tendon Insertion Associated With Isotretinoin.** *J Nucl Med* 1993, 34:455–457.

24. Hughes RA: **Arthritis Precipitated by Isotretinoin Treatment for Acne Vulgaris.** *J Rheumatol* 1993, 20:1241–1242.

25. Riordan CA, Anstey A, Wojnarowska F: **Isotretinoin Associated Pseudoporphyria.** *Clin Exp Dermatol* 1993, 18:69–71.

26. Bottomley WW, Cunliffe WJ: **Median Nail Dystrophy Associated With Isotretinoin Therapy.** *Br J Dermatol* 1992, 127:447–448.

27. Lerman S: **Ocular Side Effects of Accutane Therapy.** *Lens Eye Toxic Res* 1992, 9:429–438.

28. McCartney TL, Chen YK: **Marked Hyperlipidaemia and Pancreatitis Associated With Isotretinoin Therapy.** *Am J Gastroenterol* 1992, 87:1855–1858.

29. Karvonen SL: **Acne Fulminans: Report of Clinical Findings and Treatment of 24 Patients.** *J Am Acad Dermatol* 1993, 28:572–579.

30. Bottomly WW, Cunliffe WJ: **Severe Flare of Acne Following Isotretinoin: Large Closed Comedones (Macrocomedones) Are a Risk Factor.** *Acta Derm Venereol (Stockh)* 1993, 73:74.

31. Goulden V, Layton AM, Cunliffe WJ: **Long Term Safety of Isotretinoin as a Treatment for Acne Vulgaris.** *Br J Dermatol* 1994, in press.

32. Simpson NB: **Social and Economic Aspects of Acne and the Cost-Effectiveness of Isotretinoin.** *J Dermatol Treatment* 1993, 4:S6–S9.

Victoria Goulden and William J. Cunliffe, Dermatology Department, The General Infirmary at Leeds, Great George Street, Leeds LS1 3EX, UK.

Infections and infestations

Edited by

Neil A. Sadick

Cornell University Medical College
New York, New York, USA

CURRENT SCIENCE

Necrotizing soft-tissue infections

Daniel B. Dubin, MD, and Richard Allen Johnson, MD

Harvard Medical School, Boston, Massachusetts, USA

Necrotizing soft-tissue infections are characterized by varying degrees of cellulitis, tissue necrosis, septicemia, and septic shock. Unlike other types of soft-tissue infections, surgical debridement of devitalized structures is imperative in many cases. Antibiotic therapy is governed by the sensitivities of the causative microorganisms. In some instances, adjunctive hyperbaric oxygen therapy may reduce both mortality and the number of surgical debridements necessary in treating necrotizing fasciitis and bacterial myonecrosis. Without timely treatment, these infections can be lethal. Any integumental or mucous membrane disruption can facilitate introduction of microbes into the soft tissues and thus predispose to the development of deep necrotizing infection. The majority of patients who develop fulminant necrotizing infections have premorbid conditions that compromise immune defenses against microbial attack, yet these infections do, in some cases, occur in otherwise healthy patients.

Current Opinion in Dermatology 1995:235–242

Necrotizing soft-tissue infections (NSIs) differ from other variants of cellulitis because of the associated tissue necrosis, lack of response to antimicrobial treatment alone, and the need for surgical debridement of devitalized tissues. The elaboration of proteases, which degrade extracellular matrix and fat, in combination with exotoxins and endotoxins accounts for the rapid extension of these infections [1,2]. NSIs can be divided into three categories based on their depth of involvement: necrotizing cellulitis, necrotizing fasciitis (NF), and myonecrosis (Table 1) [3–5]. Because the fascial necrosis can be determined only by surgical exploration of the infected site and confirmed by histologic examination, NSIs cannot be diagnosed accurately on clinical findings alone. Rather, NF is a progression of necrotizing cellulitis, ie, necrotizing cellulitis with additional involvement of adjoining fascia; myonecrosis may represent a primary infection of muscle after traumatic injury or an extension of NF.

Pathogenesis

Trauma, surgical injury, or chronic cutaneous infection or inflammation facilitates entry of pathogenic organisms into the soft tissues. Inflammatory and bullous dermatoses have been implicated as the portal of entry for organisms causing necrotizing infections (Table 2). Diagnosis of NSI arising in a disorder such as pyoderma gangrenosum is particularly difficult. Systemic toxicity out of proportion to local skin involvement as well as the development of a putrid lesional odor should prompt urgent surgical exploration for fascial involvement beyond the margins of cutaneous ulceration.

Local tissue devitalization due to trauma is usually required to facilitate significant anaerobic bacterial growth. Other facilitating conditions for NSI include immunodeficiency syndromes, cirrhosis, diabetes mellitus, malnutrition, alcoholism, and systemic atherosclerosis. In a normal host, penetration of epithelial barriers by pathogens is usually not sufficient to initiate NSI. In some individuals, however, NSI can occur without either a clear portal of entry or a precedent predisposing disease [20].

Clinical features

Necrotizing cellulitis

Necrotizing cellulitis can be caused by a single microorganism or by several acting in synergy (Fig. 1). In immunocompetent hosts, organisms capable of acting alone in causing necrotizing cellulitis include group A β-hemolytic *Streptococcus pyogenes* (GAS), *Vibrio* species, *Aeromonas* species, and clostridia. In immunocompromised hosts, *Pseudomonas aeruginosa*, and opportunistic fungi such as *Mucor* or *Rhizopus* species can produce NSI [3]. Progressive synergistic cellulitis requires the joint action of an anaerobic streptococcal species with either *Staphylococcus aureus* or *Proteus* species, usually occurs in surgical or traumatic wounds, and is slowly but relentlessly progressive. Because fascial planes are not involved, the undermining

---

Abbreviations

EG—ecthyma gangrenosum; **GAS**—group A β-hemolytic *Streptococcus pyogenes*; **NF**—necrotizing fasciitis; **NSI**—necrotizing soft-tissue infection.

© 1995 Current Science ISBN 1-85922-686-8 ISSN 1068–381X

Table 1. Synopsis of necrotizing soft-tissue infections

Infection type	Predisposing factors	Onset; progression	Clinical findings	Systemic toxicity	Bacteriology	Pathologic findings	Tissue involvement
Cellulitis*							
Streptococcal necrotizing cellulitis	Usually arises in an epithelial break site, traumatic or surgical; GBS; patients often elderly but otherwise healthy	Rapid; may progress to NF if not treated	Fever; overlying skin becomes dusky blue ± bullae; may progress to necrosis of tissue; initially very painful; gangrenous areas become anesthetic	Severe	Usually GAS, occasionally GBS, in wound ± blood	Vasculitis, fibrin thrombi, necrosis of epidermis and dermis; heavy infiltrate of neutrophils; gram-positive cocci	Skin through fascia
Synergistic necrotizing cellulitis	Diabetes, perineal involvement, peripheral vascular disease, renal disease; may extend to involve fascia and muscle	Days; rapid	"Dishwater" pus or edema, crepitus, fever, blebs, necrosis; begins as an ulcer that gradually enlarges	Severe	Microaerophilic or anaerobic streptococi from edematous margin; Staphylococcus aureus from central ulcer	Dense leukocytic infiltration and edema of dermis and superficial muscle	Skin through muscle
Pseudomonas aeruginosa cellulitis and ecthyma gangrenosum	Neutropenia	Days; severe	Cellulitis with central necrosis in axillae or anogenital regions fever, sepsis	Moderate to severe	P. aeruginosa	Cellulitis with vasculitis	Subcutaneous tissues
Vibrio vulnificus cellulitis	Diabetes, alcoholism, cirrhosis; ingestion of raw seafood; trauma in aquatic environment	Days; severe	Fever, blebs, edema, pain	Moderate to severe	V. vulnificus and other species	Neutrophilic cellulitis and fasciitis	Skin through muscle
Aeromonas hydrophila cellulitis	Trauma; most patients are immunocompetent; 80% of patients are male	Days; severe	Cellulitis, NF, or myonecrosis	Mild to severe	A. hydrophila may be polymicrobial	Neutrophilic cellulitis and fasciitis	Skin through muscle
Clostridial cellulitis	Trauma	3–5 days; moderate	Fever, crepitus, blebs, red-brown fluid, edema, extreme wound pain	Mild	Clostridia, mixed gram-positive and -negative organisms	Dense leukocytic dermal infiltrate with necrosis of vessels and sweat glands	Subcutaneous tissues
Mucormycosis (zygomycosis, phycomycosis)	Diabetes with ketoacidosis; trauma to soft tissue; immunocompromise	Days; moderate to severe	May occur as primary cutaneous infection at site of injury or extension from deeper focus to overlying skin	Mild to severe	Mucoraceae	Large, branched, nonseptate hyphae invading blood vessel walls	Soft tissues ± deeper structures
Fasciitis†							
Necrotizing‡	Diabetes, trauma, peripheral vascular disease, decubitis ulcer, abdominal surgery, perirectal abscess, intestinal perforation, alcoholism, parenteral drug use	Hours, days; rapid	Red-purple color, blebs, edema, hypothesias, fever Sites: lower extremities, abdominal wall, perineum, operative wounds ± Crepitus	Moderate to severe	GAS or GBS; mixed infection with at least one facultative anaerobe; gram-positive cocci ± gram-negative bacilli	Intense leukocytic infiltration, focal necrosis of fascia, thrombosis of microvasculature	Skin through muscle
Myonecrosis§							
Clostridial myonecrosis	Trauma, wound contamination	Hours, days; rapid	"Bronze" erysipelas, sweet odor, fever, crepitus, necrosis, tan color	Severe	Clostridia, mixed gram-positive and -negative organisms	Dense leukocytic dermal infiltrate with hyaline necrosis of muscle and gas formation	Muscle to skin

*Cellulitis is defined as an acute, diffuse, spreading, edematous, suppurative inflammation of the deep tissues and sometimes muscle, which may be associated with abscess formation, tending to spread to tissue spaces and cleavage planes.
†Fasciitis is an inflammation of the fascia, a sheet or band of fibrous tissue such as lies deep to the skin or forms an investment for muscles and various organs of the body.
‡May represent a progression of streptococcal necrotizing cellulitis or synergistic necrotizing cellulitis. Fournier's gangrene, also known as streptococcal scrotal gangrene or perineal phlegmon, is a regional variant of NF occurring on the scrotum with spread to the penis, perineum, and abdominal wall.
§Myonecrosis is an acute, severe, and painful condition often resulting from dirty, lacerated wounds in which the muscles and subcutaneous tissues become filled with gas and serosanguineous exudate.
GAS—group A streptococcus; GBS—group B streptococcus; NF—necrotizing fasciitis.

of skin is limited to the edges of the lesion. Clostridial cellulitis is a crepitant anaerobic infection that is limited to the subcutaneous tissues and thus causes far less systemic toxicity than its cousin, clostridial myonecrosis.

Pseudomonas aeruginosa is capable of causing a cellulitis, which in some individuals may have a necrotizing component, which is referred to as ecthyma gangrenosum (EG). The most common predisposing fac-

Table 2. Mucocutaneous lesions associated with necrotizing soft-tissue infections

Mucocutaneous lesion	Study
Odontogenic infections	Reed and Annand [2], Mizuno *et al.* [6], Valko *et al.* [7]
GAS pharyngitis	Jahnson *et al.* [8]
Porphyria cutanea tarda	Wilkerson *et al.* [9]
Pyoderma gangrenosum	Jernec and Konradsen [10]
Insulin injection site in diabetic patients	Chin *et al.* [11]
Epinephrine injection site in asthmatic patients	Hallagan *et al.* [12]
Appendicitis	Jacobs *et al.* [13]
Vibrio gastroenteritis	Howard and Bennet [14•], Yuen *et al.* [15]
Carcinoma of colon	Corey [16], Wortman [17], Stevens *et al.* [1]
Chronic cutaneous lupus erythematosus, discoid lesion	Snider *et al.* [18]
Varicella (GAS)	Zittergruen and Grose [19]

GAS—group A β-hemolytic *Streptococcus pyogenes*.

tors associated with the occurrence of pseudomonal cellulitis and EG are absolute neutropenia and poor neutrophil function. The most common pathogen causing NSI in childhood is *P. aeruginosa* [21•]. Most often arising in the axillae or anogenital regions, *P. aeruginosa* gains entry into the dermis and subcutaneous tissues via adnexal epidermal structures. EG, however, has been reported to arise at nearly any cutaneous site [22]. Bacteremia occurs soon after the onset of EG, and may result in metastatic spread of *P. aeruginosa* infec-

tion to a distant site. Most cases of EG occur in primary soft-tissue infection with secondary bacteremia [23]; EG may occur secondarily, however, following hematogenous spread to the involved soft tissue. EG is characterized by a septic vasculitis, which results in progressive infarction of soft-tissues, and frequent bacteremia and septicemia. Clinically, EG is characterized by an initial cellulitis followed by infarction of the central area of the cellulitis, which occurs within the first few days (Fig. 2). If effective antibiotic therapy is not initiated promptly following onset of fever and cellulitis, the NSI may extend rapidly, with associated sepsis and shock.

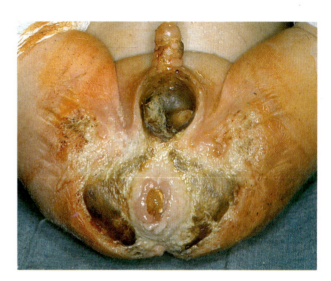

Fig. 1. Synergistic necrotizing cellulitis. Necrosis and sloughing involve much of the perineal soft tissue and extend into the muscle.

Vibrio vulnificus and other *Vibrio* species are capable of causing NSI. *V. vulnificus* is a free-living gram-negative rod that occurs naturally in the marine envi-

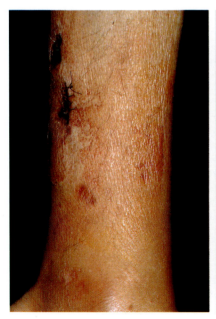
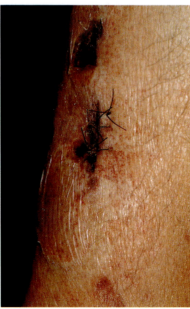

Fig. 2. Ecthyma gangrenosum. Areas of infarction are seen on the lower leg. The patient, a 65-year-old man with diabetes mellitus, had undergone amputation of the ipsilateral great toe 6 weeks previously because of peripheral vascular disease and had subsequently presented with fever and a painful cellulitis of the leg. Lesional skin biopsy showed aseptic vasculitis. *Pseudomonas aeruginosa* was isolated from the amputation stump, the necrotic tissue, and the blood.

ronment and is capable of contaminating oysters and other shellfish. Ingestion of seafood contaminated with *V. vulnificus* can result in gastroenteritis, primary septicemia, or both. *V. vulnificus* NSI can occur following septicemia and also by inoculation of the organism into breaks in the skin. During the past few years, numerous reports have documented cases of NSI caused by *V. vulnificus* [24–26] and other *Vibrio* species [27,28]. Most reported cases have occurred in Florida and the Gulf Coast (*ie*, Alabama, Louisiana, and Texas), with a peak incidence from May to October.

Aeromonas hydrophila is also found naturally in aqueous environments, and it is capable of causing soft-tissue infections with necrosis in an immunocompetent host [29,30••–32••]. *A. hydrophila* NSIs occur most often in the summertime, subsequent to injuries sustained in fresh water or the out-of-doors; the male-to-female ratio is 5:1. Other underlying conditions include AIDS, rectal cancer, stasis ulcers, and chronic osteomyelitis [33]. In one large series, 65% of cultures that contained isolates of *Aeromonas* also contained other organisms [30••]. Antibiotic selection should be based on sensitivities of the isolated organism. The third-generation cephalosporins such as cefoperazone and cefotaxime, the aminoglycosides (with the exception of streptomycin), trimethoprim-sulfamethoxazole, and the quinolones have proven to be the most active agents against *Aeromonas* species [34].

Necrotizing cellulitis has been reported with a variety of unusual pathogens especially in immunocompromised hosts. *Legionella micdadei*, primarily a pathogen of the pulmonary tract, has been reported to cause a necrotizing cellulitis beginning on the finger and extending proximally to the arm in a renal transplant recipient [35]. Amputation of the arm at the elbow was performed, and the patient survived.

Necrotizing fasciitis

Middle-aged to older patients are most likely to develop NF, although rare cases have been reported in neonates [36•]. NF can be caused by a single microorganism such as GAS [37], *Vibrio* species [14•,15], or Zygomycetes [38•]; however, the majority of cases are caused by polymicrobial infections with synergistic facultative aerobic (*Streptococcus* or Enterobacteriaceae) and anaerobic (*Bacteroides* and *Peptostreptococcus*) gas-forming organisms . In contrast to necrotizing cellulitis, in which skin changes demarcate the extent of disease, NF initially wreaks rapid destruction of fascial planes with relative sparing of the overlying dermis and epidermis.

Early cutaneous signs of bacterial NF include local erythema, marked edema, and moderate tenderness. Lymphangitis and regional lymphadenopathy are frequently absent. Later, gangrenous skin changes evolve as a consequence of thrombosis within nutrient dermal vessels, and the fasciitis spreads rapidly beyond the border of cutaneous necrosis (Fig. 3). As a consequence of cutaneous nerve necrosis, local tenderness is replaced by anesthesia (Fig. 4).

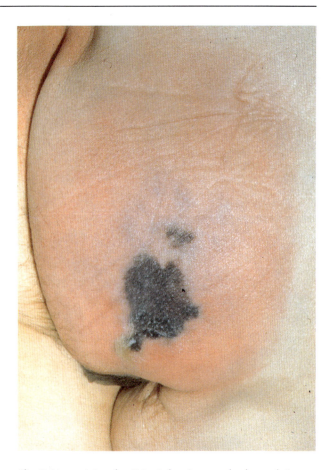

Fig. 3 Necrotizing fasciitis. Infarction on the buttock is surrounded by halo of cellulitis. (*Courtesy of* K. Wolff, Vienna, Austria.)

Synergistic polymicrobial NF is marked by a characteristic "dishwater pus" and toxicity out of proportion to the skin changes, with or without crepitation. Unlike necrotizing cellulitis, NF often requires debridement well beyond the margin of normal appearing skin.

Marine *Vibrio* species can cause sepsis and soft-tissue infections, particularly in patients with alcoholism, cirrhosis, and other chronic illnesses such as diabetes mellitus. It has been recommended that patients with cirrhosis, diabetes mellitus, and other chronic diseases avoid eating raw seafood. However, unlike *Vibrio vulnificus*, and *Vibrio alginolyticus*, which prey on compromised hosts, *Vibrio damsela* may cause fulminant necrotizing infections in immunocompetent patients. Either ingestion of raw seafood or exposure of open wounds to seawater can result in *Vibrio* bacteremia and soft tissue infection. Although most *Vibrio* infections are superficial and can be adequately treated with antibiotics, NF requiring surgical intervention does occur.

Invasive necrotizing phycomycoses of the soft tissues are an increasing cause of morbidity and mortality in patients with impaired immunity. Of the Phycomycetes, *Mucor*, *Absidia*, and *Rhizopus* organisms (family Mucoraceae) are the most common human pathogens and cause mucormycoses. Burn victims, trauma patients, and diabetic patients are partic-

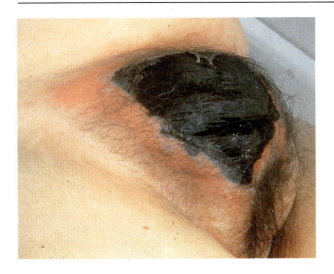

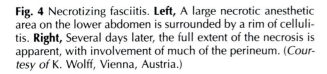

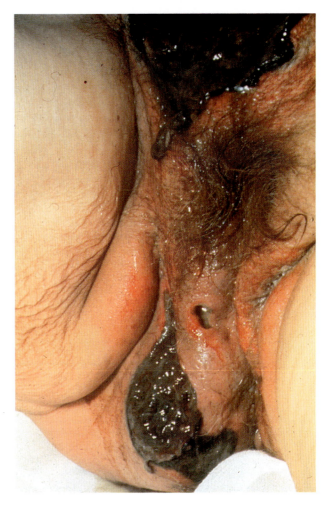

Fig. 4 Necrotizing fasciitis. **Left,** A large necrotic anesthetic area on the lower abdomen is surrounded by a rim of cellulitis. **Right,** Several days later, the full extent of the necrosis is apparent, with involvement of much of the perineum. (*Courtesy of* K. Wolff, Vienna, Austria.)

ularly susceptible to these infections. Mucormycoses are characterized by vascular invasion and occlusion, with subsequent tissue infarction and hematogenous dissemination of the invading fungus. Early diagnosis of phycomycetes can be made with a lesional biopsy specimen containing broad nonseptate hyphae, which branch at right angles. Once the condition is identified, surgical debridement and intravenous amphotericin B are indicated. As in deep necrotizing bacterial infections, mucormycoses extend rapidly and result in high mortality.

Regional variants

In contrast to necrotizing cellulitis and myonecrosis, NF has been classified according to the anatomic sites involved, such as Fournier's gangrene, or NF of the scrotum with or without involvement of the perineum (Table 3). In order of decreasing frequency of anatomic sites involved, NF arises on the extremities, trunk, perineum, and head and neck. On the extremities, the most common predisposing conditions are trauma, drug injection, and burns. In the absence of any obvious break in the skin, sites within the body should be sought, usually breaks in the gastrointestinal or urinary tract mucosa.

Necrotizing fasciitis of the penis with or without perineal involvement, also known as Fournier's gangrene, has been reported to occur following breaks of the skin, *ie*, a human bite injury of the penis [42], as well as breaks in the rectal mucosa, *ie*, a perirectal abscess [43]. NF of the vulva with or without perineal involvement has followed infected Bartholin's cysts and any perineal surgical procedure [44•]. Women with diabetes mellitus are particularly susceptible to necrotizing infections of the vulva [45•]. Vulvar NF has also been reported to have been complicated by the staphylococcal toxic shock syndrome [46].

Necrotizing fasciitis involving the head and neck most frequently occurs following odontogenic infections, but it may also occur following a variety of traumatic injuries [47]. The deep fascia of the neck invests the great vessels and communicates with the mediastinal and pleural compartments, providing a conduit for NF associated with mediastinitis, arterial erosion, jugular venous thrombosis, and empyema. NF of the head and neck can also spread superiorly along a relatively avascular fascial plane extending from the platysma to the galea aponeurotica. Anterior cervical NF may mimic acute thyroiditis [48]. NF of the eyelid, which might be better classified as a necrotizing cellulitis, may follow injury to the facial skin [49] and remain fairly well lo-

Table 3. Conditions predisposing to necrotizing fasciitis in various anatomic regions

Condition	Study
Extremities	Wang and Shih [39]
Trauma	
Drug injection	
Burns	
Chronic ulcers	
Abdomen	
Laparoscopy, gastrostomy tube placement, tubal ligation	Arhenholz [5]
Perforated appendix	Woodburn et al. [40•], Wang and Shih [39]
Peritonitis	
Perforation of colon	Woodburn et al. [40•], Jayatunga et al. [41•]
Omphalitis	Ryan et al. [36•]
Scrotum and perineum (Fournier's gangrene)	
Human bite of the penis	Wolf et al. [42]
Perirectal abscess	Bem [43]
Vulva and perineum	
Infected Bartholin's cysts and any perineal surgical procedure	Nolan et al. [44•]
Diabetes mellitus	Stephenson et al. [45•]

calized to the orbital tissue. The most commonly cultured organisms from periorbital NF cases are GAS alone or in combination with *S. aureus.* Dermatologists should be cautioned that necrotizing eyelid infections can complicate simple forehead epidermal cyst excision [49].

Bacterial myonecrosis

Bacterial myonecrosis has been classified into two etiologic types: clostridial and nonclostridial. *Clostridium perfringens*, *Clostridium novyi*, and *Clostridium septicum*, the etiologic agents of clostridial myonecrosis, thrive in the devitalized tissue of traumatized wounds, elaborating exotoxins that mediate the severe accompanying toxicity. The clinical course of infection progresses rapidly, with high morbidity and mortality in spite of adequate treatment. The earliest clinical lesion of myonecrosis is characterized by tenderness and tense edema with little epidermal change. A distinctively foul-smelling, serosanguineous discharge exudes from eroded areas within the infected site. Crepitation is often present, but it may be masked by the tense edema. Older lesions may have areas of yellow-bronze or green-black necrosis, at times with bulla formation.

Nonclostridial crepitant myonecrosis may be caused by anaerobic streptococci, other anaerobes acting in synergy, and *A. hydrophilia.* Unlike clostridial myonecrosis, streptococcal myonecrosis presents with overlying cutaneous erythema. Synergistic anaerobic myonecrosis, which is caused by the same organisms that cause polymicrobial NF, begins as a cellulitis, which extends

to involve the underlying muscle. Deep-penetrating, fresh water–associated trauma can rarely result in a crepitant *A. hydrophila* myonecrosis. Independent of the etiologic agent of bacterial myonecrosis, the prognosis is grave even with aggressive management.

Diagnosis

Both knowledge of the degree of systemic toxicity and the results of an integument examination may help differentiate superficial necrotizing cellulitis from an established, deeper NSI. Given the necessity to treat NSIs early, however, a low threshold for proceeding with surgical investigation should be maintained. Ahrenholtz [5] detailed indications for at least an open biopsy: confusion, tachycardia, tachypnea, ketoacidosis and hyperglycemia, gangrenous skin changes, bronzing of the skin, severe pain or spreading areas of anesthesia, thin reddish discharge with undermining of wound edges, crepitus, an abscess with multiple tracks, and cellulitis that either progresses despite antibiotics, has extensive surrounding edema, or complicates a surgical wound.

Early deep incisional lesional biopsy and histopathologic examination on frozen sections have been shown to improve mortality in NF by expediting treatment [50]. Necrosis and dense polymorphonuclear infiltration confined to the deep dermis and fascia in association with obliterative vascular thrombosis are classic for NF. Surgical exploration of NF with a gloved finger or metal probe reveals inordinately facile undermining of adjacent superficially uninvolved skin. In contrast, the surrounding fascial planes in necrotizing cellulitis maintain their normal resistance to blunt dissection.

Because incisional biopsy in young children may require general anesthesia, some have proposed serial magnetic resonance imaging to diagnose NF [19]. Although this approach may appear humane, early surgical intervention is preferable if NF is suspected. The risks and inconvenience of general anesthesia are far outweighed by a potential delay in diagnosis, which can result in disfiguring resections and loss of life. However, initial radiographic studies do have a role in identifying soft-tissue air and detecting extensive soft-tissue involvement.

Bacteriologic evaluation of wound exudate, bulla fluid, excised tissue, needle soft-tissue aspirates, and blood is essential. Isolation of pathogens from a clinical specimen usually takes days; however, Gram stains and fungal wet preparations of specimens are often helpful in arriving at an evaluation within minutes. A wound exudate with gram-positive rods and few polymorphonuclear leukocytes is nearly pathognomonic of clostridial infection. Fungal wet preparation of crushed tissue can identify hyphal forms and prompt the early administration of antifungal therapy. Gram stains may also be useful in tailoring antibiotic therapy for polymicrobial necrotizing infections, although broad coverage would be prudent until culture data are available.

Differential diagnosis

The differential diagnosis of dermal gangrene includes vasculitis, thromboembolic phenomenon, peripheral vascular disease, warfarin necrosis, calciphylaxis, traumatic injury, and toxin exposure. A careful history may be useful in excluding envenomation by the brown recluse spider, *Loxosceles reclusa*, which can induce a sterile, progressive necrotic cutaneous ulcer up to 30 cm in diameter, fever, and hemolysis [51]. Necrosis associated with a brown recluse spider bite may be attenuated by systemic corticosteroids or dapsone [52].

Treatment and prognosis

The mortality rate for NF has been reported to be 39%, and early diagnosis and aggressive treatment are the most important factors in determining outcome [53,54••]. Risk factors that can negatively affect outcome include age of more than 50 years, diabetes mellitus, malnutrition, hypertension, and intravenous drug abuse. Premorbid diabetes mellitus alone and the presence of three or more of these risk factors have been reported to be predictive of a significantly higher mortality rate [55••]. Overall, clostridial infections have an attendant mortality of 19% to 70%. Spontaneously occurring myonecrosis has a more ominous mortality of 67% to 100% owing to its insidious onset and high association with underlying malignancy. Death is usually due to sepsis, multisystem organ failure, or invasion of major vessels.

Treatment of NSI centers on early and complete surgical debridement of necrotic tissue in combination with high-dose antibiotics. Until bacteriologic data identify the causative pathogens, broad coverage is recommended. Vancomycin, gentamicin, and either metronidazole or clindamycin have constituted an effective initial regimen for treating suspected nonclostridial NSI. While clostridia are susceptible to penicillin, clindamycin, and chloramphenicol, optimal treatment has not been established. High-dose penicillin either alone or in combination with clindamycin or chloramphenicol may be adequate.

Although prospective studies are lacking, retrospective data indicate that adjunctive hyperbaric oxygen therapy may reduce morbidity and mortality in both clostridial and nonclostridial necrotizing infections [56••,57,58]. Proposed mechanisms by which hyperbaric oxygen could improve outcome include enhancement of leukocyte production of bactericidal free radicals, direct inhibition of anaerobic bacterial growth, preservation of poorly perfused tissue, and promotion of wound healing.

Further important considerations in the treatment of these often critically ill patients include nutritional support, fecal diversion, and surgical drains when serosal lined cavities are involved. Debridement defects should never be repaired primarily. Healing by second intention or delayed closure is acceptable. Secondary plastic surgery should be considered for correction of functional or cosmetic defects.

Conclusions

Necrotizing soft-tissue infections are associated with high morbidity and mortality. The incidence is increasing in the expanding population of iatrogenically immunocompromised individuals. Early diagnosis and initiation of effective treatment, which includes antibiotics and surgical debridement, improve the prognosis of affected individuals.

References and recommended reading

Papers of particular interest, published within the annual period of review, have been highlighted as:
•   Of special interest
•• Of outstanding interest

1. Stevens DL, Musher DM, Watson DA, Eddy H, Hamill RJ, Gyorkey F, Rosen H, Mader J: **Spontaneous, Nontraumatic Gangrene Due to Clostridium septicum.** *Rev Infect Dis* 1990, 12:286–296.

2. Reed MJ, Annand VK: **Odontogenic Cervical Necrotizing Fasciitis With Intrathoracic Extension.** *Otolaryngol Head Neck Surg* 1992, 104:596–600.

3. Swartz MN: **Skin and Soft Tissue Infections.** In *Principles and Practice of Infectious Diseases*, edn 3. Edited by Mandell GL, Douglas RG, Bennet JE. New York:Churchill Livingstone; 1990:796–817.

4. Patino JF, Castro D: **Necrotizing Lesions of Soft Tissues: A Review.** *World J Surg* 1991, 15:235–239.

5. Arhenholtz DH: **Necrotizing Soft Tissue Infections.** *Surg Clin North Am* 1988, 68:199–214.

6. Mizuno I, Mizutani H, Ueda M, Kaneda T: **Temporal Necrotizing Infection of Dental Origin.** *J Oral Maxillofac Surg* 1993, 51:79–81.

7. Valko PC, Barrett SM, Campbell JP: **Odontogenic Cervical Necrotizing Fasciitis.** *Ann Emerg Med* 1990, 19:568–571.

8. Jahnson L, Axelsson JE, Berggren L, Bjorsell-Ostling E, Bonnerstig J, Holmberg H: **Streptococcal Myositis.** *Scand J Infect Dis* 1992, 24:661–665.

9. Wilkerson R, Paull W, Coville FV: **Necrotizing Fasciitis.** *Clin Orthop* 1987, 216:187–192.

10. Jernec G, Konradsen L: **Pyoderma Gangrenosum Complicated by Necrotizing Fasciitis.** *Cutis* 1994, 53:139–141.

11. Chin RL, Martinez R, Garmel G: **Gas Gangrene From Subcutaneous Insulin Administration.** *Am J Emerg Med* 1993, 11:622–625.

12. Hallagan LF, Scott JL, Hrowitz BC, Feied CF: **Clostridial Myonecrosis Resulting From Subcutaneous Epinephrine Suspension.** *Ann Emerg Med* 1992, 21:434–436.

13. Jacobs P, van der Sluis R, Tack C, Wobbes T: **Necrotizing Fasciitis of the Lower Limb Caused by Undiagnosed Perforated Appendicitis, Which Necessitated Disarticulation of the Hip.** *Eur J Surg* 1993, 159:307–308.

14. Howard RJ, Bennet NT: **Infections Caused by Halophilic Marine Vibrio Bacteria.** *Ann Surg* 1993, 217:525–531.
•
Marine *Vibrio* bacteria can cause necrotizing soft-tissue infections, especially in patients with severe liver disease and other chronic illnesses such as diabetes mellitus. Both ingestion of raw seafood and direct exposure to seawater can introduce *Vibrio* species into the soft tissues.

15. Yuen K, Ma L, Wong S, Ng W: **Fatal Necrotizing Fasciitis Due to Vibrio Damsela.** *Scand J Infect Dis* 1993, 25:659–661.

16. Corey EC: **Nontraumatic Gas Gangrene: Case Report and Review of the Literature.** *J Emerg Med* 1991, 9:431–436.

17. Wortman PD: **Bacterial Infections of the Skin.** *Curr Probl Dermatol* 1993, 5:195–224.

18. Snider JM, McNabey WK, Pemberton LB: **Necrotizing Fasciitis Secondary to Discoid Lupus Erythematosus.** *Am Surg* 1993, 59:164–169.

19. Zittergruen M, Grose C: **Magnetic Resonance Imaging for Early Diagnosis of Necrotizing Fasciitis.** *Pediatr Emerg Care* 1993, 9:26–28.

20.   Rich RS, Salluzzo RF: **Spontaneous Clostridial Myonecrosis in a Non-immunocompromised Patient.** *Ann Emerg Med* 1993, 22:1477–1480.

21.   Boisseau AM, Sarlangue J, Perel Y, Hehunstre JP, Taieb A, Maleville
•   J: **Perineal Ecthyma Gangrenosum in Infancy and Early Childhood: Septic and Nonsepticemic Forms.** *J Am Acad Dermatol* 1992, 27:415–418.
Case reports of six neutropenic children with anogenital perineal EG, one of whom died of the infection.

22.   Sevinsky LD, Viecens C, Ballesteros DO, Stengel F: **Ecthyma Gangrenosum: A Cutaneous Manifestation of *Pseudomonas aeruginosa* Sepsis.** *J Am Acad Dermatol* 1992, 29:106–108.

23.   Fergie JE, Patrick CC, Lott L: ***Pseudomonas aeruginosa* Cellulitis and Ecthyma Gangrenosum in Immunocompromised Children.** *Pediatr Infect Dis J* 1991, 10:496–500.

24.   ***Vibrio vulnificus* Infections Associated With Raw Oyster Consumption: Florida, 1981–1992.** *MMWR Morbid Mortal Wkly Rep* 1993, 42:405–407.

25.   Levine WC, Griffin PM, Gulf Coast *Vibrio* Working Group: **Vibrio Infections on the Gulf Coast: Results of First Year of Regional Surveillance.** *J Infect Dis* 1993, 167:479–483.

26.   Raza H, Cutrona AF: ***Vibrio vulnificus* Septicemia Should Prompt the Search For Liver Disease.** *Infect Dis Clin Pract* 1993, 2:273–274.

27.   Rabinowitch BL, Nam MH, Levy CS, Smith MA: ***Vibrio parahaemolyticus* Septicemia Associated with Water Skiing [Letter, Comment].** *Clin Infect Dis* 1993, 16:339–340.

28.   Perez-Tirse J, Levine JF, Mecca M: ***Vibrio damsela*: A Cause of Fulminant Septicemia.** *Arch Intern Med* 1993, 153:1838–1840.

29.   **Aeromonas Wound Infections Associated With Outdoor Activities: California.** *MMWR Morbid Mortal Wkly Rep* 1990, 39:334–335.

30.   Voss LM, Rhodes KH, Johnson KA: **Musculoskeletal and Soft Tissue
••   Aeromonas Infection: An Environmental Disease.** *Mayo Clin Proc* 1992, 67:422–427.
Report of 28 cases of *Aeromonas* infection from the Mayo Clinic; 13 of 23 cases followed an acute open or penetrating water-related injury. All *Aeromonas* isolates were sensitive to gentamycin sulfate, cefuroxime sodium, and the third-generation cephalosporins. Surgical debridement was an integral part of therapy.

31.   Gold WL, Salit IE: ***Aeromonas hydrophila* Infections of Skin and
••   Soft Tissue: Report of 11 Cases and Review.** *Clin Infect Dis* 1993, 16:69–74.
Report of 11 cases of skin and soft-tissue *A. hydrophila* infections, nine of which were community-acquired and two nosocomial. Underlying systemic diseases including alcoholism and chemotherapy for metastatic breast cancer were present in three individuals. The extent of infection ranged from abscess formation to myonecrosis with subcutaneous gas.

32.   Kelly KA, Koehler JM, Ashdown LR: **Spectrum of Extraintestinal Disease Due to Aeromonas Species in Tropical Queensland, Australia.**
••   *Clin Infect Dis* 1993, 16:574–579.
Report of 56 cases of extraintestinal *Aeromonas* infection occurring during a 12-month period; 46 patients had community-acquired infection, and 6 had nosocomial infection. Of the 46 patients with community-acquired infections, 22 required hospitalization, and 27 had trauma-associated infections (63% of which were on the hands or feet exposed to surface water or soil).

33.   Bonatus TJ, Alexander AH: **Posttraumatic *Aeromonas hydrophila* Osteomyelitis.** *Orthopedics* 1990, 13:1158–1163.

34.   Baddour LM: **Extraintestinal *Aeromonas* Infections: Looking for Mr. Sandbar.** *Mayo Clin Proc* 1992, 67:496–498.

35.   Kilborn JA, Manz LA, O'Brien M, Douglass MC, Horst HM, Kupin W, Fisher EJ: **Necrotizing Cellulitis Caused by *Legionella micdadei*.** *Am J Med* 1992, 92:104–106.

36.   Ryan CA, Fischer J, Gayle M, Wenman W: **Surgical and Postoperative
•   Management of Two Neonates With Necrotizing Fasciitis.** *Can J Surg* 1993, 36:337–341.
Case reports of two neonates with NF complicating omphalitis treated with surgical debridement of the anterior abdominal wall. One child survived, and the other died of sepsis.

37.   Weinbren MJ, Perinpanayagam RM: **Streptococcal Necrotizing Fasciitis.** *J Infect* 1992, 25:299–302.

38.   Virden CP, Lynch FP, Hansbrough JF: **Invasive Necrotizing Phycomycoses.** *Infect Med* 1993, 10:30–33.
•
Invasive necrotizing phycomycotic infections usually occur in immunocompromised patients and cause high morbidity and mortality.

39.   Wang K, Shih C: **Necrotizing Fasciitis of the Extremities.** *J Trauma* 1992, 32:179–182.

40.   Woodburn KR, Ramsay G, Gillespie G, Miller DF: **Retroperitoneal
•   Necrotizing Fasciitis.** *Br J Surg* 1992, 79:342–344.
Five cases of retroperitoneal NF not amenable to adequate debridement were uniformly fatal.

41.   Jayatunga AP, Caplan S, Paes TRF: **Survival After Retroperitoneal
•   Necrotizing Fasciitis.** *Br J Surg* 1993, 80:981.
Early diagnosis and treatment saved the life of one patient with retroperitoneal NF. Treatment included fecal diversion, high-dose antibiotics, and peritoneal drainage, but surgical debridement was limited owing to anatomical constraints.

42.   Wolf JS, Gomez R, McAninch JW: **Human Bites to the Penis.** *J Urol* 1992; 147:1265–1267.

43.   Bem C: **Necrotizing Fasciitis: 10 Years' Experience in a District General Hospital [Letter, Comment].** *Br J Surg* 1992, 79:1247.

44.   Nolan TE, King LA, Smith RP, Gallup DC: **Necrotizing Surgical In-
•   fection and Necrotizing Fasciitis in Obstetrical and Gynecologic Patients.** *South Med J* 1993, 86:1363–1367.
Case reports of five patients with underlying obstetric or gynecologic problems and NF. Underlying problems were diabetes mellitus, Bartholin's gland abscess, and recent surgical procedures (including episiotomy).

45.   Stephenson H, Dotters DJ, Vatz V, Droegemueller W: **Necrotizing
•   Fasciitis of the Vulva.** *Am J Obstet Gynecol* 1992, 166:1324–1327.
Delays in recognition of vulvar NF were associated with increased morbidity and mortality. Twenty of the 29 patients studied were diabetic, and they accounted for 11 of the 14 deaths reported.

46.   Farley DE, Katz VL, Dotters DJ: **Toxic Shock Syndrome Associated
•   With Vulvar Necrotizing Fasciitis.** *Obstet Gynecol* 1993, 82:660–662.
One patient developed toxic shock syndrome 3 days after successful surgical treatment of a vulvar NF caused by multiple organisms including *S. aureus*.

47.   Kaddour HS, Smelt FR: **Necrotizing Fasciitis of the Neck.** *J Laryngol Otol* 1992, 106:1008–1010.

48.   Gillis AR, Gillis TM: **Necrotizing Cervical Fasciitis of Unknown Origin.** *J Otolaryngol* 1992, 21:171–173.

49.   Overholt EM, Flint PW, Overholt EL, Murakami CS: **Necrotizing Fasciitis of the Eyelids.** *Otolaryngol Head Neck Surg* 1992, 106:339–344.

50.   Stamenkovic I, Lew PD: **Early Recognition of Potentially Fatal Necrotizing Fasciitis: The Use of Frozen-Section Biopsy.** *N Engl J Med* 1984, 310:1689–1693.

51.   Hobbs GD, Harrell RE: **Brown Recluse Spider Bite.** *Am J Emerg Med* 1989, 7:309–312.

52.   Ingber A, Trattner A, Cleper R, Sandbank M: **Morbidity of Brown Recluse Spider Bites.** *Acta Derm Venereol (Stockh)* 1991, 71:337–340.

53.   Ward RG, Walsh MS: **Necrotizing Fasciitis: 10 Years' Experience in a District General Hospital.** *Br J Surg* 1991, 78:488–489.

54.   Voros D, Pissiotis C, Georganta D, Katsargakis S, Antoniou S, Pa-
••   padimitriou J: **Role of Early and Extensive Surgery in the Treatment of Severe Necrotizing Soft Tissue Infection.** *Br J Surg* 1993, 80:1191–1192.
Of 30 patients with NSI, only two died following early diagnosis and treatment, whereas delayed surgical intervention in 12 patients led to 9 deaths.

55.   Francis KR, Lamute HR, Davis JM, Fizzi WF: **Implications of Risk
••   Factors in Necrotizing Fasciitis.** *Am Surg* 1993, 59:304–308.
Of 25 patients with NF, those who died exhibited a significantly higher percentage of diabetes mellitus than those who survived. Malnutrition, hypertension, old age, and intravenous drug abuse are also implicated as predictors of poor outcome.

56.   Kindwall   EP: **Hyperbaric   Oxygen.**   *BMJ*   1993,   307:515–
••   516.
This article details the current indications for hyperbaric oxygen therapy.

57.   Riseman JA, Zamboni WA, Curtis A, Graham DR, Konrad HB, Ross DS: **Hyperbaric Oxygen Therapy for Necrotizing Fasciitis Reduces Mortality and the Need for Debridements.** *Surgery* 1990, 108:847–850.

58.   Burge TS, Zamboni WA, Kindwall EP: **Hyperbaric Oxygen: Still Unproved in Necrotizing Fasciitis.** *BMJ* 1993, 307:936.

Daniel B. Dubin, MD, and Richard A. Johnson, MD, New England Deaconess Hospital, Harvard Medical School, Department of Dermatology, 110 Francis Street, Suite 7H, Boston, MA 02115, USA.

Dermatologic infections in the world traveler

Diana N. J. Lockwood, MRCP, and Francisco Kerdel-Vegas, MD

Northwick Park Hospital, Harrow, Middlesex, UK, and
National Academy of Medicine, Caracas, Venezuela

Tropically acquired dermatoses are an increasing problem as global travel becomes more common. The most common lesion acquired in the tropics is a secondarily infected insect bite, but clinicians should be aware of other potential diagnoses. A careful history focusing on the type of travel, the areas visited, and the risk factors for infections such as cutaneous leishmaniasis and cutaneous larva migrans is crucial in making the correct diagnosis. Herein we discuss the etiology, diagnosis, and management of tropically acquired papules, linear lesions, ulcers, and myiasis. Although the likely range of diagnoses is quite small, it is important that these conditions should be borne in mind because misdiagnosis and delayed diagnosis are common.

Current Opinion in Dermatology 1995:243–248

The dermatologist faced with a skin condition in someone who has traveled abroad needs to be a geographically, ecologically, and culturally aware detective. The etiology of such a lesion will be determined by where patients have traveled, how long they have traveled, and what type of travel, sport, and leisure pursuits they have followed. A careful travel history, noting not just the main locations visited but also short stops en route, is vital to making a diagnosis. A chronic ulcerating lesion appearing after residence in Southern Africa, for example, will be difficult to recognize as leishmaniasis until the supplementary history of prior residence in the Middle East is obtained. The length of stay is also a critical determinant of the range of diagnostic possibilities; the Peace Corps worker who resides in rural South America for 2 years is at far greater risk of contracting trypanosomiasis than the adviser who visits villages for 1 or 2 days. The most important variable is the type of travel; businessmen visiting capital cities in the tropics are unlikely to acquire tropical skin complaints, but field workers, anthropologists, construction workers, and adventurous tourists on treks through remote areas are at risk of acquiring exotic dermatoses.

The ecology of areas visited is important, because altitude and climate have a profound effect upon the flora and fauna of a location. Many tropical conditions are metoxenous, ie, they require two hosts for the full life cycle. These diseases usually have a vertebrate reservoir that may carry the disease either passively or in a chronic pathological form. The other reservoir is usually invertebrate, and in this host sexual multiplication of the parasite occurs. Old World cutaneous leishmaniasis (CL) is a good example of this life cycle, with dogs being the vertebrate host and sandflies the invertebrate host for the parasite *Leishmania tropica*. Humans are infected accidentally when bitten by an infected sandfly. Many parasitic diseases that have an extrahuman reservoir and need a vector for transmission occur only in rural environments where both the vertebrate reservoir and insects thrive, providing the ecological niche for the parasite. One may regard humans as invaders of this ecosystem and therefore at risk for bites by parasite-infested insects. Zoonoses, infections of animals that are transmitted to humans, are another important category of conditions to be aware of, and animal contact should be specifically inquired about.

It is difficult to obtain published data on the frequency and types of skin lesions occurring after tropical travel. This lack of data is partly due to the fact that straightforward conditions are managed by family doctors, only those lesions causing diagnostic difficulty are referred to dermatologists, and only a very small subset of lesions reach dermatologists with tropical expertise. The development of chronic tropical dermatoses in visitors to the tropics is a rare event. Short-term travelers (<3 weeks) very rarely acquire diseases such as leprosy, yaws, filariasis, Buruli ulcers, or cysticercosis. These disorders are usually only seen in immigrants and are unusual even in long-stay travelers (>3 months) or overseas workers. When Lockwood and Keystone [1••] reviewed the dermatoses presenting to the Tropical Disease Unit at Toronto Hospital, secondarily infected insect bites, pyoderma, cutaneous larva migrans (CLM), and nonspecific dermatitis were the most frequently diagnosed conditions. Preexisting chronic dermatoses

---

Abbreviations
CL—cutaneous leishmaniasis; **CLM**—cutaneous larva migrans.

such as eczema are frequently worsened by hot, humid climates.

A useful approach to the diagnosis of a presumed tropically acquired lesion is to consider the appearance of the lesion. Our discussion focuses on common tropical skin conditions and is grouped by type of lesion. Table 1 summarizes the conditions discussed.

Papules

The most frequent papular lesions seen in returning travelers are arthropod bites caused by mosquitoes, midges, sandflies, and fleas, all of which have a worldwide distribution. The appearance of individual bite reactions is usually nondiagnostic, but the configuration of multiple bites may provide useful clues as to the etiology. Bites caused by fleas, bedbugs, and reduviid (kissing) bugs are often grouped in clusters or have a linear distribution. Most arthropod bites are pruritic, but the bites of deer, tsetse, and black flies are usually painful.

Bites from stinging arthropods such as scorpions, brown recluse spiders, and hymenopterans (bees, wasps, and fire ants, for example) must also be considered in the differential diagnosis of painful bites. In coastal travelers, stings from venomous jellyfish and sea urchins should be considered.

It is not uncommon for patients to complain of pruritic insect bites that come and go for weeks or months after return from the tropics. These prolonged reactions are most often associated with bedbug and flea bites. The Venezuelan Caripito itch, characterized by intense itching with wheals, may be produced by contact with swarms of migrating *Hylesia urticans* adult moths [2].

Scabies, caused by the mite *Sarcoptes scabiei*, is extremely common in the tropics. It is usually seen in the backpacking adventurous traveler. The mite's burrow, a gray or skin-colored linear, raised ridge measuring a few millimeters to 1.5 cm, is most frequently found on the finger webs, wrists, genitalia, axillary folds, and female nipples. Generalized pruritic urticarial papules due to parasite sensitization appear 6 to 8 weeks after the initial infestation. Scabies is diagnosed by unroofing a burrow with a needle or scalpel blade coated with oil and examining scrapings microscopically for mites and their ova.

Miliaria rubra (prickly heat), a frequent disorder in travelers to tropical environments, results from sweat gland blockage. It is characterized by a discrete, erythematous, papular, or vesicular eruption that spares hair follicles and is usually confined to covered areas of the body. The lesions are usually pruritic or stinging.

In long-stay travelers, particularly those from West and Central Africa, onchocerciasis and streptocerciasis are two forms of filariasis that may present with a pruritic papular rash, most often on the trunk or lower extremity. These patients are usually lightly infected with only pruritus or a mild rash. One does not see the advanced skin atrophy of oncocercal dermatitis that is reported from populations in the endemic area. In travelers, 18 months or more may pass before the first symptoms appear [3•]. The diagnosis is made by searching for microfilaria that migrate out of skin snips made with a corneal scleral punch biopsy.

Contact with insects should be considered when diagnosing vesicles and blisters. Both the Spanish fly (*Lytta*

Table 1. Common causes of skin lesions in returning travelers

Lesion type	Etiology	Clinical features
Papules		
Insect bites	Mosquito	Pruritic wheal, flare, or papule
	Flea	Discrete pruritic papule with central hemorrhagic punctum
	Tick	Painful swelling with central necrosis and erythematous margin
	Bedbug	Pruritic papules in a linear configuration
Scabies	*Sarcoptes scabiei*	Raised linear burrows
Prickly heat	None	Erythematous, vesicular eruption around sweat glands
Onchocerciasis	*Onchocerca volvulus*	Pruritic, papular rash
Linear lesions		
Cutaneous larva migrans	Animal hookworm	Severely pruritic serpiginous track
Larva currens	*Strongyloides stercoralis*	Pruritic, fast-moving erythematous band
Ulcers		
Ecthyma	*Staphylococcus aureus*, β-hemolytic *Streptococcus*	Vesicle or crusted pustule
Leishmaniasis	*Leishmania*	Indolent, slow-healing ulcer
Rickettsial eschar	*Rickettsia conorii*	Small ulcer with black center, systemic illness
Myobacterial infection	*Mycobacterium marinum*	Violaceous nodule, late ulceration
Subcutaneous swellings		
Myiasis	*Dermatobia hominis* larva, *Cordylobia anthropophaga* larva	Larva protruding from subcutaneous cavity

vesicatoria) and the rove beetle (genus *Paederus*) contain toxic materials in their body fluids that produce blisters on contact with human skin [4].

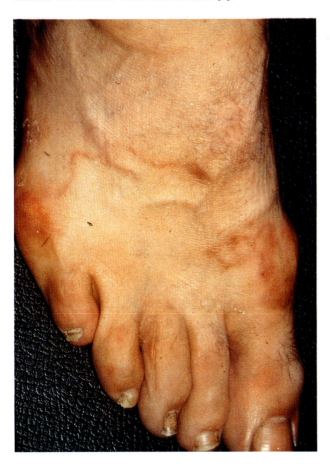

Fig. 1. Cutaneous larva migrans on the foot of a traveler who had been on a beach holiday in the Caribbean.

Linear lesions

Cutaneous larva migrans is the most frequent linear lesion seen in travelers. Lesions are produced by the migration of the larval stage of the dog hookworm (*eg, Ankylostoma caninum*). Production of proteolytic enzymes accompanies larval migration through the skin, resulting in local inflammation, and the migration is marked by an intensely pruritic, linear serpiginous lesion (Fig. 1). It is exceedingly rare for these dog hookworms to establish infection in the human host, so the condition is not as alarming as first appears. Davies *et al.* [5••] have reviewed cases of CLM seen at a Canadian tropical disease unit. The majority of patients had recently vacationed in the tropics, particularly the Caribbean. The mean time from arrival in the tropics to onset of the lesion was 14 days (range 2 to 50 days), and 48% of the patients had returned home by the time the lesion developed. Ninety-five percent had visited a beach and there exposed the subsequently affected part. In 87%, the plantar aspect of the foot was affected; other affected sites included elbows, breasts,

and buttocks. The lesions were characteristic of CLM, with 98% of patients complaining of pruritus and 96% having a linear, serpiginous track. Fifty-eight percent of these Canadian patients had been either misdiagnosed or treated inappropriately before referral to a specialist unit. Local application of 15% thiabendazole cream twice daily cured 98% of the patients in the Canadian study. Albendazole has also been shown to be very efficacious in the treatment of CLM when given orally as a single 400-mg dose or at a dosage of 200 mg twice daily for 3 days [6–8]. A French group recently reported their experience in using ivermectin (the current drug of choice for onchocerciasis) for the treatment of CLM [9]. In a small, open prospective study, 12 patients with CLM were given a single 12-mg oral dose of ivermectin; in all cases the pruritus resolved completely, and the progression of the larval tracks stopped within 48 hours. No side effects related to the ivermectin were reported.

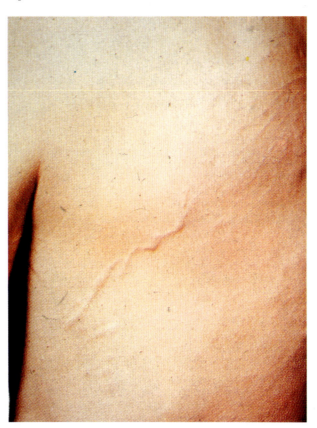

Fig. 2. The transient urticarial rash of larva currens in chronic strongyloidiasis acquired in Thailand.

The migratory path of *Strongyloides stercoralis* larvae produces a faster-moving track, larva currens, moving at a rate of 5 to 10 cm per hour, compared with 2 to 3 cm per day for the dog hookworm. This urticarial wheal surrounded by a flare is intensely itchy and often transient (Fig. 2), lasting only a few hours. The lesions are seen on the buttocks, groin, and trunk, tending to occur in crops over a few days with weeks of freedom in between. Vague gastrointestinal pain or diarrhea often accompanies the rash, as does eosinophilia. The parasite can remain in the same host for many years by autoinfection. Infections have gone undiagnosed in ex–World War II Far East prisoners of war for 30 years after their liberation [10]. A recent study on these veterans showed that albendazole is the treatment of choice for chronic strongyloidiasis [11•].

Ulcers

The most frequent cutaneous ulcer in a returning traveler is ecthyma, a shallow, painful, purulent ulcer, resulting from skin trauma or insect bites that have become infected with pyogenic organisms, particularly *Staphylococcus aureus* or group A streptococci. Erysipelas, cellulitis, furuncles, and carbuncles are all common in the tropics.

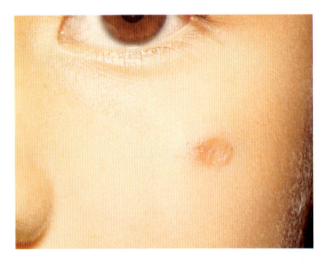

Fig. 3. A typical New World cutaneous leishmaniasis lesion in a Venezuelan child.

All other types of tropical ulcers are rare. Although rare, CL should be considered in the differential diagnosis of an ulcerating skin lesion. Herwaldt *et al.* [12••] have reviewed 59 US civilians who acquired New World leishmaniasis requiring treatment with sodium stibogluconate. Fifty-six percent of this group had been infected in Mexico or Central America, and 46% were conducting field studies. Travel in forested areas was an important risk factor, with 98% of the travelers having spent time in forests. The time spent in forests varied from 2 to 180 days and lesions appeared from day 1 onward. Seventeen percent of patients did not notice lesions for at least 1 month after returning. Patients consulted one to seven physicians (mean 2.1) before a diagnosis was reached. Overall, the median time from noticing lesions to treatment was 112 days, and even in patients unusually knowledgeable about leishmaniasis it was 55 days. The calculated risk of US travelers acquiring CL ranges from one per 1000 visitors to Surinam to less than one per million visitors to Mexico. A series of American civilians with CL treated at the National Institutes of Health covers the whole spectrum of CL [13••]. Cutaneous lesions acquired in the New World usually consisted of one or two lesions (Fig. 3), whereas multiple lesions often characterized Old World infections. Chronic relapsing and diffuse cutaneous disease were only seen in patients native to endemic areas who had been infected at an early age. Old World leishmaniasis has been reported in Fijian soldiers stationed in Sinai as part of the multinational peacekeeping force, emphasizing the importance of a careful travel history [14]. Leishmaniasis in soldiers has also been featured in reports of New World CL in British soldiers stationed in Belize [15•]. In all these series typical leishmanial ulcers have been described, being indolent with a granulomatous or crusted base and heaped-up margins. Leishmaniasis may occasionally present in a linear fashion, with ulcers spreading along lymphatics similarly to sporotrichosis or *Mycobacterium marinum* infections.

Optimal treatment of CL has not yet been agreed upon. The options for treatment and future drug development have been well reviewed by Olliaro and Bryceson [16••]. Treatment of CL is complex because several different species of *Leishmania* parasites cause CL and in many cases the lesions are self-healing. The World Health Organization recommends that for Old World disease, uncomplicated lesions in inconspicuous sites do not require treatment, whereas sodium stibogluconate is recommended either intralesionally for early inflamed nodular lesions or systemically for complicated lesions [17]. The only reported placebo-controlled trial for Old World CL was unable to show superiority of antimonials over placebo [18]. Ketoconazole has been used successfully in all New and Old World and mucocutaneous leishmaniasis but has not been subjected to placebo-controlled trials [14]. The lack of new, efficacious, nontoxic drugs for a common tropical problem reflects the relative lack of interest by the major pharmaceutical companies in developing therapies for unprofitable markets in the Third World.

Certain clues in the history or examination may point to the cause of an ulcer. The granulomatous ulcer seen in *M. marinum* infection (fish tank granuloma), for example, is associated with exposure to water, particularly swimming pools, and grows as a nodular, hyperkeratotic growth on the extremities.

Tick eschars due to *Rickettsia conorii* are not infrequently seen in people who have visited game parks in Southern Africa or walked in the bush. The eschar starts as an erythematous macule at the bite site and progresses through papular, vesicular, and necrotic stages to form a painless, small, black lesion surrounded by an erythematous halo. Regional adenopathy is common and the generalized illness is accompanied by fever, a macular rash, and intense headaches.

The investigation of a cutaneous ulcer from the tropics begins with a swab of the base for bacterial culture. Mycobacterial and fungal disorders are diagnosed by histology or culture of the viable ulcer edge. *Leishmania* amastigotes may be detected by Giemsa stain of biopsy or a touch preparation of the ulcer edge or culture of ulcer material.

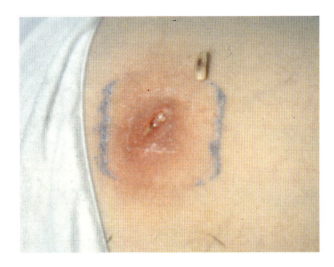

Fig. 4. Abdominal myiasis in an expatriate from the UK who had resided in West Africa. (*Courtesy of* R. N. Davidson, Harrow, Middlesex, UK.)

Subcutaneous swellings

Myiasis is the most common subcutaneous swelling and is caused by infestation of the skin with larvae of the South American botfly *Dermatobia hominis* and the African Tumbu fly *Cordylobia anthropophaga*. The larvae develop in a subcutaneous space with a central sinus. This orifice serves as an air source for the larvae, and the larval respiratory spiracles periodically protrude through the sinus (Fig. 4). Patients with myiasis often feel movement within the larval burrow and experience intermittent sharp, lancinating pains. The diagnosis of myiasis is made on clinical grounds and should be suspected in any furuncular lesion accompanied by pain and a crawling sensation in the skin. Pallai *et al.* [19•] reported four cases in travelers to Central America and noted the importance of differentiating between myiasis and early leishmaniasis. Treatment has traditionally relied on extruding the larva by squeezing gently on the burrow and catching the larva with tweezers. A variety of methods for suffocating the larva have been proposed, most notably occluding the respiratory orifice with raw bacon fat [20,21]. Nunn [22•] has reported the problems that may occur with injudicious attempts at removal of these larvae and advocates the traditional tweezer method or sticking plaster. Secondary infection of myiasis is remarkably infrequent and rapid healing follows removal of intact larvae. *Loa loa* infection may present with transient subcutaneous swellings and pruritus. The diagnosis is made by finding microfilariae in daytime blood specimens.

Conclusions

Skin problems in travelers to the tropics constitute a small but important problem. In this review we have focused on the skin lesions alone, but it is useful to remember that skin rashes may be a feature of travel-associated systemic infectious diseases such as the rose spots of typhoid and the blanching macular rash of dengue fever. We have shown here that the range of likely diagnoses is quite small but it is important that patients should be diagnosed promptly and referred to tropical specialists where appropriate.

Acknowledgments

We would like to thank Dr. R. N. Davidson and Professor G. Pasvol for their constructive critical readings of this review.

References and recommended reading

Papers of particular interest, published within the annual period of review, have been highlighted as:
• Of special interest
•• Of outstanding interest

1. Lockwood DNJ, Keystone JS: **Skin Problems in Returning Travelers.**
•• *Med Clin North Am* 1992, 76:1393–1411.
A comprehensive review of the common skin lesions found in travelers to the tropics. It is particularly useful because it is arranged on a lesion-by-lesion basis and has numerous helpful tables for each diagnostic group.

2. Dinehart SM, Archer ME, Wolf JE: **Caripito Itch: Dermatitis From Contact With Hylesia Moths.** *J Am Acad Dermatol* 1985, 13:743–747.

3. Pryce D, Behrens R, Davidson RN, Bryceson ADM: **Onchocerciasis**
• **in Members of an Expedition to Cameroon: Role of Advice Before Travel and Long Term Follow Up.** *BMJ* 1992, 304:1285–1286.
Members of an expedition to Cameroon were offered follow-up to detect onchocerciasis. Twenty-six percent of respondents were diagnosed as having disease on the basis of either a positive skin snip test or a positive Mazotti test. Pruritus, rash, and swellings were reported in 77%, 68%, and 41% respectively of those diagnosed as having onchocerciasis.

4. Kerdel-Vegas F, Goihman M: *Paederus* **Dermatitis.** *Arch Dermatol* 1966, 94:175–185.

5. Davies HD, Sakuls P, Keystone JS: **Creeping Eruption: A Review of**
•• **Clinical Presentation and Management of 60 Cases Presenting to a Tropical Disease Unit.** *Arch Dermatol* 1993, 129:588–591.
Cutaneous larva migrans due to nonhuman hookworm migration through the skin is a regular problem acquired in the tropics. Sixty cases presenting to a Canadian tropical disease unit are reviewed here. Fifty-eight percent of patients had been misdiagnosed or inappropriately treated; notably, 12% had been treated with liquid nitrogen. Ninety-eight percent of patients were cured with topical thiabendazole.

6. Williams H, Monk B: **Creeping Eruption Stopped in Its Tracks by Albendazole.** *Clin Exp Dermatol* 1989, 14:355–356.

7. Jones S, Reynolds N, Oliwiecki S, Harman R: **Oral Albendazole for the Treatment of Cutaneous Larva Migrans.** *Br J Dermatol* 1990, 122:99–101.

8. Sanguigni S, Marani M, Teggi A, De Rosa F: **Albendazole in the Therapy of Cutaneous Larva Migrans.** *Trans R Soc Trop Med Hyg* 1990, 84:83.

9. Caumes E, Datry A, Paris L, Danis M, Gentilini M: **Efficacy of Ivermectin in the Therapy of Cutaneous Larva Migrans.** *Arch Dermatol* 1992, 128:994–995.

10. Gill GV: *Strongyloides stercoralis* **Infection in Former Far East Prisoners of War.** *BMJ* 1979, 2:572–574.

11. Archibald LK, Beeching NJ, Gill GV, Bailey JW, Bell DR: **Albendazole**
• **Is Effective Treatment for Chronic Strongyloidiasis.** *Q J Med* 1993, 86:191–195.
Three hundred one British ex–Far East prisoners of war were screened for strongyloidiasis. Fifty-two were found to have chronic strongyloidiasis, and 50% of this group described a characteristic larva currens rash. Seventy-five percent were cured with a single course of albendazole.

12. Herwaldt BL, Stokes SL, Juranek DD: **American Cutaneous Leishma-**
•• **niasis in US Travelers.** *Ann Intern Med* 1993, 118:779–784.
This paper reviews a series of patients treated for CL with sodium stibogluconate and focuses on the epidemiologic risk factors for disease, the time taken for the development of lesions, and the delays in diagnosis and treatment.

13. Melby PC, Kreutzer RD, McMahon-Pratt D, Gam AA, Neva FA: **Cu-**
••   **taneous Leishmaniasis: Review of 59 Cases Seen at the National**
     Institutes of Health. *Clin Infect Dis* 1992, **15**:924–937.
A detailed review of 59 cases of CL seen at the National Institutes of Health. The
disease types seen represent all types of CL. The majority of patients acquired
disease through work-related activities. The paper includes a comprehensive
discussion of the diagnosis and treatment of CL.

14. Norton SA, Frankenburg S, Klaus SN: **Cutaneous Leishmaniasis Ac-**
     quired During Military Service in the Middle East. *Arch Dermatol*
     1992, **128**:83–87.

15. Hepburn NC, Tidman MJ, Hunter JAA: **Cutaneous Leishmaniasis in**
•   **British Troops From Belize.** *Br J Dermatol* 1993, **128**:63–68.
One hundred eighty-seven British soldiers developed CL after a tour of duty in
Belize. *Leishmania braziliensis braziliensis* and *Leishmania mexicana mexi-
cana* were cultured from 78 and 29 cases, respectively. Treatment with sodium
stibogluconate was effective.

16. Olliaro PL, Bryceson ADM: **Practical Progress and New Drugs**
••   **for Changing Patterns of Leishmaniasis.** *Parasitology Today* 1993,
     9:323–328.
A magisterial review of currently available therapies for both cutaneous and
visceral leishmaniasis.

17. *Control of the Leishmaniases: Report of a WHO Expert Committee.*
     Geneva: World Health Organization; 1990. [World Health Organiza-
     tion Technical Report Series 793.]

18. Belazzoug S, Neal RA: **Failure of Meglumine Antimoniate to Cure**
     Cutaneous Lesions Due to *Leishmania major* **in Algeria.** *Trans R
     Soc Trop Med Hyg* 1986, **80**:670–671.

19. Pallai L, Hodge J, Fishman SJ, Millikan LE, Phelps RG: **Case Report:**
•   **Myiasis. The Botfly Boil.** *Am J Med Sci* 1992, **303**:245–248.
Four patients with myiasis after travel to Central America are reported on. The
pathology of myiasis and the treatment options are considered.

20. Brewer TF, Wilson ME, Gonzalez E, Felsenstein D: **Bacon Therapy**
     and Furuncular Myiasis. *JAMA* 1993, **270**:2087–2088.

21. Bernhard JD: **Bringing on the Bacon for Myiasis.** *Lancet* 1993,
     342:1377–1378.

22. Nunn P: **Tangling With Tumbu Larvae.** [Letter]. *Lancet* 1994, **343**:
•   676.
A letter outlining the difficulties in extracting tumbu fly larvae and suggesting
that bacon fat might not be the revolutionary answer to the problem. The author reminds readers of the value of preventing tumbu fly infestation by ironing
clothes dried in open air in Africa.

Diana Lockwood, MRCP, Department of Infection and Tropical
Medicine, St. Mary's Hospital Medical School, Imperial College of Sci-
ence, Technology and Medicine, Northwick Park Hospital, Harrow,
Middlesex HA1 3UJ, UK.

Francisco Kerdel-Vegas, MD, National Academy of Medicine, Apar-
tada 804, Caracas 1010-A, Venezuela.

The reemergence of tuberculosis and atypical mycobacterial diseases

Nathalie Franck, MD,* and André Cabié, MD†

*Hôpital Tarnier-Cochin and †Hôpital Bichat-Claude Bernard, Paris, France

The reemergence of tuberculosis in the 1990s seems to be associated with the spread of HIV infection. The emergence of multidrug-resistant tuberculosis is a real problem because of its very high overall mortality and because of its interhuman transmission. Immunocompromised patients are at risk for developing atypical mycobacterial infections, such as disseminated *Mycobacterium avium* complex infection in AIDS. Recently, a cluster of *Mycobacterium haemophilum* infections has been reported. Clarithromycin has given promising results in disseminated *M. avium* complex infection in AIDS patients and seems to be the drug of choice for disseminated cutaneous disease due to *Mycobacterium chelonae*.

Current Opinion in Dermatology 1995:249–253

Whereas the beginning of the 1980s was marked by the appearance of AIDS, the beginning of the 1990s is witnessing the reemergence of tuberculosis in developed countries and its outright eruption in developing countries. This reemergence of tuberculosis is distinguished by the association of tuberculosis with HIV infection and by the emergence of multidrug-resistant (MDR) tuberculosis. Certain atypical mycobacterial infections that had been only infrequently encountered now appear in some immunocompromised patients. The discovery of drugs such as clarithromycin and rifabutin makes it possible to fight these atypical mycobacterial infections.

Tuberculosis

Reemergence of tuberculosis

In 1990, the World Health Organization estimated that 1.7 billion people were or had been infected by the tuberculosis bacillus [1]. In addition, 4 million people had coinfection with HIV and the tuberculosis bacillus; three fourths of these people (77.8%) lived in sub-Saharan Africa [2]. In the United States between 1985 and 1991, in addition to the cases expected, 39,000 additional cases of tuberculosis were recorded (Fig. 1) [3]. This rise in the US tuberculosis rate is due mainly to the arrival of immigrants from countries having high rates of tuberculosis, to coinfection with HIV, and to epidemics in different communities and health care centers [3]. Once infected with HIV, patients have a higher risk of developing tuberculosis [3]. Finally, a nosocomial tuberculosis epidemic has emerged since 1990.

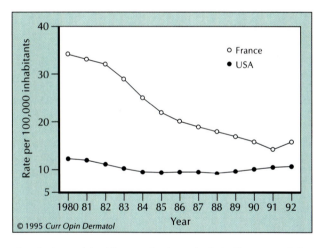

Fig. 1. Annual incidence of tuberculosis in France and the United States, 1980 to 1992.

Emergence of multidrug-resistant tuberculosis

Epidemics of nosocomial MDR tuberculosis broke out in several US cities, in particular New York City and Miami, as well as in New Jersey [4–7]. The tuberculosis bacilli were resistant to isoniazid and rifampin and often to other antituberculous drugs. Interhuman transmission of the tuberculosis bacilli was demonstrated in most cases by DNA restriction fragment length polymorphism analysis [8]. In more than 80% of cases, the patients were infected with HIV. The emergence of MDR strains of tuberculosis bacilli is mainly the result of poor observance of antituberculous treatment in the index cases.

Abbreviations
MAC—*Mycobacterium avium* complex; **MDR**—multidrug-resistant.

Multidrug-resistant tuberculosis is generally seen in patients with advanced HIV infection. In a study of 62 patients by Fischl *et al.* [9], the median survival time was 2.1 months in patients with MDR tuberculosis, versus 14.6 months in those with drug sensitive tuberculosis. The overall mortality rate in patients with MDR tuberculosis was 80%. A study carried out by the Centers for Disease Control during the third quarter of 1991 assessed the level of tuberculosis resistance in the United States [10]. The overall rate of resistance to at least one drug was 14%; the rates of resistance were 9.1% to isoniazid, 3.9% to rifampin, 5.8% to pyrazinamide, and 2.4% to ethambutol. The average incidence of MDR tuberculosis was 3.5%, but the incidence reached 13.9% in New York City.

The treatment of MDR tuberculosis involves the use of six to nine antituberculous drugs. Even with this type of treatment, many failures occur [11]. The real means of fighting the MDR tuberculosis epidemics is prevention. In a case study of an MDR tuberculosis epidemic involving *Mycobacterium bovis*, the authors showed that nosocomial transmission can be effectively avoided by measures for respiratory isolation [12]. Since 1990, the Centers for Disease Control has set forth guidelines for preventing tuberculosis transmission in treatment units [13].

New diagnostic methods

The significant delay in diagnosing tuberculosis is a factor facilitating nosocomial tuberculosis epidemics. The BACTEC (Becton Dickinson Diagnostic Instrument Systems, Sparks, MD) system makes it possible to shorten the period required for the culture and the antibiogram by 30% [14].

Numerous studies have assessed the use of the polymerase chain reaction for making a rapid diagnosis of tuberculosis based on various pathologic specimens (*eg*, sputum, medullar biopsy, and hepatic biopsy specimens). It has a specificity of nearly 100% and a sensitivity of higher than 95% for positive smear results, although the sensitivity is only 50% in the case of negative smear (and positive culture) findings [3]. Some reports have demonstrated the utility of the PCR in the investigation of cases believed to represent cutaneous tuberculosis, especially in tuberculids [15], lupus vulgaris [16–18], and erythema induratum of Bazin [19,20].

Rapid detection of resistance

Detection of genes coding for resistance

The resistance mechanisms and the genes involved in resistance are still little known. For rifampin, resistance is due to changes in a gene zone (rpo B) coding for subunit β of the RNA polymerase. Telenti *et al.* [21••] showed that there were mutations affecting the eight amino acids in the rpo B gene strains of *Mycobacterium tuberculosis* resistant to rifampin. Such mutations were found in 64 of 66 strains resistant to rifampin but in none of 56 strains sensitive to rifampin. In 1992, Zhang *et al.* [22] showed that the disappearance or

deletion of a gene coding for a catalase (KatG) was associated with resistance to isoniazid. However, a deletion of KatG was found in only two of eight strains of *M. tuberculosis* resistant to isoniazid. Thus, this mechanism of resistance is not the only one. In 1994, Banerjee *et al.* [23] showed that the target of isoniazid could be a protein (InhA protein) involved in the synthesis of fatty acids (mycolic acids). A mutation or the presence of a multicopy form of gene coding for this protein (InhA) gives an initially nonresistant bacteria resistance to isoniazid and ethionamide (Fig. 2).

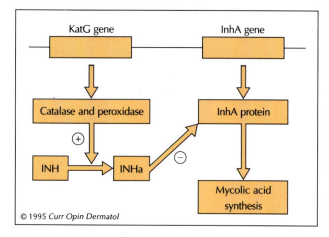

Fig. 2. Isoniazid (INH) is transformed into an active derivative (INHa) by a catalase and peroxidase enzyme, a product of the KatG gene. INHa acts by inhibiting the InhA protein, a product of the InhA protein gene. InhA protein is responsible for mycolic acid synthesis. This synthesis is suspended by INHa. A mutation or deletion of the KatG gene or a mutation or the presence of a multicopy of the InhA gene is responsible for giving bacteria resistance to INH.

Use of phages with a luciferase

Resistance can also be detected with the use of mycobacteriophages to which has been added a gene coding for an enzyme (luciferase) that in the presence of ATP produces light [3]. When a strain of mycobacteria infected by this phage is placed in the presence of an antituberculous drug, this method quickly differentiates between a resistant strain (light is produced) and a nonresistant strain (no light is produced). This same method allows the screening of potentially active drugs.

Treatment

The treatment of tuberculosis is now well codified and is based on the bacteriologic criteria of the length of time for the doubling of bacilli and the various bacilli populations [24]. The first phase of treatment is aimed at eliminating the multiplying bacteria. Three or four antituberculous drugs are taken for 2 months (isoniazid, rifampin, pyrazinamide, and ethambutol). The second phase is intended to sterilize the lesions. For this, isoniazid and rifampin are used for 4 months (in HIV infected patients, for 7 months, or for 6 months after negative culture results). Complete guidelines are given in an article by Hopewell [25]. The cure rate is identical for HIV-positive and -negative patients [26].

Mycobacterium avium complex infection

Before 1980, *Mycobacterium avium* complex (MAC) was a rare pathogen. By the beginning of the 1990s in the United States, 15% to 40% of HIV-infected patients had disseminated MAC disease [27•]. *M. avium* complex is found in the environment. It is transmitted through the air into the respiratory system, through water and food products into the digestive system, or in both ways, without interhuman transmission. In HIV-infected patients, infection occurs only in cases of severe immunodepression (most frequently at less than 50 CD4 cells/mm^3) [27•].

Symptoms of disseminated MAC disease include fever, night sweating, weight loss, diarrhea, and abdominal pains. Intra-abdominal adenopathies associated with hepatosplenomegaly are frequently noted. Anemia and a high alkaline phosphatase level are generally present [27•]. Horsburgh *et al.* [28] found a survival time of 4 months in patients with MAC infection, as opposed to 11 months in comparable patients without MAC infection. The diagnosis is made by a single positive blood culture result or a positive MAC culture finding from an osteomedullar or hepatic biopsy specimen.

Treatment

In vitro studies of the responsiveness of MAC infection to various antibiotics have shown a correlation to clinical response only with the macrolides, and clarithromycin in particular. Strains with a minimal inhibitory concentration of greater than 32 μg/mL are resistant, whereas those with a minimal inhibitory concentration of less than 2 μg/mL are not. Between these two levels, *in vivo* activity is not predictable [29]. A randomized study comparing clarithromycin with a four-drug treatment regimen clearly showed that clarithromycin was superior to the other drugs [30•]. The best dosage seems to be between 1500 and 2000 mg/d [30•]. Acquired resistance to clarithromycin appeared 2 to 7 months after the start of therapy [30•].

A single trial with azithromycin, which involved 16 patients, showed promising results [31]. Masur and the Public Health Service Task Force on Prophylaxis and Therapy for *Mycobacterium avium* Complex [29] recommended the use of clarithromycin or azithromycin in association with ethambutol and one of the following drugs: clofazimine, rifampin, rifabutin, ciprofloxacin, or eventually amikacin. This treatment must be continued for life. When it is effective, a clinical response can be expected in 4 to 6 weeks, and a bacteriologic response in 4 to 12 weeks [29].

Prophylaxis

Two randomized, double-blind studies assessed the value of rifabutin versus placebo for preventing MAC infections [32•]. Rifabutin (300 mg/d) was given to 1146 patients with at least 200 CD4 lymphocytes/mm^3. The results are given in Table 1. Although rifabutin reduced the risk of MAC bacteremia by half, it did not reduce mortality. Rifabutin at a daily dose of 300 mg could be proposed as prophylaxis for disseminated MAC disease for patients with fewer than 100 CD4 lymphocytes/mm^3 and in whom an MAC infection or tuberculosis can be formally ruled out [29].

Mycobacterium haemophilum infection

During a 20-month period, 13 sporadic cases of *Mycobacterium haemophilum* infection were diagnosed in New York City [33•]. The principal risk group is composed of immunocompromised patients, including

Table 1. Incidence and relative risk of *Mycobacterium avium* complex bacteremia among AIDS patients in two randomized, double-blind trials*

	Placebo-treated patients, *n*	Rifabutin-treated patients, *n*	Relative risk† (95% CI)	*P* value
Group 1				
Total patients	298	292		
Intention-to-treat analysis§	51	24	0.43 (0.26–0.70)	<0.001
Double-blind analysis¶	41	16	0.36 (0.20–0.64)	<0.001
Group 2				
Total patients	282	274		
Intention-to-treat analysis§	51	24	0.47 (0.29–0.77)	0.002
Double-blind analysis¶	48	19	0.41 (0.24–0.70)	<0.001

*From Nightingale *et al.* [32•]; with permission.
†Data are shown for the rifabutin group compared with the placebo group.
§Patients developing *M. avium* complex bacteremia.
¶Excludes those patients in whom *M. avium* complex bacteremia developed more than 30 days after the last dose of the study drug given during the blinded phase.

AIDS patients (11 of 13) with a low CD4 count (<25 cells/mm^3).

Cutaneous lesions are the most common manifestation of the disease. They are multiple, tender, violaceous nodules and ulcerations most frequently found on the extremities and overlying the joints. They may realize an acute pustular eruption [34]. *M. haemophilum* also causes disease of bones, joints, lymphatics, and lungs.

M. haemophilum was isolated from cutaneous lesions, bone, sputum, synovial fluid, blood, and lung biopsy specimens. *M. haemophilum* grows on enriched chocolate agar or heme-supplemented media, and the optimal incubation temperature is reported to be 32°C.

The mode of transmission is unknown. No standardized susceptibility tests and no recommended therapy are yet available. This pathogen should be considered in evaluating an immunocompromised patient who has cutaneous joint, or bone manifestations.

Mycobacterium genavense infection

Böttger *et al.* [35] reported disseminated infection with an acid-fast microorganism in 18 AIDS patients with fever, diarrhea, and weight loss. *Mycobacterium genavense* does not grow on solid media, although limited growth was observed in liquid blood culture. No susceptibility tests and no recommended therapy are yet available.

Mycobacterium chelonae infection

Mycobacterium chelonae, a rapidly growing environmental mycobacterium, is a recognized cause of community-acquired disease (posttraumatic skin, soft-tissue, and bone infections and disseminated cutaneous infections) and sporadic nosocomial infections (infections after plastic surgery, infections after injection abscesses, and catheter-related infections) [36•].

Disseminated cutaneous disease is the most common manifestation, with multiple nodular subcutaneous erythematous lesions [36•]. These lesions predominate on the distal surfaces of a single extremity and may have a sporotrichoid pattern [37]. Another type of disease is localized cellulitis, subcutaneous abscess, and osteomyelitis, which usually occurred after a skin injury [36•].

Wallace *et al.* [36•] showed that 62% of 100 patients with *M. chelonae* skin infection were receiving corticosteroids that and 72% were immunosuppressed. Disseminated infection is rare. HIV infection appeared to carry no risk for infection with *M. chelonae*. Wallace *et al.* showed that 100% of isolates were inhibited by low concentrations of clarithromycin *in vitro*.

A man receiving prednisone and methotrexate for a rheumatoid arthritis was successfully treated with clar-

ithromycin (500 mg twice a day) for a disseminated sporotrichoid *M. chelonae* skin infection without withdrawal of the immunosuppressive therapy [37]. In an open-label noncomparative trial, 14 patients with *M. chelonae* disease were treated with clarithromycin (500 mg twice daily for 6 months) and had good clinical and bacteriologic responses to therapy [38]. One relapse was seen with an isolate that had become resistant to clarithromycin. Tolerance to clarithromycin was excellent, and the use of this agent produced very few side effects (including bitter taste, nausea, vomiting, central nervous system symptoms, and elevated liver enzyme levels) [39••]. It seems that clarithromycin may be the drug of choice for cutaneous disseminated disease due to *M. chelonae*, although acquired drug resistance is a risk with monotherapy for mycobacterial species. The best dosage and duration of therapy have not yet been studied.

Conclusions

The beginning of the 1990s was marked by the return of tuberculosis, which was sometimes MDR, and by the emergence of atypical mycobacterial infections, particularly MAC infections. These two events are strongly linked to the pandemic rise of AIDS. Simultaneously, the considerable progress in molecular biology on mycobacteria and their resistance mechanisms makes it possible to use new diagnostic and epidemiologic tools to fight these infections. Finally, the discovery of clarithromycin and, to a lesser extent, of rifabutin represents a significant advance in the treatment and prevention of atypical mycobacterial infections, in particular MAC infections.

References and recommended reading

Papers of particular interest, published within the annual period of review, have been highlighted as:
- •   Of special interest
- •• Of outstanding interest

1. Kochi A: **The Global Tuberculosis Situation and the New Control Strategy of the World Health Organization.** *Tubercle* 1991, 72:1–6.
2. DeCock K, Soro B, Coulibaly I, Lucas S: **Tuberculosis and HIV Infection in Sub-Saharan Africa.** *JAMA* 1992, 268:1581–1587.
3. Ellner J, Hinman A, Dooley S, Fischl M, Sepkowitz K, Goldberger M, Shinnick T, Iseman M, Jacobs W: **Tuberculosis Symposium: Emerging Problems and Promise.** *J Infect Dis* 1993, 168:537–551.
4. Pearson M, Jereb J, Frieden T, Crawford J, Davis B, Dooley S, Jarvis W: **Nosocomial Transmission of Multidrug-Resistant *Mycobacterium tuberculosis*: A Risk to Patients and Health Care Workers.** *Ann Intern Med* 1992, 117:191–196.
5. Centers for Disease Control: **Nosocomial Transmission of Multidrug Resistant Tuberculosis to Health Care Workers and HIV-Infected Patients in an Urban Hospital: Florida.** *MMWR Morb Mortal Wkly Rep* 1990, 39:718–722.
6. Centers for Disease Control: **Nosocomial Transmission of Multidrug Resistant Tuberculosis Among HIV Infected Persons: Florida and New York, 1988–1991.** *MMWR Morb Mortal Wkly Rep* 1991, 40:585–591.
7. Fischl M, Uttamchandani R, Daikos G, Poblete R, Moreno J, Reyes R, Boota A: **An Outbreak of Tuberculosis Caused by Multidrug Resistant Tubercle Bacilli Among Patients With HIV Infection.** *Ann Intern Med* 1992, 117:177–183.
8. Edlin B, Valway S, Onorato I: **Clusters of Multidrug Resistant Tuberculosis.** *Ann Intern Med* 1993, 118:77.

9.   Fischl M, Daikos G, Uttamchandani R, Poblete R, Moreno J, Reyes R, Boota A, Thompson L, Clearly T, Oldham S, Saldana M, Lai S: **Clinical Presentation and Outcome of Patients With HIV Infection and Tuberculosis Caused by Multiple-Drug-Resistant Bacilli.** *Ann Intern Med* 1992, 117:184–190.

10.   Bloch A, Cauthen G, Onorato I, Dansbury K, Kelly G, Driver C, Snider D: **Nationwide Survey of Drug-Resistant Tuberculosis in the United States.** *JAMA* 1994, 271:665–671.

11.   Iseman M: **Treatment of Multidrug-Resistant Tuberculosis.** *N Engl J Med* 1993, 329:784–791.

12.   Bouvet E, Casalino E, Mendoza-Sassi G, Lariven S, Valée E, Pernet M, Gottot S, Vachon F: **A Nosocomial Outbreak of Multidrug Resistant *Mycobacterium bovis* Among HIV-Infected Patients: A Case-Control Study.** *AIDS* 1993, 7:1453–1460.

13.   Dooley S, Castro K, Hutton M, Mullan R, Polder J, Snider D: **Guidelines for Preventing the Transmission of Tuberculosis in the Era of Multidrug Resistance: Recommendations of the Advisory Council for the Elimination of Tuberculosis.** *MMWR Morb Mortal Wkly Rep* 1990, 39:1–29.

14.   Huebner R, Good R, Tokars J: **Current Practice in Mycobacteriology: Results of a Survey of State Public Health Laboratories.** *J Clin Microbiol* 1992, 31:771–775.

15.   Victor T, Jordaan HF, Van Niekerk DJT, Louw M, Jordaan A, Van Helden PD: **Papulonecrotic Tuberculid Identification of *Mycobacterium tuberculosis* DNA by Polymerase Chain Reaction.** *Am J Dermatopathol* 1992, 14:491–495.

16.   Marcoval J, Servitje O, Moreno A, Jucglá A, Peyri J: **Lupus Vulgaris: Clinical, Histopathologic, and Bacteriologic Study of 10 Cases.** *J Am Acad Dermatol* 1992, 26:404–407.

17.   Degitz K, Steidl M, Neubert U, Plewig G, Volkenandt M: **Detection of Mycobacterial DNA in Paraffin-Embedded Specimens of Lupus Vulgaris by Polymerase-Chain Reaction.** *Arch Dermatol Res* 1993, 285:168–170.

18.   Serfling U, Penneys NS, Leonardi CL: **Identification of *Mycobacterium tuberculosis* DNA in a Case of Lupus Vulgaris.** *J Am Acad Dermatol* 1993, 28:318–322.

19.   Schneider JW, Geiger DH, Rossouw DJ, Jordaan HF, Victor T, Van Helden PD: ***Mycobacterium tuberculosis* DNA in Erythema Induratum of Bazin.** *Lancet* 1993, 342:747–748.

20.   Penneys NS, Leonardi CL, Cook S, Blauvelt A, Rosenberg S, Eells LD, Konwiser, Aaronson CM: **Identification of *Mycobacterium tuberculosis* DNA in Five Different Types of Cutaneous Lesions by Polymerase Chain Reaction.** *Arch Dermatol* 1993, 129:1594–1598.

21.   Telenti A, Imboden P, Marchesi F, Lowrie D, Cole S, Colston M, Matter L, Schopfer K, Bodmer T: **Detection of Rifampicin-Resistance Mutations in *Mycobacterium tuberculosis*.** *Lancet* 1993, 341:647–650.
••
This paper points out the genetic basis for rifampin resistance in 96% of resistant isolates of *M. tuberculosis*.

22.   Zhang Y, Heym B, Allen B, Young D, Cole S: **The Catalase-Peroxidase Gene and Isoniazid Resistance of *Mycobacterium tuberculosis*.** *Nature* 1992, 358:591–593.

23.   Banerjee A, Dubnau E, Quemard A, Balasubramanian V, Um K, Wilson T, Collins D, deLisle G, Jacobs W: **InhA, a Gene Encoding a Target for Isoniazid and Ethionamide in *Mycobacterium tuberculosis*.** *Nature* 1994, 263:227–231.

24.   Grosset J: **Present Status of Chemotherapy for Tuberculosis.** *Rev Infect Dis* 1989, 11:S347–S352.

25.   Hopewell P: **Impact of Human Immunodeficiency Virus Infection on the Epidemiology, Clinical Features, Management, and Control of Tuberculosis.** *Clin Infect Dis* 1992, 15:540–547.

26.   Grosset J: **Treatment of Tuberculosis in HIV Infection.** *Tuber Lung Dis* 1992, 73:378–383.

27.   Benson C, Ellner J: ***Mycobacterium avium* Complex Infection and AIDS: Advances in Theory and Practice.** *Clin Infect Dis* 1993, 17:7–20.
•
A good review of disseminated *M. avium* infections.

28.   Horsburgh C, Havlick J, Ellis E: **Survival of Patients With Acquired Immune Deficiency Syndrome and Disseminated *Mycobacterium avium* Complex Infection With and Without Antimycobacterial Chemotherapy.** *Am Rev Respir Dis* 1991, 144:557–559.

29.   Masur H, Public Health Service Task Force on Prophylaxis and Therapy for *Mycobacterium avium* Complex: **Recommendations on Prophylaxis and Therapy for Disseminated *Mycobacterium avium* Complex Disease in Patients Infected With the Human Immunodeficiency Virus.** *N Engl J Med* 1993, 329:898–904.

30.   Dautzenberg B, SaintMarc T, Meyohas M, Eliaszewitch M, Haniez F, Rogues A, DeWit S, Cotte L, Chauvin J, Grosset J: **Clarithromycin and Other Antimicrobial Agents in the Treatment of Disseminated *Mycobacterium avium* Infections in Patients With Acquired Immunodeficiency Syndrome.** *Arch Intern Med* 1993, 153:368–372.
•
This large series evaluates the efficacy of clarithromycin for disseminated MAC infections in AIDS patients.

31.   Young L, Wiviott L, Wu M, Kolonoski P, Bolan R, Inderlied C: **Azithromycin for Treatment of *Mycobacterium avium-intracellulare* Complex Infection in Patients With AIDS.** *Lancet* 1991, 338:1107–1109.

32.   Nightingale S, Cameron D, Gordin F, Sullam P, Cohn D, Chaisson R, Eron L, Sparti P, Bihari B, Kaufman D, Stern J, Pearce D, Weinberg W, LaMarca A, Siegal F: **Two Controlled Trials of Rifabutin Prophylaxis Against *Mycobacterium avium* Complex Infection in AIDS.** *N Engl J Med* 1993, 329:828–833.
•
This multicenter trial shows that rifabutin (300 mg/d) allows a 50% decrease in MAC bacteremia in HIV-infected patients with a CD4 count of less than 200 lymphocytes/mm³.

33.   Straus WL, Ostroff SM, Jernigan DB, Kiehn TE, Sordillo EM, Armstrong D, Boone N, Schneider N, Kilburn JO, Silcox VA, LaBombardi V, Good RC: **Clinical and Epidemiologic Characteristics of *Mycobacterium haemophilum*, an Emerging Pathogen in Immunocompromised Patients.** *Ann Intern Med* 1994, 120:118–125.
•
Thirteen immunocompromised patients with *M. haemophilum* infection are reported on. The clinical characteristics are well described, although standard therapy is not yet known.

34.   Joly P, Picard-Dahan C, Bamberger N, Bouvet E, Salmon D, Grossin M, Belaich S: **Acute Pustular Eruption: An Unusual Clinical Feature of Disseminated Mycobacterial Infection in Patients With Acquired Immunodeficiency Syndrome.** *J Am Acad Dermatol* 1993, 28:264–266.

35.   Böttger EC, Teske A, Kirshner P, Bost S, Chang HR, Beer V, Hirschel B: **Disseminated "*Mycobacterium genavense*" Infection in Patients With AIDS.** *Lancet* 1992, 340:76–80.

36.   Wallace RJ, Brown BA, Onyi GO: **Skin, Soft Tissue, and Bone Infections Due to *Mycobacterium chelonae chelonae*: Importance of Prior Corticosteroid Therapy, Frequency of Disseminated Infections, and Resistance to Oral Antimicrobials Other Than Clarithromycin.** *J Infect Dis* 1992, 166:405–412.
•
This review points out the frequency of prior corticosteroid therapy in *M. chelonae* infection. One hundred percent of isolates were inhibited by low concentrations of clarithromycin *in vitro*.

37.   Franck N, Cabié A, Villette B, Amor B, Lessana-Leibowitch M, Escande JP: **Treatment of *Mycobacterium chelonae*-Induced Skin Infection With Clarithromycin.** *J Am Acad Dermatol* 1993, 28:1019–1021.

38.   Wallace RJ, Brown BA, Griffith DE: **Drug Intolerance to High-Dose Clarithromycin Among Elderly Patients.** *Diagn Microbiol Infect Dis* 1993, 16:215–221.

39.   Wallace RJ, Tanner D, Brennan PJ, Brown BA: **Clinical Trial of Clarithromycin for Cutaneous (Disseminated) Infection Due to *Mycobacterium chelonae*.** *Ann Intern Med* 1993, 119:482–486.
••
This clinical trial showed that clarithromycin was effective for *M. chelonae* cutaneous infection.

Nathalie Franck, MD, Department of Dermatology, Hôpital Tarnier-Cochin, Pavillon ACHARD 5ᵉ etage, 27 Rue de Faubourg, St. Jacques, 75014 Paris, France

The hair follicle revisited: infectious considerations

Wilma F. Bergfeld, MD, and Thomas N. Helm, MD

Cleveland Clinic Foundation, Cleveland, Ohio, and State
University of New York at Buffalo, Williamsville, New York, USA

Although human hair has no vital physiologic function, it is a visible part of the body that is important in defining the self-image. Many disorders of the hair are infectious in origin, and as our understanding of diseases such as HIV-1 infection evolves, we are often surprised by the array of responses possible from the hair follicle and pilosebaceous unit. Not only can infectious processes cause hair loss and straightening of previously curly hair, but other changes, such as premature canities and trichomegaly, to name only a few, can also be seen. The astute observer can learn a great deal by inspecting a person's pelage. The recent observations of most interest are the changes seen in HIV infection, although many other recent developments, such as the role of drug-resistant bacteria in acne, have immediate relevance to the dermatologist's practice. This article revisits some well-known entities such as acne keloidalis, which has been suspected of having infectious causes. Knowledge of the disorders of the hair follicle and pilosebaceous unit is continually evolving, and evaluation and management in clinical practice must continue to grow simultaneously. This presentation is a current 2-year review of useful clinical information that considers infectious disorders of the hair follicle.

Current Opinion in Dermatology 1995:254–259

HIV infection and the pilosebaceous unit

The HIV-1 epidemic continues to gain momentum in the United States and clinicians in all parts of the United States and the United Kingdom have now probably encountered at least a few patients with HIV-1 infection. The experience with HIV-1 infection in Africa is great because of the large proportion of people infected in sub-Saharan Africa. Observers in endemic areas have noted that people with otherwise curly or kinky hair develop a straightening of the hair after HIV-1 infection. The straightening of otherwise curly hair has a high predictive value for HIV-1 infection. In one recent study, patients on a medical ward in Rwanda were evaluated with regard to their hair. Of the 400 patients in the study, 30 of the 209 seropositive patients and one of the 122 seronegative patients acquired straight hair. The specificity of this sign was 99%, and the predictive diagnostic value was 97% [1]. In a population with a high incidence of HIV infection, this sign appears to have practical utility. The clinician already has many markers that may raise the suspicion of HIV-1 infection, such as oral thrush, prurigo, psoriasiform dermatitis, severe seborrheic dermatitis, herpes zoster, weight loss, cytomegalovirus retinitis, and others. None of these signs is specific, but when multiple markers are present simultaneously, their utility increases substantially. In areas with limited resources, such as many parts of Africa, useful bedside indicators are of great help. Treatment for this sign is not needed because it is an asymptomatic finding.

Pityriasis rubra pilaris is a chronic papulosquamous disorder of the skin and pilosebaceous apparatus in which follicular plugging and the histologic finding of psoriasiform epidermal hyperplasia and alternating orthokeratosis and parakeratosis are found. Although it is most often idiopathic, pityriasis rubra pilaris with elongated follicular spines has been linked to HIV-1 infection, along with acne conglobata [2]. Childhood pityriasis rubra pilaris has also been associated with HIV-1 infection [3]. Whether these observations will be borne out by larger studies remains to be seen. We have encountered psoriasiform dermatitis, Reiter's syndrome, and other widespread papulosquamous disease in the setting of HIV-1 infection. Retinoids may be helpful for treatment; methotrexate and systemic corticosteroids are best avoided because of the further immunosuppression that results and its inherent complications.

Alopecia universalis has also been noted as a sign of HIV infection [4], although the incidence of HIV-1 infection in patients with extensive alopecia areata appears to be very low. Epidemic alopecia has been noted in the past, and the presence of clusters of students with alopecia in schools, such as in the original reports of alopecia parvimacularis, have led investigators to suspect infectious cofactors. The knowledge that certain HLA antigen groupings are more common in alopecia areata patients and the finding of viral particle–like inclusions in autoimmune diseases such as lupus erythematosus have led to speculation that infection in a susceptible host may lead to alopecia areata. Reports of altered T helper and suppressor ratios in alopecia areata have further bolstered this notion. In a pilot study of 30 patients with extensive alopecia areata, HIV-1 antibodies were not detected in a single case by enzyme-linked immunosorbent assay [5]. Although the link of HIV-1 with alopecia areata is probably another association and may even be coincidence, the possibility that other viral infections may trigger alopecia areata needs to be further explored.

Trichomegaly is the enlargement of hairs, and the term is typically used to refer to the enlargement of eyelashes. The trichomegaly that is seen in the setting of HIV-1 infection is not a subtle sign but is quite obvious to the affected individual, his or her family and loved ones, and the evaluating physician. This sign is yet another useful predictor of HIV infection [6]. We have encountered patients with eyelashes so long that they touch the lenses of their eyeglasses. Although this sign is uncommon in our experience, it is quite specific. Treatment with cyclosporine can cause a similar change in the eyelashes, but a brief history taking usually rapidly helps to differentiate the patient with an untoward reaction to medication from the person with HIV-1 infection.

Telogen effluvium; loose anagen syndrome; premature canities; brittle, lusterless hair with trichorrhexis nodosa; and necrotizing folliculitis are yet other manifestations of HIV-1 infection [7••,8••]. The necrotizing folliculitis is usually unresponsive to steroid and antibiotic therapy [7••]. The disorders of the hair described previously are all difficult to manage. As overall well-being improves, telogen effluvium often remits. Loose anagen hairs and trichorrhexis nodosa are best managed by gentle hair care and the avoidance of further trauma to the hair by treatments such as permanents. Canities is best handled by dying the hair.

Pustular eruptions of the hair follicle are common in HIV-1 infection. Many times, the etiology is never fully elucidated. At other times, Gram's stain of pustule contents confirms the clinical suspicion of *Staphylococcus aureus* folliculitis. When culture results are negative and antibiotics are not helpful, eosinophilic pustular folliculitis should be suspected. Papules and pustules occur in the head and neck area, on the trunk, and on the extremities and are quite pruritic. The circinate arrangement of pustules seen in classic Ofuji's disease is not as often encountered in HIV-1 infection in our experience.

Eosinophilic pustular folliculitis is an idiopathic condition that can be mimicked clinically and histologically by fungal infection [9]. Because this disorder is seen in much greater frequency in HIV infection, an infectious rather than an immunologic cause has been suspected. Thus far, studies have not been able to pinpoint a pathogenic trigger. A study of nine patients with eosinophilic pustular folliculitis failed to reveal bacterial or fungal pathogens [10]. In patients with eosinophilic pustular folliculitis who were seronegative for HIV infection, indomethacin has proved to be helpful [11]. It remains to be seen if this therapeutic modality will be helpful in the HIV-1–positive population. Ultraviolet B phototherapy is efficacious in many patients and has been the most successful therapeutic modality for eosinophilic pustular folliculitis of HIV-1 infection in our opinion, although some patients do not seem to respond to treatment no matter what treatment approach is taken.

Scopulariopsis brevicaulis is an organism known to dermatologists because it may affect nails. In the setting of HIV-1 infection, *S. brevicaulis* infection may also affect the scalp and cause hair loss [7••,12].

Demodex mites have also been implicated in some of the eruptions of HIV infection [7••]. People with HIV-1 infection manifest rosacea-like reactions and papulonodular demodicidosis, as well as generalized prurigo. What the role of *Demodex* mites is in this setting remains to be determined.

Papillomavirus infection

Although papillomavirus infection may occur anywhere on the integument, infection in an epidermal inclusion cyst has only recently been reported. The epidermal inclusion cyst has its origin from the follicular infundibulum. Koilocytes and parakeratotic keratin within a cyst led Elston *et al.* [13] to suspect human papillomavirus infection. Whether the papillomavirus infection induced the development of the cyst or whether the epidermal inclusion cyst became secondarily infected by virus was unclear. The presence of human papillomavirus in a cyst echoes the recent findings of human papillomavirus in blood and a report of transplacental transmission [14]. This virus may be able to affect the hair follicle and other areas dermatologists have previously thought unlikely.

Tinea infections

The role of different types of dermatophytes in tinea capitis is changing. In Saudi Arabia, *Trichophyton schoenleinii* infection is now rare, but *Microsporum canis* infection (Fig. 1) is of great importance [15]. *Trichophyton violaceum* is the second most prevalent agent after *M. canis* in this part of the world. Black-dot ringworm is the most common form of tinea capitis encountered in the United States. Whereas *T. violaceum* is the most common cause in Taiwan, *Trichophyton tonsurans* is commonly encountered in the United States. Histologic study has shown that the causative fungi in *T. violaceum* infection enter the proximal cortex of the hair; they then colonize the keratinized cortex and form arthrospores. The hair is almost entirely replaced by spores at the level of the infundibulum and breaks off there, giving the characteristic black-dot appearance [16]. Opportunistic fungal agents such as

Scopulariopsis species can also cause scaling alopecic lesions [7••].

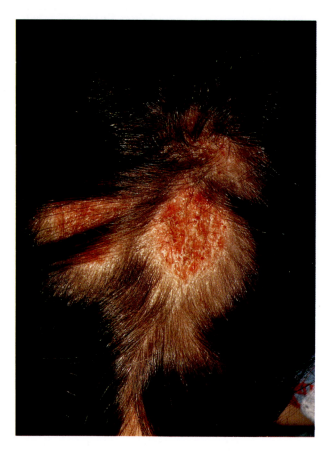

Fig. 1. Patchy alopecia with an inflammatory crust in tinea capitis. Culture findings revealed *Microsporum canis* to be the causative agent.

Even neoplastic disorders must be considered in the clinical differential diagnosis because they can exactly mimic tinea infection. For example, Langerhans cell histiocytosis often manifests as a seborrheic dermatitis–like eruption of the scalp. Dermatophytosis of the scalp may be coexistent in some cases of Langerhans cell histiocytosis, making diagnosis difficult [17]. The reason that Langerhans cell histiocytosis may so closely resemble dermatophytosis and seborrheic dermatitis is that histiocytosis X typically has periappendageal involvement histologically [18]. Performing appropriate cultures in cases not responding to treatment is critical for arriving at a correct diagnosis.

Yeast infection of the pilosebaceous unit

Pityrosporum ovale is a lipophilic yeast that has been implicated as the cause of seborrheic dermatitis. The location of this condition on the trunk and face has provided circumstantial evidence that sebaceous glands are important in its etiology: all of these affected areas are rich in sebaceous gland activity. The use of selenium sulfide shampoos and lotions has been the main-

stay of treatment in the past, along with the judicious use of topical corticosteroid preparations.

The treatment of seborrheic dermatitis has been advanced by the addition of ketoconazole shampoo to the clinicians' therapeutic armamentarium. *P. ovale* is thought to be important in the pathogenesis of seborrheic dermatitis, and ketoconazole is highly effective in eradicating this organism. A randomized, double-blind, placebo-controlled study showed that both 2% ketoconazole shampoo and 2.5% selenium sulfide shampoo controlled the itching and discomfort of seborrheic dermatitis. Although both products were similar in efficacy, patients treated with ketoconazole shampoo had fewer adverse side effects [19]. The mechanism by which ketoconazole shampoo produces this effect is not entirely clear.

Pityrosporum species can also cause widespread folliculitis on the upper trunk and shoulders. Affected individuals may have extensive seborrheic dermatitis also. Underlying immunosuppression from lymphoproliferative disorders has been associated with *Pityrosporum* folliculitis, and this association should be investigated in atypical or widespread cases [20•].

Trichosporosis

White piedra is a disorder of hair that is usually limited to temperate climates. The organism *Trichosporon beigelii* causes white concretions on hair. The concretions are softer and are less adherent to the hair shaft than are those of black piedra. Spontaneous remission is common, and shaving the affected hairs is usually curative. Disseminated trichosporosis has been reported as yet another emerging opportunistic infection in the setting of HIV-1 infection. Widespread papules and nodules that have a purpuric appearance may be seen when this infection disseminates. Histologic findings and culture allow accurate diagnosis [21]. As with other disseminated fungal infections, oral or parenteral treatment with imidazole antifungal agents is required.

Acne and the pilosebaceous unit

Acne, a multifactorial disorder of the pilosebaceous unit, is perhaps the most common disorder of the skin encountered by dermatologists. Bacteria contribute to acne through complex mechanisms. *Staphylococcus epidermidis*, micrococci, and the anaerobic *Propionibacterium acnes* all produce lipases, which result in the production of fatty acids. The irritating effects of fatty acids were previously thought to be important in the pathogenesis of acne, but current theories suggest that other factors, such as the chemoattractive effects of *P. acnes* cell wall components for neutrophils and monocytes, may be more important. Open and closed comedones, erythematous papules, pustules, and cysts of the face, chest, and back occur. Oral antibiotics are the mainstay of treatment in cases in which pustular and cystic lesions predominate, although their precise mechanism of action is not entirely clear. In many cases, some antibiotics are strikingly more effective than others. The importance of antibiotic resistance to treatment failure has recently become more clear. Antibiotic resistance may occur in up to 38% of acne patients [22••]. Erythromycin resistance is most common. Tetracycline resistance was present in 61 of 468 patients, and all of the patients with tetracycline resistance had resistance to doxycycline as well. Interestingly, minocycline resistance was not noted in the study [22••]. A minocycline dosage of 100 mg twice daily seems to be most helpful in controlling acne in patients with tetracycline-resistant propionibacteria [23]. Although some physicians have advocated the use of occasional screening laboratory studies, current information suggests that this is a needless practice that does not provide useful information. Patients receiving long-term antibiotic treatment do not benefit from routine laboratory monitoring [24•], and in the absence of any specific symptoms or complaints, we do not order such studies in our patients receiving long-term therapy.

Erythema migrans and alopecia

Lyme disease is the most common vector-borne disease in the United States [25]. Erythema migrans, with its annular appearance and central clearing, often allows the diagnosis. Alopecia in the same distribution as erythema migrans has been noted in *Borrelia burgdorferi* infection. The diagnosis can be made by characteristic clinical findings, tissue culture, and serologic findings. Warthin-Starry staining may reveal spirochetes on biopsy material. Polymerase chain reaction studies are very sensitive and have great promise in helping diagnose *B. burgdorferi* infection. Treatment with doxycycline is curative in early cases, but alopecia may require months before resolution is noted.

Idiopathic conditions

Pyoderma faciale
Pyoderma faciale is a fulminant disorder seen most commonly in young women. Erythematous papules, plaques, and cysts occur on the face and may lead to severe disfigurement. Without treatment, severe scarring may result. Bacterial agents have been suspected of being pathogenic. A thorough study by Plewig *et al.* [26], however, revealed only resident bacteria such as *S. epidermidis* and propionibacteria. These findings make an infectious cause seen unlikely. Treatment with corticosteroids is helpful initially. Isotretinoin is the treatment of choice in many cases, but it must be used with extreme caution in women of childbearing potential.

Folliculitis decalvans and acne keloidalis nuchae
Folliculitis decalvans is a chronic scarring alopecia characterized by boggy areas of follicular pustules that eventuate into cicatricial plaques. Palpation of active areas causes purulent exudate to be extruded. Cultures

may reveal *S. aureus*, although the role of infectious organisms is not clear. Histologic study reveals extensive infiltration of polymorphonuclear leukocytes in the follicular structures. Oral zinc sulfate and topical fusidic acid appear to be helpful in treatment [27].

When both superficial and deep abscesses are seen, dissecting folliculitis of the scalp may be the best diagnosis. Staphylococci, streptococci, and pseudomonads may be cultured from lesions, but antibiotic therapy is not uniformly effective. In our experience, corticosteroid treatments have sometimes had an equally beneficial effect.

Acne keloidalis is a common disorder in the black population. Papules and pustules are found in the occipital scalp and at the nape of the neck (Fig. 2). Hair granulomas and a mixed inflammatory response with lymphocytes, plasma cells, histiocytes, and neutrophils are encountered. Despite the name *acne keloidalis*, keloidal scarring is not always encountered. The incidence in dermatologic clinics in Nigeria is up to 1.4% of all patients visiting the dermatologist [28]. Because the disorder is largely asymptomatic, patients often delay in seeking treatment. A seborrheic constitution, male gender, and increased serum testosterone levels may all contribute to acne keloidalis. Increased mast cell density in the occipital scalp and capillary dilatation may help to explain the localization to the occipital scalp [28]. Retinoic acid analogues and antiandrogens may be the most promising avenues of treatment to pursue [28].

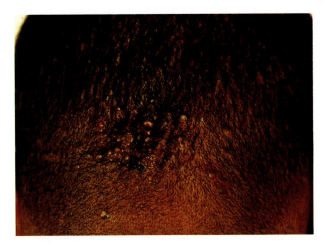

Fig. 2. Papules, pustules, and keloidal papules of the posterior scalp in acne keloidalis.

Pseudopelade of Brocq
Pseudopelade of Brocq has been suspected of being the cicatricial end-stage of various infections of the scalp (Fig. 3) because perifollicular erythema is noted that may mimic bacterial or fungal folliculitis. Recent evidence suggests that pseudopelade of Brocq may be a late stage of lichen planopilaris [29]. Unfortunately, the treatment of lichen planopilaris is usually unsuccessful. Intralesional corticosteroid injections are most

helpful in our experience. Biopsy for routine histology and direct immunofluorescence is helpful in establishing the diagnosis. Deposition of IgA and IgM on cytoid bodies and fibrinogen deposition are characteristically encountered [30]. Light microscopic study reveals a lymphocytic inflammatory response closely apposed to the follicular epithelium. Apoptosis of individual follicular epithelial cells is seen [30].

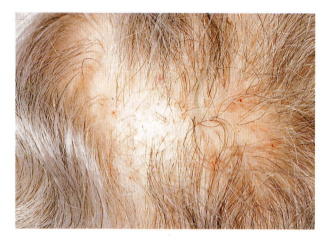

Fig. 3. Perifollicular hyperkeratosis and scarring; biopsy results are consistent with lichen planopilaris.

Erosive pustular dermatosis

Erosive pustular dermatosis of the scalp is a peculiar disorder seen in elderly women especially [31]. Erosive and pustular lesions are seen to enlarge centrifugally on the scalp. Antibiotic treatment is only intermittently helpful. We suspect that a minor immunodeficiency plays a role in this disorder by impairing the host response to common bacteria such as *S. aureus*.

Folliculitis

Follicular pustules are commonly encountered in *S. aureus* infection or as the result of gram-negative infection. Hot tub folliculitis from *Pseudomonas aeruginosa* is characterized by pustules with a striking erythematous halo. Infectious folliculitis is treated with the appropriate antibiotics.

Pseudofolliculitis from home epilation devices needs to be considered in the differential diagnosis of bacterial folliculitis. Biopsy reveals extrafollicular hair shafts in the dermis and granulomatous inflammation. Treatment with antibiotics is not helpful, and recovery may require many months [32].

Infestations

Pediculosis

Pediculosis capitis remains a problem for school-age children worldwide. The peak incidence appears to be around 7 years of age, and girls are affected more frequently than boys [33]. Parents are most often the ones to detect infection, and pyrethrins are now the most commonly used treatment in many areas [33]. Pruritus may be reported by as few as 14.2% of affected children. Careful inspection of the hair in all schoolmates is therefore important. If clinicians rely on students to present with symptoms, many affected children will be overlooked. Permethrin, malathion, and topical crotamiton are all effective in treating pediculosis. In cases of pediculosis corporis, the proper treatment of clothing by tumble drying is essential in killing lice and eggs.

Scabies mimicking seborrheic dermatitis of the scalp

Sarcoptes scabiei infestation is not usually expected in the head and neck area, and many clinicians advise patients to apply scabicidal agents from the neck down only. A report of scabies infestation of the scalp mimicking seborrheic dermatitis highlights the need to be aware of unusual manifestations of scabies in the immunocompromised host. Both patients in our report had acute lymphoblastic leukemia [34]. Scabies is treated by applying 5% permethrin cream, lindane, malathion, or benzyl benzoate for 8 hours.

Demodicidosis

Demodex mites are seen with greater frequency in patients with papular pustular rosacea [35,36]. Interestingly, patients with HIV-1 infection were not noted to have higher *Demodex* mite counts than did a control population. Patients with steroid rosacea are noted to have the highest *Demodex* counts [36]. The link between demodicidosis and rosacea is not quite clear, but it is suspected that *Demodex* mites may provoke inflammatory or allergic reactions, cause mechanical blockage of follicles, or act as vectors for microorganisms. In such cases, 5% permethrin cream appears to be helpful in controlling the papular and pustular lesions [37].

Conclusions

The scope of infections of the hair and pilosebaceous apparatus is broad. The epidemic of HIV-1 infection has led to the greatest number of recent observations, ranging from trichomegaly to hair straightening. The role of *Pityrosporum* species and *Demodex* mites in dermatologic disease is still unclear, but yeast, mites, and saprophytic fungi can clearly play an important role in human disease if given the proper opportunity. With the increase in immunodeficiency (from HIV-1 infection and from iatrogenic causes such as organ transplantation) and the increasing incidence of malignancy [38], new and unexpected presentations of hair infection are being encountered. The hair follicle and pilosebaceous unit provide one avenue by which our body mirrors underlying infections. Careful observation of the hair and pilosebaceous unit provides rewarding information to the practitioner with a careful eye.

References and recommended reading

Papers of particular interest, published within the annual period of review, have been highlighted as:
•   Of special interest
••   Of outstanding interest

1.   Saraux A, Taelman H, Batungwanayo J, Guillet G: **Haute Valeur predictive des Cheveux defrises pour Infection à HIV chez l'Adulte en Afrique centrale.** *Ann Dermatol Venereol* 1993, 120:395–396.

2.   Auffret N, Quint L, Domart P, Dubertret L, Lecam JY, Binet O: **Pityriasis Rubra Pilaris in a Patient With Human Immunodeficiency Virus Infection.** *J Am Acad Dermatol* 1992, 27:260–261.

3.   Menni S, Brancaleone W, Grimalt R: **Pityriasis Rubra Pilaris in a Child Positive for the Human Immunodeficiency Virus.** *J Am Acad Dermatol* 1992, 27:1009.

4.   Ostlere LS, Langley JAA, Staughton RCD, Samrasinghe PL: **Alopecia Universalis in a Patient Seropositive for the Human Immunodeficiency Virus.** *J Am Acad Dermatol* 1992, 27:630–631.

5.   Helm TN, Bergfeld WF, Yen-Lieberman B: **Alopecia Universalis in a Patient Seropositive for the Human Immunodeficiency Virus.** *J Am Acad Dermatol* 1993, 29:283–284.

6.   Daneschfar A, Davis CP, Trueb RM: **Trichomegalie bei HIV-Infektion.** *Schweiz Med Wochenschr* 1993, 123:1941–1949.

7.   Sadick NS: **Clinical and Laboratory Evaluation of AIDS Trichopathy.**
••   *Int J Dermatol* 1993, 32:33–38.
This article, together with that of Prose (*Int J Dermatol* 1992, 31:453–457), provides a comprehensive review of hair and nail changes found in HIV infection. Well-written and helpful in the accurate diagnosis of hair and nail disorders in HIV-infected persons, these articles constitute an outstanding resource.

8.   Prose NS, Abson KG, Scher RK: **Disorders of the Nails and Hair As-**
••   **sociated With Human Immunodeficiency Virus Infection.** *Int J Dermatol* 1992, 31:453–457.
This article, together with that of Sadick (*Int J Dermatol* 1993, 32:33–38), provides a comprehensive review of hair and nail changes found in HIV infection. Well-written and helpful in the accurate diagnosis of hair and nail disorders in HIV-infected persons, these articles constitute an outstanding resource.

9.   Haupt HM, Stern JB, Weber CB: **Eosinophilic Pustular Folliculitis: Fungal Folliculitis?** *J Am Acad Dermatol* 1990, 23:1012–1014.

10.   Duarte A, Kramer J, Yusk JW, Paller A, Schachner LA: **Eosinophilic Pustular Folliculitis in Infancy and Childhood.** *Am J Dis Child* 1993, 147:197–200.

11.   Lee ML, Tham SN, Ng SK: **Eosinophilic Pustular Folliculitis (Ofuji's Disease) With Response to Indomethacin.** *Dermatology* 1993, 186:210–212.

12.   Dhar J, Carey PB: ***Scopulariopsis brevicaulis* Skin Lesions in an AIDS Patient [Letter].** *AIDS* 1993, 7:1283–1284.

13.   Elston DM, Parker LU, Tuthill RJ: **Epidermoid Cyst of the Scalp Containing Human Papillomavirus.** *J Cutan Pathol* 1993, 20:184–186.

14.   Tseng CJ, Lin CY, Wang RL, Chen LJ, Chang YL, Hsieh TT, Pao CC: **Possible Transplacental Transmission of Human Papillomaviruses.** *Am J Obstet Gynecol* 1992, 166:35–40.

15.   Venugopal P, Venugopal T: **Tinea Capitis in Saudi Arabia.** *Int J Dermatol* 1993, 32:39–40.

16.   Lee JY, Hsu ML: **Pathogenesis of Hair Infection and Black Dots in Tinea Capitis Caused by *Trichophyton violaceum*: A Histopathological Study.** *J Cutan Pathol* 1992, 19:54–58.

17.   Pakula AS, Paller AS: **Langerhans Cell Histiocytosis and Dermatophytosis.** *J Am Acad Dermatol* 1993, 29:340–343.

18.   Helm KF, Lookingbill DP, Marks JG: **A Clinical and Histological Study of Histiocytosis-X in Adults.** *J Am Acad Dermatol* 1993, 29:166–170.

19.   Danby FW, Maddin WS, Margesson LJ, Rosenthal D: **A Randomized, Double-Blind, Placebo Controlled Trial of Ketoconazole 2% Shampoo Versus Selenium Sulfide 2.5% Shampoo in the Treatment of Moderate to Severe Dandruff.** *J Am Acad Dermatol* 1993, 29:1008–1012.

20.   Helm KF, Lookingbill DP: **Pityrosporum Folliculitis and Severe Pru-**
•   **ritus in Two Patients With Hodgkin's Disease.** *Arch Dermatol* 1993, 129:380–381.

This brief report illustrates that *Pityrosporum* folliculitis may be a sign of internal disease. In retrospect, we realize that we have encountered patients with *Pityrosporum* folliculitis and lymphoproliferative disease and have not made the connections between the two. This report highlights the need to be vigilant with patients who have widespread *Pityrosporum* folliculitis.

21.   Nahass GT, Rosenberg SP, Leonardi CL, Penneys NS: **Disseminated Infection With *Trichosporon beigelii*: Report of a Case and Review of the Cutaneous and Histologic Manifestations.** *Arch Dermatol* 1993, 129:1020–1023.

22.   Eady EA, Jonnes CE, Tipper JL, Cove JH, Cunliffe WJ, Layton AM:
••   **Antibiotic Resistant Propionibacteria in Acne: Need for Policies to Modify Antibiotic Usage.** *BMJ* 1993, 306:555–556.
This article points out that resistance of propionibacteria to antibiotics can lead to failure in the treatment of acne, and that resistance testing can be helpful clinically. The authors note the increasing incidence of resistant propionibacteria, and their methods will aid the development of effective therapy in patients with this common problem.

23.   Eady EA, Jones CE, Gardner KJ, Taylor JP, Cove JH, Cunliffe WJ: **Tetracycline-Resistant Propionibacteria From Acne Patients Are Cross-Resistant to Doxycycline, but Sensitive to Minocycline.** *Br J Dermatol* 1993, 128:556–560.

24.   Driscoll M, Rothe M, Abrahamian L, Grant-Kels JM: **Long-term Oral**
•   **Antibiotics for Acne: Is Laboratory Monitoring Necessary?** *J Am Acad Dermatol* 1993, 28:595–602.
Laboratory tests rarely detect adverse effects of long-term antibiotic therapy in acne patients. This study maintains that such tests are not warranted; it is very timely in this age of cost containment.

25.   Spach DH, Shimada JK, Paauw DS: **Localized Alopecia at the Site of Erythema Migrans.** *J Am Acad Dermatol* 1992, 27:1023–1024.

26.   Plewig G, Jansen T, Kligman A: **Pyoderma Faciale: A Review and Report of 20 Additional Cases: Is It Rosacea?** *Arch Dermatol* 1992, 128:1611–1617.

27.   Abeck D, Korting HC, Braun-Falco O: **Folliculitis Decalvans: Long-Lasting Response to Combined Therapy With Fusidic Acid and Zinc.** *Acta Derm Venereol (Stockh)* 1992, 72:143–145.

28.   George AO, Akanji AO, Nduka EU, Olasade JB, Odusan O: **Clinical, Biochemical and Morphologic Features of Acne Keloidalis in a Black Population.** *In J Dermatol* 1993, 32:714–716.

29.   Silvers DN, Katz BE, Young AW: **Pseudopelade of Brocq is Lichen Planopilaris: A Report of Four Cases That Support This Nosology.** *Cutis* 1993, 51:99–105.

30.   Mehregan DA, Van Hale HM, Muller SA: **Lichen Planopilaris: Clinical and Pathologic Study of Forty-five Patients.** *J Am Acad Dermatol* 1992, 27:935–942.

31.   Caputo R, Veraldi S: **Erosive Pustular Dermatosis of the Scalp.** *J Am Acad Dermatol* 1993, 28:96–98.

32.   Wright RC: **Traumatic Folliculitis of the Legs: A Persistent Case Associated With Use of a Home Epilating Device.** *J Am Acad Dermatol* 1992, 27:771–772.

33.   Courtiade C, Labreze C, Fontan I, Taieb A, Maleville J: **La Pediculose du Cuir chevelu: Enquete par Questionaire dans quatre Groupes scholaires de l'Academie de Bordeux en 1990–1991.** *Ann Dermatol Venereol* 1993, 120:363–368.

34.   Duran C, Tamayo L, de la Luz Orozco M, Ruiz-Maldonado R: **Scabies of the Scalp Mimicking Seborrheic Dermatitis in Immunocompromised Patients.** *Pediatr Dermatol* 1993, 10:136–138.

35.   Forton F, Seys B: **Density of *Demodex folliculorum* in Rosacea: A Case-Control Study Using Standardized Skin-Surface Biopsy.** *Br J Dermatol* 1993, 128:650–659.

36.   Bonnar E, Eustace P, Powell FC: **The Dermodex Mite Population in Rosacea.** *J Am Acad Dermatol* 1993, 28:443–448.

37.   Sahn EE, Sheridan DM: **Demodicidosis in a Child With Leukemia.** *J Am Acad Dermatol* 1992, 27:799–801.

38.   Boring CC, Squires TS, Tong T, Montgomery S: **Cancer Statistics, 1994.** *CA Cancer J Clin* 1994, 44:7–26.

Wilma F. Bergfeld, MD, Department of Dermatology A61, Head, Section of Dermatopathology, Cleveland Clinic Foundation, 9500 Euclid Avenue, Cleveland, OH 44195, USA.

Index to subjects

Abecarnil, in psychodermatologic disorders, 85
Abscess, *Mycobacterium chelonae*, 252
Absidia, in necrotizing infections, 238
Acetaminophen, in erythema multiforme, 28
Acitretin, in cancer prevention, 41
Acne
  in corticosteroid therapy, 196
  in obsessive-compulsive disorders, 86
  pathogenesis of, 256
  treatment of, 181, 256
    isotretinoin in, 231–234
Acne conglobata, 71
Acne fulminans, treatment of, 233
Acne keloidalis, 257
Acne rosacea, in HIV infection, in children, 127
Acquired immunodeficiency syndrome *see* Human immunodeficiency virus infection
Acrivastine, in atopic dermatitis, 8
Acrodermatitis enteropathica, necrolytic migratory erythema in, 89
Actinic keratosis, treatment of, 41–42
Actinic porokeratosis, treatment of, 202
Acyclovir
  in erythema multiforme, 28
  in herpes simplex virus infection, 126
  in varicella-zoster virus infection, 125
Adnexal disorders
  follicular occlusion tetrad, 69–74
  see also Follicle, hair
Adrenal suppression, in corticosteroid therapy, 195–196
Aeromonas species, in necrotizing infections, 237, 239
AGM-1470 (angiogenesis inhibitor), in neurofibromatosis, 102
AIDS *see* Human immunodeficiency virus infection
Albendazole
  in larva migrans, 244
  in strongyloidiasis, 245
Alexandrite laser, in tattoo removal, 157
Allergen-antibody complexes, in atopic dermatitis, 7–8
Allergic contact dermatitis, patch testing for, 10–17
Allergic reactions
  to corticosteroids, 196–197
  to sunscreens, 139, 176
Aloe barbadensis extract, in ultraviolet exposure protection, 228
Alopecia
  in dissecting cellulitis of scalp, 69–70
  in folliculitis decalvans, 257
  in HIV infection, 254–255
  in incontinentia pigmenti, 55
  in Lyme disease, 256–257
  in pediatric patients, biopsy of, 143
Alopecia areata, treatment of, 194
Alopecia mucinosa, 34–35
Alprazolam, in psychodermatologic disorders, 84
Aminoaciduria, necrolytic migratory erythema in, 90–91
5-Aminolevulinic acid, in squamous cell carcinoma, 39
Amithiozone, hypersensitivity reaction to, in HIV infection, 127
Amitriptyline, in psychodermatologic disorders, 85
Amphotericin B, in candidiasis, 124
Anaerobic infections, necrotizing, 237, 239
ANCA (antineutrophil cytoplasmic antibody), in vasculitis, 75–80
Anesthesia
  for pediatric patients, 149
  tumescent, for liposuction, 130–131, 162–163

Angiomatosis, bacillary, in HIV infection, in children, 126–127
Ankylostoma caninum infestation, 244
Anogenital lesions
  interferon therapy for, 146, 185–187
  in pediatric patients, 142
Antianxiety agents, in psychodermatologic disorders, 85–86
Antibiotics, 179–184
  in acne, 256
  cephalosporins, 180
  dosage of, 180
  fusidic acid, 71, 182, 257
  gentamicin, 182
  macrolides, 180–181
  mupirocin, 182
  in necrotizing infections, 240
  neomycin, 182
  new applications for, 179
  quinolones, 179–181
  resistance to, 179–180
    in acne, 256
    in tuberculosis, 249–250
  rifamycins, 181
  tetracyclines, 23, 181, 256
  topical, 181
  toxic epidermal necrolysis from, 29
  in toxic epidermal necrolysis treatment, 29–30
Antibodies
  anti–endothelial cell, in vasculitis, 75–80
  in vitiligo, 105–108
Anticoagulants, in calciphylaxis, 95
Anticonvulsants
  erythema multiforme from, 27–28
  toxic epidermal necrolysis from, 29
Antidepressants, in psychodermatologic disorders, 86–87
Antihistamines
  in atopic dermatitis, 8
  for pediatric surgery, 149
Antimalarials, 204–209
  in children, 207–208
  in erythema multiforme, 28
  in lactation, 208
  in lichen planus, 206
  in lupus erythematosus, 205
  mechanism of action of, 204
  in pemphigus foliaceus, 206
  in photodermatoses, 205–206
  in porphyria cutanea tarda, 205
  in pregnancy, 207–208
  in psoriatic arthritis, 206
  in sarcoidosis, 206
  toxicity of, 206–208
Antimony compounds, in leishmaniasis, 246
Antineutrophil cytoplasmic antibodies, in vasculitis, 75–80
Anti–obsessive-compulsive agents, in psychodermatologic disorders, 87
Antioxidants, dietary, in ultraviolet exposure protection, 228
Antipsychotic agents, in psychodermatologic disorders, 86
Anxiety
  in dermatologic disorders, treatment of, 85–86
  in pediatric patients, management of, 147–149
Apocrine glands, occlusion of, treatment of, 69–74
Argon laser
  for facial hyperpigmentation removal, 64–65

Permethrin cream, in hair follicle infestations, 258
Phenolic thioethers, in facial hyperpigmentation, 64
Photodermatoses, antimalarials in, 205–206
Photodynamic therapy, in squamous cell carcinoma, 38–40
Photopheresis
    in pemphigus, 23
    psoralen in, 168, 170
Photoreceptors, for ultraviolet B radiation, 227
Photosensitivity
    in erythropoietic protoporphyria, 219
    in quinolone therapy, 181
Phototherapy
    for atopic dermatitis, 5
    for eosinophilic pustular folliculitis, 255
    mechanism of action of, 170–171
    psoralen in, 5, 106, 167–172
    for psoriasis, calcipotriol with, 201
    for vitiligo, 106–107
Phycomycoses, necrotizing, 238
Physical therapy, in toxic epidermal necrolysis, 29
Pigmentation disorders
    in antimalarial therapy, 206–207
    facial hyperpigmentation, 61–68
    incontinentia pigmenti, 55–60
    vitiligo, 105–108
Pigmented lesion dye laser, in facial hyperpigmentation, 66
Pigmented lesions, laser surgery for, 156–157
Pilomatrixoma, excision of, 144
Pilonidal sinus, 72–73
Pilosebaceous unit see Follicle, hair
Pimozide, in psychodermatologic disorders, 85
Pityriasis lichenoides, 33–34
Pityriasis rubra pilaris
    in HIV infection, 254
    treatment of, 202
Pityrosporum ovale infections, of hair follicle, 256
Plaques
    in alopecia mucinosa, 34–35
    in incontinentia pigmenti, 55
    in mycosis fungoides, 36
    in parapsoriasis, 33–34
    urticarial, in pregnancy, 18–19
Plasma cell balanitis, treatment of, 182
Plasmapheresis
    in bullous pemphigoid, 23
    in toxic epidermal necrolysis, 30
Poikiloderma vasculare atrophicans, 34
Polyarteritis nodosa, antineutrophil cytoplasmic antibodies in, 76–78
Polydioxanone sutures, evaluation of, 131
Polyglactin sutures, evaluation of, 131
Polyglycolic acid sutures, evaluation of, 131
Polyglyconate sutures, evaluation of, 131
Polymorphic eruption of pregnancy, 18–19
Polymorphous light eruption, antimalarials in, 205–206
Polypropylene sutures, evaluation of, 131
Porokeratosis, actinic, treatment of, 202
Porphyria cutanea tarda, antimalarials in, 205
Port wine stains, laser surgery for, 145, 155–156
Potassium iodide, in erythema multiforme, 28
Prednicarbate, pharmacology of, 193
Prednisolone, in hemangioma, 110
Prednisone
    in bullous pemphigoid, 23
    in cicatricial pemphigoid, 24
    in epidermolysis bullosa acquisita, 24
    in hemangioma, 110
    in herpes gestationis, 20
    in pemphigus, 22–23

Pregnancy
    antimalarials in, 207–208
    inflammatory diseases of, 18–21
    isotretinoin in, 233
    recurrent cholestasis of, 20
Premalignant melanosis of Dubreuilh, 46–47
Prickly heat, in travelers, 244
Progesterone dermatitis, autoimmune, 20
Progressive nodular histiocytosis, 54
Proliferating cell nuclear antigen, in histiocytosis X, 51
Propionibacterial infections, treatment of, 181
Prostaglandins, for surgical flap survival, 135
Protein C deficiency, calciphylaxis in, 95
Protein deficiency, necrolytic migratory erythema in, 90
Proteinases, antibodies to, in vasculitis, 77–79
Proteus species, in necrotizing infections, 235
Protoporphyria, erythropoietic, 219–224
Prurigo gravidarum, 20
Pruritic urticarial papules and plaques of pregnancy, 18–19
Pruritus
    in herpes gestationis, 19–20
    in prurigo gravidarum, 20
    in travelers infections, 244–245
Pseudofolliculitis, 258
Pseudomonas aeruginosa infections
    folliculitis, 258
    in HIV infection, in children, 126
    necrotizing, 237
Pseudopelade of Brocq, 257
Psoralen, 167–172
    in atopic dermatitis, 5
    bioavailability of, 167–168
    cancer risk from, 170
    derivatives of, 169
    mechanism of action of, 170–171
    ultraviolet radiation wavelength for, 168–169
    in vitiligo, 106
Psoriasis
    nummular, treatment of, 194
    treatment of, 169, 181, 194
        vitamin D$_3$ analogues in, 198–202
Psoriatic arthritis, antimalarials in, 206
Psychopharmacology, in dermatologic practice, 83–86
Psychosis, in dermatologic disorders, treatment of, 86
Pulsed dye laser, for vascular lesion removal, 155–156
Purpura, in calciphylaxis, 94–95
Pustules
    in acne keloidalis, 257
    in erosive pustular dermatosis, 257–258
    of hair follicle, in HIV infection, 255
    in pregnancy, 20
PUVA therapy
    in atopic dermatitis, 5
    psoralen in, 167–172
    in psoriasis, calcipotriol with, 201
    in vitiligo, 257
Pyoderma faciale, 257
Pyogenic granuloma, excision of, 144
Pyrazinamide, in tuberculosis, 250
Pyridoxine deficiency, necrolytic migratory erythema in, 91
Pyruvic acid, in cancer prevention, 41

Q-switched lasers, in pigmented lesion removal, 156–157
Quinacrine, in skin diseases, 204–209
Quinine, in skin diseases, 204–209
Quinolones, 179–181

Radiation therapy, cancer from, 143
ras genes mutations, in ultraviolet radiation exposure, 226
Rash
    in Kawasaki syndrome, 115

List of journals scanned

The *Index Medicus* abbreviation is given in parentheses.

Acta Dermato-Venereologica (Acta Derm Venereol (Stockh))
AIDS (AIDS)
Allergologie (Allergologie)
Allergy (Allergy)
American Journal of Clinical Pathology (Am J Clin Pathol)
American Journal of Contact Dermatitis (Am J Contact Dermatitis)
American Journal of Dermatopathology (Am J Dermatopathol)
Archives of Pediatrics & Adolescent Medicine (Arch Pediatr Adolesc Med)
American Journal of Human Genetics (Am J Hum Genet)
American Journal of Medicine (Am J Med)
American Journal of Obstetrics and Gynecology (Am J Obstet Gynecol)
American Journal of Surgery (Am J Surg)
American Review of Respiratory Disease (Am Rev Respir Dis)
Annales de Dermatologie et de Venereologie (Ann Dermatol Venereol)
Annals of Emergency Medicine (Ann Emerg Med)
Annals of Internal Medicine (Ann Intern Med)
Annals of the Rheumatic Diseases (Ann Rheum Dis)
Annals of Surgery (Ann Surg)
Antimicrobial Agents and Chemotherapy (Antimicrob Agents Chemother)
Archives of Dermatology (Arch Dermatol)
Archives of Dermatological Research (Arch Dermatol Res)
Archives of Internal Medicine (Arch Intern Med)
Archives of Surgery (Arch Surg)
Arthritis and Rheumatism (Arthritis Rheum)
Australasian Journal of Dermatology (Australas J Dermatol)
British Medical Journal (BMJ)
British Journal of Dermatology (Br J Dermatol)
British Journal of Rheumatology (Br J Rheumatol)
British Journal of Surgery (Br J Surg)
Cancer (Cancer)
Cancer Research (Cancer Res)
Cell (Cell)
Cellular Immunology (Cell Immunol)
Clinical and Experimental Allergy (Clin Exp Allergy)
Clinical and Experimental Dermatology (Clin Exp Dermatol)
Clinical and Experimental Immunology (Clin Exp Immunol)
Clinical and Experimental Rheumatology (Clin Exp Rheumatol)
Clinical Immunology and Immunopathology (Clin Immunol Immunopathol)
Clinical Infectious Diseases (Clin Infect Dis)
Clinical Pharmacology and Therapeutics (Clin Pharmacol Ther)
Clinical Research (Clin Res)
Clinical Rheumatology (Clin Rheumatol)
Contact Dermatitis (Contact Dermatitis)
Cutis (Cutis)
Dermatology (Dermatology)
Diabetes (Diabetes)
Drugs (Drugs)
EMBO Journal (EMBO J)
European Journal of Dermatology (Eur J Dermatol)
European Journal of Immunology (Eur J Immunol)
Experimental Dermatology (Exp Dermatol)
FASEB Journal (FASEB J)
Giornale Italiano di Dermatologia e Venereologia (G Ital Dermatol Venereol)
Gastroenterology (Gastroenterology)
Genitourinary Medicine (Genitourin Med)
Gut (Gut)

Hautarzt (Hautarzt)
Human Genetics (Hum Genet)
Infection Control and Hospital Epidemiology (Infect Control Hosp Epidemiol)
Infection and Immunity (Infect Immun)
International Archives of Allergy and Immunology (Int Arch Allergy Immunol)
International Journal of Dermatology (Int J Dermatol)
Journal of Allergy and Clinical Immunology (J Allergy Clin Immunol)
Journal of the American Academy of Dermatology (J Am Acad Dermatol)
Journal of the American College of Surgeons (J Am Coll Surg)
Journal of Antimicrobial Chemotherapy (J Antimicrob Chemother)
Journal of Autoimmunity (J Autoimmun)
Journal of Cell Biology (J Cell Biol)
Journal of Clinical Endocrinology and Metabolism (J Clin Endocrinol Metab)
Journal of Clinical Investigation (J Clin Invest)
Journal of Clinical and Laboratory Immunology (J Clin Lab Immunol)
Journal of Clinical Microbiology (J Clin Microbiol)
Journal of Clinical Oncology (J Clin Oncol)
Journal of Clinical Pathology (J Clin Pathol)
Journal of Cutaneous Pathology (J Cutan Pathol)
Journal of Dermatology (J Dermatol)
Journal of Dermatologic Surgery and Oncology (J Dermatol Surg Oncol)
Journal of Dermatological Treatment (J Dermatol Treat)
Journal of the European Academy of Dermatology and Venereology (J Eur Acad Dermatol Venereol)
Journal of Experimental Medicine (J Exp Med)
Journal of Hospital Infection (J Hosp Infect)
Journal of Infectious Diseases (J Infect Dis)
Journal of Investigative Dermatology (J Invest Dermatol)
Journal of Laboratory and Clinical Medicine (J Lab Clin Med)
Journal of Leukocyte Biology (J Leukoc Biol)
Journal of Pediatrics (J Pediatr)
Journal of Rheumatology (J Rheumatol)
JAMA — Journal of the American Medical Association (JAMA)
Lancet (Lancet)
Mycologia (Mycologia)
New England Journal of Medicine (N Engl J Med)
Nature (Nature)
Nippon Hifuka Gakkai Zasshi—Japanese Journal of Dermatology (Nippon Hifuka Gakkai Zasshi)
Obstetrics and Gynecology (Obstet Gynecol)
Pediatric Dermatology (Pediatr Dermatol)
Pediatric Infectious Disease Journal (Pediatr Infect Dis J)
Pediatrics (Pediatrics)
Photodermatology, Photoimmunology and Photomedicine (Photodermatol Photoimmunol Photomed)
Plastic and Reconstructive Surgery (Plast Reconstr Surg)
Proceedings of the National Academy of Sciences of the United States of America (Proc Natl Acad Sci U S A)
Scandinavian Journal of Immunology (Scand J Immunol)
Science (Science)
Seminars in Dermatology (Semin Dermatol)
Sexually Transmitted Diseases (Sex Transm Dis)
Skin Pharmacology (Skin Pharmacol)
Surgery (Surgery)

© 1995 Current Science ISBN 1-85922-686-8 ISSN 1068–381X